W9-BHU-293

Handbook of
Urban Health

Handbook of **Urban Health**

Populations, Methods, and Practice

Edited by

Sandro Galea

Center for Urban Epidemiologic Studies, New York Academy of Medicine
Department of Epidemiology, Mailman School of Public Health, Columbia University
New York, New York

and

David Vlahov

Center for Urban Epidemiologic Studies, New York Academy of Medicine
Department of Epidemiology, Mailman School of Public Health, Columbia University
New York, New York

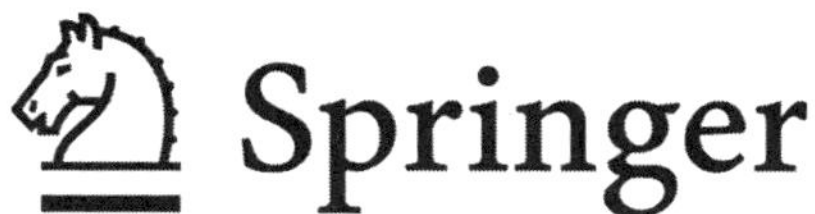

Library of Congress Cataloging-in-Publication Data

Handbook of urban health: populations, methods, and practice/edited by
Sandro Galea, David Vlahov.
p. cm.
Includes bibliographical references and index.
ISBN 0-387-23994-4
1. Urban health–Handbooks, manuals, etc. I. Galea, Sandro. II. Vlahov, David.

RA566.7.H36 2005
362.1′042–dc22

ISBN-10: 0-387-23994-4 Printed on acid-free paper.
ISBN-13: 978-0387-23994-1

Printed in the United States of America. (SPI/EB)

9 8 7 6 5 4 3 2 1

springeronline.com

Acknowledgments

We would like to thank our colleagues throughout the world who participated in the Second International Conference on Urban Health in New York City in October 2003. Discussions during the conference shaped our early thoughts about the topics covered in this volume and sowed the seeds for this book. We are grateful to all the authors who have contributed chapters to this book. We have learned a tremendous amount from them, both through our discussions as this book was taking shape, and through reading the chapters themselves. We are particularly indebted to Dr. Nicholas Freudenberg. Our ongoing conversations with Dr. Freudenberg about the health of urban populations have contributed immeasurably to our evolving thoughts about urban health. We would like to thank Dr. Jeremiah Barondess, President of the New York Academy of Medicine, for embracing urban health as a mission for the Academy and for fostering an environment of learning and research which has encouraged us to develop the ideas discussed here. This book would not have been possible without the editorial assistance of Ms. Emily Gibble and Ms. Sasha Rudenstine who have shown dedication to this work that is above and beyond the call of duty. Finally, we owe our spouses, Dr. Margaret Kruk and Dr. Robyn Gershon, a debt of gratitude for their patience and forbearance as we worked on this book over the past year.

SANDRO GALEA
DAVID VLAHOV

Contributors

Joseph H. Abraham, Department of Epidemiology at the Johns Hopkins Bloomberg School of Public Health, Baltimore, Maryland

Frances K. Barg, Department of Family Practice and Community Medicine, University of Pennsylvania School of Medicine, and the Department of Anthropology, University of Pennsylvania School of Arts and Sciences, Philadelphia, Pennsylvania

Jeremy Barron, Department of Medicine in the Division of Geriatric Medicine and Gerontology at the Johns Hopkins University, Baltimore, Maryland

Mary T. Bassett, Deputy Commissioner of the Division of Health Promotion and Disease Prevention at the New York City Department of Health and Mental Hygiene, New York, New York

Ahmed M. Bayoumi, Center for Research on Inner City Health, St.Michael's Hospital at the University of Toronto, Toronto, Ontario, Canada

Marlon G. Boarnet, School of Social Ecology, Department of Planning, Policy, and Design at the University of California at Irvine, Irvine, California

Luisa N. Borrell, Department of Epidemiology at the Mailman School of Public Health and the School of Dental and Oral Surgery at Columbia University, New York, New York

Kisha Braithwaite, Division of General Pediatrics and Adolescent Medicine in the Department of Mental Health and School of Medicine in the Bloomberg School of Public Health at the Johns Hopkins University, Baltimore, Maryland

Deborah R. Deitcher, Health Promotion and Disease Prevention at the New York City Department of Health and Mental Hygiene, New York, New York

James R. Dunn, Center for Research on Inner City Health, St. Michael's Hospital at the University of Toronto, Toronto, Ontario, Canada

Alex C. Ezeh, The African Population and Health Research Centre, Nairobi, Kenya, Africa

Nicholas Freudenberg, Hunter College Center on AIDS, Drugs and Community Health at Hunter College at the City University of New York, New York

Linda Fried, Center on Aging and Health, Department of Medicine at the Johns Hopkins University, Baltimore, Maryland

Thomas R. Frieden, New York City Commissioner of Health and Mental Hygiene at the New York City Department of Health and Mental Hygiene, New York, New York

Ruth Finkelstein, Office of Special Populations at the New York Academy of Medicine, New York, New York

Crystal Fuller, Center for Urban Epidemiologic Studies at the New York Academy of Medicine and Department of Epidemiology at the Mailman School of Public Health at Columbia University, New York, New York

Sandro Galea, Center for Urban epidemiologic Studies at the New York Academy of Medicine and Department of Epidemiology at the Mailman School of Public Health at Columbia University, New York, New York

M. Chris Gibbons, Johns Hopkins Urban Health Institute at the Johns Hopkins Medical Institutions, Baltimore, Maryland

Michael K. Gusmano, The World Cities Project at the International Longevity Center-USA, New York, New York

Bernard Guyer, Department of Population and Family Health Sciences, Bloomberg School of Public Health at the Johns Hopkins University, Baltimore, Maryland

Stephani L. Hatch, Department of Epidemiology at the Mailman School of Public Health, Columbia University, New York, New York

Donald Hoover, Department of Statistics, Institute of Biostatistics at Rutgers University, Piscataway, New Jersey

Stephen W. Hwang, Center for Research on Inner City Health, St. Michael's Hospital at the University of Toronto, Toronto, Ontario

Tej Kumar Karki, Kathmandu Valley Town Development Plan Implementation Committee, Kathmandu, Nepal

Jane Kauer, Department of Anthropology at the University of Pennsylvania School of Arts and Sciences, Philadelphia, Pennsylvania

Susan Klitzman, Urban Public Health Program and the Department of Environmental and Occupational Health Sciences at Hunter College at the City University of New York, New York

Roderick J. Lawrence, Centre for Human Ecology and Environmental Sciences at the Faculty of Social and Economic Sciences at the University of Geneva, Geneva, Switzerland

Sana Loue, Department of Epidemiology and Biostatistics at the School of Medicine at Case Western Reserve University, Cleveland, Ohio

Thomas D. Matte, Division of Health Promotion and Disease Prevention, New York City Department of Health and Mental Hygiene, New York, New York

Nancy Mendez, Department of Epidemiology and Biostatistics at the School of Medicine at Case Western Reserve University, Cleveland, Ohio

Mark R. Montgomery, Policy Research Division, Population Council at the State University of New York, New York, New York, and Department of Economics, State University of New York at Stony Brook, Stony Brook, New York

Julie Netherland, Office of Special Populations at the New York Academy of Medicine, New York, New York

Patricia O'Campo, Center for Research on Inner City Health, St. Michael's Hospital at the University of Toronto, Toronto, Ontario, Canada

Danielle Ompad, Center for Urban Epidemiologic Studies at the New York Academy of Medicine, New York, New York

Anita Palepu, St. Paul's Hospital at the University of British Columbia, Vancouver, British Columbia, Canada

Wendy C. Perdue, Georgetown University Law Center, Georgetown University, Washington, D.C.

Victor G. Rodwin, Health Policy and Management, Robert F. Wagner Graduate School of Public Policy at the New York University, New York, New York

Johnathan M. Samet, Department of Epidemiology at the Johns Hopkins Bloomberg School of Public Health, Baltimore, Maryland

Jan C. Semenza, School of Community Health at the Portland State University, Portland, Oregon

Vijay Singh, Department of Family Medicine, University of California in Los Angeles, Santa Monica, California

Joseph A. Soares, Department of Sociology at Wake Forest University, Winston-Salem, North Carolina

Lois M. Takahashi, Department of Urban Planning at the University of California at Los Angeles, Los Angeles, California

Mark W. Tyndall, the British Columbia Centre for Excellence in HIV/AIDS at the University of British Columbia, Vancouver, British Columbia, Canada

David Vlahov, Center for Urban Epidemiologic Studies at the New York Academy of Medicine and Department of Epidemiology at the Mailman School of Public Health at Columbia University, New York, New York

Michael Yonas, Department of Population and Family Health Studies at the Johns Hopkins Bloomberg School of Public Health, Baltimore, Maryland and Kellogg Community Health Scholars Fellowship at the University of North Carolina, Chapel Hill, North Carolina

Contents

Handbook of
Urban Health

Chapter 1

Urban Health

Populations, Methods, and Practice

Sandro Galea and David Vlahov

1.0. WHAT IS A CITY AND WHAT IS "URBAN HEALTH"?

We all know what cities are; or at least we think we do. However, it is more likely that each of our personal experiences has shaped what we think of when we discuss "cities" and that each of us has a different image of "city" in our own head. We may be in good company. Saul Bellow, the novelist and Nobel Prize laureate, in discussing how Americans think of New York City, suggested: " That is perhaps like asking how Scotsmen feel about the Loch Ness monster. It is our legendary phenomenon, our great thing, our world-famous impossibility . . . New York is stirring, insupportable, agitated, ungovernable, demonic. No single individual can judge it adequately" (New York Times, 1970). Indeed, cities can defeat definition and challenge the imagination. Cities are elegant, sophisticated places. Think of Piccadilly Circus in London, the Arc de Triomphe in Paris, or the Copacabana in Rio De Janeiro. But cities are also dense, teeming, and dangerous places. Think of the squatter colonies of Lagos and parts of Los Angeles or New York City. Cities can be distinctive (there is only one Paris) or can look monotonously alike (think of any number of North American mid-size cities). Cities can be small, compact areas that are immediately walkable, and can be vast, extensive, automobile-dependent metropolitan areas that are disconnected, homogenous, and pedestrian-hostile. In short, cities, and by extension the urban experience, can represent diverse conditions within which people live, and represent a range of human experiences.

What then do we mean when we write about "urban health"? In its broadest sense urban health refers to the study of the health of urban populations. We consider urban health inquiry to include two principal aspects: the description of the health of urban populations, both as a whole and as particular subgroups within cities, and an understanding of the determinants of population health in cities, with particular attention to how characteristics of cities themselves may affect the health of urban populations. The practice of urban health can then include a range of clinical, planning, or policy work that aims to improve the health of urban populations. While both aspects suggested here are broad, they arguably represent a distinct body of inquiry that builds on a long tradition of interest in the role of cities in shaping the health of urban populations. We suggest in this chapter and throughout the book that the study of urban health, nested within the larger parameters of "public health," has much to contribute, both in terms of helping us understand population health, but also in guiding local and global interventions that can improve the health of the public.

There are two primary reasons why we suggest that we should concern ourselves with thinking of urban health as a field of inquiry and practice. First, there is the growing importance, and influence, of cities worldwide. As we discuss in the next section of this chapter, city living is becoming the norm for an ever growing proportion of the world's population. Second, after more than two centuries of organized public health as an intellectual and practical discipline, we are in many ways returning to the roots of the profession and understanding once again that context, including the social, physical, political, or policy environments within which we live, matters. As such, as cities increasingly shape the context within which we live, understanding the urban context, and its possible role in shaping population health, becomes imperative. It is the role of this book to bring together work from different disciplines that can contribute to different aspects of urban health inquiry and practice.

This chapter aims to set the stage for the book. First we discuss the growing importance of cities worldwide and the role they play in shaping population health. Second, we will summarize what we think can be achieved by considering urban health as a cogent field of inquiry and practice, what that field of inquiry can look like, and the challenges it might face. We conclude this chapter by orienting readers to the book itself, discussing its structure and what each of the three principal sections have to offer. We note that we do not attempt to offer either a broad theoretical framework for urban health, nor to be comprehensive in our discussion of the determinants of the health of urban populations. Other work, and the rest of this book, fill these functions (Northridge and Sclar, 2003; Vlahov and Galea, 2002; Galea and Vlahov, 2004; Freudenberg *et al.*, in press). Rather, we intend this chapter to summarize the rationale behind this book and to summarize the gap this book aims to fill. We hope that the chapters that follow will provide the reader with a basis on which to make up her or his own mind about the role of urban health research and practice and how this may contribute to healthier urban populations.

2.0. GROWTH OF CITIES WORLDWIDE

At the beginning of the nineteenth century, only five percent of the world's population was living in urban areas. By 2003, about forty-eight percent of the world's population was living in urban areas (United Nations, 2004). By 2007 it is estimated that more than half the world's population will be living in urban areas and by 2030, up to sixty percent of the world's population will live in cities (Guidotti, *et al.*, 2001; United Nations, 2004). Overall, the world's urban population is expected to grow from 2.86 billion in 2000 to 4.98 billion in 2030 (United Nations, 2004). In addition, current estimates suggest that the trend toward an urbanizing world will continue well into the twenty-first century and that the pace of urbanization may well accelerate. For example, although London took 130 years to grow from 1 million to 8 million inhabitants, it took Bangkok, Dhaka, and Seoul 45, 37, and 25 years respectively to achieve similar population growths. Overall global population growth in the next thirty years will be primarily in cities; approximately 1 million city residents (a city approximately the size of Pittsburgh) will be added to the world's population weekly.

The pace of increase in urban areas is projected to differ by region of the world and by initial city size. In particular, most global population growth will occur in less wealthy regions of the world, with the most rapid pace of growth expected to occur in Asia and Africa. In the next thirty years more wealthy countries will account for only 28 percent of the predicted growth in the world's urban population. While North America and Europe have the highest proportion of the population living in urban areas (approximately 79.1% in North America in 2000 and in Europe 72.7% in the year 2000), the absolute number of urban dwellers in the least urbanized region, Asia, was already in the year 2000 greater than the urban population in North America and Europe combined (1.36 billion inhabitants in Asia compared to 249 million inhabitants in North America and 529 million inhabitants in Europe).

There are approximately 50,000 urban areas in the world today with close to 400 cities with a population of a million people or more (Satterthwaite, 2002). The first urban area to become a "mega-city" with more than 10 million inhabitants was the New York City metropolitan area around 1940. Today there are more than 15 mega-cities world-wide (Satterthwaite, 2000; 2002). Although, in the coming decades, mega-cities will grow, most of the world's population growth will happen in smaller cities. The proportion of people living in mega-cities is expected to rise from 4.3% of the global population in 2000 to 5.2 % in 2015 (Satterthwaite, 2002). The growth rate of mega-cities in the developing world will be much higher. For example the anticipated growth rate for Calcutta, India between 2000 and 2015 is 1.9%, compared to an anticipated growth rate of 0.4% for New York City, U.S. However, while the growth of large cities in developing countries will account for approximately a fifth of the increase in the world's population, small cities will account for almost half of this increase. Therefore, a growing number of relatively small cities throughout the world will contain most of the world's population in the twenty-first century. The three figures in this chapter provide a summary of world population growth overall and in urban areas between 1950 and 2003. Figure 1 showing the total number of people living in urban areas in different world regions, Figure 2 shows the proportion of regional populations living in urban areas, and Figure 3 shows the proportion of the world's urban population living in specific world regions (United Nations, 2004).

3.0. THE HEALTH OF URBAN POPULATIONS

Why then should we concern ourselves with cities and their relationship to population health? In some ways, having established that cities are the predominant circumstance of living in the twenty-first century one can argue that cities are ubiquitous, and their impact so pervasive, that it is difficult to consider any aspect of health without thinking of the role of cities. Arguably, multiple academic disciplines produce research that is essentially premised on the existence and the importance of cities. For example, epidemiologic research that concerns itself with the health of homeless populations does not generally dwell on urban living conditions as a determinant of either homelessness or of the health of the homeless, but undoubtedly, urbanism, and urbanization are primary determinants both of homelessness

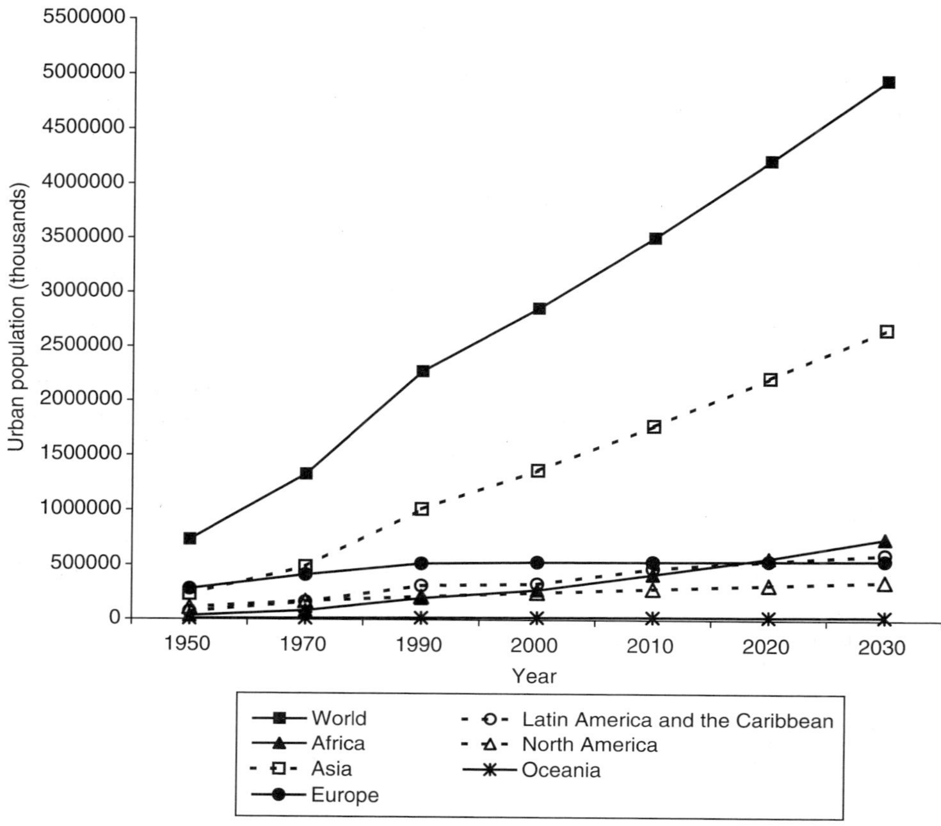

Figure 1. World Urban Population 1950-2030, by Region (*Source*: Data from United Nations Department of Economic and Social Affairs/Population Division. [2004] *World Urbanization Prospects: the 2003 Revision*. Report No. ESA/P/WP.190 [March 2004]).

rates and of the conditions of particular homeless persons in different cities. Therefore, research that considers cities as a backdrop for analyses about health does little to shed light on fundamentally *how* cities may affect health. In order to better understand the relations between features of urban living and health we must then identify the features of urban living and the urban condition that have implications for health. The diversity of cities worldwide naturally means that there is no single form of "urban living", but rather a range of living conditions with shared features.

When we think about how cities may affect health, fundamentally we must recognize that cities are places, locations, where large numbers of people live in close proximity. Therefore, we can consider the impact of cities in two primary ways. First, and most obviously, as a growing proportion of the world's population lives in cities, the health of urban populations contributes increasingly to overall population health worldwide. Therefore, factors that influence health in cities gain in importance in influencing global population health. Second, as more of us live in urban areas, it becomes increasingly likely that aspects of the urban environment in which we live will affect our health. We find it useful to think of three broad categories of theories and mechanisms that may explain how city living can affect health – the

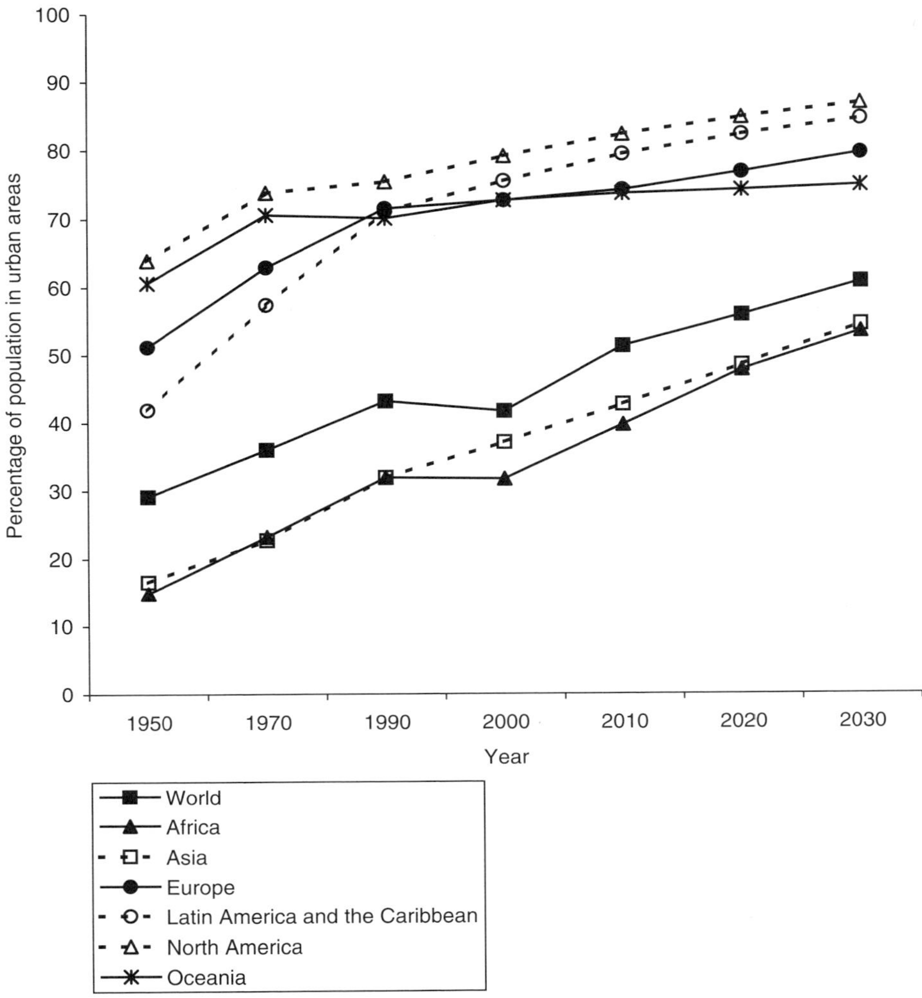

Figure 2. Proportion of Population in Urban Areas, by Region, 1950-2030 (*Source*: Data from United Nations Department of Economic and Social Affairs/Population Division. [2004] *World Urbanization Prospects: the 2003 Revision*. Report No. ESA/P/WP.190 [March 2004]).

physical environment, the social environment, and availability of and access to health and social services.

We discuss each of these briefly here and refer the reader to other work that discusses each of these mechanisms in more detail (Galea, *et al.*, 2005; Freudenberg, *et al.*, in press).

The **urban physical environment** includes, among many other aspects, the built environment, air and water quality, noise levels, parks, and climate conditions in cities; all aspects of cities that urban dwellers come in contact with on a daily basis and all having the potential to affect health. The literature on the relation between features of the physical environment and health is vast and we summarize it here briefly. The human *built environment* can influence both physical and mental health; empiric evidence about the relation between the built environment and health

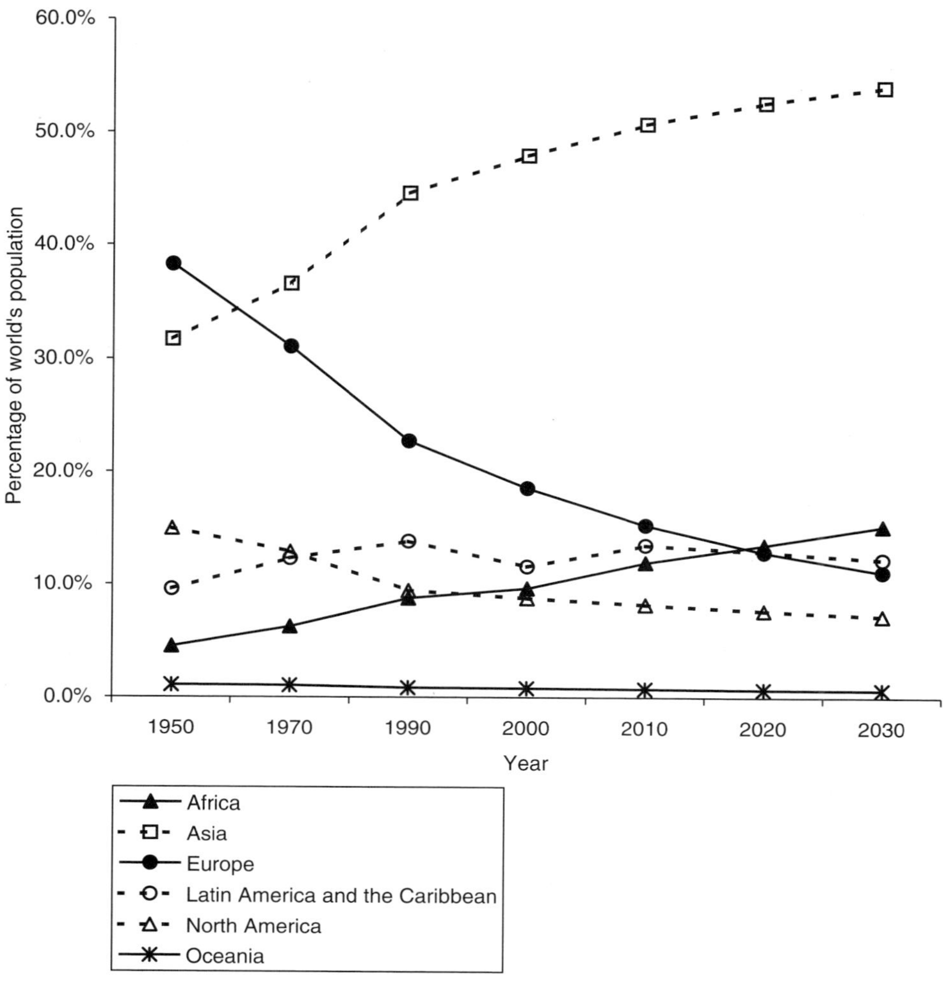

Figure 3. Percent of World's Urban Population Living in Different Regions, 1950-2003 (*Source*: Data from United Nations Department of Economic and Social Affairs/Population Division. [2004] *World Urbanization Prospects: the 2003 Revision.* Report No. ESA/P/WP.190 [March 2004]).

conditions includes, among others, asthma and other respiratory conditions, injuries, psychological distress, and child development (Evans, *et al.*, 2000; Krieger, 2002; Northridge, *et al.*, 2003). Different aspects of the built environment have been linked to specific health outcomes. For example, specific features of the built environment including density of development, mix of land uses, scale of streets, aesthetic qualities of place, and connectivity of street networks, may affect physical activity (Handy, *et al.*, 2002). In turn, low levels of physical activity are a well-established risk factor for cardiovascular disease and all-cause mortality in urban areas (Diez-Roux, 2003; Pate, *et al.*, 1995). There is substantial literature on the relation between housing and health (Kingsley, 2003, Thomson, *et al.*, 2003). Urban design may also affect health behaviors, crime, and violence rates (Berrigan and Troiano, 2001; Newman, 1986; Sampson, *et al.*, 1997) suggesting close interactions among the urban physical and social environments.

Urban infrastructure determines how a city provides water, disposes of garbage, and provides energy (Melosi, 2000). Water scarcity and water pollution are serious urban problems, particularly in less wealthy countries. It is estimated that nearly 1.5 billion people lack safe drinking water and that at least 5 million deaths per year can be attributed to waterborne diseases (Krants and Kifferstein, 1998). In longstanding urban areas, the decline of an aging infrastructure, coupled with frequently declining municipal resources, may challenge cities' ability to continue to provide safe water and sanitation for urban residents. In rapidly urbanizing areas, frequently in less wealthy countries, cities are often challenged to maintain adequate fresh water supply to growing numbers of urban residents and transporting accumulating sewage and other waste. (Rodgers, 1979). Inadequate provision for solid waste collection frequently results in contamination of water bodies, which, coupled with the population density inherent to cities, presents a substantial risk for rapidly spreading epidemics (Alexander and Ehrlich, 2000; Chanthikul, *et al.*, 2004; Satterthwaite, 2000).

Although *pollution* in cities in wealthy countries has improved during the past half century, cities still generate close to 80% of global carbon dioxide emissions and account for three-quarters of industrial wood use worldwide (O'Meara, 1999). As late as the mid-1990s, it has been estimated that air pollution contributed to 30,000 to 60,000 deaths per year in the US (Dockery, 1993; Samet, 2000). Indoor and outdoor air pollution are thought to contribute to 3 million deaths globally a year, with 90% of these deaths being in less wealthy countries (World Health Organization, 1997). Worldwide, atmospheric pollution is thought to affect more than a billion people, mostly in cities (Environmental Software and Services, 2002; Roodman, 1998). Recent work has shown that living in areas with walkable *green spaces* was associated with greater likelihood of physical activity (Booth, *et al.*, 2000), higher functional status (Guralnik, *et al.*, 1994), lower cardiovascular disease risk (Lee, *et al.*, 2001) and longevity among the elderly independent of personal characteristics (Takano, *et al.*, 2002; Takana, 1996). Ultimately, *climate* in cities can affect population health. On warm days, urban areas can be more than 5° F warmer than surrounding areas, an effect known as the urban "heat island" effect (Frumkin, 2002). This is primarily due to dark surfaces absorbing heat and the limited ability of urban areas (with relatively few trees), to cool the air through transpiration. Global climate change may exacerbate this effect. Heat is a concern in urban areas in several ways and ambient air temperature is shown to be associated with a large number of hospitalizations and deaths yearly (Basu, *et al.*, 2002; Mackenbach, *et al.*, 1997). Particular groups may be most at risk of the effects of heat in urban areas. Epidemic heat-related deaths have been particularly pronounced among socio-economically disadvantaged and socially isolated elderly persons (Kilborne, *et al.*, 1982; Semenza, 1999).

Other features of the urban physical environment that may have specific relations to human health include the vulnerability of urban structures to natural or human-made disasters, as recent earthquakes in Japan and Iran and the September 11, 2001 terrorist attacks on New York City demonstrated respectively, hazardous waste landfills, often located in or near urban areas, which may be associated with risks of low birth weight, birth defects, and cancers (Vrijheid, 2000), and noise exposure, a common urban problem, that may contribute to hearing impairment, hypertension, and ischemic heart disease (Passchier-Vermeer and Passchier, 2000).

There are multiple ways in which the *urban social environment* may affect health (Barnett and Casper, 2001). Contemporary *social strain* theories suggest that there are sources of strain in modern living, including confrontation with unpleasant stimuli that may be associated both with deviant behavior and with poor health (Agnew, 1992; Cohen, *et al.*, 2003). A substantial body of research has established a relation between stress and social strain and mental and physical health (e.g., Elliot, 2000; Latkin and Curry, 2003; Pealin, *et al.*, 1981), and newer work has posited that features of the urban neighborhood context are associated with social strain, and adverse health behaviors (Boardman, *et al.*, 2001; Galea, *et al.*, 2003). Separate from social strain, *individual social resources* also may be important determinants of health in cities. For example, limited social support may predispose persons to poorer coping and adverse health (Kawachi and Berkman, 2001; McLeod and Kessler, 1990). In the context of cities, the greater spatial proximity of one's immediate network may well accentuate the role of networks in shaping health. Social networks have been shown to be importantly associated with a range of health behaviors (Kafka and London, 1991; Madianos *et al.*, 1995). Models of social influences on biological contagion, particularly in the context of infectious disease are well established. For example, in recent years, group practices and social norms have been considered particularly important in transmission of sexually transmitted diseases and the transmission of human immunodeficiency virus (HIV) (Pick and Obermeyer, 1996; Wellington *et al.*, 1997). Importantly, newer theories include the possibility of *contagiousness of ideas and social examples.* In epidemiology it is understood that all things being equal, urban populations, characterized by high population density are at higher risk of transmission of biological organisms. Also, because concentrated urban populations share common resources (e.g., water) the practices of one group can affect the health of others. These observations may be extended to behavior and to health. For example, media representations of suicide may have an influence on the suicide of those exposed to them such that suicide becomes more likely (Phillips, 1974).

Spatial segregation of different racial/ethnic and socioeconomic groups may also be an important determinant of health in cities. Many cities worldwide are highly segregated with multiple historical, logistical, and practical barriers to mixing of social groups. Spatial segregation can have multiple effects, including the enforcing of homogeneity in resources and social network ties, suppressing diversity that may benefit persons of lower socio-economic status. Persons who live in segregated communities may have disproportionate exposure, susceptibility, and response to economic and social deprivation, toxic substances, and hazardous conditions (Williams and Collins, 2002). One study of infectious disease transmission suggested that residential segregation contributes to the transmission of tuberculosis through concentrated poverty resulting in conditions such as dilapidated housing and inadequate access to health care (Acevedo-Garcia, D., 2000). Conversely, it is worth noting that spatial segregation, by virtue of keeping persons who are different apart from one another, may serve to minimize social strain (Sampson, 2003).

Although related to many of the other features of the urban social environment, *inequality* potentially is an important determinant of health in urban areas in its own right. While there is ample evidence for the relation between poor individual and group socio-economic status and health (Adler and Newman, 2002), in the urban context, rich and poor populations live in physically proximate neighborhoods. Empiric and theoretical work suggests that this inequality in distribution of income and other resources may in and of itself shape health through multiple mechanisms (Wilkinson, 1992; Kaplan, *et al.*, 1996, Lynch, *et al.*, 2001; Ross, *et al.*, 2000). It has been suggested that perceived and actual inequity, caused by the discrepancies in income distribution, erodes social trust and diminishes the social capital that shapes societal well-being and individual health (Kawachi, *et al.*, 1997). Therefore, inequalities in urban areas may be important modifiers of the role of several of the other features of the social environment discussed here.

The relation between provision of *health and social services* and urban living is complicated and varies between cities and countries. In wealthy countries, cities are characterized by a rich array of health and social services (Casey, *et al.*, 2001; Felt-Lisk, 2002). However, as discussed earlier, many cities are characterized by sharp disparities in wealth between relatively proximate neighborhoods (Wilkinson, 1992). These disparities are often associated with disparities in the availability and quality of care (Andrulis, 2000; Wan and Gray, 1978). The presence of well-equipped, lucrative, practice opportunities in the same city decreases the likelihood that service providers will work in lower paid, public service clinics, particularly when these latter services face limited resources and wavering political commitment (Franks and Fiscella, 2002). Also, low-income urban residents continue to face significant obstacles in finding health care both in wealthy and less-wealthy countries (Hoffman *et al.*, 1997). In the U.S. context, persons with lower socio-economic status are more likely to lack health insurance coverage (Grumbach *et al.*, 1997; Williams and Rucker, 2000). In turn, uninsured persons face barriers to care, receive poorer quality care, and are more likely to use emergency systems (Merzel, 2000). Recent immigrants, homeless people, inmates released from jail or prison, all disproportionately represented in urban areas, also face specific obstacles in obtaining health care (Acosta and Toro, 2002; Guttmacher, 1984; Hammet, *et al.*, 1998; Kalet, *et al.*, 2002). In turn, these populations put a burden on health systems not adequately funded or prepared to care for them (Felt-Lisk, *et al.*, 2002; Pagano and Hoene, 2004). Internationally, several studies have highlighted the potential inadequacies of health systems in preventing and treating conditions such as malaria, dengue, and tuberculosis, whose spread is facilitated by high-density living that is characteristic of cities (Knudsen and Slooff, 1992; Molbak, *et al.*, 1992; Sodermann, 1997).

In summary, there are multiple mechanisms that may explain how cities affect health, with different mechanisms being potentially important for different morbidities. As discussed here, several characteristics of cities may be associated with poor health, but several others may confer an urban health "advantage" (Vlahov, *et al.*, 2005). Indeed, a "big picture" perspective on the relation between the urban context and health would suggest that these relations are undoubtedly complicated and that any single analysis that isolates a feature of urban living and health is just "scratching the surface". While specific features of cities may affect specific diseases adversely, other features may offer protection. Interrelationships between features of the urban environment further make generalization difficult. For example, further refinements on social strain theory in urban areas include an appreciation of the fact that in urban areas persons with different socio-economic status may be differentially faced with stressors and have differential access to resources that may help them cope with stressors. In particular, in urban areas, formal local resources can complement or substitute for individual or family resources for transient urban populations. Therefore, the relation between urban stressors and health is likely buffered by salutary resources (e.g., health care, social services) that are frequently more prevalent in urban compared to non-urban areas (Galea, *et al.*, 2004). Although these resources may be available to urban residents, socio-economic disparities in cities are linked to differential access to these resources, suggesting that persons at different ends of the socio-economic spectrum may have different opportunities to benefit from the resources available in cities.

4.0. URBAN HEALTH INQUIRY AND PRACTICE

Having established then that the world is rapidly urbanizing, and that this phenomenon will be an important determinant of population health both by virtue of the growing number of persons who will be living in cities and by the very characteristics of cities themselves that may affect health, we return to the central idea raised in this chapter, and indeed in this book–to what extent may we benefit from the explicit study of the health of urban populations and how may different disciplinary perspectives contribute to this inquiry?

The brief summary offered here about how the urban environment may affect health readily illustrates that cross-disciplinary work will be needed to improve our understanding, both general and specific, of the role urban context plays in shaping population health. For example, it will take the contribution of urban planners, medical geographers, and epidemiologists (to name but a few) to fully understand how the availability of green spaces and parkland within cities affects population health and how we may use this knowledge to design healthier cities. Similarly, it will take sociologists, anthropologists and health services researchers to understand how services that are available to urban residents are accessed (or not) and how these services can be implemented in a cost-effective fashion to cope with the ever growing numbers of urban residents who depend on them. However, the challenges inherent in cross-disciplinary work are legion. Speaking different "languages", diverse disciplines frequently rely on different theoretical perspectives and use methods that, while frequently complementary, may be challenging for researchers and practitioners schooled in disparate disciplinary traditions to understand.

What then are key considerations in the study of urban health as a distinct field of inquiry and practice? Urban health may draw upon the theoretical, empiric, and practical contributions of researchers and practitioners who have, thus far, been schooled in different disciplinary traditions. As such, as a coherent theoretical framework emerges for the study of urban health it can build on insights drawn from the multiple theoretical perspectives that inform currently extant disciplines. This makes it possible for urban health to consider the diverse possible roles of, for example, characteristics of the social environment and availability of (and access to) health and social services, from perspectives that include qualitative methods that enable an appreciation of motive and rationalization for behavior coupled with availability and cost-effectiveness of resources. In addition, combining the strengths of different disciplines will enable those trained in urban health to understand, and use, research methods that draw on qualitative and quantitative methodologic traditions, providing a solid empiric base for the emerging field.

Contemplating urban health, either as a subject of inquiry by multiple disciplines or as a cogent discipline in its right is fraught with challenges and in many ways presents a daunting prospect for researchers and practitioners interested in the area (Galea and Vlahov, 2004). One of these key challenges includes the development of more precise definitions of cities and essential concepts to urban health such as "urbanization." Currently there is no definition of urban places that has been universally adopted by national governments and as such, multiple, inconsistent definitions of urban are used by different countries. Similarly, although urbanization, at its simplest level, may be calculated as the change in the proportion of the national population that is urban, this change in proportion is dependent both on the urban population growth, and on the relative growth of the rest of the country. Thus, while countries of vastly different sizes can share urbanization rates, these urbanization rates can represent vastly different absolute numbers of urban residents.

The adequate specification of research questions that address how and why the urban context may affect health is another challenge in the study of urban health. As much of what may be considered urban health research in the literature thus far has arisen from different disciplines, it has used different theoretical frameworks, and applied different disciplinary orientations and terminologies. Importantly, many questions in urban health research do not meaningfully exist in isolation.

Understanding how the urban context affects health also requires consideration of multiple, often competing, influences. As is discussed throughout this book, cities are complex communities of heterogeneous individuals and multiple factors may be important determinants of population health in cities. Assessing how the urban context may affect health raises challenges and introduces complexity that is often not easily addressed through the application of simple analytic methods.

Cities are different from one another and may change over time. Empiric inquiry in health presupposes that there are identifiable factors that influence health and that these factors can usefully be identified (and potentially intervened upon). The complexity of cities and of city living may mean that urban characteristics that are important in one city may not be important in others, limiting the generalizations that can be drawn about how urban living influences health. Further complicating this task is the fact that cities change over time with implications for the relative contribution of different factors in determining health in cities. As such, in considering urban characteristics that affect health it may be important to note both the prevailing context within which such characteristics operate, and that the role of these characteristics may change over time.

Ultimately we note that we appreciate the perspective of "interest specialization" that has made tremendous contributions to overall population health. It is precisely for this reason that in this book we bring some of these perspectives of different specialties together in order to provide the reader an opportunity to think between and within these perspectives in problem identification and problem solving in the complex environment of cities. The book does not and cannot yet outline integrated approaches that might represent the foundations of an urban health "discipline", but bringing together experts in different areas to share vocabulary, methods, and perspectives represents a hope that the goal of enhancing healthy living in cities can be better articulated and achieved.

5.0. THIS BOOK

This book is intended to be one step toward the systematic study of urban health and a bridge between urban health inquiry and public health practice. As such, this book is divided into three sections. The first section discusses some specific populations in urban areas, providing both descriptions of their health status and discussions about the urban determinants of the health of these groups. It was the charge of the authors of these chapters to consider the health of specific populations in urban areas. In so doing these chapters aim both to describe the health of subpopulations that make up urban populations as a whole but also to consider how features of the urban environment may affect health of these populations. The second section focuses on different disciplinary methods that may be relevant to urban health research. Therefore, different authors comment, for example, on aspects of statistics and demography that may be suitably applied to urban health. While these chapters are not meant to suggest that these methods integrate easily into one coherent methodologic armamentarium, they are intended to highlight the different methods that may contribute to an improved understanding of urban health and in the process to identify common trends that together can shed light on a larger picture. Finally, the third section deals with the practice of urban health. We consider the practice of urban health to include diverse elements, ranging from the public health considerations that underlie the building of healthy cities, to the clinical considerations that may underlie the delivery of health services to marginalized urban populations. Chapter authors come from a broad range of disciplines and backgrounds and we offer brief editors' comments at the end of each section that are intended to help draw lessons and commonalities from these chapters that may guide our thinking toward a cogent study and practice of urban health. We note that although this book predominantly has a North American focus, a few chapters bring a global perspective. These chapters are intended to round out the picture of city living and population health as a truly global phenomenon. We hope that future work can build on this book and integrate both disciplinary and regional perspectives in the study of urban health.

REFERENCES

Acevedo-Garcia, D. (2000). Residential segregation and the epidemiology of infectious disease. *Soc. Sci. Med.* 51:1143–1161.

Acosta, O., and Toro, P.A. (2000). Let's ask the homeless people themselves: a needs assessment based on a probability sample of adults. *Am. J. Community Psychol.* 28(3):343–66.

Adler, N., and Newman, K. (2002). Socioeconomic disparities in health: pathways and policies. Inequality in education, income, and occupation exacerbates the gaps between the health "haves" and "have-nots." *Health Aff.* 21(2):60–76.

Agnew, R. (1992). Foundation for a general strain theory of crime and delinquency. *Criminology* 30(1):47–87.

Alexander, S.E., and Ehrlich, P.R. (2000). Population and the environment. In: Ernst, W.G. (ed.), *Earth Systems: processes and issues.* Cambridge University Press: Cambridge, UK.

Andrulis, D.P. (2000). Community, service, and policy strategies to improve health care access in the changing urban environment. *Am. J. Public Health* 90:858–862.

Barnett, E., and Casper, M. 2001. A Definition of "Social Environment". *Am. J. Public Health* 91(3):465.

Basu, R., and Samet, J.M. (2002). Relation between elevated ambient temperature and mortality: A review of the epidemiologic evidence. *Epidemiol. Rev.* 24:190–202.

Berrigan, D., and Troiano, R.P. (2001). The association between urban form and physical activity in U.S. adults. *Am. J. Prev. Med.* 23(2S):74–79.

Boardman, J.D., Finch, B.K., Ellison, C.G., Williams, D.R., and Jackson, J.S. (2001). Neighborhood disadvantage, stress, and drug use among adults. *J. Health Soc. Behav.* 42(2):151–65.

Booth, M.L., Owen, N., Bauman, A., Clavisi, O., and Leslie, E. 2000. Social-cognitive and perceived environment influences associated with physical activity in older Australians. *Prev. Med.* 31:15–22.

Casey, M.M., Thiede, C.K., and Klingner, J.M. (2001). Are rural residents less likely to obtain recommended preventive healthcare services? *Am. J. Prev. Med.* 21(3):182–188.

Chanthikul, S., Qasim, S.R., Mukhopadhyay, B., and Chiang, W.W. (2004). Computer simulation of leachate quality by recirculation in a sanitary landfill bioreactor. *Environ. Sci. Health Part A Tox. Hazard Subst. Environ. Eng.* 39(2):493–505.

Cohen, D.A., Farley , T.A., and Mason, K. (2003).Why is poverty unhealthy? Social and physical mediators. *Soc. Sci. Med.* 57(9):1631–41.

Diez-Roux, A.V. (2003). Residential environments and cardiovascular risk. *J. Urban Health* 80(4): 569–89.

Dockery, D.W., Pope, C.A. 3rd., Xu, X., Spengler, J.D., Ware, J.H., Fay, M.E., Ferris, B.G. Jr., and Speizer, F.E. (1993). An association between air pollution and mortality in six U.S. *N. Engl. J. Med.* 329(24):1753–9.

Elliott, M. (2000). The stress process in neighborhood context. *Health Place* 6:287–299.

Environmental Software and Services GmbH, Austria, 2002, (September 23, 2004); http://www.ess.co.at/AIR-EIA/LECTURES/L001.html.

Evans, G.W., Wells, N.M., Chan, H.Y., and Saltzman, H. (2000). Housing quality and mental health. *J. Consult. Clin. Psychol.* 68(3):526–30.

Felt-Lisk, S., McHugh, M., and Howell, E. 2002. Monitoring local safety-net providers: do they have adequate capacity? *Health Aff. (Millwood)* 21(5):277–283.

Franks, P., and Fiscella, K. (2002). Effect of patient socioeconomic status on physician profiles for prevention, disease management, and diagnostic testing costs. *Med. Care* 40(8):717–24.

Freudenberg, N., Galea, S., and Vlahov, D. (eds.). Cities and the health of the public. Forthcoming from Vanderbilt Press; 2006.

Frumkin, H. (2002). Urban sprawl and public health. *Public Health Rep.* 117:201–217.

Galea, S., Ahern, J., Vlahov, D., Coffin, P.O., Fuller, C., Leon, A.C., and Tardiff, K. (2003). Income distribution and risk of fatal drug overdose in New York City neighborhoods. *Drug Alcohol Depend.* 70(5):139–148.

Galea, S., Freudenberg, N., and Vlahov, D. (2005). Cities and population health. *Soc. Sci. Med.* 2005; 60(5): 1017-1033.

Galea, S., and Vlahov, D. (2004). Urban Health: Evidence, challenges and directions. *Ann. Rev. Pub. Health.* Epub instead of print, (August 18, 2004); http://arjournals.annualreviews.org/doi/abs/10.1146/annurev.publhealth.26.021304.144708.

Grumbach, K., Vranizan, K., and Bindman, A.B. (1997). Physician supply and access to care in urban communities. *Health Aff.* 16(1):71–86.

Guidotti, T.L., de Kok, T., Kjellstrom, T., and Yassi, A. (2001). Human Settlement and Urbanization. In: *Basic Environmental Health.* New York, NY: Oxford University Press, pp 293.

Guralnik, J.M., Seeman, T.E., Tinetti, M.E., Nevitt, M.C., and Berkman, L.F. (1994). Validation and use of performance measures of functioning in a non-disabled older urban population: MacArthur studies of successful aging. *Aging* 6:410–419.

Guttmacher, S. (1984). Immigrant workers: health, law, and public policy. *J. Health Polit. Policy Law* 9(3):503–14.

Hammett, T.M., Gaiter, J.L., and Crawford, C . (1998). Reaching seriously at-risk populations: health interventions in criminal justice settings. *Health Educ. Behav.* 25(1):99–120.

Handy, S.L., Boarnet, M.G., Ewing, R., and Killingsworth, R.E. (2002). How the built environment affects physical activity: Views from urban planning. *Am. J. Prev. Med.* 23(2S):64–73.

Hoffman, M., Pick, W.M., Cooper, D., and Myers, J.E. (1997). Women's health status and use of health services in a rapidly growing peri-urban area of South Africa. *Soc. Sci. Med.* 45(1):149–157.

Kafka, R.R., and London, P. (1991). Communication in relationships and adolescent substance use: the influence of parents and friends. *Adolescence* 26:587–98.

Kalet, A., Gany, F., and Senter, L. (2002). Working with interpreters: an interactive Web-based learning module. *Acad. Med.* 77(9):927.

Kaplan, G.A., Pamuk, E.R., Lynch, J.W., Cohen, R.D., and Balfour, J.L. (1996). Inequality in income and mortality in the United States: analysis of mortality and potential pathways. *B. Med. J.* 312: 999–1003.

Kawachi, I., and Berkman, L.F. (2001). Social ties and mental health. *J. Urban Health* 78(3):458–67.

Kawachi, I., Kennedy, B.P., Lochner, K., and Prothrow-Stith, D. (1997). Social capital, income inequality and mortality. *Am. J. Public Health* 87: 1491–1498.

Kilbourne, E.M., Choi, K., Jones, T.S., and Thacker, S.B. (1982). Risk factors for heatstroke. A case-control study. *JAMA.* 247(24):3332–6.

Kingsley, G.T. (2003). Housing, health, and the neighborhood context. *Am. J. Prev. Med.* 24(3S):6–7.

Knudsen, A.B., and Slooff, R. (1992). Vector-borne disease problems in rapid urbanization: New approaches in vector control. *Bulletin of the World Heath Organization* 70(1):1–6.

Krants, D., and Kifferstein, B, 1998, Water Pollution and Society (September 23, 2004); http://www.umich.edu/~gs265/society /waterpollution.htm

Krieger, J., and Higgins, D.L. (2002). Housing and health: time again for public health action. *Am. J. Public Health* 92:758–768.

Latkin, C.A., and Curry, A.D. (2003). Stressful neighborhoods and depression: a prospective study of the impact of neighborhood disorder. *J. Health Soc. Behav.* 44(1):34–44.

Lee, I.M., Rexrode, K.M., Cook, N.R., Manson, J.E., and Buring, J.E. 2001. Physical activity and coronary heart disease in women: is "no pain, no gain" passé? *JAMA.* 285:1447–1454.

Lynch, J., Smith, G.D., Hillemeier, M., Shaw, M., Raghunathan, T., and Kaplan, G. (2001). Income inequality, the psychosocial environment and health: Comparisons of wealthy nations. *Lancet* 358:1285–1287.

Mackenbach, J.P., Borst, V., and Schols, J.M. (1997). Heat-related mortality among nursing-home patients. *Lancet* 349:1297–1298.

Madianos, M.G., Gefou-Madianou, D., Richardson, C., and Stefanis, C.N. (1995). Factors affecting illicit and licit drug use among adolescents and young adults in Greece. *Acta. Psychiatr. Scand.* 4:258–64.

McLeod, L., and Kessler, R. (1990). Socioeconomic status differences in vulnerability to undesirable life events. *J. Health Soc. Behav.* 31:162–172.

Melosi, M. (2000). *The sanitary city: urban infrastructure in America from colonial times to the present.* Baltimore: Johns Hopkins Press.

Merzel, C. (2000). Gender differences in health care access indicators in an urban, low-income community. *Am. J. Public Health* 90(6):909–916.

Molbak, K., Aaby, P., Ingholt, N., Hojyling, N., Gottschau, A., Andersen, H., Brink, L., Gansted, U., Permin, A., Vollmer, A., and Jose da Silva, A.P. (1992). Persistent and acute diarrhea as the leading cause of child mortality in Urban Guidea Bissau. *Trans. R. Soc. Trop. Med.* 86(2):216–220.

New York Times. (December 6, 1970). *World famous impossibility.* Bellows, S. New York, New York:115.

Newman, O. (1986). *Defensible space: crime prevention through urban design.* McMillan: New York.

Northridge, M.E., and Sclar, E. (2003). A joint urban planning and public health framework: contributions to health impact assessment. *Am. J. Public Health* 93(1):118–21.

Northridge, M.E., Sclar, E., and Biswas, P. (2003). Sorting out the connections between the built environment and health: a conceptual framework for navigating pathways and planning healthy cities. *J. Urban Health* 80(4):556–68.

O'Meara, M. (1999). *Reinventing cities for people and the planet.* Worldwatch Institute: Washington D.C.

Pagano, M.A., and Hoene, C.W., 2004, Washington D.C. (September 23, 2004); City Fiscal Conditions in 2004 http://www.nlc.org/nlc_org/site/files/pdf/City%20Fiscal%20Conditions%20in%202004.pdf.

Passchier-Vermeer, W., and Passchier, W.F. (2000). Noise exposure and public health. *Environ. Health Perspec.* 108 Suppl 1: 123–131.

Pate, R.R., Pratt, M., Blair, S.N., Haskell, W.L., Macera, C.A., Bouchard, C., Buchner, D., Ettinger, W., Heath, G.W., King, A.L., Krisda, A., Leon, A.S., Marcus, B.H., Morris, J., Paffenbarger, R.S., Patrick, K., Pollock, M.L., Rippe, J.M., Sallis, J., and Wilmore, J.H. (1995). Physical activity and public health: A recommendation from the Centers for Disease Control and Prevention and the American College of Sports Medicine. *JAMA.* 273:402–407.

Pearlin, L., Lieberman, M., Menaghan, E., and Mullan J. (1981). The stress process. *J. Health Soc. Behav.* 22:337–356.

Phillips, D.P. (1974). The influence of suggestion on suicide: substantive and theoretical implications of the Werther effect. *Am. Sociol. Rev.* 39(3):340–54.

Pick, W.M., and Obermeyer, C.M. 1996. Urbanization, household composition, and the reproductive health of women in a South African City. *Soc. Sci. Med.* 43(1):1431–1441.

Rodgers, G.B. (1979). Income and inequality as determinants of mortality: an international cross section analysis. *Int. J. Epidemiol.* 31:182–191.

Roodman, D. (1998). The natural wealth of nations: Harnessing the market for the environment. WW Norton & Company: New York.

Ross, N.A., Wolfson, M.C., Dunn, J.R., Berthelot, J.M., Kaplan, G.A., and Lynch, J.W. (2000). Relation between income inequality and mortality in Canada and in the United States: cross sectional assessment using census data and vital statistics. *BMJ.* 1:30(7239):898–902.

Samet, J.M., Dominici, F., Curreriro, F.C., Coursac, I., and Zeger, S.L. (2000). Fine Particulate Air Pollution and Mortality in 20 US Cities, 1987-1994. *N. Engl. J. Med.* 343:1742–1749.

Sampson, R.J. (2003). Neighborhood-level context and health: lessons from sociology. In: Kawachi, I., and Berkman, L.F. (eds.). *Neighborhoods and health.* Oxford University Press; New York. pp. 193

Sampson, R.J., Raudenbush, S.W., and Earls, F. (1997). Neighborhoods and violent crime: a multilevel study of collective efficacy. *Science.* 277:918-924.

Satterthwaite, D. (2000). Will most people live in cities? *BMJ.* 321:1143–1145.

Satterthwaite, D. (March 16, 2004); http://www.rics.org/downloads/research_reports/urban_growth.pdf.

Semenza, J.C., McCullough, J.E., Flanders, W.D, McGeehin, M.A., and Lumpkin, J.R. (1999). Excess hospital admissions during the July 1995 heat wave in Chicago. *Am. J. Prev. Med.* 16(4):269–77.

Sodermann, M., Jakobsen, M.S., Molbak, K., Aaby, I.C.A., and Aaaby, P. (1997). High mortality despite good care-seeking behavior: A community study of childhood deaths in Guinea-Bissau. *Bulletin of the World Health Organization* 75(3):205–212.

Takano, T., Nakamura, K., and Watanabe, M. (2002). Urban residential environments and senior citizens' longevity in mega-city areas: the importance of walkable greenspaces. *J. Epidemiol. Community Health* 56:913–918.

Tanaka, A., Takano, T., Nakamura, K., and Takeuchi, S. (1996). Health levels influenced by urban residential conditions in a megacity-Tokyo. *Urban Stud.* 33(6):879–894.

Thomson, H., Pettricrew, M., Douglas, M. (2003). Health impact assessment of housing improvement: incorporating research evidence. *J. Epidemiol. Comm. Health* 57:11-16.

United Nations Department of Economic and Social Affairs/Population Division. (2004) *World Urbanization Prospects: the 2003 Revision.* Report No. ESA/P/WP.190 (March 2004).

Vlahov, D., and Galea, S. (2002). Urbanization, urbanicity, and health. *J. Urban Health* 79 Suppl 1:S1–S12.

Vlahov, D., Galea, S., Freudenberg, N. (2005) An Urban Health Advantage. *J. Urban Health 82*(1):1-4.

Vrijheid, M. (2000). Health effects of residence near hazardous waste landfill sites: A review of the epidemiologic literature. *Environ. Health. Perspect.* 108(Suppl 1):101–112.

Wan, T.T.H., and Gray, L.C. (1978). Differential access to preventive services for young children in low-income urban areas. *J. Health. Soc. Behav.* 19:312–324.

Wellington, M., Ndowa, F., and Mbengeranwa, L. (1997). Risk factors for sexually transmitted disease in Harare: A case-control study. *Sex. Transm. Dis.* 24(9):528–532.

Wilkinson, R.G. (1992). Income distribution and life expectancy. *BMJ.* 304:165-168.

Williams, D.R., and Collins, C. (2002). Racial Residential Segregation: a Fundamental Cause of Racial Disparities in Health. In: LaVeist, T. (ed.). *Race, ethnicity and health a public health reader.* Jossey Bass, San Francisco, pp. 369–90.

Williams, D.R., and Rucker, T.D. (2000). Understanding and addressing racial disparities in health care. *Health Care Financ. Rev.* 21(4):75–90.

World Health Organization, press release, 1997, Geneva, (September 23, 2004); http://www.who.int/archives/inf-pr-1997/en/pr97-47.html.

Part I

Populations

Chapter 2

Homeless People

Stephen W. Hwang and James R. Dunn

1.0. INTRODUCTION

Over the last quarter century, homelessness has become one of the symbols of urban blight. Regardless of the accuracy of this perception, homelessness is indeed a serious issue in many cities. More than 800,000 Americans are homeless in a given week, and 3.5 million are homeless over the course of a year (Burt, 2001). About 2-3% of the U.S. population, or 5-8 million people, have experienced at least one night of homelessness in the past five years (Link, *et al.*, 1994). About 70% of homeless people in the U.S. live in urban areas (Burt, 2001). Within the countries of the European Union, estimates of the number of homeless people in 1997 were 580,000 in Germany, 166,000 in the United Kingdom, 30,000 to 40,000 in the Netherlands, 10,000 in Finland, 8,000 in Sweden, and 6,000 in Norway (Menke, *et al.*, 2003).

Contrary to stereotypes, a broad range of people experience homelessness, including not only single men, but also single women, runaway adolescents, and families with young children. In the U.S., these subgroups represent about 60%, 16%, 9%, and 15% of the homeless population, respectively (Burt, 2001). In the European Union, substantial numbers of homeless families with children are found only in Germany and the United Kingdom (Menke, *et al.*, 2003). Here and throughout this chapter, we define homeless people as individuals who lack a fixed, regular, and adequate night-time residence, including those who are living in emergency or transitional shelters, in motels or hotels due to lack of alternative adequate accommodations, or in private or public places not intended for human habitation (such as cars, parks, public spaces, abandoned buildings, or bus or train stations).

The health of the homeless and the role of cities in their health present an important challenge. The relationship between urban living and the health of the homeless raises two intertwined questions. First, how does the urban environment influence the creation and perpetuation of homelessness, especially among (but not limited to) individuals with pre-existing health problems such as mental illness and substance abuse? Second, how does the urban environment affect the health of people after they have become homeless? At first glance, these two questions appear almost identical in terms of the specific characteristics and attributes of the urban environment that warrant scrutiny. For example, both questions will lead to a consideration of the availability of low-cost housing and the ability of the health care system to care for patients with severe mental illness. However, the distinction between these two questions is important as they distinguish factors associated with the likelihood of being homeless due to health reasons versus the likelihood of consequences given homelessness. At another level, it is also important to distinguish if outcomes and their associated factors vary between cities, both in terms of the structural factors that generate homelessness and (given homelessness) health of those who are homeless. These questions frame the issue of the impact of the urban environment on the health of disadvantaged populations.

In the course of such discussions, disagreement often arises as to whether homelessness should be considered primarily the consequence of individual vulnerabilities and failings, or the result of structural inequities in the social, economic, housing, and health care systems. Rather than creating an either/or distinction, we will approach homelessness as the result of a complex interaction between individual vulnerabilities and structural forces in the urban environment. In most cases, the relative importance of these factors in determining the health of homeless people and the prevalence of homelessness remains the subject of ongoing debate.

2.0. KEY HEALTH ISSUES FOR HOMELESS PEOPLE

The burden of illness and disease is extremely high among homeless people (Levy and O'Connell, 2004). However, any consideration of the common health problems of homeless people must first recognize the large degree of heterogeneity among people who are homeless. Among street youth, single men, single women, and mothers with children, the patterns of illness differ notably. Adolescents suffer from high rates of suicide attempts, sexually transmitted diseases, and pregnancy (Greene and Ringwalt, 1996; Greene and Ringwalt, 1998; Greene, *et al.*, 1999; Feldmann and Middleman, 2003). Female heads of homeless families tend to have far fewer health problems than single homeless women, although their health is poorer than their counterparts in the housed general population (Robertson and Winkleby, 1996). Homeless single men have a higher prevalence of alcohol abuse and drug abuse, whereas single women have a higher prevalence of serious mental illness (Fischer and Breakey, 1991).

Health status also tends to be correlated with a person's history of homelessness. Individuals with severe mental illness, substance abuse, and medical conditions are overrepresented among the chronically homeless, whereas those who are homeless for a transient period lasting only a few weeks or months are more likely to be relatively healthy (Kuhn and Culhane, 1998). Although chronically homeless people make up only about 10% of all individuals who experience homelessness in a given year, they account for a disproportionately large share of the demand for shelter beds and health care services for homeless people (Burt, 2001). In addition, the public's perception of homeless people often reflects a stereotyped image of this highly visible subgroup.

Cross-national comparisons of disease patterns among homeless people reveal the strong effect of social factors within each country. Among homeless men in Tokyo, Japan, morbidity due to alcohol dependence (but not drug use) is common, as are musculoskeletal injuries incurred doing construction work (Takano, *et al.*, 1999b). In contrast, 60% of homeless people in Amsterdam, the Netherlands, suffer from drug abuse or dependence (primarily heroin), and most are chronically homeless (Sleegers, 2000c).

2.1. Mental Illness and Substance Abuse

The prevalence of serious mental illness and substance abuse is high among homeless persons. In a nationwide U.S. survey of homeless people, 39% had mental health problems, 50% had an alcohol and/or drug problem, and 23% had concurrent mental health and substance use problems (Burt, 2001). Common psychiatric diagnoses among homeless people include major depression, bipolar disorder, schizophrenia, and personality disorders. A systematic review of the prevalence of schizophrenia in homeless persons found rates ranging from 4 to 16% and a weighted average of 11% in the ten methodologically strongest studies (Folsom and Jeste, 2002). Characteristics associated with a higher prevalence of schizophrenia were younger age, female sex, and chronic homelessness. Marked cross-national variation is seen in the prevalence of schizophrenia, with prevalence rates of 23-46% reported among homeless people in Sydney, Australia (Teesson, *et al.*, 2004).

The prevalence of substance abuse is extremely high among homeless single adults. In a study from St. Louis, Missouri, large increases were seen in the prevalence of drug use among homeless men and women between 1980 and 2000. In 2000, 84% of men and 58% of women had an alcohol or drug use disorder (North, *et al.*, 2004). In another study, about three-quarters of homeless adults met criteria for substance abuse or dependence (O'Toole, *et al.*, 2004). Homelessness increases the risk of adverse health outcomes among substance abusers: in five Canadian cities, the risk of a non-fatal overdose was twice as high among illicit opiate users who were homeless compared to those who were housed (Fischer, *et al.*, 2004).

Homeless adolescents also have very high rates of mental health problems and substance abuse. In a study from Seattle, 83% of street youths had been physically and/or sexually victimized after leaving home, and 18% met criteria for post-traumatic stress disorder (Stewart, *et al.*, 2004). Across the U.S., 55% of street youth and 34% of shelter youth had used illicit drugs other than marijuana since leaving home, in comparison to 13% of youth who had never been runaway or homeless (Greene, *et al.*, 1997). Street youth use a wide range of drugs, including hallucinogens, amphetamines, sedative/tranquilizers, inhalants, cocaine, and opiates. Unfortunately, the initiation of injection drug use is quite common, with an incidence rate of 8.2 per 100 person-years among street youth in Montreal (Roy, *et al.*, 2003).

2.2. Infectious Diseases

Infectious diseases are a common cause of health problems in homeless people (Raoult, *et al.*, 2001). The most serious of these infections include tuberculosis (TB), human immunodeficiency virus (HIV) infection, viral hepatitis, and other sexually transmitted infections. Outbreaks of TB among homeless people have been reported frequently, especially in individuals co-infected with HIV (Barnes, *et al.*, 1999; McElroy, *et al.*, 2003; Morrow, *et al.*, 2003). The incidence of active TB in a cohort of homeless people in San Francisco between 1992 to 1996 was 270 per 100,000, or 40 times higher than that seen in the U.S. general population in 1998 (Moss, *et al.*, 2000). Homeless people with TB require more hospital-based care than non-homeless people with TB, resulting in average hospital costs that are higher by $2,000 per patient.(Marks, *et al.*, 2000) Contact tracing in the homeless population is difficult, and in one study only 44% of identified contacts completed treatment for latent TB infection (Yun, *et al.*, 2003). Among street youth, latent tuberculosis is more common than in the general population, but probably less prevalent than among homeless adults. In a study conducted in Sydney, Australia, 9% of homeless young people aged 12-25 years had latent TB infection (Kang, *et al.*, 2000).

Homeless people are at increased risk of HIV infection. Data from an older U.S. survey conducted from 1989 to 1992 in 14 cities found median HIV seroprevalence rates of 4.0% in adult men, 1.8% in adult women, and 2.3% in youths (Allen, *et al.*, 1994). In more recent studies, HIV seroprevalence was 10.5% among homeless and marginally housed adults in San Francisco in 1996, a rate five times higher than in San Francisco generally (Robertson, *et al.*, 2004). HIV infection was present in 1.8% of homeless veterans admitted to residential programs from 1995-2000 (Cheung, *et al.*, 2002). Female street youth and young homeless women who are involved in prostitution are at increased risk of HIV infection, due to both injection drug use and risky sexual behaviors (Weber, *et al.*, 2002). In one study of homeless adolescents, the HIV infection rate was alarmingly high at 16% (Beech, *et al.*, 2003). Among substance users, homelessness is associated with higher rates of HIV seroprevalence (Surratt and Inciardi, 2004; Smereck and Hockman, 1998). Among HIV-infected persons, those who are unstably housed (homeless or temporarily staying with friends or family) are less likely to receive adequate health care than those who are stably housed (Smith, *et al.*, 2000).

Homeless people are at increased risk of viral hepatitis, primarily due to high rates of injection drug use. Infection with hepatitis C was found in 22% of homeless men in Los Angeles (Nyamathi, *et al.*, 2002), 32% of individuals using a mobile medical van in New York City (Rosenblum, *et al.*, 2001), and 27% of homeless persons in Oxford, England (Sherriff and Mayon-White, 2003). In a Veterans Affairs population, the prevalence of anti-hepatitis C virus antibody was 41.7% and the prevalence of hepatitis B surface antigen was 1.2% (Cheung, *et al.*, 2002). Among street youth, the prevalence of these markers of infection was also high: 12.6% and 1.6%, respectively, in Montreal (Roy, *et al.*, 1999; 2001) and 5.0% and 3.6%, respectively, in a northwestern U.S. city (Noell, *et al.*, 2001b).

Sexually transmitted diseases (STDs) are a particularly serious problem among street youth. In a longitudinal study of homeless adolescents, the annual incidence of *Chlamydia trachomatis* infection was 12.1% in females and 7.4% in males; the annual incidence of herpes simplex virus type 2 was 25.4% in females and 11.7% in males. (Noell, *et al.*, 2001) A study of street youth and sex workers in Quebec City, Canada found that 13% of women less than 20 years old were infected with *Chlamydia trachomatis* and 1.7% had *Neisseria gonorrhoeae* (Poulin, *et al.*, 2001). Newer urine-based screening tests make it easier to screen homeless youth for STDs in outreach settings (Van Leeuwen, *et al.*, 2002).

2.3. Chronic Diseases

Common chronic diseases, including hypertension, diabetes, chronic obstructive pulmonary disease (COPD), seizures, and musculoskeletal disorders, are often undiagnosed or inadequately treated in homeless adults. Relatively little research has focused on these medical conditions in the homeless population. The prevalence of hypertension was higher among homeless clinic patients than among non-homeless patients at an inner-city primary care clinic (65% vs. 52%) (Szerlip and Szerlip, 2002). The prevalence of diabetes is similar in homeless and non-homeless individuals, but homeless people with diabetes face a number of serious barriers to appropriate disease management, including lack of access to a suitable diet and difficulties coordinating medication administration with meal times (Hwang and Bugeja, 2000b). Glycemic control was found to be inadequate in 44% of homeless diabetics in Toronto (Hwang and Bugeja, 2000b).

Smoking rates are extremely high (about 70%) among homeless people (Connor, *et al.*, 2002). As a result, COPD is a common health problem among older adults. In a study of shelter residents in San Francisco, the prevalence of COPD based on spirometry was 15%, or more than twice the prevalence in the general population (Snyder and Eisner, 2004). Smoking also contributes to the high risk of cancer, especially among homeless single men. In a study from Scotland that adjusted for age and socioeconomic deprivation, the incidence of cancer of the oral cavity and pharynx, larynx, esophagus, and lung in homeless men was 139%, 87%, 61%, and 23% higher than expected, respectively (Lamont, *et al.*, 1997). Homeless people are also less likely to receive recommended cancer screening than the general population: among homeless women age 40 and over in Los Angeles County, only 55% had undergone a Pap smear and only 32% had undergone a mammogram within the last year (Chau, *et al.*, 2002). Thus, interventions such as smoking cessation treatment and routine preventive health services may provide significant benefit.

Although it is not surprising that homeless people with mental illness often receive inadequate care for medical comorbidities, the adequacy of care differs according to type of mental illness. Homeless people with schizophrenia receive less detailed physical examinations, fewer primary care visits, and less preventive health services than homeless people with major depression (Folsom, *et al.*, 2002). While it is unknown if these differences are due to patient factors, provider factors, or both, careful attention clearly needs to be paid to the physical health needs of homeless people with psychoses.

2.4. Trauma and Injuries

Trauma and injuries are significant hazards associated with life on the street (Staats, *et al.*, 2002). In a sample of homeless and marginally housed people in San Francisco, 32% of the women and 27% of the men had been sexually or physically assaulted in the last year (Kushel, *et al.*, 2003). Among women, being homeless (compared to being marginally housed) was associated with a more than 3-fold increase in the risk of sexual assault. In Sydney, Australia, 58% of shelter residents reported experiencing a serious physical assault in their lifetime, and half of the women reported having been raped (Buhrich, *et al.*, 2000). Among homeless youth in Los Angeles, reported exposure to violence was found to be equally high among males and females (Kipke, *et al.*, 1997).

2.5. Other Health Conditions

Foot problems are very common among homeless adults due to prolonged standing, long-term exposure to cold and damp, ill-fitting footwear, and inadequate foot hygiene. Problems can range in severity from mild blisters and fungal infections to debilitating chronic venous stasis ulcers, cellulitis, diabetic foot infections, and frostbite. Other common skin problems include sunburn and bites due to infestations by head lice, body lice, scabies, or bedbugs (Stratigos and Katsambas, 2003). The prevalence of serious dermatologic conditions, while probably quite high among street-dwellers, appears to be relatively low among homeless people living in shelters that provide adequate clothing, laundry facilities, bathing facilities, and medical care. In a study of men staying at such a shelter in Boston, the majority of individuals had relatively normal findings on skin examinations (Stratigos, *et al.*, 1999).

Dental problems are an extremely prevalent and troubling but often-neglected problem for many homeless people. Common conditions include advanced caries, periodontal disease, and ill-fitting or missing dentures. These problems may be related to poverty, lack of access to dental care, and substance use, rather than homelessness *per se*. In a study comparing homeless and domiciled veterans in Veterans Affairs rehabilitation programs for substance abusers, the two groups had similarly poor oral health (Gibson, *et al.*, 2003).

2.6. Mortality

Given the high prevalence of illness among homeless people and the adverse health effects of homelessness itself, it is not surprising that homeless people have very high mortality rates. Men using homeless shelters are 2 to 8 times more likely to die than age-matched men in the general population (Barrow, *et al.*, 1999; Hwang, 2000a). Homeless women 18-44 years of age have mortality rates that are 5 to 31 times higher than in the general population (Cheung and Hwang, 2004). Common causes of death among homeless people under the age of 45 are unintentional injuries, drug overdoses, AIDS, suicide, and homicide (Hwang, *et al.*, 1997; 2000a). In a longitudinal cohort study of street youth in Montreal, the standardized mortality ratio was 11.4; HIV infection, daily alcohol use in the last month, homelessness in the last 6 months, drug injection in the last 6 months, and male sex were independent predictors of mortality (Roy, *et al.*, 2004).

2.7. Pregnancy

Among homeless women, major barriers to contraception include cost, fear of side effects or potential health risks, and the partner's dislike of contraception (Gelberg, *et al.*, 2002). Pregnancy is particularly common among homeless adolescents. In a U.S. survey of runaway females age 14-17 years, 12% of street-dwelling youths and 10% of those residing in shelters were currently pregnant (Greene and Ringwalt, 1998). In a group of pregnant homeless women, the risk of low birth weight (less than 2,500 gm) was 17%, compared to the national average of 6% (Stein, *et al.*, 2000). Lack of prenatal care and severity of homelessness (homelessness in the first trimester of pregnancy, number of times homeless, and percentage of life spent homeless) were independent risk factors for low birth weight.

2.8. Children in Homeless Families

The health of children in homeless families has been the focus of relatively little research. Some but not all studies of these children have found an increased prevalence of behavioral and mental health problems compared to children in housed low-income families (Bassuk, *et al.*, 1997; Vostanis, *et al.*, 1998). Infectious diseases are a significant concern in these children (Ligon, 2000). Up to 40% of children in homeless families in New York City suffer from asthma, a rate six times higher than the national rate in children (McLean, *et al.*, 2004c).

3.0. DIMENSIONS OF THE URBAN ENVIRONMENT THAT AFFECT THE PREVALENCE OF HOMELESSNESS AND THE HEALTH OF HOMELESS PEOPLE

The medical literature has usually examined health problems from the perspective of the individual homeless person, and has given relatively little attention to the urban environment within which these health problems arise and must be ameliorated. This section addresses this gap by highlighting dimensions of the urban environment that affect, through interaction with individual vulnerabilities, the prevalence of homelessness and/or the health of homeless people. The following is not intended to be a comprehensive listing, but rather a selection of important determinants about which at least some information is available. These determinants have been grouped into categories encompassing the demographic and physical characteristics of urban centers (population and climate), their socioeconomic and service-delivery structures (income and poverty, social welfare systems, and health care systems), and their spatial and political organization (urban geography and urban governance). Although these dimensions may have differential effects on the health of various subgroups of homeless people (e.g., youths, single adults, and families), these differences are not discussed in depth here.

3.1. Population Size and Migration

Homelessness is a problem in cities across the U.S., as demonstrated by the fact that federally-funded Health Care for the Homeless Programs exist in 161 cities in all 50 states, the District of Columbia, and Puerto Rico (Health Care for the Homeless Information Resource Center). There is limited information on the relationship between population size and prevalence of homelessness in different urban centers. One reason for this paucity of data is the logistical difficulty of conducting an accurate count of homeless persons, particularly those living on the street. Another reason is that point-prevalence counts of the homeless population cannot be used to determine how many individuals are homeless in a city over an entire year, especially given seasonal fluctuations in the homeless population and the fact that homelessness is a transient state.

Counts of shelter users are particularly informative when all shelters contribute to a common administrative database, because this makes it possible to determine the total number of individuals who use shelters in a particular city over the course of a year, rather than simply the number of shelter users at a single point in time (Metraux, *et al.*, 2001). In 1992, an estimated 1.0% of the 1.5 million residents of Philadelphia and 1.2% of the 7.2 million inhabitants of New York City stayed at a homeless shelter at least once (Culhane, *et al.*, 1994). In Toronto, Canada, 1.3% of the city's total population of 2.5 million used a homeless shelter during 2002. These figures are remarkably similar and strikingly high. Thus, homelessness is quite common in large urban centers, although for many individuals the duration of homelessness is quite brief. In a U.S. survey of homeless people, 28% had been homeless for only 3 months or less, 26% had been homeless for 4-12 months, and 46% had been homeless for more than one year (Burt, 2001).

Cross-sectional counts of the number of shelter residents provide an important but somewhat less accurate picture of the homeless population. The maximum size of a city's shelter population is obviously determined by the number of available shelter beds. In a city with few shelters, this can create the illusion of a smaller homeless population than is actually the case. In addition, shelter beds may be less widely available in cities that do not experience severe cold weather in the winter. In the nine largest metropolitan areas in Canada, the number of shelter beds per capita ranges more than four-fold, from 21 to 97 per 100,000 population (Hwang, 2001). The number of shelter beds per capita is not significantly correlated with population size. Interestingly, the lowest number of shelter beds per capita in Canada was observed in Vancouver, a city with a very mild climate, and the highest figure was seen in Calgary, a city with extremely cold winters. Overall, this evidence suggests that episodes of homelessness are quite common among residents of major urban centers, but there is significant variation in the prevalence of homelessness across cities that does not necessarily correlate with population size.

A related question is the role of migration in determining the size of the homeless population in urban centers. Whereas some homeless people are migrants who were homeless before or upon their arrival in the city, others are local residents who have become homeless. In a nationwide U.S. survey, 56% of homeless people reported living in the same city where they became homeless (Burt, 2001). Among the 44% of individuals who had moved from one location to another during their current episode of homelessness, the most common pattern was a net flux from urban fringes and medium-sized cities into large central cities. The most commonly cited reasons for these moves were lack of available jobs, lack of affordable housing, and eviction (Burt, 2001).

3.2. Climate

Climate is an interesting example of a characteristic of the urban environment that affects both the prevalence of homelessness and the health of homeless people. Certain cities in warm regions may become a preferred destination for people who are homeless or at high risk for homelessness. As noted above, in cities with warmer climates, a larger proportion of the homeless population is likely to be found on the street rather than in shelters. People living on the street are more likely to be disengaged from the health care and social service systems, and typically these individuals have poorer health than shelter-dwelling homeless people (Cousineau, 1997). In colder climates, exposure to the elements has an obvious adverse impact on the health of homeless people, who face serious risks from trench foot, frostbite, and injury or death from hypothermia (Tanaka and Tokudome, 1991). Conversely, in hot weather, homeless people may experience severe sunburn, heat exhaustion, or heat stroke.

3.3. Income and Housing

The prevalence of severe poverty among the residents of an urban area is certainly an important factor affecting the prevalence of homelessness. Poverty alone, however, does not necessarily lead to homelessness. Data from nine U.S. cities demonstrate wide variation in the proportion of a city's poor residents that stays at a homeless shelter over the course of one year, ranging from a low of 1.3% to a high of 10.2% (Metraux, *et al.*, 2001). Some have argued, based on historical data, that an increase in the number of unmarried men with very low income is a particularly important explanatory factor for adult homelessness (Jencks, 1994). During the latter half of the twentieth century, the earning potential of men with limited education was greatly diminished by the decline of manufacturing jobs in urban centers (Wilson, 1987; 1996). At the same time, the availability of open-market sources of low-cost housing such as single-room occupancy hotels and rooming houses shrank steadily due to gentrification and urban renewal (Hasson and Ley, 1994). In this setting, the level of government support for subsidized rental housing plays a key role in determining the availability of units that a low-income individual or family can afford; the 1980's saw a decline in this support in both the U.S. and the United Kingdom (Cohen, 1994).

Some have suggested that income distribution, specifically the ratio of middle-income to low-income households within a given city, is an important determinant of homelessness among both single adults and families (O'Flaherty, 1996). O'Flaherty argues that because the construction of new rental housing for low-income individuals is economically unattractive, the main source of housing for poor people is deteriorating housing stock that has been vacated by middle-income people. O'Flaherty theorized that cities with fewer middle-class people relative to the number of poor people have higher rents at the bottom of the market (because middle-income housing is not being "handed down" to the poor), resulting in higher rates of homelessness.

Members of ethnic and racial minorities are disproportionately represented in the homeless population (e.g., blacks and latinos in the U.S., and Aboriginal people in Canada) (Burt, 2001; Hwang, 2001). The higher prevalence of poverty in these disadvantaged groups may explain this observation. However, other race-related factors in the urban environment may contribute to the excess risk of homelessness among people of color, including discrimination in the housing market and segregation of low-income minorities in neighborhoods with fewer economic opportunities than neighborhoods in which low-income whites reside.

Any discussion of the role that urban poverty plays in causing homelessness also raises questions about nature of the causal relationship between homelessness and poor health. Poverty is consistently and strongly associated with poor health (Marmot, *et al.*, 1997). Thus, the poor health observed among homeless people may be explained in large part by the fact that they experience extreme poverty and deprivation, rather than the fact that they happen to be homeless at the present time. This is particularly likely to be the case for individuals who have only recently become homeless, and less so for the chronically homeless, who have been subjected to the adverse health effects of lack of housing for a lengthy period. To extend this concept further, homelessness is a marker for severe poverty in the urban environment, and it may be this level of poverty, rather than the negative impact of homelessness itself, that has the greatest effect on population health in urban centers. This issue is discussed further in section 4 of this chapter.

3.4 Social Welfare System

Social welfare systems in urban centers have a major impact on both the prevalence of homelessness and the health of homeless people. However, these systems are usually governed at the state or national level, rather than at the municipal level. Wide variation is seen in the scope of social welfare programs, with more generous benefits typically seen in countries or regions that have less tolerance for high levels of income inequality and place a higher value on social cohesion (Sleegers, 2000b).

For example, eligibility criteria for welfare benefits in the U.S. vary significantly from state to state. Some states allow single men to collect welfare, whereas others exclude them. These policies would likely affect the risk of homelessness among low-income single men living in any city within a given state. In addition,

U.S. federal funds may not be used to provide Temporary Aid to Needy Families (TANF) if an adult in the family has received assistance for more than 60 months, but individual states may elect to continue providing assistance to these families using state funds (State Policy Documentation Project). In coming years, as families that are unable to become self-supporting begin reaching the 60-month federal time limits on benefits, their risk of becoming homeless may be greatly affected by the policies of the state in which they live. In contrast, most European Union countries have extensive social welfare and public housing systems that make family homelessness less common.

One area of controversy is whether the provision of cash entitlements or disability benefits has significant effects on the health of homeless people. On one hand, the health of homeless people should improve if public benefits allow them to obtain food, housing, and other essentials of life. On the other hand, increased income could be detrimental to health if the money is used to purchase alcohol or drugs. One of the few studies on this issue examined 173 homeless mentally ill veterans who applied for Social Security Disability Insurance (SSDI) or Supplemental Security Income (SSI). The 50 individuals who were eventually awarded benefits did not differ in their past history of substance use from the 123 individuals who were eventually denied benefits. Three months after the decision to award or deny benefits, the group that was awarded benefits had significantly higher average total income (by $277 per month) and higher quality of life than the group that was denied benefits. There was no evidence of increased alcohol or drug use or deterioration in psychiatric status among those who received benefits (Rosenheck, *et al.*, 2000).

Most homeless people depend on their city's shelter system for housing, food, and other social services, and these shelters can therefore have a significant impact on the health of homeless people. The availability and quality of homeless shelters vary greatly. As noted previously, homeless people in cities with few shelter beds are more likely to live on the street or other places not intended for human habitation, with potentially adverse health effects. In addition, the staff at homeless shelters can play an important role in connecting homeless people to social services, job training, housing applications, and substance abuse treatment. The quantity and quality of food provided at shelters determines to a large extent the nutritional value of homeless people's diets, with potential downstream health effects (Dachner and Tarasuk, 2002). Finally, the physical environments at shelters range from extremely crowded, poorly ventilated, and unsanitary facilities to modern, clean, and well-run establishments. Adverse shelter conditions have an impact on the transmission of tuberculosis and viral respiratory infections and the prevalence of health conditions such as skin infestations and asthma exacerbations. Shelter conditions could also plausibly have an effect on mental and emotional well-being among residents. To date, however, little research has examined the effects of the physical shelter environment on the health of homeless persons, with the exception of the relationship between crowding and poor ventilation in shelters and the transmission of tuberculosis (Advisory Council for the Elimination of Tuberculosis, 1992b).

3.5. Health Care System

The organization and financing of the urban health care system has an enormous impact on the health of homeless people, and to some extent on the prevalence of homelessness as well. In the U.S., 55% of homeless people lack health insurance, creating a significant barrier to obtaining care (Kushel, *et al.*, 2001). These individuals are dependent on state- or city-based systems designed to provide care for the indigent. In many large urban centers in the U.S., a designated public, county, or charity hospital provides the majority of hospital-based health care for homeless people. Some cities have free-care clinics or community health centers that provide ambulatory services for homeless persons as well as other low-income residents. In 161 U.S. cities, federally-funded Health Care for the Homeless Programs have established multidisciplinary teams of physicians, nurses, social workers, and outreach workers that provide care to homeless people on the street and in shelters. This limited set of health care providers is typically the only source of care available to homeless people in urban areas in the U.S., and the local funding and staffing level of these organizations is a critical determinant of access to health care. For homeless veterans, the proximity and availability of Veterans Health Administration services is also an important factor.

In countries such as Canada and the United Kingdom that have systems of universal health insurance, homeless people still face non-financial barriers to care. Many access problems stem from the fact that a health care system designed to meet the needs of the general population may not accommodate the unique requirements of homeless people(Crane and Warnes, 2001; Hwang and Bugeja, 2000a, 2000b). For example, the provision of universal health insurance does not necessarily result in the establishment of outreach programs for homeless people, appropriate treatment programs for homeless persons with mental illness or substance abuse, or an adequate supply of health care providers who are willing, able, and trained to work with this challenging population (Buchanan, *et al.*, 2004). In the United Kingdom, individuals must register with a general practitioner to obtain primary care, and some physicians are reluctant to accept homeless people into their practice because of their complex needs and the extra workload entailed (Wood, *et al.*, 1997). Health insurance does not protect against the fragmentation and discontinuity of care that homeless people often experience, nor does it eliminate the daily struggle to meet basic survival needs that may cause homeless people to place a lower priority on seeking health care (Gelberg, *et al.*, 1997).

Inadequate access to primary health care may result in uncontrolled disease progression and frequent emergency department visits and hospitalizations (Han and Wells, 2003). Emergency department visits by homeless people should be seen as an indicator of high levels of unmet health needs, rather than inappropriate health care utilization (Kushel, *et al.*, 2002). About 50% of homeless children with severe persistent asthma have had at least one emergency department visit in the last year, a finding indicative of inadequate access to health care and undertreatment of their disease (McLean, *et al.*, 2004).

Because individuals with severe mental illness who do not receive appropriate health care are at high risk of becoming homeless, the health care system can have a direct impact on the prevalence of homelessness. The role of deinstitutionalization in contributing to the problem of homelessness has been discussed extensively. Beginning in the 1960's and 1970's, the advent of effective anti-psychotic medications to treat schizophrenia and an understandable desire to move people out of chronic mental hospitals, where conditions were sometimes horrendous, led to the discharge of tens of thousands of long-term psychiatric patients (Dear and Wolch, 1987; Jencks, 1994). The number of beds at psychiatric institutions fell precipitously. In theory, these patients were supposed to receive mental health care and social support in the community. In reality, many of these patients received little if any services and ended up swelling the ranks of the homeless population in the 1970's and 1980's.

Today, many decades after these events took place, "deinstitutionalization" is no longer the major cause of homelessness among people with serious mental illness. It is now uncommon for people with psychiatric disorders to have ever been institutionalized for an extended period, and any admissions tend to be quite brief. Not surprisingly, individuals with severe illness, few social supports, and/or inadequate access to appropriate outpatient psychiatric care often become homeless. In a sense, homeless shelters have assumed the role that was played by chronic psychiatric hospitals fifty years ago.

For these homeless people with severe mental illness, the delivery of appropriate health care is challenging but essential to improving their health and housing status. The Assertive Community Treatment (ACT) model attempts to address this problem through a team of psychiatrists, nurses, and social workers who follow a small caseload of homeless mentally ill clients, seeking them out in the community to provide high-intensity mental health treatment and case management. Studies have found that mentally ill homeless people receiving ACT spend fewer days hospitalized as a psychiatric inpatient and have somewhat greater improvement in symptoms than those receiving usual care (Lehman, *et al.*, 1997). However, ACT is labor-intensive and costly, and its availability is often quite limited.

The availability and type of addictive substances in the urban environment have an important effect on the prevalence of homelessness and on the health of homeless people (Munoz, *et al.*, 1998). The advent of crack cocaine has been clearly implicated in the rise of homelessness in the U.S. in the 1980's (Jencks, 1994). In Japan, alcoholism is the predominant addiction contributing to homelessness and morbidity among homeless people, whereas in the Netherlands, homelessness is closely linked to chronic heroin addiction (Takano, *et al.*, 1999a; Sleegers, 2000a).

Access to addiction treatment is therefore a vital issue for a large proportion of homeless people. A number of treatment modalities for adults have been shown to be effective in controlled studies: admission to a post-detoxification stabilization program results in longer periods of abstinence than direct release into the shelter system (Kertesz, *et al.*, 2003), and abstinence-contingent work therapy in a long-term residential setting has been shown to improve outcomes (Milby, *et al.*, 2000). Studies have examined the effectiveness of case management for homeless people with addictions, with mixed results (Morse, 1999).

3.6. Urban Geography

The forces underlying the urban geography of homelessness are aptly described in the seminal work of Dear and Wolch (Dear, *et al.*, 1987). They examined how deinstitutionalization, rollbacks in entitlements to social assistance, and changes in the global economy in the late 1970s and early 1980s combined to create complex problems of poverty, inequality, and homelessness in North American cities that persist to this day. Dear and Wolch (1987) argued that these problems manifested themselves in the specific urban form of the "service-dependent ghetto," which refers to the spatial concentration in the inner city of service-dependent populations (such as people with mental illness, physical handicaps, addictions, or recent incarceration) and the organizations that assist them. While on one hand these can be characterized as areas of "urban blight," Dear and Wolch (1987) argued that they serve as a supportive environment and adaptive coping mechanism that can have a positive effect on the health and well-being of residents who have few other options. Service-dependent ghettos are often the object of antagonism from surrounding communities. Paradoxically, however, these more affluent communities often perpetuate the forces that create the service-dependent ghetto and entrench processes of inner-city decay through citizen resistance to housing and services for low-income people and exclusionary land use policies and zoning practices (Dear and Taylor, 1982).

In some cities, the tendency has been to isolate high-poverty urban neighborhoods rather than attempt to destroy them. Davis argues that in Los Angeles and other cities, a conscious effort has been made to create geographic and physical barriers (such as expressways) that circumscribe poor and minority neighborhoods and cut them off from the rest of the city (Davis, 1990). This spatial isolation can further heighten the marginalization of these communities and limit residents' access to goods, services, and economic opportunities that are vital to health.

Since homeless people spend a great deal of their time in public spaces, the nature of these spaces can have a significant impact on their quality of life. Some cities have numerous well-tended public spaces such as parks and squares that are conducive to those who wish to linger or rest, including homeless people. These spaces can serve a socially cohesive function if urban dwellers of diverse backgrounds perceive them to be safe "neutral" spaces in which to gather and socialize. In contrast, other cities have built environments that lack such public spaces and are instead dominated by privatized quasi-public spaces such as shopping malls. Non-purposeful lingering, which would be generally acceptable in a public space such as a park, is perceived as "loitering" in such places. In a relatively trivial but very specific expression of hostility toward homeless people, some cities have installed "bum-proof" benches that are designed to prevent reclining or sleeping on the seat. While these elements of the urban environment seem relatively minor, they may reflect a city's prevailing sentiment towards homeless and poor people that sets the tone of their daily existence (Davis, 1990).

3.7. Urban Governance

Homelessness is often perceived as having a negative effect on the quality of life in urban centers. Some consider the visible presence of homeless people in parks, street corners, and other public spaces to be a manifestation of "urban disorder" and a barrier to the successful promotion of commerce and tourism. In response to these concerns, a number of cities have enacted by-laws against panhandling, loitering or sleeping in public places, public intoxication, or possession of shopping carts. Some cities have instituted aggressive policing strategies to remove homeless people from public spaces (Graser, 2000). Efforts to displace street youth and homeless people rather than offer them any meaningful help might have negative effects on health and in fact increase high-risk behaviors such as survival sex and unsafe injection drug use practices (O'Grady and Greene, 2003; Wood, *et al.*, 2004).

Homeless people frequently interact with both police and paramedics, but they have much lower levels of trust in police than in paramedics (Zakrison, *et al.*, 2004). By inhibiting homeless people from calling for needed emergency assistance, this distrust could result in serious harms to health. In a study of injection drug users in San Francisco, 56% of those who had been present with an unconscious heroin overdose victim did not call for emergency services due to fear of police involvement (Davidson, *et al.*, 2002). Police action can also have direct adverse effects on the health through the excessive use of force (Cooper, *et al.*, 2004). In a study in

Toronto, 9% of homeless people reported having been assaulted by a police officer in the last 12 months (Zakrison, *et al.*, 2004).

On a larger scale, issues of urban governance such as fiscal disparities affect all urban dwellers, but have the potential to have a particularly severe impact on homeless and poor people. Fiscal disparities typically occur when an older central city with a significant number of high-poverty neighborhoods is surrounded by a ring of higher-income municipalities. The central city's primary revenue stream from property taxes is limited by a weak tax base, but at the same time the city is confronted by a high and rising demand for social services, some of which is driven by the downloading of 'unfunded mandates' by states onto central city municipalities (Drier, *et al.*, 2001). Meanwhile, the nearby ring communities have a strong property tax base and face a lower demand for social services, while at the same time its residents work in the central city and benefit from its economic activities and services (the so-called "free-rider" effect) (Orfield, 1998; Drier, *et al.*, 2001). These fiscal disparities greatly exacerbate the adverse effects of racial and economic segregation on homeless people and others living in extreme poverty in the central city.

In an example of an effort to redress this problem, state legislation in Minnesota, the Fiscal Disparities Act, mandates the sharing of commercial property tax between outlying, high tax base municipalities to central city municipalities to assist in the provision of social services. Enacted in 1971 by the Minnesota legislature, the plan pools 40% of the increase in all communities' commercial/industrial property valuation. All cities and townships keep their pre-1971 tax bases plus 60% of the annual growth. The pool is then taxed at a uniform rate and redistributed among all local government entities. Although this redresses some of the intra-metropolitan disparities, it does little to reduce the payoffs of "externalizing" social problems with tools like exclusionary zoning in typically more affluent communities. Moreover, the Minneapolis-St. Paul example depends on the existence of a strong regional-metropolitan level of governance, the Met Council, which although heavily studied (Orfield, 1998; Rusk, 1999; Katz and Bradley, 1999), is still a concept that is strongly resisted by homeowners' associations, gated communities, and affluent municipalities (McKenzie, 1994; Boudreau and Keil, 2001). An alternative solution is to create cities that encompass lower and higher income areas, rather allowing them to separate into different jurisdictions. In Toronto, Ontario, this was effectively accomplished through the amalgamation of five contiguous cities into a single urban entity, although the amalgamation was motivated by a desire to increase operating efficiency rather than concern regarding fiscal disparities (Boudreau, 2000).

4.0. THE EFFECTS OF HOMELESSNESS ON POPULATION HEALTH

Does homelessness have a sizeable effect on population health? This question raises a number of complex issues. Homeless people, especially those who are chronically homeless, tend to have poor health. However, homelessness is a temporary state, not a permanent trait. As many as 8 millions Americans experience homelessness over a five year period, but most of these episodes of homelessness are quite brief (Link, *et al.*, 1994). Thus, at any single point in time only a very small proportion of a city's population is without a home. Homeless people would therefore be expected to have a minimal impact on indicators of overall population health, such as health status or mortality rates. Of course, this assumption may be incorrect in urban centers in the developing world, where extremely large numbers of people often live on the street or in encampments.

Some have suggested that homelessness may have an adverse effect on public health through the spread of infectious diseases, such as tuberculosis. Compared to the general population, homeless people are clearly at increased risk of developing latent tuberculosis, which is not infectious to others, as well as active tuberculosis, which can infect those who come in close contact with the individual. During tuberculosis outbreaks, shelter residents, shelter staff, and health care providers are at increased risk of becoming infected (Advisory Council for the Elimination of Tuberculosis, 1992a). To date, however, outbreaks of tuberculosis among homeless people have not spread widely within the general population. The threat of tuberculosis is therefore an important health problem for homeless people, but one that has demonstrated relatively limited potential to affect overall population health in urban areas.

The outbreak of Severe Acute Respiratory Syndrome (SARS) in 2003 has raised the specter of rapid and uncontrolled spread of acute respiratory infections through the homeless population. The 2003 SARS outbreak in Toronto was almost entirely confined to travelers returning from abroad, health care workers, and their household contacts (Svoboda, *et al.*, 2004). No homeless person became infected with SARS. If this had happened, the large, transient, and difficult-to-locate shelter population would have made it almost impossible for Toronto public health officials to implement their core strategy of identifying and quarantining all "household contacts" of patients with SARS. Such a situation could have had devastating effects on efforts to prevent the outbreak from spreading into the city's general population. Given the threat of a recurrence of SARS or the possible emergence of other new and potentially deadly respiratory infections, infection control measures to deal with a severe acute infectious disease outbreak in the homeless population require serious consideration. Although this scenario is currently hypothetical, the potential implications for population health are considerable.

Homelessness may have major implications for population health, for reasons other than those discussed above. Emphasis on the direct impact of homelessness on population health may be misplaced. Instead, homelessness may be viewed as a sentinel event, a marker for dysfunction in multiple sectors including the housing market, job market, health care system, and social welfare system. Homelessness represents the extreme end of a larger distribution of socioeconomic status and housing status, and it attracts attention precisely because of its dire nature.

This conceptualization has been well-described in work by Rose (1985). As shown in Figure 1, the curve shown with a solid line represents the distribution of housing quality within a hypothetical population. Homelessness represents the extreme low point along the dimension of housing quality. This approach views one's housing situation as a continuum and avoids creating a simple dichotomy between being homeless and being housed. For the sake of this discussion, we assume that housing conditions have an impact on health, an assertion for which there is ample support (Fuller-Thomson, *et al.*, 2000; Krieger and Higgins, 2002). Figure 1 also illustrates two different approaches to improving health through improving housing conditions. The greatest effect in terms of population health may be gained through approach A (shifting the entire population distribution for the factor upwards slightly, to the distribution curve indicated by a dotted line) rather than approach B (focusing on improving conditions for the highest-risk

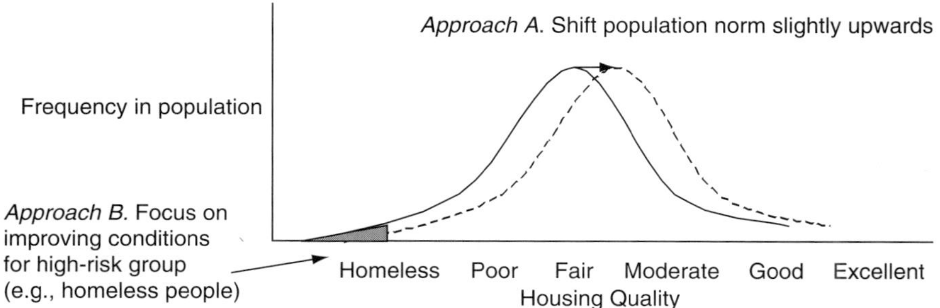

Figure 1. The Distribution of Housing Quality within a Hypothetical Population, and the Effect of Two Different Approaches to Improving Health Through Improving Housing Conditions.

group at the worst extreme of the distribution). A similar argument could be applied to the relationship between poverty and health, where the x-axis on the diagram would represent income rather than housing quality.

The case of asthma is an excellent example of this dilemma. About 40% of children staying at homeless shelters in New York City have asthma (McLean, *et al.*, 2004a). Although this is a disturbingly high rate, the prevalence of asthma is also very high among inner-city children living in substandard housing (Malveaux and Fletcher-Vincent, 1995). Because homeless children represent a relatively small proportion of all children living in poverty in a given city, the population health effect of asthma among homeless children is likely to be far smaller than the population health effect of asthma in the much larger number of children who are housed but living in decrepit buildings. While homeless children are a distressing manifestation of urban poverty, they represent "the tip of the iceberg" of the broader issue of poverty and poor housing. Thus, the problem of asthma among homeless children may be regarded as an extreme example of a much larger population health concern that may be a more appropriate target for intervention.

5.0. POTENTIAL STRATEGIES TO IMPROVE THE HEALTH OF HOMELESS PEOPLE

A consideration of strategies to improve the health of homeless people raises the question of whether our first concern should be to attempt to deal with the problem of homelessness itself, or to intervene to relieve illness among homeless youths, single adults, or families. Of course, this is not an either/or proposition. Nonetheless, an excessive emphasis on the latter approach might result in producing healthier homeless people, yet fail to recognize that homelessness is the result not only of individual vulnerabilities, but also of deeper structural problems within our society. On the other hand, a focus on the former approach may founder on the assumption that providing homeless people with stable housing will necessarily improve their health.

An example of this tension is the emergence of two contrasting service delivery models to meet the needs of chronically homeless adults with concurrent mental illness and substance abuse (Tsemberis, *et al.*, 2004; Hopper and Barrow, 2003). The first model, known as the "Continuum of Care," attempts to move homeless people from the street into transitional congregate housing, in conjunction with a requirement that the individual engage in treatment for their mental illness and addictions. Under this model, the person is allowed to make the transition to permanent housing only after they achieve abstinence from alcohol and drugs and their clinical status has been stabilized. In contrast, the "Housing First" model is based on the belief that homeless people should be afforded permanent housing as a basic human right, not as a reward contingent on participating in treatment. In this model, homeless people can obtain housing in individual apartments without any preconditions, and they are then offered an array of harm reduction and treatment services through an ACT team (see section 3.5. above). A recent randomized controlled trial assigned 225 homeless adults with concurrent severe mental illness and substance abuse to one of these two approaches. Individuals treated under the "Housing First" model spent significantly less time homeless over the follow-up period, and at the end of 24 months about 80% were in stable housing as compared to only 30% in the "Continuum of Care" model. However, there were no significant differences between the two groups in terms of alcohol use, drug use, or psychiatric symptoms. This study highlights the need to acknowledge that ending homelessness is a worthwhile goal in and of itself, but that it is not synonymous with improving the health of homeless people.

Other strategies include adapting the health care system to better meet the unique needs of homeless adolescents, single men and women, or families. As discussed in Section 3.5 above, a cornerstone of this effort is the use of multidisciplinary teams providing coordinated care at outreach sites, in combination with more traditional clinic-based health care services. For homeless people with severe mental illness, the availability of ACT services is vital, but the effectiveness of less resource-intensive systems of mental health care for homeless people needs to be assessed. For those with addictions, the availability of detoxification beds, post-detoxification stabilization programs, and longer-term (6 to 12 month) residential addiction treatment programs are important issues. In designing these services, the heterogeneous needs of different subgroups of homeless people (e.g., street youth, single men, single women, and mothers with young children) must be taken into account.

While improving conditions at shelters is by no means the preferred route to better health for homeless people, it is important that shelters not contribute to ill health. Certainly, the availability of adequate capacity to accommodate everyone who seeks a shelter bed is a reasonable first step towards protecting homeless adults from the elements. Adherence to basic standards of cleanliness, nutrition, and food hygiene within shelters and the avoidance of overcrowding and inadequate ventilation are mandatory. Perhaps equally important is the creation of a safe and welcoming environment that encourages clients to engage with service providers.

At a broader level, interventions are needed to decrease the prevalence of homelessness and address the systemic issues that contribute to homelessness. These efforts may at least in some cases have health benefits as well. For homeless families, there is compelling evidence that the provision of subsidized housing is both necessary and sufficient to end their homelessness (Shinn, *et al.*, 1998). The "Housing First" strategy appears to be more effective in moving homeless people with concurrent mental illness and substance abuse into stable housing; further research is needed to examine the effectiveness of this approach with other subgroups of homeless people.

Serious attention needs to be paid to the impact of the social welfare system on homelessness and health. Restrictions in eligibility for Temporary Aid for Needy Families and state-run welfare programs threaten to contribute to a potential rise in homelessness among families and single adults in coming years. Further research is needed in this area and on the impact of receipt of welfare or disability benefits on the health of homeless people.

Finally, upstream from the distinctive and visible issue of homelessness is the larger problem of urban poverty. The existence of entire communities and groups who are cut off from a decent education, employment opportunities, housing, and access to health care should raise extremely troubling questions for anyone who cares about the health of our urban centers. While the adverse health effects of homelessness are clearly severe, this phenomenon is only a specific and extreme example of the larger problem of the effects of poverty and inadequate housing on population health.

REFERENCES

Advisory Council for the Elimination of Tuberculosis. (1992b). Prevention and control of tuberculosis among homeless persons. Recommendations of the Advisory Council for the Elimination of Tuberculosis. *Morbidity & Mortality Weekly Report, Recommendations & Reports* 4: 13–23.

Advisory Council for the Elimination of Tuberculosis (1992a). Prevention and control of tuberculosis among homeless persons. Recommendations of the Advisory Council for the Elimination of Tuberculosis. *Morbidity & Mortality Weekly Report, Recommendations & Reports* 4:13–23.

Allen, D. M., Lehman, J. S., Green, T. A., Lindegren, M. L., Onorato, I. M., and Forrester, W. (1994). HIV infection among homeless adults and runaway youth, United States, 1989-1992. Field Services Branch. *AIDS.* 8:1593-1598.

Barnes, P. F., Yang, Z., Pogoda, J. M., Preston-Martin, S., Jones, B. E., Otaya, M., Eisenach. K,D,, Knowles, L., Harvey, S., and Cave, M.D. (1999). Foci of tuberculosis transmission in central Los Angeles. *American Journal of Respiratory & Critical Care Medicine* 159: 1081–1086.

Barrow, S. M., Herman, D. B., Cordova, P., and Struening, E. L. (1999). Mortality among homeless shelter residents in New York City. *Am. J. Public Health* 89: 529–534.

Bassuk, E. L., Weinreb, L. F., Dawson, R., Perloff, J. N., and Buckner, J. C. (1997). Determinants of behavior in homeless and low-income housed preschool children. *Pediatrics* 10: 92–100.

Beech, B. M., Myers, L., Beech, D. J., and Kernick, N. S. (2003). Human immunodeficiency syndrome and hepatitis B and C infections among homeless adolescents. *Semin. Pediatr. Infect. Dis.* 14:12–19.

Boudreau, J. A. (2000). *The Megacity Saga: Democracy and Citizenship in This Global Age.* Montreal: Black Rose Books.

Boudreau, J. A. and Keil, R. (2001). Seceding from Responsibility? Secession Movements in Los Angeles. *Urban Studies* 38:1701–1731.

Buchanan, D., Rohr, L., Kehoe, L., Glick, S. B., and Jain, S. (2004). Changing attitudes toward homeless people. *J. Gen. Intern. Med.* 19:566–568.

Buhrich, N., Hodder, T., and Teesson, M. (2000). Lifetime prevalence of trauma among homeless people in Sydney. *Australian & New Zealand Journal of Psychiatry* 34: 963–966.

Burt, M. R. (2001). *Helping America's Homeless.* Washington, DC: Urban Institute Press.

Chau, S., Chin, M., Chang, J., Luecha, A., Cheng, E., Schlesinger, J. Veena, R., Huang, D., Maxwell, A.E., Usatine, R., Bastani, R., and Gelberg, L. (2002). Cancer risk behaviors and screening rates among homeless adults in Los Angeles County. *Cancer Epidemiology, Biomarkers & Prevention* 11: 431–438.

Cheung, A. M., and Hwang, S. W. (2004). Risk of death among homeless women: a cohort study and review of the literature. [see comment]. [Review] [40 refs]. *CMAJ Canadian Medical Association Journal* 170:1243–1247.

Cheung, R. C., Hanson, A. K., Maganti, K., Keeffe, E. B., and Matsui, S. M. (2002). Viral hepatitis and other infectious diseases in a homeless population. *Journal of Clinical Gastroenterology* 34: 476–480.

Cohen, C. I. (1994). Down and out in New York and London: A cross-national comparison of homelessness. *Hospital & Community Psychiatry* 45(8): 769—776.

Connor, S. E., Cook, R. L., Herbert, M. I., Neal, S. M., and Williams, J. T. (2002). Smoking cessation in a homeless population: there is a will, but is there a way? *Journal of General Internal Medicine* 17: 369–372.

Cooper, H., Moore, L., Gruskin, S., and Krieger, N. (2004). Characterizing perceived police violence: implications for public health. *Am. J. Public Health* 94: 1109–1118.

Cousineau, M. R. (1997). Health status of and access to health services by residents of urban encampments in Los Angeles. *Journal of Health Care for the Poor & Underserved* 8:70–82.

Crane, M., and Warnes, A. M. (2001). The responsibility to care for single homeless people. *Health & Social Care in the Community* 9: 436–444.

Culhane, D., Dejowski, E. F., Ibanez, J., Needham, E., and Macchia, I. (1994). Public shelter admission rates in Philadelphia and New York City: The implications of turnover for sheltered population counts. *Housing Policy Debate* 5: 107–140.

Dachner, N., and Tarasuk, V. (2002). Homeless "squeegee kids": food insecurity and daily survival. *Soc. Sci. Med.* 54:1039–1049.

Davidson, P. J., Ochoa, K. C., Hahn, J. A., Evans, J. L., and Moss, A. R. (2002). Witnessing heroin-related overdoses: the experiences of young injectors in San Francisco. *Addiction* 97:1511–1516.

Davis, M. (1990). *City of Quartz.* New York: Vintage Books.

Dear, M. J., and Taylor, S. M. (1982). *Not on Our Street: Community Attitudes to Mental Health Care.* Pion, London.

Dear, M. J., and Wolch, J. R. (1987). *Landscapes of Despair: From Deinstitutionalization to Homelessness.* Princeton University Press, Princeton, NJ.

Drier, P., Mollenkopf, J., and Swanstrom, T. (2001). *Place Matters: Metropolitics for the Twenty-first Century.* University Press of Kansas, Kansas City

Feldmann, J., and Middleman, A. B. (2003). Homeless adolescents: common clinical concerns. *Semin. Pediatr. Infect. Dis.* 14:6–11.

Fischer, B., Brissette, S., Brochu, S., Bruneau, J., el Guebaly, N., Noel, L., Rehm, M., Tyndall, C., Wild, P., Mun, E., Haydon, E., and Baliunas, D. (2004). Determinants of overdose incidents among illicit opioid users in 5 Canadian cities. *CMAJ.* 171: 235–239.

Fischer, P. J., and Breakey, W. R. (1991). The epidemiology of alcohol, drug, and mental disorders among homeless persons. *American Psychologist. Special Issue: Homelessness* 46(11):1115–1128.

Folsom, D., and Jeste, D. V. (2002). Schizophrenia in homeless persons: a systematic review of the literature. [Review] *Acta Psychiatrica Scandinavica* 105: 404–413.

Folsom, D. P., McCahill, M., Bartels, S. J., Lindamer, L. A., Ganiats, T. G., and Jeste, D. V. (2002). Medical comorbidity and receipt of medical care by older homeless people with schizophrenia or depression. *Psychiatr. Serv.* 53: 1456–1460.

Fuller-Thomson, E., Hulchanski, J. D., and Hwang, S. W. (2000). The housing/health relationship: what do we know? *Reviews on Environmental Health* 15: 109–133.

Gelberg, L., Gallagher, T. C., Andersen, R. M., and Koegel, P. (1997). Competing priorities as a barrier to medical care among homeless adults in Los Angeles. *Am. J. Public Health* 87: 217–220.

Gelberg, L., Leake, B., Lu, M. C., Andersen, R., Nyamathi, A. M., Morgenstern, H., and Browner, C. (2002). Chronically homeless women's perceived deterrents to contraception. *Perspectives on Sexual and Reproductive Health* 34: 278–285.

Gibson, G., Rosenheck, R., Tullner, J. B., Grimes, R. M., Seibyl, C. L., Rivera-Torres, A. Goodman, H.S., and Nunn, M.E. (2003). A national survey of the oral health status of homeless veterans. *J. Public Health Den.* 63: 30–37.

Graser, D. (2000). Panhandling for change in Canadian law. *Journal of Law and Social Policy* 15: 45–91.

Greene, J. M., Ennett, S. T., and Ringwalt, C. L. (1999). Prevalence and correlates of survival sex among runaway and homeless youth. *Am J. Public Health* 89: 1406–1409.

Greene, J. M., Ennett, S. T., and Ringwalt, C. L. (1997). Substance use among runaway and homeless youth in three national samples. *Am. J. Public Health* 87:229–235.

Greene, J. M., and Ringwalt, C. L. (1996). Youth and familial substance use's association with suicide attempts among runaway and homeless youth. *Subst. Use Misuse* 31: 1041–1058.

Greene, J. M., and Ringwalt, C. L. (1998). Pregnancy among three national samples of runaway and homeless youth. *J. Adolesc. Health* 23: 370–377.

Han, B., and Wells, B. L. (2003). Inappropriate emergency department visits and use of the Health Care for the Homeless Program services by Homeless adults in the northeastern United States. *J. Public Health Manag. Pract.* 9: 530–537.

Hasson, S., and Ley, D. (1994). The limits of neighbourhood empowerment: Gentrification, resistance, and burn-out in Kitsilano. In: *Neighbourhood Organizations and the Welfare State* University of Toronto Press, Toronto, Ontario, pp. 239–270.

Health Care for the Homeless Information Resource Center. Bureau of Primary Health Care. Bethesda, Maryland, (September 10, 2004); http://www.bphc.hrsa.gov/Hchirc.

Hopper, K., and Barrow, S. M. (2003). Two genealogies of supported housing and their implications for outcome assessment. *Psychiatr. Serv.* 54: 50–54.

Hwang, S. W. (2000a). Mortality among men using homeless shelters in Toronto, Ontario. *JAMA*. 283: 2152–2157.

Hwang, S. W., and Bugeja, A. L. (2000b). Barriers to appropriate diabetes management among homeless people in Toronto.[comment]. *CMAJ*. 163: 161–165.

Hwang, S. W. (2001). Homelessness and health. *CMAJ*. 164: 229–233.

Hwang, S. W., Orav, E. J., O'Connell, J. J., Lebow, J. M., and Brennan, T. A. (1997). Causes of death in homeless adults in Boston. *Ann. Intern. Med.* 126:625–628.

Jencks, C. (1994). *The Homeless*. Harvard University Press, Cambridge, MA.

Kang, M., Alperstein, G., Dow, A., van, B., I, Martin, C., and Bennett, D. (2000). Prevalence of tuberculosis infection among homeless young people in central and eastern Sydney. *Journal of Pediatrics & Child Health* 36: 382–384.

Katz, B., and Bradley, J. (1999). Divided We Sprawl. *The Atlantic Monthly* 284:26-42.

Kertesz, S. G., Horton, N. J., Friedmann, P. D., Saitz, R., and Samet, J. H. (2003). Slowing the revolving door: stabilization programs reduce homeless persons' substance use after detoxification. *J. Subst. Abuse Treat.* 24:197–207.

Kipke, M. D., Simon, T. R., Montgomery, S. B., Unger, J. B., and Iversen, E. F. (1997). Homeless youth and their exposure to and involvement in violence while living on the streets. *J. Adolesc. Health* 20:360–367.

Krieger, J., and Higgins, D. L. (2002). Housing and health: time again for public health action. *Am. J. Public Health* 92:758–768.

Kuhn, R., and Culhane, D. P. (1998). Applying cluster analysis to test a typology of homelessness by pattern of shelter utilization: results from the analysis of administrative data. *Am. J. Community Psychol.* 26:207–232.

Kushel, M. B., Evans, J. L., Perry, S., Robertson, M. J., and Moss, A. R. (2003). No door to lock: victimization among homeless and marginally housed persons. *Arch. Intern. Med.* 163: 2492–2499.

Kushel, M. B., Perry, S., Bangsberg, D., Clark, R., and Moss, A. R. (2002). Emergency department use among the homeless and marginally housed: results from a community-based study. *Am. J. Public Health* 92: 778–784.

Kushel, M. B., Vittinghoff, E., and Haas, J. S. (2001). Factors associated with the health care utilization of homeless persons. *JAMA*. 285: 200–206.

Lamont, D. W., Toal, F. M., and Crawford, M. (1997). Socioeconomic deprivation and health in Glasgow and the west of Scotland–a study of cancer incidence among male residents of hostels for the single homeless. *Journal of Epidemiology & Community Health* 51: 668–671.

Lehman, A. F., Dixon, L. B., Kernan, E., DeForge, B. R., and Postrado, L. T. (1997). A randomized trial of assertive community treatment for homeless persons with severe mental illness. *Arch. Gen. Psychiatry* 54: 1038–1043.

Levy, B. D., and O'Connell, J. (2004). Health care for homeless persons. *N. Engl. J. Med.* 350: 2329–2332.

Ligon, B. L. (2000). Infectious diseases among homeless children and adolescents: a national concern. *Seminars in Pediatric Infectious Diseases* 11: 220–226.

Link, B. G., Susser, E., Stueve, A., Phelan, J., Moore, R. E., and Struening, E. (1994a). Lifetime and five-year prevalence of homelessness in the United States. [comment]. *Am. J. Public Health* 84:1907-1912.

Malveaux, F. J. and Fletcher-Vincent, S. A. (1995). Environmental risk factors of childhood asthma in urban centers. *Environ. Health Perspect.* 103(Suppl 6): 59–62.

Marks, S. M., Taylor, Z., Burrows, N. R., Qayad, M. G., and Miller, B. (2000). Hospitalization of homeless persons with tuberculosis in the United States. *Am. J. Public Health* 90: 435–438.

Marmot, M., Ryff, C. D., Bumpass, L. L., Shipley, M., and Marks, N. F. (1997). Social inequalities in health: next questions and converging evidence. *Soc. Sci. Med.* 44: 901–910.

McElroy, P. D., Southwick, K. L., Fortenberry, E. R., Levine, E. C., Diem, L. A., Woodley, C. L., Williams, P.M., McCarthy, K.D., Ridzon, R., and Leone, P.A. (2003). Outbreak of tuberculosis among homeless persons coinfected with human immunodeficiency virus. *Clin. Infect. Dis.* 36: 1305–1312.

McKenzie, E. (1994). *Privatopia: Homeowner Associations and the Rise of Residential Private Government.* Yale University Press, New Haven.

McLean, D. E., Bowen, S., Drezner, K., Rowe, A., Sherman, P., Schroeder, S., Redlener, K., and Redlener, I. (2004). Asthma among homeless children: undercounting and undertreating the underserved. *Arch. Pediatr. Adolesc. Med.* 158: 244-249.

Menke, R., Streich, W., Rossler, G., and Brand, H. (2003). *Report on Socio-Economic Differences in Health Indicators in Europe: Health inequalities in Europe and the situation of disadvantaged groups.* Bielefeld, Institute of Public Health, NRW, Germany

Metraux, S., Culhane, D., Raphael, S., White, M., Pearson, C., Hirsch, E. Ferrell, P., Rice, S., Ritter, B., and Cleghorn, J.S. (2001). Assessing homeless population size through the use of emergency and transitional shelter services in 1998: results from the analysis of administrative data from nine US jurisdictions. *Public Health Rep.* 116: 344–352.

Milby, J. B., Schumacher, J. E., McNamara, C., Wallace, D., Usdan, S., McGill, T., and Michael, M. (2000). Initiating abstinence in cocaine abusing dually diagnosed homeless persons. *Drug Alcohol Depend.* 60(1):55–67.

Morrow, C. B., Cibula, D. A., and Novick, L. F. (2003). Outbreak of tuberculosis in a homeless men's shelter. *Am. J. Prev. Med.* 24:124–127.

Morse, G. (1999). A review of case management for people who are homeless: Implications for practice, policy, and research. In: Fosburg, L.B., and Dennis, D.L. (eds.), *Practical Lessons: The 1998 National Symposium on Homelessness Research* (pp. 7-1-7-34). U.S. Dept. of Housing and Urban Development and U.S. Dept. of Health and Human Services, Washington D.C.

Moss, A. R., Hahn, J. A., Tulsky, J. P., Daley, C. L., Small, P. M., and Hopewell, P. C. (2000). Tuberculosis in the homeless. A prospective study. *American Journal of Respiratory & Critical Care Medicine* 162:460–464.

Munoz, M., Vazquez, C., Koegel, P., Sanz, J., and Burnam, M. A. (1998). Differential patterns of mental disorders among the homeless in Madrid (Spain) and Los Angeles (USA). *Social Psychiatry & Psychiatric Epidemiology* 33(10):514–520.

Noell, J., Rohde, P., Ochs, L., Yovanoff, P., Alter, M. J., Schmid, S., Bullard, J., and Black, C. (2001). Incidence and prevalence of chlamydia, herpes, and viral hepatitis in a homeless adolescent population. *Sex Transm. Dis.* 28:4–10.

North, C. S., Eyrich, K. M., Pollio, D. E., and Spitznagel, E. L. (2004). Are rates of psychiatric disorders in the homeless population changing? *Am. J. Public Health* 94:103–108.

Nyamathi, A. M., Dixon, E. L., Robbins, W., Smith, C., Wiley, D., Leake, B., Longshore, D., and Gelberg, L. (2002). Risk factors for hepatitis C virus infection among homeless adults. *J. Gen. Intern. Med.* 17: 134–143.

O'Flaherty, B. (1996). *Making Room: The Economics of Homelessness.* Harvard University Press, Cabridge, MA.

O'Grady, B., and Greene, C. (2003). A Social and Economic Impact Study of the Ontario Safe Streets Act on Toronto Squeegee Workers. *Online Journal of Justice Studies, 1.*

O'Toole, T. P., Gibbon, J. L., Hanusa, B. H., Freyder, P. J., Conde, A. M., and Fine, M. J. (2004). Self-reported changes in drug and alcohol use after becoming homeless. *Am. J. Public Health* 94:830–835.

Orfield, M. (1998). *Metropolitics: A regional agenda for community and stability.* Washington, DC: Brookings Institution Press and the Lincoln Institute of Land Policy.

Poulin, C., Alary, M., Bernier, F., Carbonneau, D., Boily, M. C., and Joly, J. R. (2001). Prevalence of Chlamydia trachomatis and Neisseria gonorrhoeae among at-risk women, young sex workers, and street youth attending community organizations in Quebec City, Canada. *Sex Transm. Dis.* 28:437–443.

Raoult, D., Foucault, C., and Brouqui, P. (2001). Infections in the homeless. *The Lancet Infectious Diseases* 1:77–84.

Robertson, M. J., Clark, R. A., Charlebois, E. D., Tulsky, J., Long, H. L., Bangsberg, D. R., and Moss, A.R. (2004). HIV seroprevalence among homeless and marginally housed adults in San Francisco. *Am. J. Public Health* 94:1207–1217.

Robertson, M. J., and Winkleby, M. A. (1996). Mental health problems of homeless women and differences across subgroups. [Review] [74 refs]. *Annu. Rev. Public Health.* 17:311–336.

Rose, G. (1985). Sick individuals and sick populations. *Int. J. Epidemiol.* 14: 32–38.

Rosenblum, A., Nuttbrock, L., McQuistion, H. L., Magura, S., and Joseph, H. (2001). Hepatitis C and substance use in a sample of homeless people in New York City. *J. Addict. Dis.* 20:15–25.

Rosenheck, R. A., Dausey, D. J., Frisman, L., and Kasprow, W. (2000). Outcomes after initial receipt of social security benefits among homeless veterans with mental illness. *Psychiatr. Serv.* 51: 1549–1554.

Roy, E., Haley, N., Leclerc, P., Boivin, J. F., Cedras, L., and Vincelette, J. (2001). Risk factors for hepatitis C virus infection among street youths. *CMAJ.* 165:557–560.

Roy, E., Haley, N., Leclerc, P., Cedras, L., Blais, L., and Boivin, J. F. (2003). Drug injection among street youths in Montreal: predictors of initiation. *J. Urban Health* 80:92–105.

Roy, E., Haley, N., Leclerc, P., Sochanski, B., Boudreau, J. F., and Boivin, J. F. (2004). Mortality in a cohort of street youth in Montreal. *JAMA*. 292: 569–574.

Roy, E., Haley, N., Lemire, N., Boivin, J. F., Leclerc, P., and Vincelette, J. (1999). Hepatitis B virus infection among street youths in Montreal. *CMAJ*. 161:689–693.

Rusk, D. (1999). *Inside Game/Outside Game:Winning Strategies for Saving Urban America*. Brookings Institution Press, Washington D.C.

Sherriff, L.C. and Mayon-White, R. T. (2003). A survey of hepatitis C prevalence amongst the homeless community of Oxford. *J. Public Health Med.* 25:358–361.

Shinn, M., Weitzman, B. C., Stojanovic, D., Knickman, J. R., Jimenez, L., Duchon, L., James, S., and Krantz, D.H. (1998). Predictors of homelessness among families in New York City: from shelter request to housing stability. *Am. J. Public Health* 88:1651–1657.

Sleegers, J. (2000a). Similarities and differences in homelessness in Amsterdam and New York City. *Psychiatr. Serv.* 51:100–104.

Sleegers, J. (2000c). Similarities and differences in homelessness in Amsterdam and New York City. *Psychiatr. Serv.* 51:100–104.

Sleegers, J. (2000b). Similarities and differences in homelessness in Amsterdam and New York City. *Psychiatr. Serv.* 51:100–104.

Smereck, G. A. D., and Hockman, E. M. (1998). Prevalence of HIV Infection and HIV Risk Behaviors associated with Living Place: On-the-Street Homeless Drug Users as a Special Target Population for Public Health Intervention. *Am. J. Drug Alcohol Abuse* 24:299–319.

Smith, M. Y., Rapkin, B. D., Winkel, G., Springer, C., Chhabra, R., and Feldman, I. S. (2000). Housing status and health care service utilization among low-income persons with HIV/AIDS. *J. Gen. Intern. Med.* 15: 731–738.

Snyder, L. D., and Eisner, M. D. (2004). Obstructive lung disease among the urban homeless. *Chest* 125: 1719–1725.

State Policy Documentation Project. Center for Law and Social Policy and the Center on Budget and Policy Priorities. Washington D.C. (September 10, 2004); http://www.spdp.org.

Staats, P. N., Jumbelic, M. I., and Dignan, C. R. (2002). Death by compaction in a garbage truck. *Journal of Forensic Sciences* 47:1065–1066.

Stein, J. A., Lu, M. C., and Gelberg, L. (2000). Severity of homelessness and adverse birth outcomes. *Health Psychology* 19:524–534.

Stewart, A. J., Steiman, M., Cauce, A. M., Cochran, B. N., Whitbeck, L. B., and Hoyt, D. R. (2004). Victimization and posttraumatic stress disorder among homeless adolescents. *J. Am. Acad. Child. Adolesc. Psychiatry* 43: 325–331.

Stratigos, A. J., and Katsambas, A. D. (2003). Medical and cutaneous disorders associated with homelessness. *Skinmed* 2:168–172.

Stratigos, A. J., Stern, R., Gonzalez, E., Johnson, R. A., O'Connell, J., and Dover, J. S. (1999). Prevalence of skin disease in a cohort of shelter-based homeless men. *J. Am. Academy Dermatology* 41:197–202.

Surratt, H. L., and Inciardi, J. A. (2004). HIV risk, seropositivity and predictors of infection among homeless and non-homeless women sex workers in Miami, Florida, USA. *AIDS Care* 16:594–604.

Svoboda, T., Henry, B., Shulman, L., Kennedy, E., Rea, E., Ng, W. Wallington, T., Yaffe, B., Gournis, E., Vicencio, E., Basrur, S., and Glazier, R.H. (2004). Public health measures to control the spread of the severe acute respiratory syndrome during the outbreak in Toronto. *N. Engl. J. Med.* 350:2352–2361.

Szerlip, M. I., and Szerlip, H. M. (2002). Identification of cardiovascular risk factors in homeless adults. *Am. J. Med. Sci.* 324:243–246.

Takano, T., Nakamura, K., Takeuchi, S., and Watanabe, M. (1999b). Disease patterns of the homeless in Tokyo. *J. Urban Health.* 76:73-84.

Takano, T., Nakamura, K., Takeuchi, S., and Watanabe, M. (1999a). Disease patterns of the homeless in Tokyo. *J. Urban Health.* 76:73-84.

Tanaka, M., and Tokudome, S. (1991). Accidental hypothermia and death from cold in urban areas. *Int. J. Biometeorol.* 34:242–246.

Teesson, M., Hodder, T., and Buhrich, N. (2004). Psychiatric disorders in homeless men and women in inner Sydney. *Aust. N. Z. J. Psychiatry* 38:162–168.

Tsemberis, S., Gulcur, L., and Nakae, M. (2004). Housing first, consumer choice, and harm reduction for homeless individuals with a dual diagnosis. *Am. J. Public Health* 94:651–656.

Van Leeuwen, J. M., Rietmeijer, C. A., LeRoux, T., White, R., and Petersen, J. (2002). Reaching homeless youths for Chlamydia trachomatis and Neisseria gonorrhea screening in Denver, Colorado. *Sex Transm. Infect.* 78:357–359.

Vostanis, P., Grattan, E., and Cumella, S. (1998). Mental health problems of homeless children and families: longitudinal study. *BMJ.* 316:899–902.

Weber, A. E., Boivin, J. F., Blais, L., Haley, N., and Roy, E. (2002). HIV risk profile and prostitution among female street youths. *J. Urban Health* 79:525–535.

Wilson, W. J. (1996). *When Work Disappears: The World of the New Urban Poor.* Random House, New York.

Wilson, W. J. (1987). *The truly disadvantaged : the inner city, the underclass, and public policy.* University of Chicago Press, Chicago.

Wood, E., Spittal, P. M., Small, W., Kerr, T., Li, K., Hogg, R. S., Tyndall, M. W., Montaner, J. S. G., and Schechter, M. T. (2004). Displacement of Canada's largest public illicit drug market in response to a police crackdown. *CMAJ.* 170:1551–1556.

Wood, N., Wilkinson, C., and Kumar, A. (1997). Do the homeless get a fair deal from general practitioners? *J. Royal Soc. Health* 117:292–297.

Yun, L. W., Reves, R. R., Reichler, M. R., Bur, S., Thompson, V., Mangura, B. Mangura, B., and Ford, J. (2003). Outcomes of contact investigation among homeless persons with infectious tuberculosis. *Int. J. Tuberc. Lung Dis.* 7:S405–S411.

Zakrison, T. L., Hamel, P. A., and Hwang, S. W. (2004). Homeless people's trust and interactions with police and paramedics. *J. Urban Health* In Press.

Chapter 3

Health of Economically Deprived Populations in Cities

Patricia O'Campo and Michael Yonas

1.0. INTRODUCTION

In this chapter we discuss economically deprived populations residing in urban environments in industrialized countries. While we draw heavily from the experiences of the U.S. in terms of our descriptions of the populations that comprise the economically deprived, the structural factors producing economic deprivation, and the policy solutions for this growing population, the issues discussed here are relevant for all industrialized settings.

One prominent feature of the current U.S. economy is the growing wealth and income inequality among the population. The U.S. leads the industrialized world in the income gap between its rich and poor. Currently, 1% of the wealthiest households control approximately 38% of the nation's wealth, while the lowest 80% of the households account for only 17% (Mishel, *et al.*, 2003). During the 1980s and 1990s, the income of those in the 95th percentile grew approximately 20 percentage points, while incomes in the middle- and low-income groups grew very little over this same time period (Mishel, *et al*,. 2003). These trends persist as families at the top of the income distribution gather unprecedented wealth as the sole beneficiaries of the "strong" U.S. economy (Mishel, *et al.*, 1999; 2003).

The American dream of working hard and making your dreams come true remains motivating and inspirational to many. Yet, this remains just a dream for a growing proportion of the U.S. population. With falling wages for the middle and lower classes, a shrinking public service sector, and a diminishing safety net for those at the very bottom, too many families, despite working full time, are not making ends meet.

In this chapter we explore the health problems of the economically and socially deprived residing in urban settings. We consider those who are economically deprived not only the populations living at or below the poverty line, but also those who are above the poverty line yet are struggling to maintain a basic living standard such as those persons or families earning less than a living wage. We seek to cover four questions in this chapter: (1) who are the economically deprived populations residing in urban environments; (2) what are the structural and policy factors that contribute to and maintain the plight and/or well-being of the economically deprived in urban environments; (3) what are some of the health burdens experienced by the economically and socially deprived urban populations; and (4) what are potential policies and strategies for improving the health of economically deprived populations and individuals in urban settings?

2.0. ECONOMICALLY DEPRIVED POPULATIONS RESIDING IN URBAN ENVIRONMENTS

While the first impression of economically deprived populations are those residing in poverty, there are a number of subpopulations comprising the economically deprived including those who are residing in poverty, the working poor, and even those who reside above the poverty level. These groups are described in this section.

2.1 Poverty

In 2003, approximately 35.8 million people (12.5% of the U.S. population) were living below the federal poverty level, an increase of 1.3 million people, from 12.1%, in 2002 (U.S. Census Bureau, 2004). The poverty threshold, in 2004, for a family of four was $18,979 and for one person was $9,573. For example, a family of four, one adult and three children, this would equal $8.89 an hour or $3.74 more than the current federal minimum wage level, assuming a full-time position of 40 hours a week. An increasingly important measure of severe economic deprivation is 'deep poverty' or the group of persons whose incomes are at half (50%) of the official poverty line. Fully half of those residing in poverty reside in deep poverty; for a family of 4 that would represent an income of $9,489 or less. The proportion of those residing in deep poverty is increasing rapidly as only seven years ago (1997) about 30% of the poor were in deep poverty (Mishel, *et al.*, 2003). Recent research has shown that the social policies designed to help the impoverished engage the job markets are less likely to reach these individuals thereby perpetuating the cyclic nature of disadvantage and marginalization (Mishel, *et al.*, 2003).

These numbers tell only part of the story as poverty varies significantly by race and gender. Women have about 40% higher poverty rates than men, 12.3%, and 8.7% in 2002, respectively. Similar increases are seen for women and men residing in deep poverty in 2002, 5% for women and 3.5% for men (Casey, 2003). Poverty rates in 2002 were more than double for single households headed by women (33%) versus men (16%). While these trends are concerning, what is not stated in most poverty discussions is the fact that the pathways to and out of poverty differ significantly for women versus men (O'Campo and Tang, 2001). While men can more reliably depend upon employment as a way of escaping poverty, women cannot. Women's disproportionate share of family, children, and household responsibilities precludes employment alone as a means for climbing out of poverty and economic hardship (Pearce, 1990; O'Campo and Rojas-Smith, 1998; O'Campo and Tang, 2001). Economic deprivation varies considerably by race. In 1996 poverty rates for blacks and latinos (28.4% and 29.4%) were almost three times that of whites (11.2%) (US Census Bureau, 1997).

2.2. The Working Poor

One feature of the economy that affects the majority of workers is falling wages. Since the 1970s, growth in family income has slowed considerably, especially in comparison to the growth in the U.S. following World War II. Average annual family income growth during the period 1947-1973 was 2.7%. Annual growth in family income following that period averaged 0.6%, 0.4%, and 0.1% for the periods 1973-79, 1979-89, and 1989-97, respectively. In other words, the wage increase their parents received in a single year would take today's families half their working lives to achieve. Falling wages are not a reflection of falling worker productivity. In fact, from 1968 to 2001, worker productivity has risen 75%. Had the average hourly wage kept pace with productivity since 1968, the hourly wage in 2001 would be $25.39 and not $14 as it was in 2001; moreover, minimum wage would be $14.15 (all values are 2001 dollars) (Sklar, *et al.*, 2001).

Additionally, the increase in underemployment, contingent work, and job insecurity, piled upon reduction of shrinking social aid policies, has meant that families can more easily slide into poverty, and remain there longer. Although tempting as a set of explanations, there are no data to support that changing demographics (i.e., growth in female-headed households) and lack of human capital (i.e., insufficient educational level or skills) contribute significantly to increasing poverty. Rather, recent social policies, including an eroding safety net for low-income families, "wealthfare" (laws that allow the rich to keep a greater portion of their earnings), along with falling wages, and growing inequalities, calcify the economic plight of those at the bottom (Aldelba and Folbre, 1996; Mishel, *et al.*, 1999). From 1974-1995, there was a steady increase in the proportion of individuals earning poverty-level wages while working full-time, 50 hours per week year round. Poverty rates remain consistent with those in 1973 with 20% of black families and 33% of families headed by single mothers living in poverty in the year 2000. More importantly, if contemporary measures of poverty were adopted, it is certain that the rates of poverty would be even higher (Mishel, *et al.*, 2003).

2.3. Working but Struggling: Earning a "Living Wage"

Having an annual income above a poverty level wage is no guarantee that families can make ends meet. Increasingly, there is focus on levels of income needed for economic sufficiency or a 'living' wage (Boushey, *et al.* 2001; Sklar, *et al.*, 2001; Mishel, *et al.*, 2003). While this wage varies substantially by region of the country, the range is between $6.25 and $12.00 dollars per hour.

While not recognized by the federal government as having unacceptably low incomes, the struggles to provide for basic needs within these families are real and tragic. Twenty-nine percent of working families in the U.S. with one to three children under age twelve do not earn enough income to afford basic necessities such as food, housing, healthcare, and childcare, even during the economic "boom" of the mid to late 1990's (Boushey, *et al.*, 2001). Families with incomes between the poverty line and twice the poverty line were just as likely to experience hardships and economic struggle as those families living below the federal poverty level with the reported shares of each family type as 25% and 29%, respectively (Boushey, *et al.*, 2001). The majority of these families are two-parent families with one or more workers who are again often earning incomes that are above the federally established poverty level.

3.0. STRUCTURAL AND POLICY FACTORS CREATING ECONOMIC DEPRIVATION IN URBAN ENVIRONMENTS

A conceptual framework describing how urban environments affect the health of economically deprived populations is useful for identifying determinants of, and solutions to, poorer health among this group (Heyman, 2000; Krieger, 2001). The poverty and economic deprivation noted in the earlier sections of this chapter are the consequences of historical economic, social, and political processes that have contributed to the unequal development of urban areas and to the economic and racial segregation of U.S. urban spaces. And while we emphasize the economic aspects of those with low social class position, this population experiences myriad social problems ranging from poor working conditions, substandard yet unaffordable housing, and poor quality educational systems to inaccessible health care services and daily discrimination based upon race, class, and gender.

We present a conceptual framework describing the ways in which economic, social, and political processes ultimately affect the well-being of urban populations in Figure 1. While a detailed discussion of these historical process — such as a changing economy which emphasizes a shift from manufacturing to service

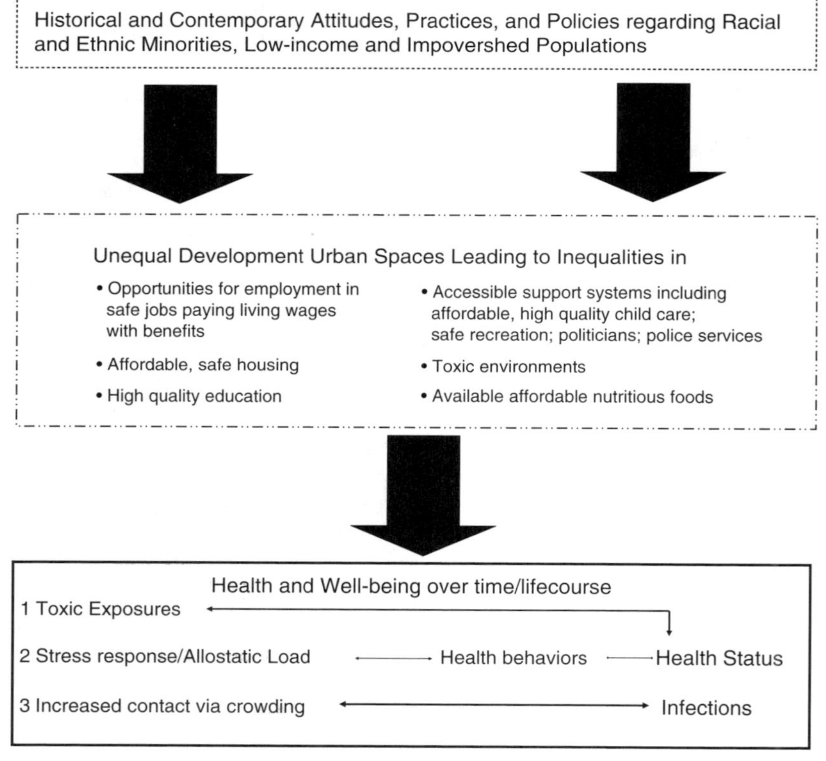

Figure 1. Social Production of Inequalities in Health and Well-Being in Urban Environments.
Note: The framework is not intended to be comprehensive but, rather, presents examples of pathways by which structural factors affect urban environments and, in turn, influence health.

oriented jobs, migration of manufacturing jobs from urban areas, employment discrimination by race and gender, housing policies including lending practices and residential segregation, demographic shifts in the composition of urban areas resulting from the migration of middle-class families to the surrounding suburbs eroding the tax base of cities, growing poverty concentration and ghetto formation, and failing educational systems – are beyond the scope of this paper, they are detailed in several excellent references published elsewhere (Wilson, 1987; Halpern, 1995; Marmot and Wilkinson, 1999; Navarro and L, 2001; Frazier, *et al.*, 2003; Hofrichter, 2003; Venkatesh, 2003; Wilson, 2003; Massey 2004; Raphael, 2004). Rather, we are only able to present selective examples of the processes and pathways by which they lead to unequal urban development and may ultimately have their impact upon the health of economically deprived populations.

While many descriptions of the inner cities of the U.S. tend to convey poor neighborhoods and urban spaces as if those characteristics are inherent in the populations or neighborhoods where low-income residents reside, we agree with Wilson and others (Frazier, *et al.*, 2003; Venkatesh, 2003; Wilson, 2003; Massey, 2004) that these deprived urban areas are the result of larger policies and practices as suggested by the top two boxes in Figure 1. A primary determinant of economic deprivation is lack of employment that pays well and provides ample benefits (e.g., health care coverage). Given the shift in the U.S. economy away from higher paying manufacturing jobs for those individuals with lower skills, jobs that often carried health, vacation, and retirement benefits have largely been eliminated. This shift has hurt those at the bottom and racial and ethnic minorities, blacks in particular, the hardest. While approximately one-third of those employed in the 1950s were in the manufacturing sector, that has dropped to just 12% in the late 1990s. There has been a growth in service-sector jobs but these jobs often have low pay, few benefits, and are less secure (Mishel, *et al.*, 2003). Those at the bottom have fewer resources to rely on during hard times, e.g., families with surplus economic resources, have access to home equity loans as a result of being a homeowner and unemployment insurance payments that cover basic costs (Leondar-Wright, 2004). The migration of jobs out of urban areas cities has particularly affected the most deprived areas of the city. As noted in Wilson's *When Work Disappears* (1996), the ghettos have gone from having a majority of adults working around the middle of the 20th Century to high rates of joblessness and only a minority of individuals in ghettos being employed at the end of the last century (Wilson, 1996). To illustrate this differential impact, one study of Illinois job migration from the cities in the 1970s showed that black job loss was 24% while white losses were only 10% (Leondar-Wright, 2004). Access to employment can be particularly challenging for women who primarily shoulder child rearing and other household responsibilities (Hanson and Pratt, 1995; Amott and Matthaei 1996; Frazier, *et al.*, 2003). Women are not able to commute as long to employment opportunities. The changes in the U.S. economy have left women in urban environments, especially those residing in areas of concentrated poverty, with fewer, and poorer, employment choices. While changes in recent decades in the national economy have contributed to the problem of access to good paying jobs for those residing in urban areas, related factors have additionally eroded the support of families including suboptimal public transportation, lack of a national child care program, and lack of a national health program.

Policies and practices that have produced racial inequalities in economic and social well being in the U.S. unfortunately are numerous (Wilson, 1987; Massey and Denton,1994; Yinger, 2001; Bonilla-Silva, 2003; Hofrichter, 2003; Leondar-Wright,

2004; Massey ,2004). These are also noted in the top box in Figure 1 as contributing to the unequal access to resources among racial and ethnic minorities residing in urban areas. Numerous examples of such practices and policies can be found in relation to housing (and the physical environment) (Squires, 1994; Evans, 2003; Frazier, *et al.*, 2003; Northridge, *et al.*, 2003; Shaw, 2004). Blatant examples of racist housing related practices by the private sector include redlining (i.e. identification of geographic neighborhoods, the residents of which are denied loans or denied insurance) (Squires, 1994; Sickinger, 1999), and steering (i.e. the practice of showing prospective home buyers homes in certain neighborhoods characterized by its racial composition). Similar to steering is the documented discrimination by race in the rental market (Massey and Lundy, 2001). All such practices serve, too often, to deny racial minorities access to higher quality housing and to one of the major sources of wealth accumulation for the middle class (e.g., home ownership in higher income neighborhoods where real estate prices escalate quickly). While policies such as the Fair Housing Act of 1968 or the Home Mortgage Disclosure Act in 1975 were designed to eliminate these practices, they have failed to achieve their goals as these practices have continued (Squires, 1994; Sickinger, 1999). Recent research has also described how after World War II, the transportation and housing industries collaborated to dramatically transform cities and suburban areas, contributing to the increased patterns of segregation in metropolitan areas (Mohl, 2002). These are examples of the historical and contemporary policies and practices that are highlighted in the top box of Figure 1.

These larger societal processes, in turn, contribute to the unequal development of cities within the U.S. Those who are struggling to make ends meet are often faced with multiple problems which collectively contribute to and help maintain the low social standing of these individuals and families, especially those residing in urban ghettos or areas of concentrated poverty. Examples of these factors and challenges are noted in the middle box of Figure 1. Our framework should not be interpreted as suggesting that all persons in deprived urban areas are homogeneous with regard to how they experience the consequences of the public and private practices and policies that affect them. Rather, there is quite a bit of heterogeneity within deprived areas and across deprived areas with regard to the characteristics listed in the middle box in Figure 1.

While urban race, class, and gender inequalities in income, quality of residential neighborhoods, access to high paying jobs, and access to supportive resources are well documented, the evidence that these factors also affect the health and well-being of urban populations is also growing (Pamuk, *et al.*, 1998; Marmot, *et al.*, 1999; Acevedo-Garcia, 2000; Evans, 2003; Massey, 2004). We illustrate these pathways in Figure 1 where we note the relationship between the policies and practices of governments and the private sector in contributing to unequal development of urban spaces and their ultimate effect upon the health of city residents. Again, while low-income urban populations experience myriad health effects due to their social and economic deprivation, we cannot fully cover these complex relationships. Rather, we mention just a few pathways as means of illustration.

Toxins in the environment can have a direct impact on health (see pathway 1 in the bottom box of Figure 1). Examples of these include pollution levels on asthma and other respiratory conditions (Schwartz, 2004), lead exposures from lead paint in the home on the cognitive performance of adults and children (Lidksy and Schneider, 2003), and toxic waste sites near residential areas on cancer rates (Lidksy and Schneider, 2003). Segregation and racial discrimination has been suggested as having significant health impacts (Polednak, 1996; Acevedo-Garcia, 2000; Krieger, 2000; Massey, 2004; Caughy, *et al.*, In press). Massey, (2004) describes in his thorough review of segregation and health, not only the contemporary face of segregation but the pathways by which experiences of segregation affect health. (see pathway 2 in the bottom box of Figure 1). For example, among blacks residing in the U.S., more than half are residing in either highly segregated or hyper-segregated environments. Moreover, the levels of segregation for many metropolitan areas in the U.S. have changed very little over the past 20 years. High segregation and hyper-segregation leads to environments with simultaneously chronic and high levels of crime, concentrated poverty, diminished basic resources, substandard housing, and high unemployment to name a few. These kinds of environments contribute to increases in negative stress or allostatic load among the residents. This in turn leads to health conditions including compromised immune function, hypertension, cardiovascular disease, asthma, Type I diabetes to name a few (Massey, 2004). Acevedo-Garcia discusses the details of how segregation directly affects the risk for infectious diseases, TB in particular, via the crowding created by adverse residential environments of segregated neighborhoods (Acevedo-Garcia, 2000) (see pathway 3 in the bottom box of Figure 1). These are but a few examples of how the health of economically and socially deprived populations is affected by their environments and the societal level policies that create those environments.

4.0 HEALTH BURDENS EXPERIENCED BY ECONOMICALLY AND SOCIALLY DEPRIVED URBAN POPULATIONS

Studies of individual and population health for those living in urban areas have consistently demonstrated the variation in health status by context, race, income, and gender. While patterns of disparity differ for various outcomes, a consistent relationship of increased morbidity and mortality has been observed for economically disadvantaged urban populations compared to their less deprived counterparts for outcomes such as cardiovascular disease, homicide, mental health, asthma, and premature mortality (Brunner and Marmot, 1999; Geronimus, *et al.* 1999; Shaw, *et al*, 1999.; Weil, 1999; Aligne, *et al.*, 2000; Grant, *et al.*, 2000; House, *et al.*, 1978; Cooper, *et al.* 2001; Geronimus, 2003; Kreuger, *et al.*, 2004; McGruder, *et al.*, 2004).

We present here data that demonstrates the health status of the economically deprived residing in urban areas. While a full understanding of health disparities requires a focus upon race/ethnicity, income, poverty, context, and gender, few past research efforts have explored and presented their findings to elucidate such health patterns. We present some data from published sources but also examined social class, race and gender inequalities using the National Health Interview Survey conducted in 2001.

4.1. Studies from the Published Literature

In an original investigation, House and colleagues (2000) provide the first estimates for the prospective impact of urban residence on mortality within a national sampling study. House, *et al.*, (2000) sought to estimate the prospective effects of urban, suburban, and rural residence on mortality for adults over the age of 25 in the U.S. In order to determine whether excess mortality among urban residents is attributed to specific urban areas or causes of death, the investigators conducted face-to-face interviews with a stratified, multi-stage sample of 3,617 individuals who were not institutionalized, with over sampling for individuals over the age of 60 and black. Deaths of participating individuals were acquired through National Death Index or through direct follow-up with study participants.

While controlling for a variety of factors such as age, race, socioeconomic status, and self-reported health status, this study found that mortality increased sharply by age and with decreasing education, income, and self reported health status. In addition, individuals living in urban areas were also likely to experience significantly higher mortality than individuals residing in small town/rural areas (Figure 2). Adjusted for sociodemographic, socioeconomic, and health predictors, multivariate analysis showed that individuals living in the city had a significantly higher hazard ratio of 1.62 (95%) times greater than those individuals living in small towns/rural areas. Although not statistically significant, participants living in suburban areas were also more likely to experience higher mortality rates of 1.15 than those living in small towns/rural areas. In addition, individuals with income less than $10,000 had significantly higher hazard ratios of 2.65 than those making more than $30,000 a year and participants making between $10,000 and $29,999 were also significantly more likely to have higher hazard ratios, 2.31 than those with a higher annual income.

One explanation for these findings is that living in the city, coupled with living within a lower income stratification often involves navigating an increased number of stressful life experiences which include increased conflict with interpersonal relations, increased sensory stimulation, noise, stress, and anxiety associated with city-life, which can often encompass situations involving increased exposure to crime and violence (Yonas, 2004; Fischer, 1984; House, 1978; Milgram, 1970). City residents often experience limited access to and ability to engage institutional resources such as nutritious food resources, healthcare, mental health counseling, and/or social support networks necessary for successfully negotiating the stresses of living in

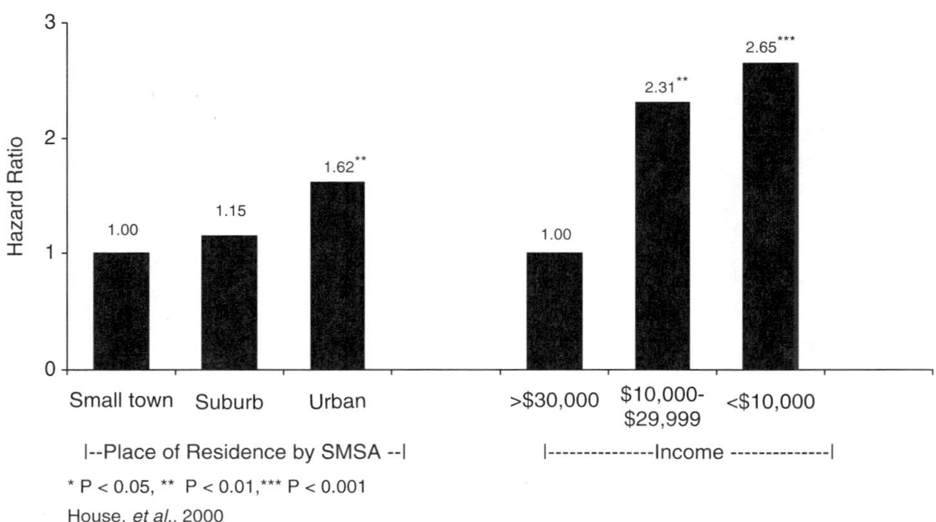

Figure 2. Adjusted Hazard Ratios for All-Cause Mortality, 1986-1994.

urban areas, as well as increased risk to other exposures such as dilapidated and vacant housing, and increased access to liquor stores and corner store markets.

In another study, Aligne, *et al.*, (2000) sought to explore if living in an urban area contributed independently to the risk for childhood asthma, after controlling for other commonly studied factors with asthma such as race/ethnicity, poverty status, and other environmental and demographic conditions. The investigators for this study again used a national database through the Child Health Supplement to the 1988 National Health Interview Survey to conduct a prospective study among a nationally representative sample of 17, 110 children between the ages of zero and 17.

Bivariate analyses and stepwise regression analyses were used to understand the relationship of numerous demographic variables, and their analyses were conducted to illustrate the role of race and poverty towards childhood asthma by adjusting for urban versus non-urban living situation (Figure 3).

Interestingly, this investigation identified that urban status alone was statistically significantly associated with an increased risk for childhood asthma for both black and white children, with odds ratios (OR) of 1.4 and 1.2, obtained respectively. While controlling for urban versus non-urban living status, results from this investigation additionally showed that both poor and non-poor children had significantly higher odds ratios than non-urban children in the sample, although poor children remained at increased risk for childhood asthma as compared to their non-poor counterparts.

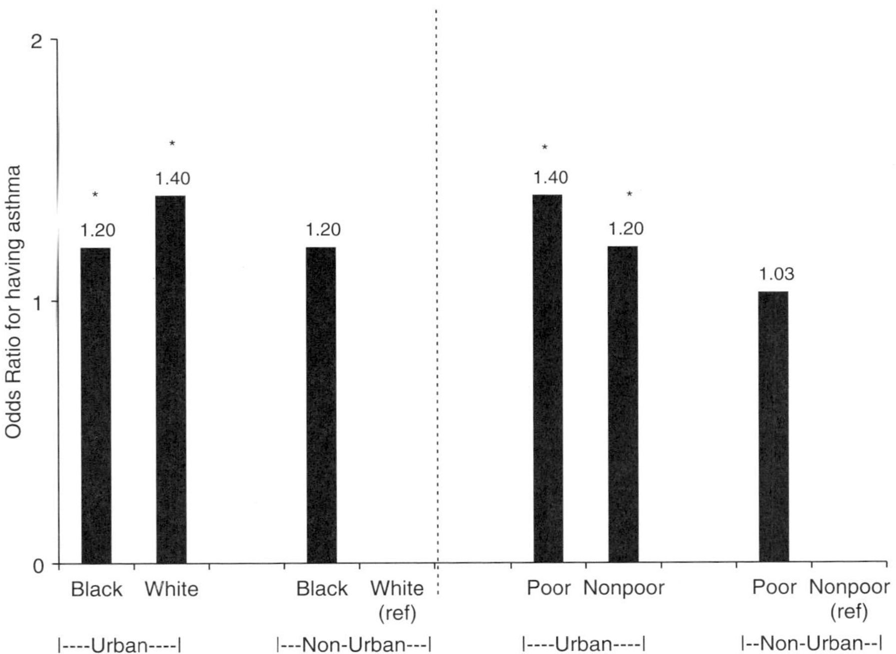

Figure 3. Urban Status with either Black Race or Poverty as Risk Factors for Childhood Asthma (ages 0-17).

Regardless of race or family income status, children living in urban areas were found to be at increased risk for childhood asthma. Since this analysis is cross sectional it does not indicate a causal relationship, but these findings do strengthen previous findings which propose an environmental link between childhood asthma and living in urban areas often attributed to individual and contextual factors such as exposure to passive smoking, substandard housing conditions, exposure to cockroaches, decreased access to healthcare and other institutional resources, poor diet, and limited care giving capacity due to stress and anxiety (Aligne, *et al.*, 2000; Eggleston, 2003).

4.2 Economic Deprivation and Health in Urban Environments

4.2.1. Evidence from the 2001 National Health Interview Survey

To more completely explore the joint effects of urban context, income, race/ethnicity, poverty, and gender on health disparities of economically and socially deprived populations, data from the 2001 National Health Interview Survey (NHIS) were examined. The NHIS is a nationally representative health survey conducted by the National Center for Health Statistics (NCHS) and the Centers for Disease Control and Prevention (CDC). The complete sample of participants for the 2001 NHIS was 38,932 households, which yielded 100,761 individuals and 39,633 families in the U.S. and we limited our sample to those residing in larger urban areas. All analysis were conducted utilizing the assigned sample weights to accurately obtain national sample survey estimates (National Health Interview Survey 2001). We limited our analyses to those residing in large metropolitan areas comprised of populations 500,000 to 5,000,000.

A variety of indices were constructed for this analysis. We created an indicator of income using, the ratio of family income to federal poverty level. This 'poverty' indicator had four continuous categories (<0.5, 0.5-1.99, 2.0-3.49, and 3.5-4.99) where a value of 1.0 indicates a family residing at the official poverty level. A dichotomous indicator was created from information on the short 6-item screening Composite International Diagnostic Interview (CIDI) to indicate mental health status (Kessler, *et al.*, 2003). Those endorsing 4 to 6 items were considered as having "Poor mental health" as they fell into the top half of the distribution for that scale, and those endorsing 3 or fewer were considered as having as "Not poor mental health". The survey also asked if the respondent had ever been told by a doctor that they had had a stroke. We used this information for those individuals over the age of 44 to examine gradients by income, race, and gender.

Cross tabulation analyses involving mental health by poverty level shows an unambiguous inverse linear relationship; 41% of individuals living at half the federal poverty level had poor mental health status compared to 23.1% of those individuals living at the highest income category of 3.5 to 4.99 times the poverty level (Figure 4).

When we stratified these analyses by gender the inverse linear relationship by poverty level remains and women consistently report higher levels of poor mental health across all poverty levels with the greatest gaps seen at lower poverty levels (Figure 5).

Forty five percent of women versus 33.7% of men were living at half the federal poverty level, 39.9% of women versus 31.5% of men were at the 0.5-1.99 poverty level, 32.9% of women versus 26.9 % of men were at the 2.0-3.49 level, and almost

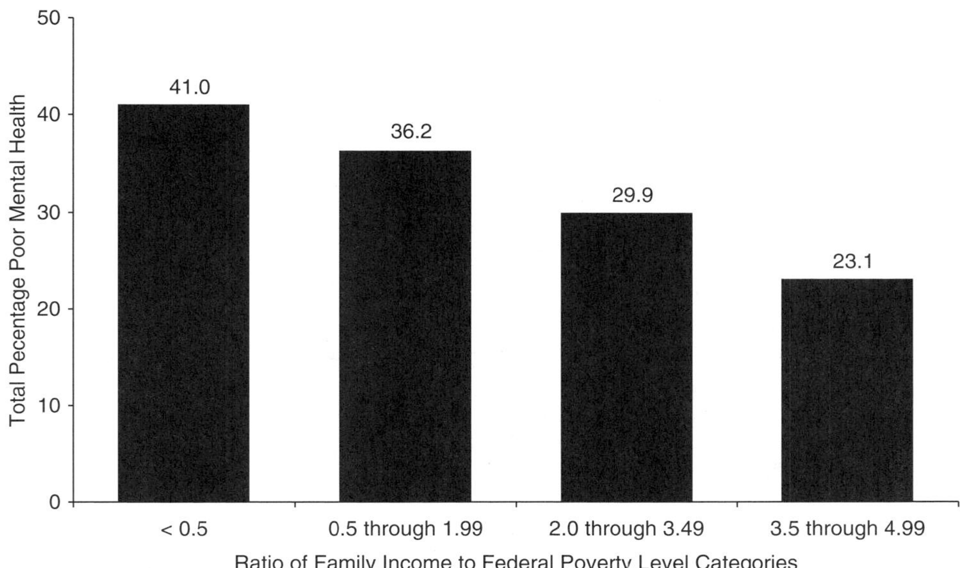

Figure 4. Self-Reported Poor Mental Health by Ratio of Family Income to Poverty Level for Metropolitan Populations.*

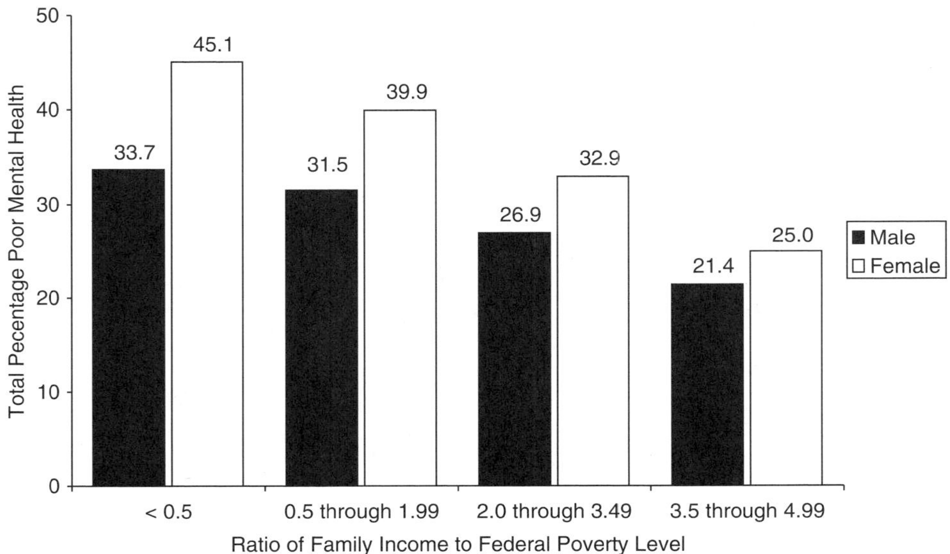

Figure 5. Self-Reported Poor Mental Health and Gender by Ratio of Family Income to Poverty Level for Metropolitan Populations.*

equal levels of poor mental health status were observed at the 3.5-4.99 level above poverty for women and men, 25% of women versus 21.4% of men, respectively.

When these same data were examined by race/ethnicity (latino, black, and white), an inverse linear relationship for poverty level remained (Figure 6), but the pattern for race/ethnicity within the poverty level categories varied.

Previous research suggests that racial/ethnic minorities report lower levels of mental health symptoms than whites even when social class is considered (Muntaner, 2004). Yet for those residing at the lowest income category of 0.5 poverty level, blacks and latino report more mental health symptoms than whites (Figure 6). Almost half of the blacks residing at 50% or less of the federal poverty level had poor mental health.

Those at the very bottom, which primarily includes racial and ethnic minorities, where the majority of blacks reside in hypersegregated areas (Massey, 2004), experience epidemic levels of contextual risk factors such as violence, drugs and illicit drug markets, dilapidated living and neighborhood conditions, lack of access to quality food resources, substandard education and day care, and decreased access to social and institutional resources such as neighborhood relationships, health care, social services, municipal services, etc. (Wirth, 1938; Milgram, 1970; House and Wolfe, 1978; Bourgois, 1995; Kawachi, *et al.*, 1999; Marmot and Wilkinson, 2001).

Cross tabulation analyses of individuals age 45 or older examined stroke by poverty status suggested an association but not necessarily a linear association as observed for poor mental health status (Figure 7).

Those residing between 50% and 200% poverty had the highest proportion of stroke at 8.4%, substantially higher than the other categories including the lowest income category of <=50% of poverty. The proportion of those experiencing stroke

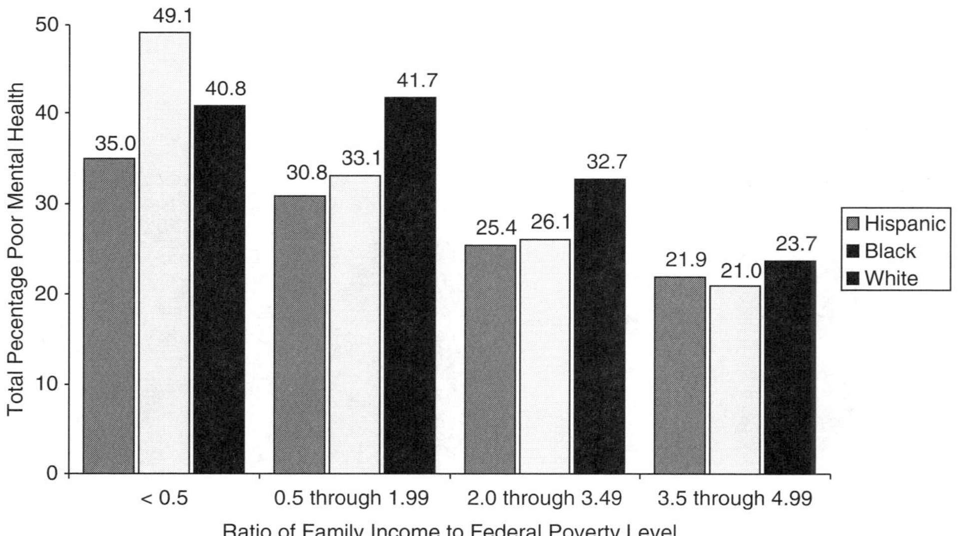

Figure 6. Self-Reported Poor Mental Health and Race/Ethnicity by Ratio of Family Income to Poverty Level for Metropolitan Populations.*

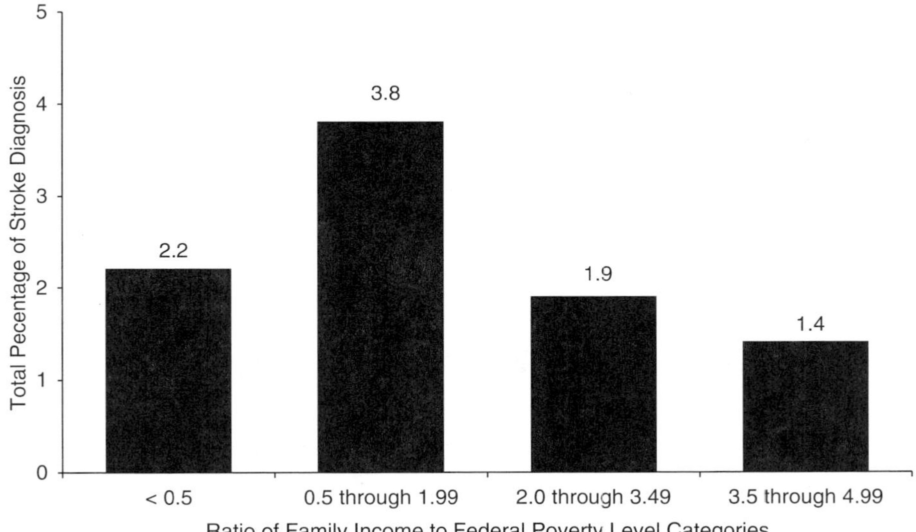

Figure 7. Stoke by Ratio of Family Income to Poverty Level for Metropolitan Populations.*

varied substantially by race within income to poverty categories (Figure 8) and the patterns by race varied across the income categories.

Within the two lowest income to poverty categories, blacks clearly had the highest proportion of reported stroke. This pattern was masked in Figure 7 when the data were presented by income only. All groups in the lowest two categories had higher proportions of stroke compared to those in the higher income brackets except the poorest whites (Figure 8).

As in previous research, this analysis found that individuals living in economically disadvantaged communities within large cities were at increased risk for incidence of stroke compared to their higher income counterparts. Higher risk for stroke among residents of economically and socially deprived communities who experience income inequality has been attributed to the negative effects of the psychosocial environment on influencing the adoption of higher prevalence of risk factors such as smoking, hypertension, stress, anxiety, and obesity (Kawachi, *et al.*, 1997; 1999; Marmot and Wilkinson, 2001; Shi, *et al.*, 2003).

5.0. POLICIES AND STRATEGIES TO IMPROVE THE WELL-BEING OF THE ECONOMICALLY DEPRIVED

While the myriad, seemingly intransigent, social and health problems facing low-income urban populations seem insurmountable, the good news is that there are solutions that can begin to alleviate the extreme deprivation experienced by this population and eventually lead to improvements in their health status. Among industrialized countries, the U.S. maintains the highest poverty and economic deprivation rates worldwide (Vleminckx and Smeeding, 2001). The solution to high levels of poverty, high levels of social problems, and poorer health status, therefore, is

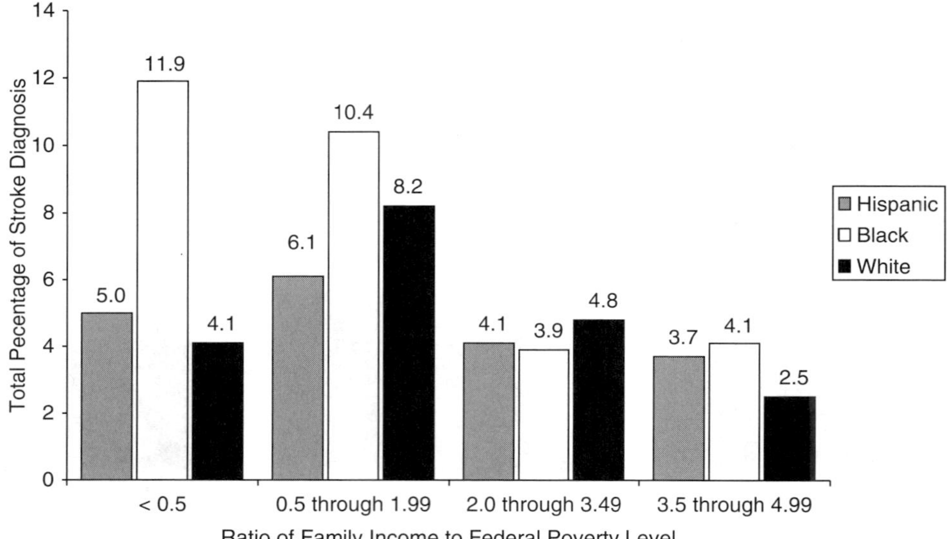

Figure 8. Stoke by Race/Ethnicity for four categories of Family Income to Poverty Ratio for Urban Residents Over Age 45.*

no mystery and is related to the amount of social spending for the lower income populations in a variety of areas including housing, child care, unemployment benefits, health care, education, and public transportation just to name a few (Navarro, 2001; Hofrichter, 2003; Raphael and Bryant, 2004). Industrialized countries with social democratic traditions such as Norway, Denmark, and Finland with higher levels of income redistribution resulting from strong welfare states, have better population health than countries with weaker welfare states (Navarro, 2001). While there is no single formula for social spending that universally alleviates income and social inequality across countries, it is clear that the U.S. lags significantly behind all other countries with lower poverty rates and higher social spending. We briefly describe in this section a few solutions to reducing economic and social deprivation in urban areas of the U.S. as space constraints keeps us from taking a comprehensive approach. And while each solution will be described separately, it is unlikely that implementation of a single intervention alone will significantly alleviate the deprivation of the urban poor or significantly improve their health. Rather, given that these economic and social problems are multifactorial in nature, there is a need to simultaneously implement multiple strategies to begin to make a difference.

One strategy, not touched upon in depth in this review, but relevant to U.S. populations that have low access to adequate health care coverage is *universal health care* coverage. Health care access and coverage have been the topics of longstanding discussions in the U.S., in part, because of the growing numbers of the uninsured which at last count was 15% of the U.S. population in 2002 or approximately 44 million persons, a number which keeps rising (Pugh, 2003). The U.S. is the exception among industrialized countries in having no universal health care coverage. A substantial proportion of uninsured are employed but do not have access to health insurance through their jobs. While treatment of health problems is less effective than primary prevention, and universal health care coverage is not likely to eliminate inequalities in health between the rich and the poor, universal access to health care treatment will allow those who suffer from chronic diseases, predominately those who are lower income, to better manage their conditions and to manage these conditions with fewer out of pocket costs. Health problems of women and their children are a major contributor to the inability to maintain employment among families participating in the Temporary Assistance to Needy Families (TANF) program (O'Campo and Rojas-Smith, 1998; Rojas-Smith, 2002). And those who are struggling economically are more likely to forego needed care (May and Cunningham, 2004). Thus, making access to health care a universal entitlement in the U.S., which is the case for every other industrialized country in the world, would facilitate an improvement in the health of the urban economically deprived populations. While universal access to health care is an important component of improving the health of low income populations, addressing the racial disparities in treatment and quality of care will be necessary to reduce inequalities. Recent evidence of the widespread 'unequal treatment' by race in the health care system is strong and must also be addressed (Smedley, *et al.*, 2003).

The *war on low wages* for those at the bottom needs to expand in favor of the working class. As noted earlier, significant losses in wages have been the norm for the majority of workers over the last several decades. Yet, there is one exception to this pattern of decreasing wages across the social class spectrum. Over the period 1989-1997, the pay of chief executive officers (CEO), who preside at the top of the income distribution, grew 44.6%. In fact, since 1965 the ratio of CEO pay to that of the average worker has doubled several times over, and it is the largest gap in the entire industrialized world. In 1965, the pay ratio of CEOs to the average worker was 20; by 1997 this ratio had leapt to 115 (Mishel, *et al.*, 1999). This occurs at a time when those at the very bottom are experiencing ever greater hardships due to national policies such as 'welfare reform' or the implementation of the Temporary Assistance for Needy Families (TANF) legislation in 1996 (O'Campo and Rojas-Smith,1998). Forcing a population who is not equipped to work—on a variety of fronts including lack of skills to earn high paying jobs, high levels of personal and family disabilities, and multiple social problems precluding stable employment—into the workplace has not resulted in the stated goal of 'economic self sufficiency'. Results from evaluations of state TANF programs indicate that only 10% of families have incomes above 185% of poverty after leaving welfare (Acs and Loprest, 1999). Moreover, even five years after leaving welfare, 42% still live in poverty (Cancian and Haveman, *et al.*, 2003). These data strongly suggest flaws in the current approaches to eliminating economic deprivation in the U.S. and the need for reversal of policies. Low minimum wages and greater support for those who are unemployed are not unique U.S. problems. Policy discussions in Canada, as one example, are also concerned with similar issues (Raphael and Curry-Stevens, 2004).

Raising the current minimum wage of $5.15 per hour to a level that is at or close to a living wage will be an important break for the large proportion of the population who are experiencing economic hardships despite working. A living wage as the minimum wage would also begin to equalize pay inequalities between race and ethnic groups as well as between men and women (O'Campo and Rojas-Smith, 1998; O'Campo and Tang, 2001). This would be particularly significant for the growing single headed families that are predominately women where poverty rates are the highest (Mishel, *et al.*, 2003). The minimum wage has not been raised for seven years and, in terms of its value, it has fallen substantially since 1968 as noted earlier. This policy is already taking hold as, by 2002, 70 living wage ordinances have been passed nationwide (Chapman, 2002).

Housing is another area where there are solutions within reach. While homelessness is discussed in a separate chapter, public and private development policies that support an increase in the availability of affordable homes would substantially reduce the growing problem of homelessness in the U.S. and is an issue facing many urban areas within industrialized countries. Also, as noted earlier, suboptimal, deteriorating, dangerous, or poorly designed housing is a source of many health problems, including asthma, lead poisoning, injuries, poor mental health, and chronic diseases. Increasing funding for lead abatement will reduce residential exposure to lead. Reviewing and refining housing codes in the areas of ventilation, moisture, injury hazards, noise, lighting, and toxic substances just to name a few examples, would promote structures that are consistent with healthier living environments. Such codes, even if improved, would have to be monitored and enforced. Increasing funds to public health departments would be necessary to begin to accomplish these particular changes. Yet, given that individuals spend much of their lives in their homes, multiple changes to improve housing quality, not to mention affordability, may have significant impacts upon the health of the economically deprived in urban areas (Northridge, *et al.*, 2003; Shapcott, 2004; Shaw, 2004).

One example of how an *integrated strategy* is necessary for addressing the health problems of the economically deprived urban populations is illustrated through the example of diet related diseases (e.g., cardiovascular disease, obesity, and hypertension) and food insecurity, all of which are experienced at high levels by the economically deprived. As noted by Robertson and McCarthy (McCarthy, 1999; Robertson, *et al.*, 1999), diet related diseases and food insecurity are complex social, political, and development issues because they involve politics (e.g., trade policies), economics (e.g., can comprise a high proportion of the GDP), socio-economic factors (e.g., 'food deserts' in poor urban areas), advertising in the food industry (e.g., most advertisements for food concern sugar products and rarely are products such as vegetables advertised), and transportation policies (e.g., provision of societal transportation options that promote walking or even cycling). While many public health practitioners and researchers tend to focus on the individual behaviors that contribute to diet-related diseases, these societal factors are important determinants of both dietary problems and food insecurity. Moreover, a change in a single practice or policy is unlikely to significantly improve the dietary patterns among the urban poor. Rather, a coordinated effort on multiple fronts will be the only way significant change will come about.

6.0. CONCLUSION

This chapter about the economically deprived in urban areas has primarily focused upon the U.S. However, many trends and processes described here are relevant for other industrialized countries. The U.S. has experienced little significant gain in the alleviation of poverty and economic hardship over the last several decades among those in the lower half of the income spectrum. Demographic and individual-level explanations are not major contributors to these trends. Rather, current U.S. policies and practices have resulted in falling wages and increasing economic hardship among a growing proportion of the U.S. population. The health of the economically deprived is far worse in several areas compared to those who are better off. Solutions to the economic deprivation that leads to poorer health are attainable for the wealthiest country in the world. Policy reversals, in such areas as welfare reform for the poor and corporate welfare and tax cuts for the rich that reduce overall funds for social spending, would be a good beginning. Multiple coordinated efforts will be required to significantly alter the well-being of the economically deprived.

REFERENCES

Acevedo-Garcia, D. (2000). Residential segregation and the epidemiology of infectious diseases. *Soc. Sci. Med.* 51:1143–1161.

Acs, G., and Loprest, P. (1999). The effects of disability on exits from AFDC. *Journal of Policy Analysis and Management* 28(1):28–49.

Aldelba, R., and Folbre, N. (1996). *The war on the poor.* Center for Popular Economics, New Press, New York, NY.

Aligne, A., Auinger, P., Byrd, R.S., and Weitzman, M. (2000). Risk Factors for Pediatric Asthma: Contributions of Poverty, Race and Urban Residence. *Am. Respri. Crit. Care Med.* 162: 873– 877.

Amott, T., and Matthaei, J. (1996). *Race, Gender and Work: A Multicultural Economic History of Women in the United States.* South End Press, Boston, MA.

Bonilla-Silva, E. (2003). Racism Without Racists: Color-Blind Racism and the Persistence of Racial Inequality in the United States, Rowman & Littlefield Publishers, Inc., New York, NY.

Bourgois, P. (1995). *In Search of Respect.* Cambridge University Press, New York, NY.

Boushey, H., Brocht, C., Gundersen, B., and Bernstein, J. (2001). *Hardships in America: The real story of working families.* Economic Policy Institute, Washington D.C.

Brunner, E., and Marmot, M. (1999). *Social Organization, Stress, and Health. Social Determinants of Health.* New York, Oxford University Press, pp.17-44.

Cancian, M., Haveman, F., Meyer, D., and Wolfe, B. (2003). The Employment, Earnings, and Income of Single Mothers in Wisconsin Who Left Cash Assistance. Comparisons among Three Cohorts. Wisconsin, Institute for Research on Poverty, Special report 85.

Casey, T. (2003). Reading between the lines: women's poverty in the United States, 2002, NOW Legal Defense Fund and Education Fund.

Caughy, M., O'Campo, P., and Muntaner, C. (2004). Individual and neighborhood correlates of experiences of racism among African American parents and effects on behavior problems of their preschool-aged children. *Am. J. Public Health* In press.

Chapman, J. (2002). Living Wage, Economic Policy Institute, New York, NY.

Cooper, R. S., Kennelly, J.F., Durazo-Arvizu, R., Oh, H., Kaplan, G., and Lynch, J. (2001). Relationship between Premature Mortality and Socioeconomic Factors in Black and White Populations of US Metropolitan Areas. *Public Health Rep.* 116:464–473.

Eggleston, P. (2003). Control of environmental allergens as a therapeutic approach. *Immunol. Allergy Clin. North Am.* 23(3): 533–547.

Evans, G. (2003). The Built Environment and Mental Health. *J. Urban Health* 80(4): 536–555.

Frazier, J., Margai, F., and Tettey-Fio, E. (2003). Race and Place: *Equity Issues in Urban America.* Westview Press, Oxford.

Fischer, C. (1984). *The Urban Experience.* Harcourt Bruce, New York, NY.

Geronimus, A. (2003). *Addressing Structural Influences on the Health of Urban Populations. Health and Social Justice: A Public Health Reader.* H. R. San Francisco, CA, Johns Wiley and Sons, pp. 542-556.

Geronimus, A. T., Bound, J., and Waidmann, T. A. (1999). Poverty, Time, and Place: Variation in Excess Mortality across Selected U.S. Populations, 1980-1990. *J. Epid. Com. Health* 53:325-334.

Grant, E. N., Lyttle, C.S., and Weiss, K.B. (2000). The Relation of Socioeconomic Factors and Racial/Ethnic Differences in US Asthma Mortality. *Am. J. Public Health* 90(12):1923-1925.

Halpern, R. (1995). Rebuilding the inner city: a history of neighborhood initiatives to address poverty in the United States. Columbia University Press, New York, NY.

Hanson, S., and Pratt, G. (1995). *Gender, Work and Space.* Routledge, New York, NY.

Heyman, J. (2000). Health and social policy. Social Epidemiology. In: Berkman, L., and Kawachi, I. Oxford University Press, New York, NY, pp. 368-382.

Hofrichter, R. (2003). *Health and Social Justice: Politics, Ideology, and Inequity in the Distribution of Disease.* John Wiley and Sons, San Francisco, CA.

House, J. S., Lepkowski, J.M., Williams, D.R., Mero, R., Lantz, P.M., Robert, R.A., and Chen, J. (2000). Excess Mortality Among Urban Residents: How Much, for Whom, and Why. *Am. J. Public Health* 90(12): 1898-1904.

House, J. S., and Wolfe, S. (1978). Effects of urban residence on interpersonal trust and helping behavior. *J. Pers. Soc. Psych.* 36:1-43.

Kawachi, I., Kennedy, B., and Glass, R. (1999). Social capital and self-rated health: a contextual analysis. *Am. J. Public Health* 89:1187-1193.

Kawachi, I., Kennedy, B., Lochner, K., and Smith, D. (1997). Social capital, income inequality, and mortality. *Am. J. Public Health* 87:1491-1498.

Kessler, R., Barker, P., Colpe, L., Epstein, J., Gfroerer, J., Hiripi, E., Howes, M., Normand, S., Manderscheid, R., Walters, E., and Zaslavsky, A. (2003). Screening for Serious Mental Illness in the General Population. *Arch. Gen. Psychiatry* 60(3):184-189.

Kreuger, P. M., Bond Huie, S.A., Rogers R.G., and Hummer, R.A. (2004). Neighborhoods and homicide mortality: an analysis of race/ethnic differences. *J. Epid. Comm. Health* 58:223-230.

Krieger, N. (2000). *Discrimination and health. Social Epidemiology.* In: Berkman, L. and Kawachi, I. Oxford University Press, Oxford.

Krieger, N. (2001). Theories for social epidemiology in the 21st century: an ecosocial perspective. *Int. J. Epid.* 30: 668-677.

Leondar-Wright, B. (2004). Black job loss deja-vu. *Dollars and Sense* (253).

Lidksy, T., and Schneider, J. (2003). Lead neurotoxicity in children: basic mechanisms and clinical correlates. *Brain* 127:5-19.

Shapcott, M. (2004) Housing. In: Raphael, D. (ed.), *Social determinants of health: Canadian perspectives* (pp. 201-215). Canadian Scholars Press Inc., Toronto, Canada.

Marmot, M., and Wilkinson, R.G. (1999). *Social Determinants of Health.* Oxford University Press, New York, NY.

Marmot, M., and Wilkinson, R. (2001). Psychosocial and material pathways in the relation between income and health: a response to Lynch. *BMJ* 322:1233-1236.

Massey, D. (2004). Segregation and stratification: a biosocial perspective. *DuBois Review* 1(1);7–25.

Massey, D., and Denton, N. (1994). *American Apartheid: segregation and the making of the underclass.* Harvard University Press, Harvard, CT.

Massey, D., and Lundy, G. (2001). Use of Black English and racial discrimination in urban housing markets: new methods and findings. *Urban Affairs Review* 36:470-496.

May, J., and Cunningham, P. (2004). Tough trade-offs: medical bills, family finances and access to care. Health System Change, Issue Brief.

McCarthy, M. (1999). Transport and Health. Social determinants of health. Oxford University Press, Oxford, England.

McGruder, H.F., Malarcher, A.M., Antoine, T.L. Greenlund, K.J., and Croft, J.B. (2004).

Racial and Ethnic Disparities in Cardiovascular Risk Factors Among Stroke Survivors: United States 1999 to 2001. *Stroke* 35:1557-1561.

Milgram, S. (1970). The Experience of living in cities. Science. *Science* 167:1461-1468.

Mishel, L., Bernstein, J., and Boushey, H. (2003). The State of Working America 2002/2003. Cornell University, New York, NY.

Mishel, L., Bernstein, J., and Schmitt, J. (1999). The State of Working America 1998-1999. Economic Policy Institute, Washington D.C.

Mohl, R. (2002). The Interstates and the Cities: Highways, Housing and the Freeway Revolt. Poverty and Race Action Council, Washington D.C.

Muntaner, C.E.W., Miech, R., and O'Campo, P. (2004). Socioconomic position and major mental disorders. *Epid. Rev.* 26:53-62.

National Health Interview Survey, 2001, Datasets, Maryland (October 8, 2004); ftp://ftp.cdc.gov/pub/Health_Statistics/NCHS/Datasets/NHIS/2001/

Navarro, V., and S. L. (2001). The political context of social inequalities in health. *Soc. Sci. Med.* 52(3): 481-491.

Northridge, M. E., Sclar, E.D., and Biswas, P. (2003). Sorting out the connections between the built environment and health: a conceptual framework for navigating pathways and planning healthy cities. *J. Urban Health* 80(4):556-68.

O'Campo, P., and Rojas-Smith, L. (1998). Welfare Reform and Women's Health: Review of the Literature and Implications for State Policy. *J. Public Health Pol.* 19(4):420-46.

O'Campo, P., and Tang, J. (2001). Poverty and Health: Gendered pathways. WHO commissioned papers on gender and health, Geneva.

Pamuk, E., D. Makuc, D., Heck, K., Reuben, C., and L. K. (1998). Socioeconomic status and health chartbook. Health, United States, 1009. National Center for Health Statistics, Hyatesville, MD.

Pearce, D. (1990). Welfare is not for women: why the war on poverty cannot conquer the feminization of poverty. In: L.Gorden. (ed.). *Women, the state and welfare.* University of Wisconsin Press, Madison, WI.

Polednak, A. (1996). Trends in US urban black infant mortality, by degree of residential segregation. *Am. J. Public Health* 86(5):723-726.

Pugh, T. (2003). Common Dreams, New York, (October 8, 2004); http://www.commondreams.org/headlines03/0930-01.htm

Raphael, D. (2004). *Social determinants of health: Canadian perspectives.* Canadian Scholars Press Inc., Toronto, Canada.

Raphael, D., and Curry-Stevens, A. (2004). *Addressing and surmounting the political and social barriers to health.* Canadian Scholars Press Inc, Toronto, pp. 345-360.

Raphael, D., and Bryant T. (2004). The welfare state as a determinant of women's health: support for women's quality of life in Canada and four comparison nations. *Health Policy* 68: 63-79.

Robertson, A., Brunner, E., and Sheiham, A. (1999). Food is a political issue. In: M. M., and W. R.G. *Social determinants of health.* Oxford University Press, Oxford, England.

Rojas-Smith L.O. C. P., and Grason, H. (2002). Welfare reform and women's health: Challenges and opportunities to advance the public response to the health needs of poor women through monitoring and collaboration. *Journal of Prevention and Intervention in the Community* 23:129-149.

Schwartz, J. (2004). Air pollution and children's health. *Pediatrics* 113:1037-1043.

Shaw, M. (2004). Housing and public health. *Ann. Rev. Public Health* 25: 397-418.

Shaw, M., Dorling, D., and Smith, G.D. (1999). Poverty, Social exclusion, and minorities. Social Determinants of Health. M. M and W. RG. Oxford University Press, New York, NY, pp. 211-239.

Shi, L., Macinko, J., Starfield, B., Xu, J., and Politzer, R. (2003). Primary Care, Income Inequality, and Stroke Mortality in the United States. *Stroke* 34:1958-1964.

Sickinger, T. (1999). *American Dream Denied: when the door is locked to buying a home.* Kansas City Star, Kansas.

Sklar, H., Mykata, L., and Wefald, S. (2001). Raise the floor. Ms Foundation for Women, New York, NY.

Smedley, B., Stith, A., Nelson, A., and Committee on Understanding and Eliminating Racial and Ethnic Disparities in Health Care. (2003). *Unequal Treatment: Confronting Racial and Ethnic Disparities in Health Care.* National Academies Press, Washington D.C.

Squires, G. (1994). *Capital and Communities in Black and White: the intersection of race, class and uneven development.* State University of New York Press, Albany, NY.

U.S. Census Bureau, 1997, Poverty rates of people by race and Hispanic origin 1995 and 1996, (October 8, 2004); http://ferret.bls.census.gov/macro/031997/pov/4_001.htm

US Census Bureau and CNN. (2004). More Americans living in poverty, August 26, 2004, (October 8, 2004); http://money.cnn.com/2004/08/26/news/economy/poverty_survey/?cnn=yes

Venkatesh, S. (2003). Whither the 'socially isolated' city? *Ethn Rac Stud.* 26(6):1058-1072.

Vleminckx, K. and Smeeding, T. (2001). Child Well-Being, Child Poverty and Child Policy in Modern Nations, Policy Press, Bristol, England.

Weil, C. M., Wade, S.L., Bauman, L.J., Lynn, H., Mitchell, H., and Lavigne, (1999). The Relationship Between Psychosocial Factors and Asthma Morbidity in Inner-City Children with Asthma. *Pediatrics* 104(6):1274-1280.

Wilson, W. (2003). Race, class and urban poverty: A rejoinder. *Ethnic and Racial Studies* 26(6):1096–1114.

Wilson, W.J. (1987). The Truly Disadvantaged: the inner city, the underclass, and public policy. University of Chicago Press, Chicago, IL.

Wilson, W.J. (1996). *When Work Disappears: the world of the new urban poor.* Alfred A. Knopf, New York, NY.

Wirth, L. (1938). Urbanism as a way of Life. *Am. J. Soc.* 44:3-24.

Yinger, J. (2001). Housing discrimination and residential segregation as causes of poverty. In: Danziger, S., and Haverman, R. (eds.). *Understanding poverty.* Russell Sage, New York, NY, pp.359-391.

Yonas, M. (2004). Exploring the contextual and individual level dynamics of urban youth violence in Baltimore City: a need assessment. Presentation of dissertation, March 2004 at the Bloomberg School of Public Health, Baltimore, MD.

Chapter 4

Racial/Ethnic Minorities and Health

The Role of the Urban Environment

Luisa N. Borrell and Stephani L. Hatch

1.0. OVERVIEW OF RACIAL/ETHIC MINORITY HEALTH

Over the course of the past century, although the health of Americans improved considerably, the rate of this progress was not shared equally by all racial/ethnic groups (Andersen, *et al.*, 1987; Cooper, 1993; Hummer, 1996; Lillie-Blanton, *et al.*, 1996; Manton, *et al.*, 1987; Miller, 1987; Williams and Collins, 1995). For example, infant mortality has been considered an important indicator of a nation's health and well-being (Nersesian, 1988) (Table 1). However, in 1999, the U.S. with a rate of 7.1 deaths per 1,000 live births as a whole ranked 28th internationally. Furthermore, when comparing infant mortality by race/ethnicity, the rates range from 5.1 deaths per 1,000 live births for Asians or Pacific Islanders to 13.9 for blacks (Freid, *et al.*, 2003). The infant mortality rates are higher for black and American Indians or Alaska Natives than for white infants. In fact, although the absolute differences between 1950 and 2003 for blacks and whites have declined dramatically, the relative differences have not. In 1950, the infant mortality rate was 43.9 deaths per 1,000 live births for blacks infants and 26.8 for white infants for a relative risk of 1.6 (Singh and Yu, 1995). By 2003, infant mortality rate for blacks infants had decreased to 13.8 which was still 2.4 times greater than the rate for white infants (5.8), a ratio higher than the one observed in 1950 (Freid, *et al.*, 2003).

Despite the fact that whites are the older group among the American population, blacks exhibit a 32% higher age-adjusted *all-cause mortality rate*, when compared to whites. American Indians or Alaska Natives, latinos and Asians or Pacific Islanders exhibit lower age-adjusted all-cause mortality rates by at least 28% than whites (Freid, *et al.*, 2003). A similar scenario can be observed for selected causes of deaths such as heart disease, cancer and diabetes (Table 1). Blacks exhibit 28% and 26% higher age-adjusted mortality rates for disease of the heart and cancer,

Table 1. Infant and Age-Adjusted Death rates* for All-Cause and Selected Cause of Deaths by Race/Ethnicity, United States, 2000

Indicator	White	Black	American Indian or Alaska Native	Asian or Pacific Islander	Latino
Infant Mortality	5.8	13.9	9.0	5.1	5.7
Age-adjusted mortality	849.8	1,121.4	709.3	506.4	665.7
All-cause	253.4	324.8	178.2	146.0	196.0
Heart disease	197.2	248.5	127.8	121.9	134.9
Cancer	9.6	49.5	41.5	16.4	36.9
Diabetes					

*Per 100,000 population.

respectively, than whites. In addition, blacks are 5.2 times more likely to die from diabetes than their white counterparts. Although some variation is observed, blacks, American Indians or Alaska Natives and latinos rate the worst for most causes of deaths when compared to the other minority groups (Freid, *et al.*, 2003). For blacks, specifically, cardiovascular disease, cancer, and infant mortality are responsible for over half of the excess mortality for adults under 70 years of age, accounting for 50% and 63% of the excess deaths for males and females, respectively (Cooper, 1993).

Minority groups also bear a higher burden of morbidity than their white counterparts (Lethbridge-Cejku, *et al.*, 2004). For example, in the most recent report card of the U.S., American Indians and Alaska Natives exhibited the highest age-adjusted prevalence of diabetes (16.0%) for adults 18 years of age or older followed by blacks (10.0%) and latinos (9.4%). Whites (5.8%) and Asians (6.3%) had the lowest age-adjusted prevalence of diabetes. For hypertension, blacks (29.9%) and American Indians and Alaska Natives (21.2%) exhibited the highest age-adjusted prevalence, whites (20.7%) having an intermediate prevalence and Asians (16.7%) and latinos (18.2%) having the lowest prevalence. Working-age blacks (12.1%) were also more likely to have a disability than their white (9.7%) and latinos peers (7.8%) (Freid, *et al.*, 2003).

In terms of *health risk behaviors*, blacks (34.8%) and American Indians and Alaska Natives (31.3%) are more likely to be obese than whites (21.9%) and latinos (25.4%) (Lethbridge-Cejku, *et al.*, 2004). Cigarettes smoking and lack of physical activity are preventable behaviors that contribute substantially to morbid conditions that lead to deaths in the U.S. population (McGinnis and Foege, 1993; Mokdad, *et al.*, 2004). Among adults 18 years or older, American Indians and Alaska Natives (34.1%) are more likely to smoke than whites (24%), blacks (21.8%), latinos (15.8%), and Asians (12.5%). In the case of physical activity, on average over half of the U.S. adults 18 years of age population are physically inactive, with latinos (71.1%) and blacks (67.5%) being the least active (Lethbridge-Cejku, *et al.*, 2004).

Other factors that may play a key role in the health disparities among racial/ethnic groups are *access and use of medical care.* Race/ethnic disparities in the quantity and quality of medical care for individuals has been pervasive over many years (Swift, 2002). For example, a third of latinos and American Indians and Alaska Natives under 65 years of age are uninsured, while 19.2% of blacks lack health insurance (Freid, *et al.*, 2003). Further, latinos (25.5%) and Asians (19.4%) are less likely to have a usual place of care than whites (11.2%), blacks (13.4%) and American

Indians and Alaska Natives (13.4%) (Lethbridge-Cejku *et al.*, 2004). The latter indicates that latinos and Asians are more likely to suffer from a lack of continuity in health care. A similar scenario is also observed for preventive care such as prenatal care among mothers and influenza vaccine among adults 65 years of age or older. Latinos (24.3% and 45.2%) and blacks (25.5% and 51.2%) are less likely to have access to these services (Freid *et al.*, 2003).

2.0. MINORITY GROUPS, URBAN LIFE, AND HEALTH

The unequal distribution of disease and disability across racial/ethnic groups accompanied with the disproportionate settlement of racial/ethnic minority groups in urban cities could have implications for urban health, specifically in terms of the contribution that minority health makes to the overall health in the city. However, in order to explain and understand the relationship between health and urban life, it is important to disentangle the effects of person and place. For example, although 73% of U.S. counties are classified as nonmetropolitan or rural areas, 80% of the American population lives in counties classified as metropolitan or urban areas (Eberhardt, *et al.*, 2001). The Northeast region, which contains the lowest percent of the U.S. population (19%), exhibits the highest percentage (90.1%) of people living in metro areas, while the Midwest, home of 23% of the U.S. population, exhibits the highest proportion of people living in non-metropolitan (26.4%) with 14.4% of those living in rural counties.

Although the association between urban areas and health has not been directly investigated, per se, findings from social science research (Coleman, 1988, 1990; Harris, 1999; Jargowsky, 1996; Massey and Denton, 1993; Sampson and Morenoff, 1997; Sampson, *et al.*, 1997; 1995; Shaw and McKay, 1969; Wilson, 1987; 1996) suggest that urban areas provide both advantages and disadvantages to their residents. Economic development and the higher levels of community resources can facilitate dissemination of health related information that potentially leads to better health. Obverse, the impact on family and community organization of the lack of resources and organization within the social milieu of urban areas could lower the health benefits of other resources and information related to health.

The overall benefit of community resources to all their residents is what Rose (1985) has called a preventive paradox, that is everybody benefits by being exposed to multiple sources of information and services (Rose, 1985). A good example of this paradox is the case of health promotion leading to positive health behaviors, such as physical activity, anti-smoking campaigns, and sexual education among adolescents. People living in urban areas are more likely to be active than those living in rural settings, regardless of their race/ethnicity, and as a result less likely to be overweight (Eberhardt, *et al.*, 2001). Cigarette smoking and birth rates among adolescents are lower in urban setting than in rural areas (Eberhardt, *et al.*, 2001). In fact, there is evidence that black adolescents in urban cities have lower rates of smoking than whites and are more likely to initiate later in life (Bachman, *et al.*, 1991; McIntosh, 1995; Nelson, *et al.*, 1995; Siegfried, 1991). However, not all resources are part of this paradox.

The impact on family and community organization resulting from the lack of resources and organization within the social milieu of urban areas could lower the health benefits of resources and information related to health. Access to care has been underscored as a reason for better health in urban areas but members of minority groups, specifically blacks and latinos are consistently among the uninsured in comparison to their white counterparts, regardless of the region where they reside in the U.S. (Freid, *et al.*, 2003). Moreover, the proportion of blacks and latinos without insurance living in urban cities is higher than the proportion living in rural areas (Eberhardt, *et al.*, 2001). Lack of insurance could limit access to care for these populations. To complicate matters, during the 1970s and 1980s, many American cities experienced the closings and relocations of hospitals, especially voluntary and public hospitals. These hospitals, in some cases, were the only source of care for minority communities. These closings had a tremendous impact on access to care and the creation of a spatial mismatch between needs and services. Furthermore, Sager (1983) found that one of the most significant predictors for hospitals closing and relocations was the proportion of blacks in the area (Sager, 1983).

Another problem of urban cities is the high proportion of people living below poverty levels. For years, poverty has been associated with poor health due to inadequate nutrition, substandard housing, exposure to environmental hazards, unhealthy lifestyles and behaviors, and decreased access to and use of health care services (Andrulis and Goodman, 1999; Pamuk, *et al.*, 1998). There is pervasive evidence that poor people exhibited more disease, disability and are more likely to die than their higher socioeconomic status (SES) counterparts (Williams and Collins, 1995). In 1999, 12.4% of Americans lived below the poverty threshold (Bishaw and Iceland, 2003). Furthermore, race/ethnicity is strongly associated with poverty in U.S. urban life. Although 54% of poor Americans belong to racial/ethnic minority groups, the distribution of poverty nationwide follows the concentration of minority population, specifically blacks and latinos. Blacks and latinos are more likely to live in urban areas with a high proportion of people living below poverty than their white counterparts (Freid, *et al.*, 2003). In 1999, 1 in 4 blacks or latinos lived below poverty level (Bishaw and Iceland, 2003). These figures have remained nearly unchanged in 2003 (DeNavas-Walt, *et al.*, 2004). For example, Figures 1, 2 and 3 show first an overlay of urban areas and poverty; and second, urban areas,

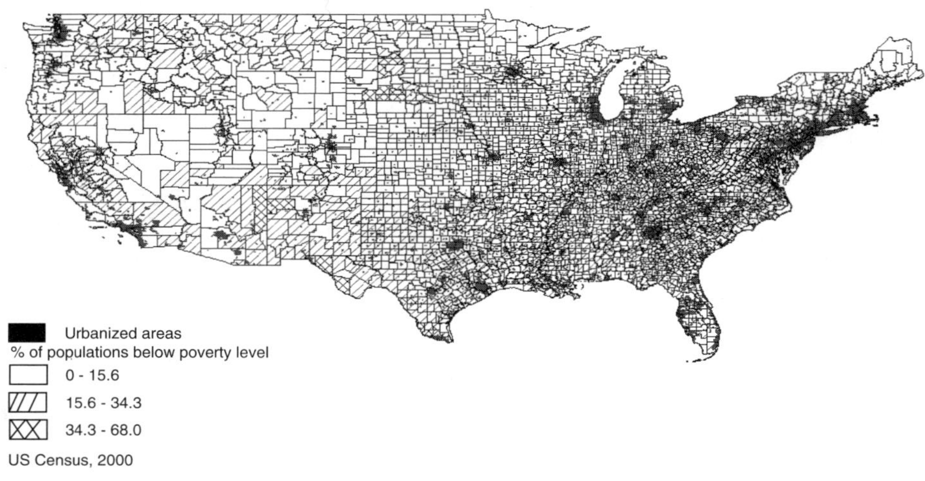

Figure 1. Poverty and Urbanized areas, 1999.

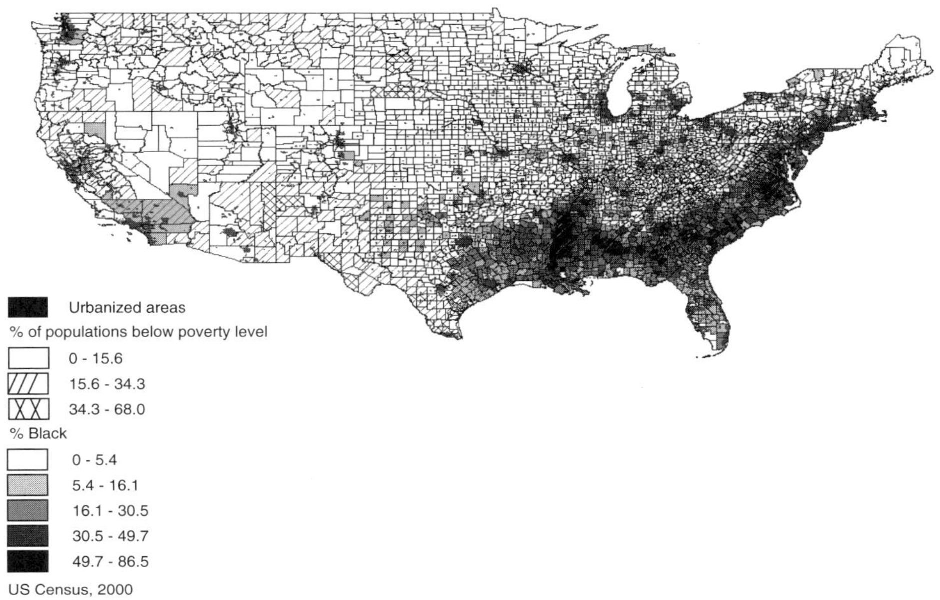

Figure 2. Blacks, Poverty, and Urbanized areas, 2000.

poverty and percent of minority. In general, urban areas, poverty areas, and concentration of blacks and latinos tend to overlap but the most striking finding is that the higher the concentration of blacks and latinos in urban areas the higher the percentage of people living below poverty in the area. Therefore, blacks and latinos are more likely to experience the "health disadvantage" associated with living in urban cities. This disadvantage in turn represents what Andrulis has called the 'urban health penalty', which refers to the accumulation of health problems in urban areas (Andrulis, 1997). The topic of poverty and health has been treated with greater detail in a separate chapter.

3.0. HEALTH DISPARITIES: THE ROLE OF RACE, SOCIOECONOMIC STATUS, AND THE URBAN ENVIRONMENT

Racial/ethnic minority populations tend to have worse health outcomes than the white majority population. However, minority groups, specifically blacks and latinos, also tend to be over represented in the lowest stratum of education and income in our society. Therefore, poverty and racial/ethnic minority status tend to cluster nationwide regardless of region and urbanization. This clustering refers to what has been coined by Williams J. Wilson as 'the concentration effects' or the concentration of the most disadvantaged segments of minority groups in a particular geographic area (Wilson, 1987). In addition, this clustering leads to social isolation from mainstream America, which in turn amplifies the effects of living in a poverty area.

Socioeconomic status (SES) is important for the health of minority populations because differentials in health status associated with SES are larger than those

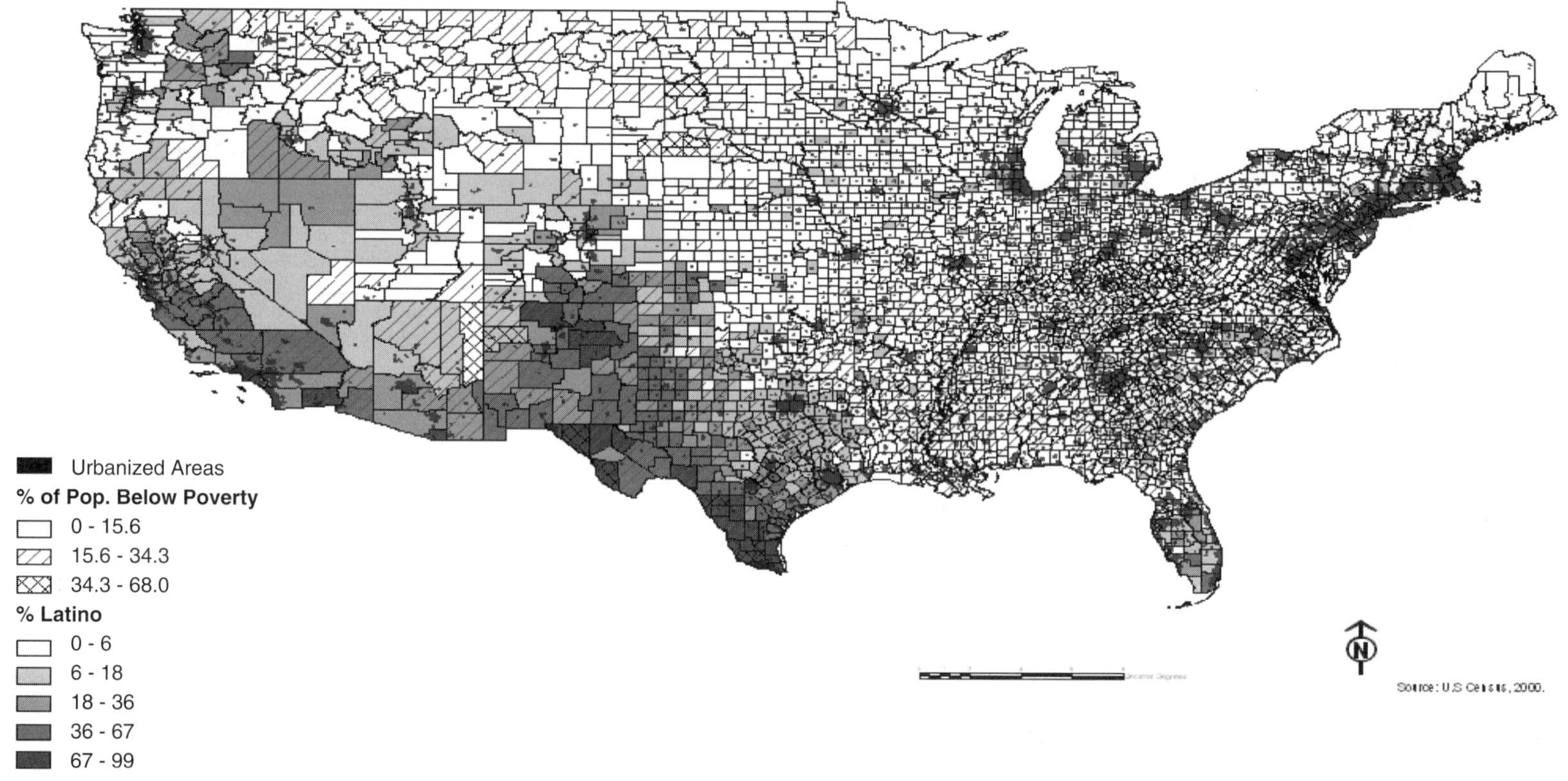

Figure 3 Latinos, Poverty and Urbanized Areas: 2000.

associated with race/ethnicity. Furthermore, SES accounts for many of the racial/ethnic differences in health. It is worth noting that race and SES are two distinct concepts: race tends to have an effect on health independent of SES, and in fact, racial/ethnic minority groups, specifically blacks, tend to have worse health outcomes in each level of SES than whites, regardless of the SES indicator use (Williams, 1999). When evaluating the contribution of SES on racial/ethnic health differences, it is important to keep in mind that socioeconomic indicators are not equivalent across racial/ethnic groups. Status inequality is maintained by many macro-structural supports, such as discriminatory access to opportunity structures. As a result, structural arrangements clearly influence many of the conditions and circumstances, including where one lives, with whom one associates, access to goods and services, and exposure to conditions associated with poverty, such as inadequate housing, joblessness, and crime (Wilson, 1999). Furthermore, being located within the lower class constricts individuals' access to quality education, primary labor market occupations, and social resources that allow for the attainment and preservation of advantaged class positions. Economic inequalities in resources and opportunities hinder a large sub-population of low-income and poor individuals and families from maintaining a basic quality of life commonly shared by mainstream society (Wilson, 1999). In fact, Reich (1994) contends that economic consequences are related to the operation of racism and discrimination in the educational system, residential location, health care, as well as the labor market (Reich, 1994).

Blacks and latinos received lower income returns for a given level of education than whites. Further, the link between education and income affects occupational attainment and the accumulation of wealth through investments, such as home ownership. Home equity is a major source of wealth. However, blacks tend to receive smaller returns on their real estate investment than whites. Purchasing power also varies by race/ethnicity. Blacks and latinos living in urban areas tend to pay more for food, groceries, auto insurance, housing and other goods and services than the running prices in more suburban areas (Williams and Collins, 2001).

To add to the lower education level of blacks and latinos, urban areas have suffered from structural economic changes by shifting from jobs which required lower education to jobs in industries that require higher levels of education, by the relocation of industries to suburban areas (or other countries) due to cost in the city, and by the decrease in the share of metropolitan jobs in the manufacturing sector. Those who remain employed in the formal labor market often do so under considerable strain, making the pursuit of income in informal sectors a viable alternative (Wilson, 1996).

Low-income communities historically have relied on informal sectors for goods and services, such as medical assistance, child care, and home maintenance (Liebow, 1967; Maher, 1997; Stack, 1974). Joblessness and absence from the formal economy often lead to the poor and lower class members to seek out non-employment income sources other than employment that are considered to be compatible with the secondary labor market, including illicit economic activities (Piore, 1994). Spatial mismatch between the education distribution of racial/ethnic minority groups living in urban cities and the existing job opportunities has led to unemployment, participation in informal economies and social disorganization such as crime, violence, teen pregnancies, drug use and distribution, etc. Participation in informal economies develops out of a need to address the lack of opportunity for economic enterprise and transactions that are available in the formal economy.

Involvement in illegitimate activity (e.g., criminal activity, illicit drug use and distribution) often emerges from experiencing periods of unemployment or exclusion from the labor force due to lack of education and skills (Rabow and Watts, 1983). When job opportunities exist, many lower income inner city neighborhoods are characterized by secondary work sectors that involve fewer attractive job opportunities, poor working conditions, low wages, and little opportunity for job mobility (Piore, 1994). The secondary labor market is differentiated by low skilled, low wage, and intermittent positions. Members of minority groups are most likely to suffer from the economics of racism and discrimination associated with operating within secondary labor markets (Piore, 1994; Reich, 1994).

Class is also closely intertwined with race and ethnicity, with minorities living in inner city areas often perceived by many to be a threat to conventional upper class orientations (MacLeod, 1994; MacLeod and James, 1999; Roberts, 1997). For example, references made to members of the lower classes as being the "underclass" refer not only to their economic positions but also to several social pathologies, such as welfare dependency, violence, drug abuse, illegitimate childbearing, and crime (Roberts, 1997). The joint effects of race and class subjugation consistently reproduce uneven economic growth and support the development of informal economies as an alternative to access to the primary labor market.

4.0. MINORITY GROUPS AND THE URBAN ENVIRONMENT

As stated throughout this chapter, minorities are more likely to live in urban cities, where features of the urban environment either enhance or negatively affect health. Individuals' characteristics have been seen as the panacea to produce and promote positive health outcomes. However, individuals live and interact with their peers in urban areas under circumstances that provide an enhancing or damaging milieu for health. Therefore, it is important to understand how features of the social environment affect individuals' behaviors differently to promote or damage health status.

Research has shown that the social milieu in which individuals interact could vary by the racial/ethnic composition of the area. For example, Sampson and Wilson found in an analysis of the 171 largest cities in the U.S. that: "The worst context in which whites reside was considerably better than the average context of Black communities" (Sampson, *et al.,* 1995). The authors also stated that the effect of concentrated poverty, male unemployment, and residential instability contribute to family disruption, which in turn contribute to higher levels of violence. These features of social disorganization at the community level could also lead to negative health-related behaviors at the individual level. For example, the burden of chronic disease in communities is directly related to individual's risk behaviors that can be preventable (Williams, 1998). However, changes in behaviors do not occur in a vacuum. Behaviors are the product of the interaction between individuals and their social environment.

Although health risk behaviors such as smoking, alcohol consumption, and diet have been viewed simply as individual characteristics, accepting this view ignores the forces and inequalities in our society that not only promote the initiation of these behaviors but also help maintain these practices. For example, alcohol and smoking have been positively associated with poverty and are frequently used to obtain relief from harsh living, working conditions and stressful environment induced by the social structures and unequal distribution of resources. In addition, there is also a strong association between availability of these products, specifically alcohol consumption (Rabow and Watts, 1983; 1984). Blacks and latinos are more likely to hold stressful jobs and live in impoverished communities. To complement that, it is well known that blacks and latinos have been targeted by these industries, and in fact, over 80% of billboards in the U.S. contain advertisements targeted to blacks and latinos with a large majority placed in the neighborhoods in which these groups live (Hacker, *et al.*, 1987; Maxwell and Jacobson, 1989). Fast food restaurants and convenience stores follow a similar pattern of product placement and advertisement in urban cities. Morland and colleagues (2002a and 2002b) found a greater number of fast food restaurants and convenience stores in black neighborhoods when compared to white neighborhoods. In addition, this type of store was more commonly located in poorer neighborhoods. Furthermore, Diez-Roux and colleagues found that living in low income neighborhoods decreased intake of fruits, vegetables and fish and increased intake of meat (Diez-Roux, *et al.*, 1999). The increase accessibility to high caloric food and the lack of healthy food could contribute to the increased prevalence of obesity among minority communities.

5.0. RESIDENTIAL SEGREGATION AND GENTRIFICATION

A major problem of urban cities is the residential segregation of minority groups, which leads to economic constraints, lack of social and material resources, and diminished social capital. Residential segregation results, in part, from two of the most dominant demographic trends in almost all cities in the U.S., suburbanization (i.e., "white flight") and metropolitan deconcentration (Browne, 2000; Immergluck, 2001; Massey and Denton, 1988). Metropolitan deconcentration reflects the process of metropolitan areas spreading past planned and established suburbs to areas more remote to those living in center cities. Both trends continue to increase both class and racial residential segregation and shift resources away from inner cities. For example, when people move to the suburbs so do the property taxes and other sources of revenue that are used for schools, infrastructure, and other essential city services (sanitation, police and fire protection, etc). Along with the relocation of individuals and families, businesses seeking cheaper commercial property with lower utility and service rates also move. This contributes to the relocation of jobs and the reduction of the property tax base of the city. Therefore, communities are heavily affected by property taxes and other sources of revenue that are used for schools, infrastructure, and other essential city services (sanitation, police and fire protection, etc) moving to the suburbs.

The impact of these disinvestments is increased by differential practices in inner city communities, such as redlining and gentrification. Redlining refers to the practice of not providing loans housing purchases and home improvements, or insurance, in what is deemed to be undesirable areas. These areas are often made up of concentrations of minorities and located in central cities. Gentrification is somewhat different in that it is thought to result from changes in the economic base of a community and typically involves the buying of older, often dilapidated, properties and turning them into middle-income condos, townhouses, single-family dwellings, lofts and apartments (Redfern, 2003). In the process, residents are displaced due to inability to pay increased rents, purchase prices, and property taxes based on raised property values.

Racial segregation refers to the composition and spatial distribution of a segment of the population, specifically blacks and low income people, across neighborhoods (Lieberson, 1980; Massey and Denton, 1993; Wilson, 1987). Latinos are also likely to be segregated from whites. Latinos are likely to live in neighborhoods similar to or near non-latino blacks' neighborhoods. Previous studies showed that Puerto Ricans were highly segregated from whites as a result of their African ancestry (Massey, 1979, 2001; Massey and Bitterman, 1985). This segregation pattern persists regardless of Puerto Ricans' economic mobility. Although racial segregation, as measured by the percent of minorities in a neighborhood, could be considered a contextual characteristic, segregation could have an effect at both individual and neighborhood levels. At the individual level, segregation would affect quality of education, employment opportunities, health-related behaviors, access to care and exposure to stress-related conditions (McLafferty, 1982; Whiteis, 1992; Wilson, 1996). At the neighborhood level, segregation can affect quality of the physical environment (i.e. pollutants, environmental hazards), targeted tobacco and alcohol advertisements, housing opportunities, and mobility as well as crime and violence (Harris, 1999; Jargowsky, 1996; Sampson and Wilson, 1995; Wallace, 1990; 1991; Wilson, 1987). Williams and Collins, building on Link and Phelan's framework, suggested that segregation could be a fundamental cause of racial disparities in health (Link and Phelan, 1995; Williams and Collins, 2001). When addressing health disparities, residential segregation could be considered as a gatekeeper for resources conducive to health and as a reservoir of disadvantages and inequalities conducive to disease. The effects of segregation are likely to be detrimental to health not only for blacks and latinos living in the area but also for other racial/ethnic groups residing in the same environment. In fact, a recent study shows an association between segregation and increased mortality risk for whites living in areas with high concentration of blacks (Collins, 1999).

Despite the deleterious direct and indirect health effect of residential segregation, it is worth noting that there are some positive effects of racial segregation on minority groups. For example, in segregated black communities two historically related social institutions that are likely to strengthen blood and fictive kinship ties are black families and church (Billingsley, 1999; Chatters and Taylor, 1988; Chatters, *et al.*, 2002; Hill, 1999). Both families and churches address many issues facing black families and communities (e.g., poverty, coping with a death of a loved one, care giving for the ill and disabled), as well as provide both instrumental and emotional social support to community members (Chatters, *et al.*, 2002). Social support is in turn linked to quality of social networks and community structure (Lin, 1999). In addition, communities with strong ties are likely to provide some type of regulation and attachment to norms and values within the community that may lead to what has been called by Sampson and colleagues as Collective Efficacy (Sampson and Morenoff, 1997). Communities with high collective efficacy are more likely to care about the common goods such as physical environment and public order. For latinos, the benefit of living in homogenous community is associated with preservation of language, traditions, and cultural norms that may be health protective. The Church, specifically the clergy, is also a source of support and a mental health resource among Mexican-Americans (Chalfant, *et al.*, 1990). Finally, factors related to culture, such as social support, religiosity/spirituality, and extended family resources have protective effects against poor mental health among blacks, Native Americans, and Latinos (Samaan, 2000).

6.0. ENVIRONMENTAL JUSTICE AND HEALTH

Environmental problems and their associated costs are often passed along to the people living in disadvantaged social contexts. Poor people and minorities in urban areas not only work in the most dangerous jobs, as mentioned above, but also live in the most polluted neighborhoods where their children are exposed to various environmental toxins in play areas and in their homes (Bryant and Mohai, 1992; Bullard, 1994).

In a report focused on environmental risk factors and health, the Institute of Medicine (Institute of Medicine, 1999) confirmed that low-income and minority communities are exposed to greater levels of pollution than more affluent white communities. Further, race, independent of SES, impacts the distribution of air pollution, the location of landfills and incinerators, abandoned toxic waste dumps, and lead poisoning in children (Bullard and Johnson, 2000; Pirkle, *et al.*, 1994). The greatest health risks for individuals living in disadvantaged communities comes from exposure to water pollution, toxins, solid and hazardous waste, raw sewage, toxic releases from industries, pesticides, air pollution, and lead (Bullard and Johnson, 2000). Pirkle and colleagues (1994) found higher rates of blood lead levels in black and Mexican-American children in comparison to white children (Pirkle, *et al.*, 1994). This study, an analysis of the NHANES III, also revealed that at every income level, black children suffer from lead poisoning at more than twice the rate of white children.

Air pollution, another environmental threat, has been identified as a risk factor for hospitalization for lung and heart disease, as well as respiratory disorder (Arif, *et al.*, 2003; Zanobetti, *et al.*, 2000). In general, results from multiple community sites suggest a positive relationship between outdoor air pollution/smog and asthma (Clean Air Task Force, 2002; National Campaign Against Dirty Power, 1999). Outdoor air pollution has been implicated as a major trigger in increased respiratory-related emergency room visits and hospital admissions (Bullard, *et al.*, 2000; National Campaign Against Dirty Power., 1999). Urban metropolitan areas, such as Atlanta, Georgia, have been found to be repeatedly in violation of the Clean Air Task Force, with cars, trucks and buses being the greatest source of air pollution (Bullard, *et al.*, 2000).

The reason why minority groups, particularly blacks and latinos, are more likely to be exposed to higher levels of environmental contaminants is not an accident, but rather a function of their position in the structure of our society (Fitzpatrick and LaGory, 2000). Minority groups are more likely to live in communities with weak political organization, and hence, are unable to fight back the location of toxic dumps and landfill in their communities (Harvey, 1997).

Environmental justice focuses on the rights of individuals to be equally protected from environmental degradation by emphasizing the utilization of congressional acts, such as the Civil Rights Act of 1964, the Fair housing act of 1968, and the Voting rights act of 1965. The preferred environmental justice strategy focuses on a public health model of prevention, specifically the elimination of threat before the occurrence of harm, and shifting the burden of proof from the racial/ethnic minorities to polluters and dischargers who act in a harmful and discriminatory manner (Bullard and Johnson, 2000). Advocates of the environmental justice framework argue for requirements that force corporations and businesses applying for operating permits (e.g., landfills, incinerators, refineries, chemical plants, etc.) to provide evidence that their operations are not harmful to human health and will not disproportionately impact racial and ethnic minorities and other protected groups. Affected communities rarely have the resources to secure and maintain the legal support, experts, and doctors needed for protection from and/or removal of environmental threats.

Social and environmental scientists involved in environmental justice are making efforts to challenge procedural equity (i.e., the standardized application of governing rules, regulations, and enforcement), geographic equity (i.e. spatial configuration of communities and their proximity to unwanted land uses and noxious facilities), and social equity (i.e., assessment of how race/ethnicity, class, culture, and political power affect environmental decision making) (Bullard, 2004).

7.0. CONCLUSION

Urban cities are polarized environments combining risks and protective behaviors. This polarization tends to follow the distribution of goods and resources in our society. Racial/ethnic minority groups occupy the lower end of our society and are concentrated in areas with a high level of people living below poverty, high unemployment, high proportion of people on pubic assistance, lack of health insurance, and limited access to health care. Therefore, minorities occupy a higher risk position in our society and particularly so in urban areas. Minority groups' exposures to health damaging circumstances and promotion of negative health behaviors are a function of their social position. Therefore, to understand the contribution of the urban environment in shaping the health of their residents, the structures and processes driving the racial/ethnic relationships of our society needs to be placed in the context of the historic, economic, and social forces creating and ultimately shaping these relationships in our day-to-day life. Specifically, the historic meaning of race, and more recently ethnicity, needs to be deconstructed to provide equal opportunities to all racial/ethnic groups in our society and to eventually eliminate the health damaging effects of the urban environment.

REFERENCES

Andersen, R. M., Mullner, R. M., and Cornelius, L. J. (1987). Black-white differences in health status: methods or substance? *Milbank Quarterly* 65 (Suppl 1):72-99.

Andrulis, D. P. (1997). The urban health penalty: New dimensions and directions in inner-city health care. (May 20, 2004); http://www.acponline.org/hpp/pospaper/andrulis.htm.

Andrulis, D. P., and Goodman, N. J. (1999). *The social and health landscape of urban and suburban America.* Health Forum, Inc., Chicago, IL

Arif, A. A., Delclos, G. L., Lee, E. S., Tortolero, S. R., and Whitehead, L. W. (2003). Prevalence and risk factors of asthma and wheezing among US adults: an analysis of the NHANES III data. *Eur. Respir. J.* 21:827-833.

Bachman, J. G., Wallace, J. M., Jr., O'Malley, P. M., Johnston, L. D., Kurth, C. L., and Neighbors, H. W. (1991). Racial/Ethnic differences in smoking, drinking, and illicit drug use among American high school seniors, 1976-89. *Am. J. Public Health* 81(3):372-377.

Billingsley, A. (1999). *Mighty like a river: The Black church and social reform.* Oxford University Press, New York.

Bishaw, A., and Iceland, J. (2003). Poverty: 1999 Census 2000 Brief. (May 29, 2004); http://www.census.gov/prod/2003pubs/c2kbr-19.pdf

Browne, I. (2000). Opportunities lost? Race, industrial restructuring, and employment among young women heading households. *Social Forces* 78(3):907-929.

Bryant, B., and Mohai, P. (1992). Race and the incidence of environmental hazards. Westview Press., Boulder, Co.

Bullard, R. D. (2004). Environmental Justice in the 21st Century. http://www.ejrc.cau.edu/ejinthe21century.htm.

Bullard, R. D. (1994). *Dumping in Dixie: Race, class, and environmental quality*. Westview Press, Boulder, CO.

Bullard, R. D., and Johnson, G. S. (2000). Environmental justice: grassroots activism and its impact on public policy decision making. *J. Soc. Issues* 56(3): 555-578.

Bullard, R. D., Johnson, G. S., and Torres, A. O. (2000). The routes of American apartheid. *Forum Appl. Res. Public Policy* 15(3): 66-74.

Chalfant, H. P., Heller, P. L., Roberts, A., Briones, D., Aguirre-Hochbaum, S., and Farr, W. (1990). The clergy as a resource for those encountering psychological distress. *Review of Religious Research* 31:305-313.

Chatters, L. M., and Taylor, R. J. (1988). Church members as a source of informal social support. *Review of Religious Research* 30:193-203.

Chatters, L. M., Taylor, R. J., Lincoln, K. D., and Schroepfer, T. (2002). Patterns of informal support from family and church members among African Americans. *J. Black Stud.* 30:66-85.

Clean Air Task Force. Air of injustice: African Americans and power plant pollution. (2002). Washington, D.C., (September 10, 2004); http://www.blackleadershipforum.org/articles/air_injustice.html.

Coleman, J. S. (1988). Social capital in the creation of human capital. *Am. J. Soc.* 94:S95-S120.

Coleman, J. S. (1990). *Foundations of Social Theory*. Harvard University Press, Cambridge, MA.

Collins, C. A. (1999). Racism and health: segregation and causes of death amenable to medical intervention in major U.S. cities. *Ann. N. Y. Acad. Sci.* 896:396-8.

Cooper, R. S. (1993). Health and the social status of blacks in the United States. *Ann. Epidemiol.* 3(2):137-44.

DeNavas-Walt, C., Proctor, B. D., and Mills, R. J. (2004). U.S. Census Bureau, Current Population Reports, P60-226, Income, Poverty, and Health Insurance Coverage in the United States: 2003. U.S. Government Printing Office, Washington D.C.

Diez-Roux, A. V., Nieto, F. J., Caulfield, L., Tyroler, H. A., Watson, R. L., and Szklo, M. (1999). Neighbourhood differences in diet: the Atherosclerosis Risk in Communities (ARIC) Study. *J. Epidemiol. Comm. Health* 53(1): 55-63.

Eberhardt, M. S., Ingram, D. D., Makuc, D. M., Pamuk, E. R., Fried, V. M., Harper, S.B., Schoenborn, C. A., and Xia, H. (2001). Urban and Rural Health Chartbook. Health, United States, 2001. National Center for Health Statistics, Hyattsville, MD.

Fitzpatrick, K., and LaGory, M. (2000). *Unhealthy Places. The ecology of risk in the urban landscape*. Routledge, New York, NY.

Freid, V. M., Prager, K., Mackay, A. P., and Xia, H. (2003). *Chartbook on Trends in the Health of Americans. Health, United States, 2003*. National Center for Health Statistics, Hyattsville, MD.

Hacker, A. G., Collins, R., and Jacobson, M. (1987). *Marketing booze to Blacks*. Center for Science in the Public Interest, Washington D.C.

Harris, D. R. (1999). All suburbs are not created equal: a new look at racial differences in suburban locations. Research Report No. 99–440. University of Michigan, Population Studies Center, Ann Arbor, MI.

Harvey, D. (1997). The environment of justice. In: Merrifield, A., and E. Swyngedouw. (eds.), The Urbanization of Justice. New York University Press, New York, pp.65-99.

Hill, R. B. (1999). The strengths of African American families: Twenty-five years later (2nd ed.). Sage, Thousands Oak, CA.

Hummer, R. A. (1996). Black-white differences in health and mortality: A review and conceptual model. *Sociol. Q.* 37(1):105-125.

Immergluck, D. (2001). The financial services sector and cities: restructuring, decentralization, and declining urban employment. *Economic Development Quarterly* 15(3): 74-288.

Jargowsky, P. A. (1996). take your money and run: economic segregation in the U.S. metropolitan areas. *Am. Sociol. Rev.* 61:984-998.

Lethbridge-Cejku, M., Schiller, J. S., and Bernadel, L. (2004). Summary health statistics for U.S. Adults: National Health Interview Survey, 2002.

Lieberson, S. (1980). *A piece of the pie: black and white immigrants since 1880*. University of California Press, Berkeley, CA.

Liebow, E. (1967). Talley's corner: A study of Negro streetcorner men. Little Brown, Boston, MA.

Lillie-Blanton, M., Parsons, P. E., Gayle, H., and Dievler, A. (1996). Racial differences in health: not just black and white, but shades of gray. *Ann. Rev. Public Health* 17:411-448.

Lin, N. Y. X. E. W. M. (1999). Social Support and Depressed Mood: A Structural Analysis. *J Health Soc. Behav.* 40(4):344-359.

Link, B. G., and Phelan, J. C. (1995). Social conditions as fundamental causes of disease. *J. Health Soc. Behav.* Supplement: 80-94.

MacLeod, J. (ed.). (1994). *Ain't no makin it: Leveled aspirations in a low income neighborhood.* Westview Press, Bouldwer, CO.

MacLeod, J., and James, N. (eds.). (1999). *Social Stratification and Inequality.* Kluwer Academics/Plenum Publishers, New York, NY.

Maher, L. (1997). *Sexed work.* Clarendon Press, Oxford.

Manton, K. G., Patrick, C. H., and Johnson, K. W. (1987). Health differentials between blacks and whites: recent trends in mortality and morbidity. *Milbank Q.* 65(Suppl 1):100-128.

Massey, D. S. (1979). Effects of Socioeconomic-Factors on the Residential Segregation of Blacks and Spanish-Americans in United-States Urbanized Areas. *Am. Soc. Rev.* 44(6):1015-1022.

Massey, D. S. (2001). Residential Segregation and neighborhood conditions in US metropolitan areas. In: Smelser, N., Wilson, W. J. and Mitchell F. (eds.), *American becoming: Racial trends and their consequences* (Vol I). National Academy of Sciences Press, Washington, pp. 391-34.

Massey, D. S., and Bitterman, B. (1985). Explaining the Paradox of Puerto-Rican Segregation. *Social Forces.* 64(2):306-331.

Massey, D. S., and Denton, N. A. (1988). Suburbanization and segregation in U S metropolitan areas. *Am. J. Soc.* 94:592-26.

Massey, D. S., and Denton, N. A. (1993). *American apartheid: segregation and the making of the underclass.* Harvard University Press, Cambridge, MA.

Maxwell, B., and Jacobson, M. (1989). *Marketing disease to Hispanics: The selling of alcohol, tobacco and junk foods.* Center for Science in the Public Interest, Washington D.C.

McGinnis, J. M., and Foege, W. H. (1993). Actual causes of death in the United States. *JAMA.* 270(18):2207-2212.

McIntosh, H. (1995). Black teens not smoking in great numbers. *J. Nat'l. Cancer Inst.* 87(8):564.

McLafferty, S. (1982). Neighborhood characteristics and hospital closures: a comparison of the public, private, and voluntary systems. *Soc. Sci. Med.* 16:1667-1674.

Miller, S. M. (1987). Race in the health of America. *Milbank Q.* 65(Suppl 2):500-31.

Mokdad, A. H., Marks, J. S., Stroup, D. F., and Gerberding, J. L. (2004). Actual Causes of Death in the United States, 2000. *JAMA.* 291(10):1238-1245.

Morland, K., Wing, S., and Diez Roux, A. (2002a). The contextual effect of the local food environment on residents' diets: the atherosclerosis risk in communities study. *Am. J. Public Health* 92(11):1761-1767.

Morland, K., Wing, S., Diez Roux, A., and Poole, C. (2002b). Neighborhood characteristics associated with the location of food stores and food service places. *Am. J. Prevent. Med.* 22(1):23-29.

Navarro, V. (1990). Race or class versus race and class: mortality differential in the United States. *Lancet* 336: 1230-1240.

Neighborhood safety and the prevalence of physical inactivity-selected states. (1999). *MMWR.* 48(7):143-146.

Nelson, D. E., Giovino, G. A., Shopland, D. R., Mowery, P. D., Mills, S. L., and Eriksen, M. P. (1995). Trends in cigarette smoking among US adolescents, 1974 through 1991. *Am. J. Public Health* 85(1):34-40.

Nersesian, W. S. (1988). Infant mortality in socially vulnerable populations. *Annu. Rev. Public Health* 9:361-377.

National Campaign Against Dirty Power. (1999). Out of Breath: Adverse health effects associated with ozone in the eastern United States. Washington, DC, (September 10, 2004); http://www.pewtrusts.com/pdf/env_out_of_breath.pdf.

Pamuk, E., Makuc, D. M., Heck, K., Reuben, C., and Lochner, K. (1998). *Socioeconomic Status and Health Chartbook. Health, United States, 1998.* National Center for Health Statistics, Hyattsville, MD.

Piore, M. (1994). The dual labor market theory: Theory and implications. In: Grusky, D. (ed.), *Social stratification: Class, race, and gender in sociological perspective.* Westview Press, Boulder, CO.

Pirkle, J. L., Brody, D. J., Gunter, E. W., Kramer, R. A., Paschal, D. C., Flegal, K. M., and Matte, T.D. (1994). The decline in blood lead levels in the United States. The National Health and Nutrition Examination Surveys (NHANES). *JAMA.* 272(4):284-291.

Rabow, J., and Watts, R. K. (1983). The role of alcohol availability in alcohol consumption and alcohol problems. *Recent. Dev. Alcohol* 1:285-302.

Rabow, J., and Watts, R. K. (1984). Alcohol availability, alcohol beverage sales, and alcohol-related problems. *Journal of Study of Alcohol* 43:767-801.

Redfern, P. A. (2003). What Makes Gentrification 'Gentrification?' *Urban Studies* 40(12):2351-2366.

Reich, M. (1994). The economics of racism. In: Grusky, D. (ed.), *Social stratification: Class, race, and gender in sociological perspective.* Westview Press, Boulder, CO.

Roberts, D. (1997). *Killing the Black Body.* Vintage Books, New York.

Rose, G. (1985). Sick individuals and sick populations. *Int. J. Epidemiol.* 14(1):32-38.

Rubio, M., and Williams, D. R. (2004). The social dimension of race. In: Beech, B. M. and Goodman, M. (eds.), Race & Research. Perspectives on minority participation in health studies (5th edition). American Public Health Association, Washington, D.C., pp. 1-26.

Sager, A. (1983). Why urban voluntary hospitals close. *Health Serv. Res.* 18(3):451-475.

Samaan, R. A. (2000). The influences of race, ethnicity, and poverty on the mental health of children. *J. Health Care Poor Underserved* 11:100-110.

Sampson, R. J., and Morenoff, J. D. (1997). Ecological perspectives on the neighborhood context of urban poverty. In: Brooks-Gunn, J., Duncan, G.J., and Aber, J. L. (eds.), *Neighborhood poverty: Context and consequences for children (Vol. II: Policy implications in studying neighborhoods).* Russell Sage, New York.

Sampson, R. J., Raudenbush, S. W., and Earls, F. (1997). Neighborhoods and violent crime: A multilevel study of collective efficacy. *Science* 277(5328): 918-924.

Sampson, R. J., and Wilson, W. J. (1995). Toward a theory of race, crime and urban inequality. In: Hagan J., and Petersen, R. D. (eds.), *Crime and inequality.* Stanford University Press, Stanford, CA, pp. 37-54.

Shaw, C., and McKay, H. (1969). *Juvenile Delinquency and Urban Areas, 2nd ed.*. University of Chicago Press, Chicago.

Siegfried, J. (1991). Black teens have low smoking rates. *J. Nat'l. Cancer Inst.* 83(24):1790-1791.

Singh, G. K., and Yu, S. M. (1995). Infant mortality in the United States: trends, differentials, and projections, 1950 through 2010. *Am. J. Public Health* 85(7):957-964.

Stack, C. (1974). *All our kin: Strategies for survival in a Black community.* Harper and Row, New York.

Swift, E. K. (2002). *Committee on Guidance for Designing a National Healthcare Disparities Report.* Institute of Medicine of the National Academies. The National Academies Press, Washington, D.C.

Institute of Medicine. (1999). Toward environmental justice: Research, education, and health policy needs. National Academy Press, Washington, D.C.

US Department of Commerce, Office of Federal Statistical Policy and Standards.(1978). *Race and Ethnic Standards for Federal Agencies and Administrative Reporting, Federal Statistical Policy Directive.* Report No. 15. US Government Printing Office, Washington, D.C.

Wallace, R. (1990). Urban desertification, public health and public order: "Planned shrinkage," violent death, substance abuse, and AIDS in the Bronx. *Soc. Sci. Med.* 31:801-813.

Wallace, R. (1991). Expanding coupled shock fronts of urban decay and criminal behavior: how U.S. cities are becoming "hollowed out". *J. Quantit. Crimin.* 7:333-356.

Whiteis, D. G. (1992). Hospital and community characteristics in closures of urban hospitals, 1987-87. *Public Health Rep.* 107:409-416.

Williams, D. R. (1998). African-American health: the role of the social environment. *J. Urban Health* 75(2):300-21.

Williams, D. R. (1999). Race, socioeconomic status, and health. The added effects of racism and discrimination. *Ann. N. Y. Acad. Sci.* 896:173-188.

Williams, D. R., and Collins, C. (1995). US Socioeconomic and Racial Differences in Health -Patterns and Explanations. *Ann. Rev. Soc.* 21:349-386.

Williams, D. R., and Collins, C. (2001). Racial residential segregation: a fundamental cause of racial disparities in health. *Public Health Rep.* 116(5):404–16.

Wilson, W. J. (1987). *The truly disadvantaged.* University of Chicago Press, Chicago.

Wilson, W. J. (1996). When work disappears: the world of the new urban poor. Alfred A. Knopf, New York.

Zanobetti, A., Schwartz, J., and Gold, D. (2000). Are there sensitive subgroups for the effects of airborne particles? *Environ. Health Persp.* 108(9):841-845.

Chapter 5

Sexual Minority Groups and Urban Health

Ruth Finkelstein and Julie Netherland

1.0. INTRODUCTION

No specific research describes either the effect of urban life on lesbian, gay, bisexual and transgender (LGBT) people or the effect of LGBT people on the overall health of cities. However, there is evidence that LGBT people live in cities in large numbers and are, in fact, clustered in many of the country's largest urban areas. Evidence also suggests (though the quality of the research leaves much to be desired) that specific health issues, including barriers to accessing care, particularly affect LGBT people. Furthermore, there is growing acknowledgement that LGBT make specific contributions to the life of cities that may impact the health of urban residents. This chapter begins with a review of the scant evidence that exists about the number, characteristics, and geographic dispersion of LGBT people, proceeds to discuss the effect of cities on LGBT health and their effect on the overall health of cities, summarizes the specific health issues affecting these populations, and proposes some basic strategies to address them.

2.0. DEMOGRAPHY OF LGBT PEOPLE

The nature, composition and size of the "gay community" have been the subject of much debate. Indeed, whether or not LGBT people constitute a community at all is often questioned. And if such a community exists, how ought it be defined? Is this a community that can be defined geographically or by its institutions and organizations? Or is this an "imagined" community that exists, not in any spatial location, but in the sense of a shared affinity and common purpose? (Woolwine, 2000) Are its members defined by claiming a LGBT identity or by engaging in same-sex behavior? Although the answers to these questions have important implications for urban public health, they remain unresolved. LGBT persons defy simple categorization, varying widely in sociodemographic characteristics, like racial and cultural background, income, age and place of residence. They also vary in their self-definition and level of affinity with other LGBT people. Furthermore, identity can change over time and "is neither static nor independent, but the result of a complex interplay between place, community and politics" (Kenney, 2001). Public health has often turned to behavioral definitions (e.g., men who have sex men or "MSM") to overcome the problems with defining groups by sexual orientation, but behavioral definitions mute the importance of identity and of LGBT cultures that thrive among a wide array of ethnic and racial groups (Meyer, 2001). Despite their differences and these definitional difficulties, LGBT people share experiences of living in a society that stigmatizes and discriminates against same-sex identity and behavior and transgressive gender expression. The social and institutional forces that sustain such stigma and discrimination are at the root of many of the health problems and health needs of this population. Cities play a key role in both intensifying and ameliorating the effects of these forces.

While LGBT people are difficult to classify and identify, what does seem clear is that they tend to cluster in large urban centers and, in some cases, have formed "gay ghettos" marked by high concentrations of LGBT people as well as social, cultural and political institutions that cater to them. The difficulty in finding and enumerating hidden or stigmatized populations is well known; nonetheless, several studies have suggested a strong association between urbanicity and gay identity (Bailey, 1999; Bradford, *et al.*, 2002; Gates and Ost, 2004; Kenney, 2001; Levay and Nonas, 1995). Throughout this chapter, the acronym we use to refer to sexual minorities changes. This is because the research on which we rely varies in how samples are defined and what groups are included. For example, almost all of the demographic research available is based on census reports of same-sex couples, and therefore, conclusions can only be drawn about gays and lesbians and those bisexuals who happen to be in a same-sex relationship. In general, "T" is excluded from this discussion, not because the issues of transgender people are any less important than those of other sexual minorities, but because of the dearth of research on transgender people. Unfortunately, bisexual people are also often excluded from research, though not to the same extent.

In 1990, when the U.S. census began collecting data on same-sex couples, 81% of same-sex couples resided in cities with populations over 700,000 versus 52% of the total U.S. population (Black, *et al.*, 2002). According to 2000 census data, though they live in 99% of all U.S. counties, same-sex couples had the highest probability of living in an urban area compared to both married and unmarried heterosexual couples. For example, same-sex couples were three times more likely to live in San Francisco and almost 50% more likely to live in New York or Los Angeles than other couples (Gates and Ost, 2004). In fact, five major metropolitan areas – New York, Los Angeles, San Francisco, Washington D.C., and Chicago – account for more than 25% of all same-sex couples but only 12% of the general population in the U.S. (Bradford, *et al.*, 2002). On average, same-sex couples tend to live in neighborhoods that are not only more urban, but also more racially and ethnically diverse, have higher crime rates, more foreign born people, and older housing stocks than neighborhoods where married heterosexual couples live (*The demographics of diversity: why cities are courting the gay and lesbian community*, 2003; Gates and Ost, 2004). In addition, same-sex couples are almost twice as likely as married couples to be of mixed race or ethnicity (Gates and Ost, 2004). Analyses of these data also show that, while both gay men and lesbians are more likely to live in metropolitan areas, they do not necessarily live in the same communities. Although gay and lesbian communities seem to overlap to a large degree, lesbians tend to be more broadly integrated into an array of neighborhoods (Bailey, 1999). Same-sex couples with children (whether gay or lesbian) tend to live in states and metropolitan areas with relatively low concentrations of same-sex couples but high concentrations of other families raising children (Gates and Ost, 2004).

Explanations as to why LGB people are drawn to cities vary widely. Some scholars root the urban nature of the LGB community in historical events, such as the discharge of gay soldiers in San Francisco following World War II (D'Emilio, 1989). Others have suggested that LGB people are drawn to areas with more favorable social and political climates. Indeed, disentangling cause from effect is difficult, yet 9 of the 12 states without a law prohibiting same-sex marriage and 11 of the 14 states that prohibit employment discrimination based on sexual orientation are also among the 20 states with the highest proportion of same-sex couples (Gates and Ost, 2004). Others have suggested that economic, not political, forces draw LGB people to cities, claiming that because same-sex couples tend to live in smaller housing units, they are able to afford housing in "high amenity" areas like cities (Black, *et al.*, 2002). More commonly, scholars have suggested that large concentrations of LGB people gather in urban communities in response to stigma and prejudice to form spaces in which they can safely express their sexual orientation and where LGB identities and relationships can be realized, acknowledge, and respected (Meyer, 2001). Cities offer support for the development and celebration of LGB identity as well as a degree of anonymity and a sense of safety (Kirkey and Forsyth, 2001; Silvestre, *et al.*, 2002). Clearly, cities also provide a critical mass of people needed to sustain social, cultural and political institutions that have become integral to LGBT life in many urban areas. Bars, bath houses, book stores, political action groups, and social service and health organizations have been born of and facilitate gay socialization and friendship networks (Green, 2002). "Gay ghettos," which tend to be predominantly white and male, are the most visible markers of gay urban life and have received the most attention, but cities also foster other forms of connectivity and community among a wide array of LGB people, including lesbians and LGB people of color (Lo and Healy, 2000). Whatever the reasons, the development of LGBT communities are clearly tied to urbanism. As Kenney explains:

> The social diversity, economic opportunity, and political exchange characteristic of modern American cities support both individual and collective growth, as well as the development of subcultures. Thus, the history of homosexuality and the development of the city in the U.S. are intertwined phenomena (2001).

Given the interdependence of urbanization and LGBT identity, understanding how urban environments shape the health of LGBT people (for good or ill) is critical.

3.0. HOW CITIES AFFECT LGBT HEALTH

Research has focused on understanding the health disparities among urban populations, though parsing out the ways in which urban life contributes to or ameliorates risk behavior and/or poor health outcomes of specific populations has proven complicated (e.g., House, *et al.*, 2000; Baquet, *et al.*, 2002; Schulz, *et al.*, 2002). We are aware of no studies that specifically address how urban characteristics affect the health of LGBT people. While most studies of LGBT health have used urban samples, they do not explore the effect of cities on health per se. Furthermore, although cities and neighborhoods vary tremendously in rates of risk behavior, health problems, and access to services, we know of no studies which map LGBT people in relation to these variables. Vlahov and Galea (2002) suggest three facets of urban life that affect health, which provide a useful framework for exploring how cities might affect LGBT health – social environment, physical environment, and the provision of health and social services. We will consider how each of these potentially affects the risk behavior, health, and access to services of urban LGBT populations. In addition, the population density of cities combined with the heterogeneity of LGBT people give rise to a number of special populations; we will briefly consider the unique health issues of some of these, including people of color, immigrants, youth, the elderly and transgender people.

3.1. Social Environment

Social environment refers to the cultural milieu, social norms and networks, and stressors that affect individual behavior and health. Many LGBT people are drawn to cities because of their perceived culture of tolerance, diversity and social acceptance (Valentine and Skelton, 2003). As will be further discussed below, some cities have actively recruited LGB tourists and residents, clearly signaling a level of tolerance and acceptance – at least by some government agencies (Rushbrook, 2002; Swope, 2003). Many cities have instituted laws and policies that either prohibit discrimination based on sexual orientation and/or recognize same-sex relationships. According to the Human Rights Campaign, 258 municipalities have passed anti-discrimination ordinances, and 130 cities have passed domestic partnerships laws (Human Rights Campaign). Although these laws have severe limitations, they do suggest that those who work and live in these cities may in fact have greater protection and more rights than their suburban and rural counterparts since few state and no federal laws protect LGBT individuals or couples. Domestic partnership laws directly affect the ability of LGBT people to access health insurance, while employment non-discrimination laws have been associated with higher income for some groups of LGB people (Gates, 2003). At the very least, such policies signal a level of acceptance and tolerance, which may help LGBT residents feel safe and supported, and could potentially impact their levels of stress and self-esteem.

Large urban areas also offer LGBT populations access to neighborhoods, cultural institutions and events that support and affirm their identity. "Gay ghettos," for example, provide spaces in which LGBT people can safely and openly express their sexual orientation. Because sexual orientation is so stigmatized and hidden elsewhere, such spaces are experienced by some LGBT people as profoundly liberating and supportive (Valentine and Skelton, 2003). Events, like Pride parades, and cultural institutions, like the Lesbian Herstory Archives in New York and LGBT newspapers, all contribute to a shared sense of community, history and identity. Dozens of cities have LGBT community centers that provide residents with an array of social services, cultural events, as well as a meeting place for groups. These centers offer both concrete assistance and as well as opportunities for LGBT people to meet and connect. On the one hand, feeling included and welcome in such spaces may well improve individuals' self-esteem and ameliorate feelings of isolation and internalized homophobia; on the other hand, feeling excluded (e.g., because of race, transgender experience appearance) may reinforce negative feelings. As Valentine and Skelton point out:

> the very notion of community tends to privilege the ideal of unity over difference . . . Communities are predicated on one identity that becomes a single rallying point to the exclusion of other aspects of participants' multiple identities. (Valentine and Skelton, 2003)

Clearly, for those who access them, these cultural institutions and events offer LGBT people greater opportunities to develop social networks than might be possible in rural settings. Because cities provide a critical mass of LGBT as well as opportunities for LGBT people to identify one another, they facilitate a greater choice of peers and romantic partners. For instance, almost 150 social and political groups use the LGBT Community Services Center in New York.

Urban social networks may provide support with potentially significant health benefits (Kimmel, *et al.*, 1998; Latkin, *et al.*, 2003; McCarthy, 2000). Given the rejection and stigma that many LGBT people face, their social networks may be particularly important sources of affirmation and support (Valentine and Skelton, 2003). Many, though certainly not all, LGBT people are estranged from their biological families, and some research suggests that GL couples perceive they have more support from their friends than from their family members (Turner, *et al.*, 1993). In one study of young people entering an urban LGB social "scene," participants described forming social connections that acted as substitutes for family relationships (Valentine and Skelton, 2003). The importance of peer networks became especially clear when friendship networks and voluntary organizations provided daily care to thousands of men living with and dying from AIDS. The social networks of gay men have also been used to disseminate HIV prevention campaigns (Kelly, *et al.*, 1992; Ross and Williams, 2002) and to reinforce norms supporting safer sex (Kelly, *et al.*, 1991). Although social networks clearly play an important role in shaping the health risk and behavior of LGBT people, studies suggest the level of attachment to gay community networks varies by race, ethnicity, and gender (Mills, *et al.*, 2001; O'Donnell, *et al.*, 2002; Valentine and Skelton, 2003).

Furthermore, social networks in any population can be a double-edged sword (Leviton, *et al.*, 2000); LGBT social networks are no exception. For example, even though many gay male social networks support safer sex, these same networks introduce men to potential partners, including HIV-infected men (O'Donnell, *et al.*, 2002). Urban centers, like New York and Los Angeles, have long been the leading edge of the HIV-epidemic, and the higher HIV-prevalence rates in urban areas increase the risk of transmission among members of those sexual networks. Similarly, the recent increase in STIs among MSM in urban centers is certainly facilitated by sexual networks of men in those cities (CDC, 1997; 1999a; 1999b; 2001a; 2002b). Networks of men in internet chat rooms, which allow men in large cities to easily find one another, have also been linked to STI transmission (Klausner, *et al.*, 2000). Some evidence suggests that these urban social networks may be especially risky for young people. Valentine and Skelton (2003) found that young people, especially those with low self-esteem or feelings of internalized homophobia, had difficulty resisting the sexual advances of older adults and often felt coerced into having sex they did not want. Furthermore, because a large portion of the "scene" focuses on bars and clubs (particularly for gay men), the social connections that form there may reinforce unhealthy drinking and/or drug use (Valentine and Skelton, 2003).

In addition to the risks posed by social networks, urban LGBT people face other stressors. One such stressor is the history of the HIV epidemic in the LGBT community, particularly in urban areas. Many LGBT people witnessed large numbers of friends and lovers suffer and die from AIDS during a time when medical treatments were few and government and social support for people living with AIDS was minimal. These experiences of care-giving and grief, which continue today, add to the overall experiences of stress and distress LGBT people face (Gluhoski, *et al.*, 1997; Morin, *et al.*, 1984; Turner and Catania, 1997). The heightened risk of HIV in urban areas and the constant vigilance that is required to prevent transmission maybe also experienced as stressful by some MSM (McKirnan, *et al.*, 1996).

While cities may offer more social support and institutional protections than other regions, experiences of prejudice, stigma, and violence continue impact urban LGBT people's health and access to health care. In fact, the very visibility of LGBT life in cities may aid perpetrators in identifying victims. Being in a "gay" neighborhood or going to a gay-identified venue, for instance, can make one a target of anti-gay violence (Valentine and Skelton, 2003). One recent study of young urban gay and bisexual men found that those who were more open about disclosing their sexual orientation experienced more anti-gay violence (Huebner, *et al.*, 2004). Transgender people and street youth may be at particular risk for violence and harassment, including from law enforcement (Dean, *et al.*, 2000). Criminal incidents and other sorts of emergencies may be exacerbated by the history of adversarial relationships between the LGBT community and the police. LGBT people may be reluctant to involve the authorities (e.g., in a case of same-sex domestic violence), and law enforcement and emergency responders may be slow to respond and/or respond inappropriately to LGBT victims.

3.2. Physical Environment

Researchers are increasingly acknowledging that, like the social environment, features of the physical environment are predictive of and may account for some of the variation in health outcomes in urban areas (Hancock, 2002; Northridge, *et al.*, 2003; Perdue, *et al.*, 2003; Schulz, *et al.*, 2000; Weich, *et al.*, 2002). Although contextual factors (like air pollution, fewer services, lack of safe places to relax and exercise, greater physical deterioration) are difficult to disentangle from individual factors (like socioeconomic status and health behavior), they appear to contribute to the unfavorable health outcomes in poor neighborhoods (Acevedo-Garcia, *et al.*, 2003; Cohen, *et al.*, 2000; Leventhal and Brooks-Gunn, 2003; Reijneveld, 2002). In many cities, residential segregation by race means that people of color bear the brunt of the health effects of residing in neighborhoods with harmful physical environments. The health of LGBT people who are poor, particularly people of color, is surely impacted by these physical spaces. Evidence, though limited, suggests that LGBT people on average are poorer than their heterosexual counterparts (Badgett, 1998). A study of 40 metropolitan areas with high gay and lesbian residential concentrations showed a slightly negative relationship between same-sex couples and household income, except in Los Angeles, Manhattan and Atlanta (Cahill, *et al.*, undated). Furthermore, the over-representation of urban same-sex couples in neighborhoods that are more ethnically/racially diverse, have higher rates of crime, and have older housing stock (Gates and Ost, 2004) may indicate that LGB people tend to settle in neighborhoods with less salutary physical environments. A growing body of research has documented the role of LGB people as urban pioneers who move into deserted or dilapidated areas (Florida, 2002; Simon, 2002). The impact of these settlement patterns on LGB health is unknown, but research increasingly suggests that urban physical environments can have deleterious health effects (Ambrose, 2001; Cohen, *et al.*, 2003; Cummins and Jackson, 2001; Krieger, *et al.*, 2000; Lawrence, 1999; Satterthwaite, 1993). Living in older, unrenovated buildings, for example, is associated with a higher prevalence of asthma (Krieger and Higgins, 2002).

3.3. Provision of Health and Social Services

While cities generally offer a wide array of medical and social services, populations that face barriers to care, including LGBT people, tend to be concentrated in cities. For instance, people of lower economic status, immigrants and minorities are less likely to have health insurance and face significant impediments to receiving high quality care (Menlo Park: Kaiser Family Foundation, 2003; National healthcare disparities report, 2004). In poor neighborhoods, particularly, service systems may be over-burdened and under-resourced (Campbell, *et al.*, 1993; Gallagher, *et al.*, 1995). Urban LGBT people who are people of color, immigrants and/or poor may face significant impediments to accessing and staying engaged in quality healthcare services. Barriers to care specific to LGBT people are discussed further below.

Despite these short-comings, cities have also afforded some LGBT communities the resources and opportunity to develop specialized services to specifically address their unique healthcare needs. Several cities now have community health clinics staffed with providers who are themselves LGBT or LGBT-sensitive and trained to ask about and address LGBT health concerns. Generally, these clinics are situated in neighborhoods where large numbers of LGBT live but serve LGBT people throughout the metropolitan area. Other LGBT-specific services (e.g., drug treatment, self-help groups, group therapy, health promotion campaigns, HIV prevention and treatment services) are also available in large cities. Although these services are tremendous resources to LGBT urban residents, they cannot serve nor do they meet the needs of all LGBT people. For instance, people who do not embrace a gay or lesbian identity may not feel comfortable going to agencies designated as such. People who reside at a distance from LGBT services may want to receive care in their own neighborhoods. And racial/ethnic minorities may feel that such services cannot address their needs in a culturally competent manner.

4.0. SPECIAL POPULATIONS OF URBAN LGBT PEOPLE

In addition to a city's social environment, physical environment, and provision of health services, the composition, diversity and density of urban populations also play a role in the health of urban LGBT residents because they include sub-populations of LGBT people facing special health needs or barriers to care. For instance, census data suggest that individuals in same-sex couples are as racially diverse as the general U.S. population (Rubenstein, *et al.*, 2003), and more than a quarter of the same-sex couples counted in the last census included a racial or ethnic minority. These couples tend to live in urban areas with large minority communities and in areas with large LG populations (Gates and Ost, 2004). Indeed, many cities have large, vibrant LGBT communities of color. In addition to being subject to health disparities associated with race, LGBT people of color must navigate multiple identities and communities and/or contend with compound layers of stigma and prejudice. Although research in this area is extremely limited, some evidence indicates that homophobia, racism, and poverty interact to compound health problems – particularly psychological distress – and health risks (Diaz and Ayala, 2001; Diaz, *et al.*, 2001; Office of Gay and Lesbian Health, 1999). In addition, an analysis of data from the National Lesbian Health Care Survey established that, within a national sample of lesbians, blacks were more likely to be uninsured than white respondents (Dean, *et al.*, 2000). In one of the most researched areas of LGBT health – HIV – the racial/ethnic disparities are profound. In a study of young MSM from 7 cities, HIV prevalence was 7% among whites, 14% among latinos, and 32% among blacks (CDC, 2001). Anti-gay prejudice may prevent communities of color from dealing effectively with HIV among MSM, while racism may prevent the LGBT community from effectively addressing the needs of people of color (Office of Gay and Lesbian Health, 1999).

Immigrants, many of whom first settle in urban areas, also face unique challenges that affect their health. While no accurate estimates of the number of LGBT immigrants in the U.S. exist, service providers have long asserted that significant numbers of LGBT people from countries less accepting of homosexuality and other gender differences strive to immigrate to the U.S. They may be barred from obtaining legal employment as well as many benefits and services. Furthermore, immigration law generally prohibits people who are HIV-infected from becoming permanent residents, citizens or otherwise upgrading their immigration status (Office of Gay and Lesbian Health, 1999). Unlike heterosexuals, LGB immigrants are barred from gaining the rights and benefits of citizenship through marrying their partner. Language barriers pose additional difficulties for immigrants. Individuals, particularly those reliant on a family or community member for interpretation, may be unwilling to disclose important health information, especially for issues that are highly stigmatized, like sexual orientation, STI risk, substance use or mental health. Those who go outside their ethnic community for care can confront lack of cultural understanding, including misunderstandings about the meanings of diagnoses and prescribed regimens (Office of Gay and Lesbian Health, 1999).

In addition to race and immigration status, the age of urban LGBT people may impact the incidence of health problems as well as their access to health care. LGBT youth leave home more often than their heterosexual peers and make up a disproportionate percentage of the homeless youth population (Cochran, *et al.*, 2002). Many of these young people are drawn to cities for the same reasons as LGBT adults. Regardless of where they live, LGBT youth face a number of challenges, including a host of elevated risk behaviors. Population-based studies of high school students have shown that LGB youth are more likely to report attempted suicide; use tobacco, alcohol, and cocaine; share syringes; and have multiple sexual partners in the past three months (Goodenow, *et al.*, 2002; Robin, *et al.*, 2002). Despite their vulnerability to health problems, LGBT young people who are estranged from the families face legal barriers to receiving benefits and health care (Office of Gay and Lesbian Health, 1999). Not under the supervision of either their families or the foster care system, street youth must find some way of establishing their status as emancipated minors and then navigate the complicated world of public benefits. Physicians may be reluctant to treat minors without parental consent or be unfamiliar with the laws governing adolescents' rights to seek health care on their own.

Although less is known about their health care needs, like youth, elder LGBT people face unique barriers to receiving quality care. Nearly one in five people in a same-sex couple is at least 55 years old (Gates and Ost, 2004), and estimates of the number of LGBT people over 65 range from one to three million (Cahill, *et al.*, undated). This number will surely increase as the baby boomer generation continues to age. Isolation and lack of mobility are problems for all seniors, and LGBT seniors, particularly those who have migrated to cities, may be without the traditional support of family and community (Office of Gay and Lesbian Health, 1999). One study of LGB seniors in New York City found that 65% were living alone compared to 36% of New York's general senior population (*Assistive housing needs for elderly gays and lesbians in New York City*, 1999). In addition to social isolation, institutional barriers, which will be discussed below, make LGB seniors particularly vulnerable to inadequate insurance and poverty.

We know of no research documenting the migration of transgender people to cities, but anecdotal evidence suggests the transgender people are drawn to urban areas for many of the same reasons as LGB people, including to build community institutions and foster social support and acceptance. Little information about the health issues and health risks of transgender people exists. Dean et al have reviewed and summarized the available health-related research on transgender issues (2000). As with LGB populations, many of the health problems of transgender people are thought to result from the prejudice, discrimination, and other culturally-based stressors (Dean, *et al.*, 2000). Transgender people face extraordinarily high rates of victimization, including sexual assault and harassment (Dean, *et al.*, 2000). Studies on the mental health issues facing transgender people suggest difficulties similar to other groups facing significant discrimination, including adjustment disorders, anxiety, post-traumatic stress and depression (Dean, *et al.*, 2000). A few studies, which have focused on sex workers, have found increased rates of HIV and other STIs among transgender sex workers compared to female sex workers (Dean, *et al.*, 2000). One such study found that 35% of transgender sex workers were HIV-positive (Clements-Nolle, *et al.*, 2001); another study of sex workers in Atlanta revealed that 68% were HIV-positive (Elifson, *et al.*, 1993); and a recent study of transgender people of color (not exclusively sex workers) in San Francisco found HIV seroprevalence rates ranging from 13% among Asian Pacific Islanders to 41% among blacks (Nemoto, *et al.*, 2004). Evidence also suggests higher rates of HIV-related risk behavior (Dean, *et al.*, 2000; Nemoto, *et al.*, 2004) and drug use among transgender people (Dean, *et al.*, 2000).

Despite these evident preventative and treatment-related health needs, pervasive prejudice against transgender individuals in American society and in medicine poses significant barriers to care (Dean, *et al.*, 2000). Studies have shown that transgender people underutilize medical and social services and may resort to self-medication or, in the case of hormones, black market medication (Dean, *et al.*, 2000). Discrimination also contributes to their social and economic marginalization, including unemployment or underemployment. This, in turn, contributes to high rates of uninsured transgender people (Dean, *et al.*, 2000). Although gender identity remains a psychiatric diagnosis in the *Diagnostic and Statistical Manual of Mental Disorders IV*, transgender individuals are explicitly excluded from the American with Disabilities Act and, therefore, do not receive its protections or benefits. Only a handful of jurisdictions prohibit discrimination based on gender identity or expression. Medicaid and many private insurers generally refuse to cover sex reassignment surgery.

Overall, sexual and gender orientation is just one dimension of identity for urban inhabitants. While these dimensions of identity may enhance specific health risks, issues and opportunities, these effects are strongly mediated by other dimensions of identity, including race, class, gender and age. The relationship between these various urban identities and populations and health is dynamic. Just as cities shape the health of LGBT people, LGBT people have shaped the health of cities.

5.0. HOW LGBT POPULATIONS AFFECT THE OVERALL HEALTH OF CITIES

The in- and out-migration of various populations is one element of urbanization likely to shape the health risks and healthcare response of cities (Vlahov and Galea, 2002). Therefore, how populations of LGBT people affect the health of cities in both negative and positive ways merits consideration, and we will begin by addressing the issues of communicable diseases, particularly HIV.

One of the major impediments to early recognition and coherent action to address the emerging epidemic of HIV was the lethal combination of homophobia and the fear of a homophobic response. The role of homophobia in shaping the response to AIDS (particularly within agencies of the federal government in the early 1980's) has been discussed exhaustively (Altman, 1987; Patton, 1990; Shilts, 1987). However, less clearly explicated is the role that fear of a homophobic response played in muting and shaping aspects of the gay community response and consequent policy framework for the epidemic. The dominant theme influencing policy issues early in the epidemic was fear of identification, blame and discrimination. The saliency of the need to protect confidentiality, enactment of anti-discrimination protections, and hesitancy regarding traditional methods of case finding and reporting were born out of the unquestioned expectation of a homophobic response if one were identified as gay or lesbian. Over time, AIDS itself became stigmatized (not, of course, unrelated to its association with the stigmatized identities of homosexual or drug user), but initial fears were of personal identification as homosexual and of further discrimination against the community.

Therefore, while it is the case that HIV infection was first identified in urban gay men in this country and has subsequently spread through sexual and blood-borne transmission beyond that population, it as also the case that the epidemic may not have become as widespread in this country had prevention and intervention efforts not been constrained by homophobia and the anticipation of homophobia. Similarly, current concerns about HIV transmission from men on the "down low" (men whose publicly identify as straight, but have sex with other men) can simultaneously be viewed as negative health consequences accruing to others via same-sex sexual activity or as negative health consequences resulting from the hidden nature of same-sex sexual activity in a society that deems such behavior unacceptable.

Despite its limitations, the response of urban LGBT population to AIDS had many positive effects, particularly in modeling new methods of healthcare activism, patient empowerment, and community-based healthcare delivery and financing paradigms. Groups, like ACT-UP, are widely credited for drawing attention to HIV/AIDS and prodding a reluctant government into action (Hunter, 1998). Using direct action tactics, including civil disobedience, they made explicit the politics behind funding for research and treatment, linking societal homophobia to the government's lack of response. Their impact on public policy has been considerable; they have: 1) forced the FDA to accelerate drug trials for AIDS; 2) successfully lobbied pharmaceutical companies to reduce drug prices; 3) publicized pharmaceutical company profits; 4) demanded redefinition of AIDS to include more women and ensure that women with AIDS received disability benefits and were included in drug trials; and 5) established some of the first needle exchange programs.

The very word "PWA" (Person Living with AIDS), now modified to "PLWH" (Person Living with HIV) is itself definitional of a different empowered relationship between the "patient" and the "disease" (Navarre, 1988). This concept and the organization of PWA's into groups, like the National Association of People with AIDS, represent a fundamental restructuring of the power relationship between patients, providers, and policy-makers.

Similarly, the voluntary AIDS service organizations, like the Gay Men's Health Crisis, the San Francisco AIDS Foundation, Health Education Resource Organization (HERO) in Baltimore, and the Whitman Walker Clinic, that sprang up in major urban centers in the early 1980's represent an indigenous response to crisis. Though later funded by the government and private foundations and staffed by professionals, these organizations were originally volunteer-driven, community-led, grass roots responses funded and resourced by individuals and local businesses. This volunteer response transformed into a service sector that then advocated for and received significant federal resources, largely through the Ryan White CARE Act. This Act, the largest disease-specific categorical federal funding for services, has numerous unusual provisions, including mandated community participation in planning and allocation decisions. All of these innovations, activism, patient empowerment, advocacy, volunteerism and community planning, have shaped policy and programmatic responses to health issues from breast cancer to diabetes.

The impact of LGBT people on the health of cities extends beyond their response to the HIV epidemic. A growing body of research indicates that LGBT populations positively affect the infrastructure, social climate, cultural life, and economies of cities (*The demographics of diversity: why cities are courting the gay and lesbian community*, 2003; Florida, 2002; Lee, 2002; Rushbrook, 2002; Swope, 2003). Improvements in these arenas may, in turn, contribute to improved health and healthcare. Analyses of the census data affirm that LGB people play a role as urban pioneers on the vanguard of urban renewal (Gates and Ost, 2004). Same-sex couples appear more likely than heterosexual couples to move into "riskier" neighborhood in return for a potentially larger payoff on their financial investments (*The demographics of diversity: why cities are courting the gay and lesbian community*, 2003). Although LGB couples do not have greater income than married couples, those attracted to urban areas are less likely to have children, and, therefore, have more income to invest in improving housing (*The demographics of diversity: why cities are courting the gay and lesbian community*, 2003). These investments not only advance property values but also result in increased taxes to cities without a corresponding demand for public school services (*The demographics of diversity: why cities are courting the gay and lesbian community*, 2003). Indeed, LGB people have been credited with revitalizing a number of urban neighborhoods (Lee, 2002; Rich, 2004). To the extent that LGBT populations improve the housing stock, living conditions and services in a neighborhood, they likely enhance the health of its residents. Although the restoration of neighborhoods is generally seen as benefiting cities and their residents, the rising housing costs that accompany such changes may displace poor families forcing them into worse living conditions. More research is needed to explore the long-term benefit and harm of these urban renewals.

In addition to being credited with revitalizing residential areas, LGBT urban populations are seen by some as a marker of a tolerant social climate, cultural creativity and cosmopolitanism (*The demographics of diversity: why cities are courting the gay and lesbian community*, 2003; Rushbrook, 2002). Social tolerance and acceptance of diversity have been linked to both the perception of an enhanced quality of life (Rushbrook, 2002) and to urban economic vitality (Swope, 2003). Richard Florida has argued that a strong and vibrant LGBT community is an indicator that a city is open to many different kinds of people (Florida, 2002, 2004). Though not empirically documented, LGBT people are also credited with enhancing the cultural life of cities through their involvement in theater, music, and fine arts. These features of city life – diversity, tolerance and culture – in turn, attract the "creative class" and fuel economic growth in the high-tech sector (Florida, 2004). Florida (2002) demonstrated a correlation between areas experiencing economic growth in the technology sector and high concentrations of LGB people. This reasoning has been accepted by several cities and companies that are now actively seeking to attract LGBT residents and workers (*The demographics of diversity: why cities are courting the gay and lesbian community*, 2003; Swope, 2003). Cincinnati-based Proctor and Gamble, for instance, has criticized the city for passing an anti-gay employment discrimination law because they feel the law detracts from the company's ability to recruit LGBT people and their allies (Swope, 2003). As manufacturing jobs continue to decline, cities are scrambling to attract the "creative class," including gays:

> The most striking new development is the growing number of blue collar cities never considered especially friendly to gays that are passing gay-rights laws anyway. They seem to be saying that if gays need cities, then cities need gays. (Swope, 2003)

The tolerance, diversity and economic growth that LGBT people are credited with enhancing in cities are likely to improve the welfare and health of minority groups in particular and city residents generally.

6.0. HEALTH ISSUES AFFECTING LGBT POPULATIONS

Almost no public health research has examined the differences in risk behavior or health outcomes between urban and suburban/rural LGBT populations. Furthermore, few studies explore the interaction between sexual orientation, sexual behavior, gender identity and membership in other groups at higher risk for morbidity and mortality (e.g., being a racial minority or belonging to a low income group). Nonetheless, a growing body of research has made clear that LGBT people are disproportionately affected by a number of health problems. This literature has been well summarized elsewhere (Dean, *et al.*, 2000), and a comprehensive review of these issues is beyond the scope of this chapter. However, knowledge and understanding of these health issues, which are certainly more concentrated in cities with large LGBT populations, are critical for planning effective urban health strategies and interventions. Some LGBT health problems are the result of unique exposures to risks related to sexual behavior, but many appear to be related to social conditions characterized by prejudice, stigmatization and discrimination (Meyer, 2001).

Of those health problems related directly to sexual behavior, HIV is currently the one most closely identified with the gay community, though it was foreshadowed by hepatitis B. The clinical and epidemiological evidence that hepatitis B was prevalent among gay men resulted in landmark hepatitis B vaccine trials in New York City in the late 70's and early 80's (Dienstag, *et al.*, 1982; Stevens and Taylor, 1986; Szmuness, *et al.*, 1980; Szmuness, *et al.*, 1981). Ironically, an epidemiological study tracking the incidence of gay hepatitis B among gay men in three gay urban areas (San Francisco, New York, and Amsterdam) provided some of the earliest evidence about the emergence and progression of HIV (Hessol, *et al.*, 1994; Van Griensven, *et al.*, 1993). HIV has profoundly affected the LGBT community, both in terms of the unprecedented loss of community members and in terms of the community mobilization and institution-building it engendered. Despite advances in treatment and a broad-based change in community norms governing sexual behavior, HIV remains a serious threat to the health of men who have sex with men. Almost 60% of all cases of HIV among men are due to exposure through sex with other men (CDC, 2003). In addition to HIV, men who have sex with men are at increased risk for other sexually transmitted infections (STIs), including viral hepatitis (Dean, *et al.*, 2000; Schreeder, *et al.*, 1982). Some communities, in fact, are reporting recent increases incidence of other STIs among MSM (CDC, 1997; 1999a; 1999b; 2001; 2001a; 2002b). The impact of HIV and other STIs on lesbians and bisexual women remains under-researched, although most studies suggest a higher HIV seroprevalance among women who have sex with women compared to heterosexual women (Office on Women's Health, 2000). While female-to-female transmission of HIV is a biological possibility, transmission is more likely a result of injecting drug use and/or sex with men (Young, *et al.*, 1992). HPV, bacterial vaginosis and candidiasis do occur in lesbians and can be transmitted between women; in general, however, lesbians appear to be at less risk for STIs than any other sexually active group (Dean, *et al.*, 2000).

Some preliminary studies have suggested that gay men and lesbians may be at increased risk for certain types of cancer (Dean, *et al.*, 2000), though the reasons for these elevated risks are generally due to variables other than sexual behavior. For instance, the higher incidence of breast cancer among lesbians is likely attributable to increased rates of obesity, alcohol consumption, nulliparity and smoking and lower rates of breast cancer screening, gynecological care, and hormone exposure through oral contraceptives (Dean, *et al.*, 2000; Office on Women's Health, 2000). Lesbians are also less likely than heterosexual women to have a Pap test (Aaron, *et al.*, 2001), although no studies have documented higher rates of cervical cancer. Studies have found higher rates of Kaposi's sarcoma, non-Hodgkins lymphoma, Hodgkin's disease, and anal cancer among gay men, but all of these, except anal cancer, have been attributed to increased incidence of HIV/AIDS (Dean, *et al.*, 2000; Hessol, *et al.*, 1992; Katz, *et al.*, 1994; Koblin, *et al.*, 1996; Lifson, *et al.*, 1990).

A number of the unique health problems facing LGBT people are related to anti-gay social and cultural forces. Anti-gay violence is perhaps the clearest example. Data on the prevalence of anti-gay hate crimes are scarce, but one report examining hate crimes generally concluded that lesbians and gay men are probably the most frequent victims (Finn and McNeil, 1987). The latest report by the National Coalition of Anti-Violence Programs, which reports hate crimes from 11 cities, shows a continuing rise of hate crimes against LGBT people (Patton, 2004), and a recent study of young urban gay and bisexual men found that 37% had experienced anti-gay verbal harassment and 4.8% reported physical violence in the past six months (Huebner, *et al.*, 2004). Obtaining accurate numbers of hate-motivated violence is complicated by the reluctance of many LGBT people to report incidents and/or disclose their sexual orientation to the police – a reluctance based on a history of police harassment and violence towards LGBT people. One review article concluded that between 16-30% of LGBT hate-crime victims has been victimized by the police (Berrill, 1992).

Intimate partner violence and sexual assault are also health concerns for LGBT people (Burke and Follingstad, 1999). Although empirical evidence is limited, one probability sample of urban MSM found that 22% had experienced physical abuse (Greenwood, *et al.*, 2002), while studies of lesbians have found rates slightly lower than those found for heterosexual women (Dean, *et al.*, 2000). Lifetime prevalence of attempted and completed rape among lesbians is comparable to that among heterosexual women, but gay men appear to be at elevated risk for sexual abuse and assault (Dean, *et al.*, 2000). Fears about homophobic reactions and laws and service systems that presume heterosexuality make it especially difficult for LGBT victims to seek legal assistance, medical treatment, emergency shelter, and support services (Dean, *et al.*, 2000). Clearly, hate crimes and experiences of intimate partner violence and/or sexual assault are likely to place individuals at greater risk for HIV and other STIs as well as impact their emotional and mental health.

Sexual orientation is not intrinsically linked to mental health problems; however, stigma, homophobia, and prejudice may negatively impact the mental health of LGBT individuals (Meyer, 2003). Furthermore, estrangement from family members, adjusting to a LGBT identity, lack of support for relationships and families may be additional stressors. Unfortunately, population-based estimates of prevalence of mental disorders among LGBT people are lacking (Dean, *et al.*, 2000). The few probability based studies that have been done found higher rates of depression, panic attacks syndrome, and psychological distress among MSM (Cochran and Mays, 2000; Cochran, *et al.*, 2003; Mills, *et al.*, 2004), especially among those who had experienced anti-gay harassment (Mills, *et al.*, 2004). Lesbian and bisexual women appear to have higher prevalence of general anxiety disorder compared to heterosexual women (Cochran, *et al.*, 2003). HIV (Bing, *et al.*, 2001; Dickey, *et al.*, 1999) as well as the stress of caring for and losing loved ones to HIV (Sikkema, *et al.*, 2003) have been associated with depressive symptoms and other mental health problems. Others studies found that sexual orientation is a significant predictor of eating disorders among men, though not among women (Dean, *et al.*, 2000). Finally, researchers have found elevated rates of suicidal ideation and attempts, but not completed suicides, among LGB people (Dean, *et al.*, 2000; Matthews, *et al.*, 2002).

In a review of the literature, the Center for Substance Abuse Treatment concluded that "gay men and lesbians were heavier substance and alcohol users than the general populations" (Center for Substance Abuse Treatment, 2001). Although many studies conducted in the past were perceived as biased because they recruited subjects from clubs and bars, some studies with less problematic samples support the finding that LGB people use drugs at higher rates than heterosexuals (Cochran and Mays, 2000; Stall, *et al.*, 2001; Stall and Wiley, 1988; Woody, *et al.*, 2001). A number of studies have also suggested that both gay men and lesbians use tobacco at much higher rates than the national average (Dean, *et al.*, 2000; Office on Women's Health, 2000). Increased rates of substance use adversely impact the health of LGBT people in myriad ways, including interactions with HIV medications and increasing rates of unsafe sexual behavior (Center for Substance Abuse Treatment, 2001; Dean, *et al.*, 2000).

7.0. BARRIERS TO HEALTH CARE

Many of the health problems that affect LGBT people disproportionately result from or are exacerbated by prejudice, discrimination and stigma (Brotman, *et al.*, 2002; Cahill, *et al.*, 2002; Dean, *et al.*, 2000; Diaz and Ayala, 2001; Meyer, 2001). In addition, such forces clearly play a role in LGBT people's willingness and ability to access health services as well as the quality of services they receive. These impediments can be rooted in the biases of providers, institutionalized in agency policies and state and federal laws, and manifest in the attitudes or behaviors of individual LGBT people who internalized the societal stigma and homophobia directed at them. Historically, the relationship between LGBT people and the medical profession has been an uneasy one. With the classification of homosexuality and transgressive gender identity/expression as pathological psychiatric disorders, medicine has been in the position of asserting social control over the lives of many LGBT people (Brotman, *et al.*, 2002). The perceived failure of government and community leaders to respond promptly to the AIDS crisis as well as sex-phobic nature of some HIV prevention campaigns exacerbated feeling of mistrust. In addition, in reviewing the literature, Dean et al concluded that LGBT people are subject to discrimination and bias in medical encounters, are likely to receive substandard care, and face significant obstacles in communicating with healthcare providers (2000). Other evidence suggests a range of provider attitudes from overt hostility (Douglas, *et al.*, 1985; Hayward and Weissfeld, 1993) and discomfort (Mathews, *et al.*, 1986) to simply not being sensitive to or knowledgeable about the particular health needs of LGBT people (Lena, *et al.*, 2002; McNair, 2000; McNair, 2003; Smith, *et al.*, 1985; Westerstahl, *et al.*, 2002).

These difficulties are further compounded by the reality that, due to fear and mistrust, many LGBT people delay seeking care, do not disclose their sexual orientation to providers, and/or may hide clinical conditions that might reveal their sexual orientation (Brotman, *et al.*, 2002; Dean, *et al.*, 2000). Intake and screening forms and institutional policies usually presume heterosexuality and normative gender expression (i.e., male or female) and provide little opportunity for the routine disclosure of alternate sexualities and gender identities. Providers who rely on stereotypes about LGBT people or assume patients are heterosexual may misdiagnose patients and/or miss important opportunities to educate patients about health risks.

Systemic barriers to healthcare for LGBT people extend far beyond the attitudes of providers or the policies of individual institutions. LGBT people also face financial and structural barriers that severely impede their ability to access high quality preventive and clinical services. Only 15 states prohibit employment discrimination based on sexual orientation and only four states prohibit discrimination based on gender identity, leaving LGBT people vulnerable to employment discrimination (*The demographics of diversity: why cities are courting the gay and lesbian community*, 2003; Gates, 2003). Furthermore, LGBT workers are at a disadvantage because many employers and insurance companies deny spousal benefits, like health insurance, to unmarried partners. Even when such benefits are offered, same-sex couples must pay tax on them, while married couples do not. In addition to having lower incomes, LGB people are more likely to be uninsured or underinsured than their heterosexual counterparts (Dean, *et al.*, 2000; Cahill, *et al.*, undated).

A number of other benefits are unavailable to same-sex couples because the federal government does not recognize their relationships. For instance, Medicaid regulations permit married couples to retain a jointly owned house without jeopardizing the other's right to Medicaid coverage, and married couples receive a spouse's Social Security benefits following his or her death. Wrongful death claims and pensions may also be unavailable to same-sex partners, and a partner's retirement benefits, if they can be claimed at all, are taxed. The Family Medical Leave Act expressly defines "family" to exclude same-sex couples hindering the ability of LGB people to care for their partners, children and other family members. The lack of recognition of same-sex partnerships poses myriad other problems, from denial of hospital visitation and medical decision-making rights to prohibiting partners from being placed in the same nursing home. Such institutional discrimination leaves LGBT seniors particularly vulnerable. Unfortunately, there are very few LGBT-specific elder services to which they can turn.

Both individual attitudes and institutional forms of discrimination contribute to a social environment that reinforces stigma against LGBT people. The stress of living with societal anti-gay attitudes and institutional discrimination as well as internalized homophobia directly impact the risk behavior and health of LGBT people (Brotman, *et al.*, 2002; Dean, *et al.*, 2000; Diaz and Ayala, 2001; Meyer, 2001). Cities, for all that they offer LGBT people, must go further in addressing barriers to care and in promoting environments which nurture and support the health of LGBT people.

8.0. POTENTIAL STRATEGIES FOR IMPROVING THE HEALTH OF SEXUAL MINORITIES GROUPS IN THE CITY

The dominant strategy adopted to improve the access of LGBT people to appropriate, non-homophobic health care has been the creation and expansion of LBGT clinics. These clinics began as special sessions (principally treating STI's) within LGBT community centers or at free or community health clinics. Over time the combination of HIV/AIDS funding and other third party reimbursement (public and private) for health services have caused these clinics to separate from (and in many cases eclipse in size) their home institutions. The largest LGBT health clinics – including Callen Lorde in New York City, Chase Brexton in Baltimore, Fenway in Boston, Howard Brown in Chicago, and the Los Angeles Gay & Lesbian Community Service Center – serve thousands of patients annually and provide services ranging from primary care and family planning to mental health and substance abuse counseling. A second, related strategy has been the development of LGBT-orientated specialty clinics – largely for HIV care and substance abuse treatment. These specialized settings are a haven for many urban LGBT people; administrative systems, institutional policies, assessments, and providers are attuned to and take into consideration the family structures and special health care needs of LGBT people.

There are, however, major limitations to the specialized clinic strategy. The first is a challenge shared by other community health centers – access may be limited for people without private insurance. To serve people covered by Medicaid (just one subset of people without private insurance) requires extensive state certification, an administrative barrier to these relatively grass roots institutions. For those who surmount it, they enter the world of inadequate reimbursement common to other providers of poverty healthcare. Thus, a trade-off exists between access for all and financial viability. The second challenge to the LGBT clinic model is that such clinics are typically centered in and largely staffed by members of the dominant gay community, which is generally white and middle class. Members of other communities express discomfort having to select among their identities in order to receive LGBT-sensitive services.

Similarly, LGBT clinics may lack appropriate services or be uncomfortable for elders. In general, the "gay culture" remains very youth oriented despite the aging of the first post Stonewall generation and the impending old age of the baby boomers. A related, but distinct problem, with using LGBT clinics to solve all health care access and quality problems for LGBT people is the need to make referrals for specialty services. With the exception of some HIV, mental health, and substance abuse services, all other specialty care must be referred out. Lastly, LGBT clinics require a critical population mass to survive, and many LGBT people live in mid-sized cities unable to sustain them.

One solution to these interlocking problems is to enhance the skills, training, and attitudes of all health care providers about LGBT health needs and issues rather than isolate care into a few specific settings. Especially for practitioners planning to practice in major urban areas, cultural competency in the health and lifestyle issues of LGBT communities seems as critical as such competency regarding ethnic minorities. Therefore, models of undergraduate, graduate, and continuing education should be adopted from other diversity and cultural competency programs. As with these other training models, factual information is merely one component; exercises and exploration that reveal and challenge people's attitudes are equally important. Another approach to helping LGBT patients feel comfortable is to make healthcare settings an appealing workplace for LGBT people so that employees feel comfortable being visible and "out" at work. The presence of "people like me" goes a long way toward dispelling discomfort.

In addition to issues of attitudes and comfort, institutional barriers that pose access barriers to LGBT people must also be addressed. For instance, institutions should develop and disseminate forms and policies that more accurately capture people's sexual orientation, gender identity, living arrangements, and families. The ubiquitous policy barrier to health care access for LGBT people is the lack of employment-based health insurance because domestic partners are less commonly covered than spouses, such coverage is typically expensive when offered, and there is some evidence that LGBT people may cluster in occupations less likely to provide health coverage (service, arts, retail, etc.). Solutions include inducements for employers to offer domestic partner coverage, such as the laws enacted by the cities of San Francisco and New York requiring such coverage for all City contractors. Further development of health insurance purchasing cooperatives for freelancers, part-time workers, and artists is another strategy to increase coverage.

The numerous policy barriers to medical decision-making, inheritance rights, and visitation options are most efficiently addressed by simply recognizing same-sex marriage, as all these rights accrue automatically to the married. In the interim, expanding access to the legal services required to execute the numerous legal documents that make the wishes of the partners clear must suffice. Obviously, affording these services is difficult for many LGBT people. These are among the legal services offered at no cost by AIDS service organizations; however, other community institutions that serve LGBT people should offer them at low or no cost.

Efforts to change the health behavior within the LGBT community have focused almost exclusively on preventing HIV and other STIs. Despite this emphasis, several steps whose effectiveness is well documented have not been fully taken. Salient among these is the widespread availability of sterile syringes, through exchanges and from pharmacies without prescription. This ongoing issue has HIV prevention significance for LGB who are injecting drug users, as well as for transgender people who use syringes to inject hormones. None of the existing syringe exchanges cater explicitly to LGB populations (though one in New York City has specific programming for transgender people). Despite extraordinarily high rates of HIV seroprevalence and the frequency of voluntary and coerced sexual behavior and drug use in prisons and jails, neither condoms nor sterile syringes are available to those incarcerated. Finally, the early conceptual divide between HIV risk due to sexual behavior and HIV risk due to drug using behavior continues to impede adequate sexual risk reduction among drug users, adequate harm reduction from drug use among those at risk due to sexual behaviors, and adequate approaches to the intersections between drug use and sex (as in the current use of crystal meth among gay men). Another preventive service that should be integrated into all standard practice for MSM is hepatitis B vaccination. Of course, to identify the people who should be vaccinated, more appropriate sexual histories are a prerequisite.

Other public health campaigns (e.g., to encourage smoking cessation, increase exercise, decrease excess weight, avoid driving while intoxicated, use seat belts and bike helmets) should include images and messages targeting LGBT people just as they do members of other minority groups. In addition, research into appropriate structural interventions to reduce smoking and other substance abuse for segments of the LGBT community are needed. Lastly, causes of poor health in the LGBT community that are related directly and indirectly to homophobia and its consequent stress (e.g., depression, substance abuse, violence) can most effectively be prevented by continued efforts to improve the social conditions, antidiscrimination protections, and acceptance of LGBT people.

9.0. CONCLUSION

LGBT history, culture and health are inextricably intertwined with cities. Cities, despite the health risks they pose, continue to play a critical role in supporting and affirming the full diversity of the LGBT community. LGBT people, in turn, have contributed much to the cultural and economic life of cities as well as to innovative approaches to health care advocacy and service delivery. Nonetheless, significant health issues and barriers to healthcare for LGBT people remain. Because of the numbers and density of LGBT people in urban areas, cities provide a unique opportunity for public health practitioners, urban planners, and policy makers to develop and test creative strategies to improve the health and well-being of sexual minorities and eliminate the barriers that persist.

REFERENCES

Aaron, D. J., Markovic, N., Danielson, M. E., Honnold, J. A., Janosky, J. E., and Schmidt, N. J. (2001). Behavioral risk factors for disease and preventive health practices among lesbians. *Am. J. Public Health* 91(6): 972–975.

Acevedo-Garcia, D., Lochner, K. A., Osypuk, T. L., and Subramanian, S. V. (2003). Future directions in residential segregation and health research: a multilevel approach. *Am. J. Public Health* 93(2): 215–221.

Altman, D. (1987). *AIDS in the mind of America.* Anchor Press, Garden City, NJ.

Ambrose, P. J. (2001). Living conditions and health promotion strategies. *J. R. Soc. Health* 121(1):9–15.

Assistive housing needs for elderly gays and lesbians in New York City. (1999). New York: Hunter College and Senior Action in a Gay Environment (October, 2004); http://www.asaging.org/networks/lgain/outword_online/1999/outnov99.cfm

Badgett, M. (1998). Income inflation: the myth of affluence among gay, lesbian and bisexual Americans. National Gay and Lesbian Task Force, Washington D.C.

Bailey, R. W. (1999). Gay politics, urban politics: Identity and economics in the urban setting. *Sage Urban Studies Abstracts* (3).

Baquet, C. R., Hammond, C., Commiskey, P., Brooks, S., and Mullins, C. D. (2002). Health disparities research–a model for conducting research on cancer disparities: characterization and reduction. *J. Assoc. Acad. Minor Phys.* 13(2):33–40.

Berrill, K. (1992). Anti-gay violence and victimization in the U.S.: an overview. In: Berrill, K. (ed.), *Hate crimes: confronting violence against lesbians and gay men.* Sage, Newbury Park, CA.

Bing, E. G., Burnam, M. A., Longshore, D., Fleishman, J. A., Sherbourne, C. D., London, A. S., Turner, B. J., Eggan, F., Beckman, R., Vitiello, B., Morton, S. C., Orlando, M., Bozzette, S. A., Ortiz-Barron, L., and Shapiro, M. (2001). Psychiatric disorders and drug use among human immunodeficiency virus-infected adults in the United States. *Arch. Gen. Psychiatry* 58(8): 721–728.

Black, D., Gates, G., Sanders, S., and Taylor, L. (2002). Why do gay men live in San Francisco? *J. Urban Economics* 51(1):54–76.

Bradford, J., Barrett, K., and Honnold, J. A. (2002). The 2000 census and same-sex households. National Gay and Lesbian Task Force, Washington D.C.

Brotman, S., Ryan, B., Jalbert, Y., and Rowe, B. (2002). The impact of coming out on health and health care access: the experiences of gay, lesbian, bisexual and two-spirit people. *J. Health Soc. Policy* 15(1):1–29.

Burke, L. K., and Follingstad, D. R. (1999). Violence in lesbian and gay relationships: theory, prevalence, and correlational factors. *Clin. Psychol. Rev.* 19(5):487–512.

Cahill, S., Ellen, M., and Tobias, S. (2002). Family policy: issues affecting gay, lesbian and bisexual transgender families. National Gay and Lesbian Task Force, Washington, D.C.

Cahill, S., South, K., and Spade, J. (undated). Outing age: public policy issues affecting gay, lesbian, bisexual and transgender elders. National Gay and Lesbian Task Force, Washington D.C.

Campbell, J. P., Gratton, M. C., Salomone, J. A., 3rd, and Watson, W. A. (1993). Ambulance arrival to patient contact: the hidden component of prehospital response time intervals. *Ann. Emerg. Med.* 22(8):1254–1257.

CDC. (1997). Gonorrhea among men who have sex with men – selected sexually transmitted disease clinics, 1993-1996. *MMWR.* 46(38): 889–892.

CDC. (1999a). Increases in unsafe sex and rectal gonorrhea among men who have sex with men – San Francisco, California, 1994-1997. *MMWR.* 48(3):45–48.

CDC. (1999b). Resurgent bacterial sexually transmitted disease among men who have sex with men – King County, Washington, 1997-1999. *MMWR.* 48(35):773–777.

CDC. (2001). HIV incidence among young men who have sex with men – seven U.S. cities, 1994–2000. *MMWR.* 50(21):440–444.

CDC. (2001a). Outbreak of syphilis among men who have sex with men – Southern California, 2000. *MMWR.* 50(7):117–120.

CDC. (2002b). Primary and secondary syphilis among men who have sex with men – New York City, 2001. *MMWR.* 51(38):853–856.

CDC. (2003). Increases in HIV diagnoses: 29 states, 1999-2002. *MMWR.* 52(47):1145–1148.

Center for Substance Abuse Treatment. (2001). *A provider's introduction to substance abuse treatment for lesbian, gay, bisexual and transgender individuals.* U.S. Department of Health and Human Services, Rockville.

Clements-Nolle, K., Marx, R., Guzman, R., and Katz, M. (2001). HIV prevalence, risk behaviors, health care use, and mental health status of transgender persons: implications for public health intervention. *Am. J. Public Health* 91(6):915–921.

Cochran, S. D., and Mays, V. M. (2000). Relation between psychiatric syndromes and behaviorally defined sexual orientation in a sample of the US population. *Am. J. Epidemiol.* 151(5):516–523.

Cochran, B. N., Stewart, A. J., Ginzler, J. A., and Cauce, A. M. (2002). Challenges faced by homeless sexual minorities: comparison of gay, lesbian, bisexual, and transgender homeless adolescents with their heterosexual counterparts. *Am. J. Public Health* 92(5):773–777.

Cochran, S. D., Mays, V. M., and Sullivan, J. G. (2003). Prevalence of mental disorders, psychological distress, and mental health services use among lesbian, gay, and bisexual adults in the United States. *J. Consult. Clin. Psychol.* 71(1):53–61.

Cohen, D. A., Mason, K., Bedimo, A., Scribner, R., Basolo, V., and Farley, T. A. (2003). Neighborhood physical conditions and health. *Am. J. Public Health* 93(3):467–471.

Cohen, D., Spear, S., Scribner, R., Kissinger, P., Mason, K., and Wildgen, J. (2000). "Broken windows" and the risk of gonorrhea. *Am. J. Public Health* 90(2): 230–236.

Cummins, S. K., and Jackson, R. J. (2001). The built environment and children's health. *Pediatr. Clin. North Am.* 48(5):1241–1252.

Dean, L., Meyer, H., Robinson, K., Sell, R., Sember, R., Silenzio, V. M., Bowen, D., Braford, J., Rothblum, E. D., Scout, Wolfe, D., and Xavier, J. (2000). Lesbian, gay, bisexual and transgender health: findings and concerns. *Journal of the Gay and Lesbian Medical Association* 4(3):101–151.

D'Emilio, J. (1989). Gay politics and community in San Francisco since World War II. In: Duberman, M., Vicinus, M., and G. Chauncey (eds.), *Hidden from history: reclaiming the gay and lesbian past.* NAL Books, New York, NY.

The demographics of diversity: why cities are courting the gay and lesbian community. (2003). The Urban Institute, Washington D.C.

Diaz, R. M., and Ayala, G. (2001). *Social discrimination and health: the case of Latino gay men and HIV risk.* National Gay & Lesbian Task Force, Washington D.C.

Diaz, R. M., Ayala, G., Bein, E., Henne, J., and Marin, B. V. (2001). The impact of homophobia, poverty, and racism on the mental health of gay and bisexual Latino men: findings from 3 U.S. cities. *Am. J. Public Health* 91(6): 927-932.

Dickey, W. C., Dew, M. A., Becker, J. T., and Kingsley, L. (1999). Combined effects of HIV-infection status and psychosocial vulnerability on mental health in homosexual men. *Soc. Psychiatry* 34(1):4–11.

Dienstag, J. L., Stevens, C. E., Bhan, A. K., and Szmuness, W. (1982). Hepatitis B vaccine administered to chronic carriers of hepatitis b surface antigen. *Ann. Intern. Med.* 96(5):575–579.

Douglas, C. J., Kalman, C. M., and Kalman, T. P. (1985). Homophobia among physicians and nurses: an empirical study. *Hosp. Community Psychiatry* 36(12):1309–1311.

Elifson, K. W., Boles, J., Posey, E., Sweat, M., Darrow, W., and Elsea, W. (1993). Male transvestite prostitutes and HIV risk. *Am. J. Public Health* 83(2): 260–262.

Finn, P., and McNeil, T. (1987). *The response of the criminal justice system to bias crime.* Abt Associates, Cambridge, MA.

Florida, R. (2002). The rise of the creative class: why cities without gays and rock bands are losing the economic development race. *Washington Monthly*, May.

Florida, R. (2004). Revenge of the squelchers. *The Next American City*, (August 30, 2004); http://www.americancity.org.

Gallagher, E. J., Lombardi, G., and Gennis, P. (1995). Effectiveness of bystander cardiopulmonary resuscitation and survival following out-of-hospital cardiac arrest. *JAMA.* 274(24):1922–1925.

Gates, G. (2003). *Workplace protection linked to higher earnings for less-educated gay men.* The Urban Institute, Washington D.C.

Gates, G., and Ost, J. (2004). *The gay and lesbian atlas.* Urban Institute Press, Washington D.C.

Gluhoski, V. L., Fishman, B., and Perry, S. W. (1997). The impact of multiple bereavement in a gay male sample. *AIDS Educ. Prev.* 9(6):521–531.

Goodenow, C., Netherland, J., and Szalacha, L. (2002). AIDS-related risk among adolescent males who have sex with males, females, or both: evidence from a statewide survey. *Am. J. Public Health* 92(2):203–210.

Green, A. (2002). "Chem friendly": the institutional basis of club drug use in a sample of urban gay men. *Deviant Behavior* 24:427–447.

Greenwood, G. L., Relf, M. V., Huang, B., Pollack, L. M., Canchola, J. A., and Catania, J. A. (2002). Battering victimization among a probability-based sample of men who have sex with men. *Am. J. Public Health* 92(12):1964–1969.

Hancock, T. (2002). Indicators of environmental health in the urban setting. *Can. J. Public Health* 93 (Suppl 1):S45–51.

Hayward, R., and Weissfeld, J.L. (1993). Coming to terms in the era of AIDS: attitudes of physicians in U.S. residency programs. *J. Gen. Internal Med.* 8:10–18.

Hessol, N. A., Katz, M. H., Liu, J. Y., Buchbinder, S. P., Rubino, C. J., and Holmberg, S. D. (1992). Increased incidence of Hodgkin disease in homosexual men with HIV infection. *Ann. Intern. Med.* 117(4):309–311.

Hessol, N. A., Koblin, B. A., van Griensven, G. J., Bacchetti, P., Liu, J. Y., Stevens, C. E., Coutinho, R.A., Buchbinder, S.P., and Katz, M.H. (1994). Progression of human immunodeficiency virus type 1

(HIV-1) infection among homosexual men in hepatitis B vaccine trial cohorts in Amsterdam, New York City, and San Francisco, 1978-1991. *Am. J. Epidemiol.* 139(11):1077–1087.

House, J. S., Lepkowski, J. M., Williams, D. R., Mero, R. P., Lantz, P. M., Robert, S. A., and Chen, J. (2000). Excess mortality among urban residents: how much, for whom, and why? *Am. J. Public Health* 90(12):1898–1904.

Huebner, M., Rebchook, G., and Kegeles, S. (2004). Experiences of harassment discrimination and physical violence among young gay and bisexual men. *Am. J. Public Health* 94(7):1200–6.

Human Rights Campaign, 2004, Washington D.C. (June 22, 2004); http://www.hrc.org.

Hunter, J. (1998). Government and activism. In: Smith R. (ed.), *Encyclopedia of AIDS: a social, cultural and scientific record of the HIV epidemic.* Fitzroy Dearborn Publishers, Chicago.

Katz, M. H., Hessol, N. A., Buchbinder, S. P., Hirozawa, A., O'Malley, P., and Holmberg, S. D. (1994). Temporal trends of opportunistic infections and malignancies in homosexual men with AIDS. *J. Infect. Dis.* 170(1):98–202.

Kelly, J. A., St Lawrence, J. S., Diaz, Y. E., Stevenson, L. Y., Hauth, A. C., Brasfield, T. L., Kalichman, S. C., Smith, J. E., and Andrew, M. E. (1991). HIV risk behavior reduction following intervention with key opinion leaders of population: an experimental analysis. *Am. J. Public Health* 81(2):168–171.

Kelly, J. A., St Lawrence, J. S., Stevenson, L. Y., Hauth, A. C., Kalichman, S. C., Diaz, Y. E., Brasfield, T. L., Koob, J. J., and Morgan, M. G. (1992). Community AIDS/HIV risk reduction: the effects of endorsements by popular people in three cities. *Am. J. Public Health* 82(11):1483–1489.

Kenney, M. (2001). *Mapping gay Los Angeles: the intersection of place and politics.* Temple University Press, Philadelphia, PA.

Kimmel, P. L., Peterson, R. A., Weihs, K. L., Simmens, S. J., Alleyne, S., Cruz, I., Umana, W.O., Alleyne, S., and Veis, J.H. (1998). Psychosocial factors, behavioral compliance and survival in urban hemodialysis patients. *Kidney Int.* 54(1):245–254.

Kirkey, K., and Forsyth, A. (2001). Men in the valley: gay male life on the suburban-rural fringe. *J. Rural Studies* 17:421-441.

Klausner, J. D., Wolf, W., Fischer-Ponce, L., Zolt, I., and Katz, M. H. (2000). Tracing a syphilis outbreak through cyberspace. *JAMA.* 284(4):447–449.

Koblin, B. A., Hessol, N. A., Zauber, A. G., Taylor, P. E., Buchbinder, S. P., Katz, M. H., and Stevens, C.E. (1996). Increased incidence of cancer among homosexual men, New York City and San Francisco, 1978-1990. *Am. J. Epidemiol.* 144(10):916–923.

Krieger, J. W., Song, L., Takaro, T. K., and Stout, J. (2000). Asthma and the home environment of low-income urban children: preliminary findings from the Seattle-King County healthy homes project. *J. Urban Health* 77(1):50–67.

Krieger, J., and Higgins, D. (2002). Housing and health: time again for public health action. *Am. J. Public Health* 92:758–768.

Latkin, C. A., Forman, V., Knowlton, A., and Sherman, S. (2003). Norms, social networks, and HIV-related risk behaviors among urban disadvantaged drug users. *Soc. Sci. Med.* 56(3):465–476.

Lawrence, R. J. (1999). Urban health: an ecological perspective. *Rev. Environ. Health* 14(1):1–10.

Lee, D. (2002). Glory days? Gay pioneers muscle in on Springsteen's turf. *New York Times,* September 6, 2002.

Lena, S. M., Wiebe, T., Ingram, S., and Jabbour, M. (2002). Pediatricians' knowledge, perceptions, and attitudes towards providing health care for lesbian, gay, and bisexual adolescents. *Ann. R. Coll. Physicians Surg. Can.* 35(7):406–410.

Levay, S., and Nonas, E. (1995). *City of friends: a portrait of gay and lesbian community on America.* MIT Press, Cambridge, MA.

Leventhal, T., and Brooks-Gunn, J. (2003). Moving to opportunity: an experimental study of neighborhood effects on mental health. *Am. J. Public Health* 93(9):1576–1582.

Leviton, L. C., Snell, E., and McGinnis, M. (2000). Urban issues in health promotion strategies. *Am. J. Public Health* 90(6):863–866.

Lifson, A. R., Darrow, W. W., Hessol, N. A., O'Malley, P. M., Barnhart, J. L., Jaffe, H. W., and Rutherford, G. W. (1990). Kaposi's sarcoma in a cohort of homosexual and bisexual men. Epidemiology and analysis for cofactors. *Am. J. Epidemiol.* 131(2):221–231.

Lo, J., and Healy, T. (2000). Flagrantly flaunting it? contesting perceptions of locational identity among urban Vancouver lesbians. *Journal of Lesbian Studies* 4(1):29–44.

Mathews, W., Booth, M., Turner, B. J., and Kessler, L. (1986). Physicians' attitudes towards homosexuality -survey of California County Medical Society. *West. J. Med.* 144(106).

Matthews, A. K., Hughes, T. L., Johnson, T., Razzano, L. A., and Cassidy, R. (2002). Prediction of depressive distress in a community sample of women: the role of sexual orientation. *Am. J. Public Health* 92(7):1131–1139.

McCarthy, M. (2000). Social determinants and inequalities in urban health. *Rev. Environ. Health* 15(1-2):97–108.

McKirnan, D. J., Ostrow, D. G., and Hope, B. (1996). Sex, drugs and escape: a psychological model of HIV-risk sexual behaviours. *AIDS Care.* 8(6):655–669.

McNair, R. (2000). Lesbian sexuality. Do GPs contribute to lesbian invisibility and ill health? *Aust. Fam. Physician* 29(6):514–516.

McNair, R. P. (2003). Lesbian health inequalities: a cultural minority issue for health professionals. *Me. J. Aust.* 178(12):643–645.

Menlo Park: Kaiser Family Foundation. (2003). Disparities in healthcare coverage, access, and quality: the impact of citizenship and language on low-income immigrants. (August 30, 2004); http://www.kff.org/uninsured/loader.cfm?url=/commonspot/security/getfile.cfm&PageID=22107

Meyer, I. (2001). Why lesbian, gay bisexual and transgender public health? *Am. J. Public Health* 91(6):856–859.

Meyer, I. H. (2003). Prejudice, social stress, and mental health in lesbian, gay, and bisexual populations: conceptual issues and research evidence. *Psychol. Bull.* 129(5):674–697.

Mills, T. C., Stall, R., Pollack, L., Paul, J. P., Binson, D., Canchola, J., and Catania, J. A. (2001). Health-related characteristics of men who have sex with men: a comparison of those living in "gay ghettos" with those living elsewhere. *Am. J. Public Health* 91(6):980–983.

Mills, T. C., Paul, J., Stall, R., Pollack, L., Canchola, J., Chang, Y. J., Moskowitz, J. T., and Catania, J. A. (2004). Distress and depression in men who have sex with men: the Urban Men's Health Study. *Am. J. Psychiatry* 161(2):278–285.

Morin, S. F., Charles, K. A., and Malyon, A. K. (1984). The psychological impact of AIDS on gay men. *Am. Psychol.* 39(11):1288–1293.

National healthcare disparities report, 2004, Rockville: Agency for Healthcare Research and Quality, (August 30, 2004); http://www.ahrq.gov/qual/nhdr04/premeasures.htm.

Navarre, M. (1988). Fighting the victim label. In: Crimp, D. (ed.), *AIDS: cultural analysis, cultural activism.* MIT Press, Cambridge, MA.

Nemoto, T., Operario, D., Keatley, J., Han, L., and Soma, T. (2004). HIV risk behaviors among male-to-female transgender persons of color in San Francisco. *Am. J. Public Health* 94(7):1193–99.

Northridge, M. E., Sclar, E. D., and Biswas, P. (2003). Sorting out the connections between the built environment and health: a conceptual framework for navigating pathways and planning healthy cities. *J. Urban Health* 80(4):556–568.

O'Donnell, L., Agronick, G., San Doval, A., Duran, R., Myint, U. A., and Stueve, A. (2002). Ethnic and gay community attachments and sexual risk behaviors among urban Latino young men who have sex with men. *AIDS Educ. Prev.* 14(6):457–471.

Office of Gay and Lesbian Health. (1999). Report on the health status of gay men and lesbians in New York City. New York: New York City Department of Health, (August 30, 2004); http://www.nyc.gov/html/doh/html/public/press99/pr37-630.html

Office on Women's Health. (2000). Scientific workshop on lesbian health 2000: steps for implementing the IOM report. Department of Health and Human Services, Washington, D.C., (September 8, 2004); http://www.glma.org/policy/swlh_report.pdf

Patton, C. (1990). *Inventing AIDS.* Routledge, New York, NY.

Patton, C. (2004). National Coalition of Anti-violence Programs 2004 report: preview edition. National Coalition of Anti-violence Programs, New York, NY.

Perdue, W. C., Stone, L. A., and Gostin, L. O. (2003). The built environment and its relationship to the public's health: the legal framework. *Am. J. Public Health* 93(9):1390–1394.

Reijneveld, S. A. (2002). Neighbourhood socioeconomic context and self reported health and smoking: a secondary analysis of data on seven cities. *J. Epidemiol. Community Health* 56(12):935–942.

Rich, M. (2004). Edged out by the stroller set. *New York Times*, May 27th, p. F1.

Robin, L., Brener, N. D., Donahue, S. F., Hack, T., Hale, K., and Goodenow, C. (2002). Associations between health risk behaviors and opposite-, same-, and both-sex sexual partners in representative samples of Vermont and Massachusetts high school students. *Arch. Pediatr. Adolesc. Med.* 156(4):349–355.

Ross, M. W., and Williams, M. L. (2002). Effective Targeted and Community HIV/STD Prevention Programs. *J. Sex. Res.* 39(1):58–62.

Rubenstein, W., Sears, B., and Sockloskie, R. (2003). *Demographic characteristics of the gay community in the United States.* Williams Project, UCLA School of Law.

Rushbrook, D. (2002). Cities, queer space, and the cosmopolitan tourist. *GLQ.* 8(1-2):183–206.

Satterthwaite, D. (1993). The impact on health of urban environments. *Environ. Urban* 5(2):87–111.

Schreeder, M.T., Thompson, S.E., Hadler, S.C., Berquistm K.R., Zaidi, A., Maynard, J.E., Ostrow, D., Judson, F.N., Braff, E.H., Nylund, T., Moore, J.N. Jr., Gardner, P., Doto, I.L., and Reynolds, G. (1982). Hepatitis B in homosexual men: prevalence of infection and factors related to transmission. *J. Infect. Dis.* 46(1):7-15.

Schulz, A., Williams, D., Israel, B., Becker, A., Parker, E., James, S. A., and Jackson, J. (2000). Unfair treatment, neighborhood effects, and mental health in the Detroit metropolitan area. *J. Health Soc. Behav.* 41(3):314–332.

Schulz, A. J., Williams, D. R., Israel, B. A., and Lempert, L. B. (2002). Racial and spatial relations as fundamental determinants of health in Detroit. *Milbank Q.* 80(4):677–707.

Shilts, R. (1987). *And the band played on, 3rd Ed.* St. Martin's Press, New York, NY.

Sikkema, K. J., Kochman, A., DiFranceisco, W., Kelly, J. A., and Hoffmann, R. G. (2003). AIDS-related grief and coping with loss among HIV-positive men and women. *J. Behav. Med.* 26(2): 165–181.

Silvestre, A. J., Arrowood, S. H., Ivery, J. M., and Barksdale, S. (2002). HIV-prevention capacity building in gay, racial, and ethnic minority communities in small cities and towns. *Health Soc. Work* 27(1): 61–66.

Simon, B. (2002). New York Avenue: the life and death of gay spaces in Atlantic City, New Jersey, 1920-1990. *J. Urban Hist.* (3):300–327.

Smith, E. M., Johnson, S. R., and Guenther, S. M. (1985). Health care attitudes and experiences during gynecologic care among lesbians and bisexuals. *Am. J. Public Health* 75(9): 1085–1087.

Stall, R., and Wiley, J. (1988). A comparison of alcohol and drug use patterns of homosexual and heterosexual men: the San Francisco Men's Health Study. *Drug Alcohol Depend.* 22(1-2):63–73.

Stall, R., Paul, J. P., Greenwood, G., Pollack, L. M., Bein, E., Crosby, G. M., Mills, T.C., Binson, D., Coates, T.J., and Catania, J.A. (2001). Alcohol use, drug use and alcohol-related problems among men who have sex with men: the Urban Men's Health Study. *Addiction* 96(11):1589–1601.

Stevens, C. E., and Taylor, P. E. (1986). Hepatitis B vaccine: issues, recommendations, and new developments. *Semin. Liver Dis.* 6(1):23–27.

Swope, C. (2003). Chasing the rainbow: is a gay population an engine of urban revival? Cities are beginning to think so. *Governing* (September 8, 2004); http://www.governing.com/articles/10gays.htm

Szmuness, W., Stevens, C. E., Harley, E. J., Zang, E. A., Oleszko, W. R., William, D. C., Sadovsky, R., Morrison, J.M., and Kellner, A. (1980). Hepatitis B vaccine: demonstration of efficacy in a controlled clinical trial in a high-risk population in the United States. *N. Engl. J. Med.* 303(15):833–841.

Szmuness, W., Stevens, C. E., Zang, E. A., Harley, E. J., and Kellner, A. (1981). A controlled clinical trial of the efficacy of the hepatitis B vaccine (Heptavax B): a final report. *Hepatology* 1(5):377–385.

Turner, H. A., Hays, R. B., and Coates, T. J. (1993). Determinants of social support among gay men: the context of AIDS. *J. Health Soc. Behav.* 34(1):37–53.

Turner, H. A., and Catania, J. A. (1997). Informal care giving to persons with AIDS in the United States: caregiver burden among central cities residents eighteen to forty-nine years old. *Am. J. Community Psychol.* 25(1):35–59.

Valentine, G., and Skelton, T. (2003). Finding oneself, losing oneself: the lesbian and gay scene as a paradoxical space. *Int. J. Urban Reg. Res.* (4): 849-866.

van Griensven, G. J., Hessol, N. A., Koblin, B. A., Byers, R. H., O'Malley, P. M., Albercht-van Lent, N., Buchbinder, S.P., Taylor, P.E., Stevens, C. E., and Coutinho, R.A. (1993). Epidemiology of human immunodeficiency virus type 1 infection among homosexual men participating in hepatitis B vaccine trials in Amsterdam, New York City, and San Francisco, 1978-1990. *Am. J. Epidemiol. 137* (8):909–915.

Vlahov, D., and Galea, S. (2002). Urbanization, urbanicity, and health. *J. Urban Health* 79 (4 Suppl 1): S1–S12.

Weich, S., Blanchard, M., Prince, M., Burton, E., Erens, B., and Sproston, K. (2002). Mental health and the built environment: cross-sectional survey of individual and contextual risk factors for depression. *Br. J. Psychiatry* 180:428–433.

Westerstahl, A., Segesten, K., and Bjorkelund, C. (2002). GPs and lesbian women in the consultation: issues of awareness and knowledge. *Scand. J. Prim. Health Care* 20(4):203–207.

Woody, G. E., VanEtten-Lee, M. L., McKirnan, D., Donnell, D., Metzger, D., Seage, G., 3rd., Gross, M., and HIVNET VPS 001 Protocol Team. (2001). Substance use among men who have sex with men: comparison with a national household survey. *J. Acquir. Immune Defic. Synd.* 27(1):86–90.

Woolwine, D. (2000). Community in gay male experience and moral discourse. *J. Homosex.* 38(4):5–37.

Young, R., Weissman, G., and Cohen, J. (1992). Assessing risk in the absence of information: HIV risk among injection drug users who have sex with women. *AIDS Public Policy* 7(3):175–183.

Chapter 6

Health and Health Access Among Urban Immigrants

Sana Loue and Nancy Mendez

1.0. MIGRATION TO THE CITIES: THE PROCESS OF IMMIGRATION

It has been estimated that the U.S. has almost 34.5 million immigrants, comprising 8% of its population (U.S. Census Bureau, 2002), and that, on average, an additional three quarters to a million new immigrants enter the country each year. Census data indicate that between 1990 and 2000, the U.S. attracted 27% of the world's migrants (U.S. Census Bureau, 2002). A portion of these individuals enter with permanent resident status ("green card" or mica holders), by virtue of their relationship to a U.S. citizen spouse, parent, child, or sibling or a permanent resident spouse or child or on the basis of a specified employment offer, enabling them to remain and work in the United States indefinitely. In 2002 alone, a total of 1,064,318 individuals received permanent resident status in the U.S. (Office of Immigration Statistics, 2003). Others enter on a temporary basis as legal nonimmigrants, holding statuses as students, tourists, journalists, sports players, and so on. Still others enter seeking refuge in the form of asylum from persecution due to their religion, political beliefs, nationality, or membership in a social group.

For many, the process of gaining legal admission is not an easy one. In recent years, the process has been rendered increasingly difficult as a result of visa quotas that result in extended delays to obtain a permanent resident status, income requirements excluding from the U.S. persons earning below a certain income level, health-related criteria barring individuals with certain conditions, such as HIV infection, sexually transmitted diseases, tuberculosis, and certain mental illnesses, among others from entering, and fears of terrorism, resulting in the exclusion of those who may have any connection to groups viewed suspiciously.

Yet another portion of these individuals, known variously as "undocumented" or "illegal," enter without legal authorization, often in search of a better life for themselves and their families. These individuals are at particularly high risk of victimization, with significant adverse health consequences, due to their legal status and concomitant fear of discovery, their unfamiliarity with our legal system, their inability to speak English, and their dependence on the individuals who helped them to enter illegally. News reports have publicized widely the hardships faced by these individuals in relatively isolated geographic areas (Greenhouse, 2002; Rodriguez, 2002). Perhaps less well-publicized or known are the abuses suffered by these individuals in urban areas, which have included confinement in crowded, unsanitary conditions (Phoenix metropolitan area) (Billeaud, 2004), the imprisonment and sale of women into prostitution (Los Angeles area) (U.S. Department of Justice, 2003), the kidnapping of individuals' infants as ransom in exchange for forced labor (New York City) (Editorial, 1997), and the sale of young girls as sex slaves and indentured servants (Anaheim, Berkeley, and Silicon Valley, California; Miami metropolitan area) (Luna and Tran, 2004; McCormick and Zamora, 2000; Pacenti, 1998).

Once in the U.S., immigrant populations have tended to congregate in or near large metropolitan areas. By the turn of the 20th century, 87% of Chicago's population, 80% of New York's population, and 84% of Detroit's and Milwaukee's population consisted of immigrants (Bodnar, 1987; Daniels, 1990). It has been estimated that, during the 1980s and 1990s, 10 metropolitan areas of the U.S., which were home to 17% of the nation's population, attracted 55% of all legal immigrants to the U.S. and an even larger percentage of those who immigrated illegally (Enchautegui, 1993). New York, Los Angeles, San Francisco, Miami, Chicago, and Washington, D.C. have been and continue to be foremost among these cities (Enchautegui, 1993; Office of Immigration Statistics, 2003; United States Census Bureau, 2002). According to the 2000 U.S. census, 874,567 of Miami-Dade County's population of 2,253,362 were foreign-born, accounting for 45.1% of the area's population. The Immigration and Naturalization Service (now the Bureau of Immigration and Customs Enforcement of the Department of Homeland Security) reported the admission of an additional 297,533 foreign-born persons in Miami (Immigration and Naturalization Service, 2000).

As residents in these urban areas, immigrants have tended to settle in ethnic enclaves of three types: suburban areas, occupied predominantly by skilled workers, mid-range professionals, and upper-level civil service workers, and consisting of single-family housing in the outer city and apartments and other units towards the center; tenement areas that are inhabited by lower-paid blue and white collar workers living in cheaper single-family homes; and relatively abandoned areas of the city, with large numbers of homeless and unemployed persons. These enclaves may provide significant employment opportunities to new immigrants (Marcuse, 1996). However, many new immigrants, and refugees in particular, confront difficult financial circumstances. A survey of 739 Hmong, Khmer, Laotian, Chinese-Vietnamese, and Vietnamese in San Diego County, California found that 75.8% were living below the poverty level (Rumbaut, *et al.*, 1988). A study of 196 Afghan immigrants in the San Francisco Bay area reported that 8% of the men were employed as professionals (professors, judges, or government officials), 27% were in skilled employment, administration, or business, and 39% were unemployed, compared to 29%, 50%, and 0%, respectively, when the men were living in Afghanistan (Lipson, *et al.*, 1995).

Despite the large numbers of immigrants residing in urban areas, we actually know relatively little about the relationship of urban residence to health status among immigrants specifically. First, many reports fail to specify the immigration status of the patients or research participants. This information may be unavailable due to individuals' unwillingness to disclose their status or author unfamiliarity with issues specifically related to immigrants, as contrasted with specific ethnic, groups. Even when reports indicate immigration status, they often fail to specify individuals' duration of residence in the U.S., or the extent of their English language ability, which may be critical to an understanding of their ability to utilize the health care system or the occurrence of specific diseases. Many other reports speak about immigrants as a homogeneous group or immigrants of a particular ethnicity or nationality without specifying their area of residence, despite the potential relevance of their urban, suburban, or rural residence to the issue under examination such as, for example, exposure to violence or incidence of asthma.

This chapter provides an overview of key issues related to health status, health care delivery, and health research among immigrants with a particular focus on immigrants in urban areas. It is critical, however, to recall that although we speak of "immigrants," immigrant communities are not homogenous. For instance, in 2002, immigrants arrived in the United States from all continents, with the exception of Antarctica; the leading source countries for new legal immigrants to the U.S. included countries as diverse as Mexico, India, China, the Philippines, and Vietnam (Office of Immigration Statistics, 2002). Some of the more obvious differences include individuals' mechanism of entry (legally or illegally, for permanent residence or a temporary time, etc.), religion, language, English language ability, and educational and economic levels, and preferred diet. Other differences may be less obvious but even more critical to their health and health care, including their level of familiarity and comfort with U.S. systems, health and disease status at entry, models of illness, and expectations about health care.

2.0. HEALTH AND DISEASE

Immigrants are affected by both communicable disease and chronic disease. They may bring these illnesses and disorders with them, or they may acquire them subsequent to their arrival in the U.S. This section focuses on those diseases that are highly prevalent among various immigrant groups in urban areas of the U.S. and that have been the focus of research. The incidence and prevalence of these diseases are discussed, as well as potential risk factors for their occurrence and the availability and utilization of screening procedures for their prevention.

2.1. Communicable Disease

The circumstances of immigrants' transit to and entry into the U.S. may have serious implications for their health and the delivery of health care. A particularly unusual case illustrates the need for health care providers in urban areas to be aware of the conditions associated with illegal immigration and the associated health risks. This case involved the Honduran-registered ship *Golden Venture*, which ran aground off the Rockaway Peninsula in Queens, New York carrying 289 Chinese passengers following a failed attempt to rendezvous with smaller ships that would carry the passengers to the shores of the U.S. illegally. Ten of the passengers died from hypothermia or drowning (Metropolitan Desk, 1993), a number disappeared after receiving treatment at local hospitals (McFadden, 1993), and the remainder were taken into custody by the INS. A few of those who were detained were ultimately granted asylum or were released through other legal mechanisms. Two of those individuals who were apprehended were found to be suffering from Reiter's syndrome, characterized by swelling and pain in the foot, ankle, and knee and, in one individual, by diarrhea and eye pain. The cause of the infection was ultimately attributed to improperly stored "thousand-year-old eggs" that were consumed on the ship during the voyage (Solitar, *et al.*, 1998). Other, less dramatic, but more frequent occurrences also merit attention from clinicians and public health practitioners.

Immigrants to the U.S. also may be at increased risk of specific communicable diseases as a result of the higher prevalence of these infections in their originating countries. An examination of data at a Minneapolis clinic from the charts of 102 recently immigrated patients from 12 different African nations, for instance, found that despite a healthy appearance, 8 patients had active tuberculosis, 10 had hepatitis B, 11 were suffering from various parasitic infections (trichuriasis, amebiasis, schistosomiasis, and ascariasis), 1 had malaria, and 2 patients had human immunodeficiency virus (HIV) (Adair and Nwaaneri, 1999). Of these patients with communicable diseases, 3 had entered illegally, in the hopes that they would be granted asylum, 1 had entered on a student visa, which does not require medical screening, and several who had active tuberculosis were improperly classified.

Another analysis of the health of immigrants was through examinations of 2,545 refugees arriving in Minnesota in 1999 from countries in Eastern Europe, Southeast Asia, and sub-Saharan Africa; this study reported that of the 2,129 (84%) of refugees with results of stool ova and parasite examinations, 8% were found to have trichuriasis; 7%, giardiasis; 3%, schistosomiasis; 3%, hookworm; 2%, amebiasis; 1%, ascariasis; and 1%, strongyloidiasis (Lifson, *et al.*, 2002). Seven percent of the individuals had a positive hepatitis B surface antigen. Although protocols are in place for screening individuals who intend to immigrate permanently to the U.S., such procedures do not encompass all possible situations and cannot be relied upon. Because of the likelihood that new immigrants to the U.S. will settle in urban areas, it is particularly important that health care providers be trained to not only recognize the signs and symptoms of commonly occurring communicable diseases, but also to conduct appropriate screening tests at the time of individuals' first visit.

Tuberculosis is an especially important concern. In 1997, it was found that 39% of all cases of tuberculosis occurred in foreign-born individuals (Centers for Disease Control and Prevention, 1998). An analysis of all incident TB cases nationwide for the period from 1985 through 1992 revealed that the number of cases among foreign-born persons in the U.S. increased by 48% and accounted for 60% of the total increase in the number of incident U.S. cases (Cantwell, *et al.*, 1994). The median interval from the time of immigration to the reporting of foreign-born cases in 1992 was 3 years; 30% of the cases were reported within one year of immigration.

Numerous cities and counties have felt the impact of increasing numbers of TB cases attributable to the immigrant populations. From 1998 through 2001, the annual number of TB cases among African immigrants and refugees in Seattle and King County increased almost three-fold compared to the period from 1993 to 1997 (Anon., 2002). Almost one-half of the individuals had extrapulmonary TB. Of the 3,364 cases of TB occurring between 1985 and 1994 among Asians in Los Angeles County, California, 98% were immigrants (Makinodan, *et al.*, 1999). The TB case rate per 100,000 foreign-born Asians living in Los Angeles County was 162.1, compared to 2.6 per 100,000 among U.S.-born Asians in the same county. A retrospective study of Tibetan immigrants evaluated in Minneapolis between 1992 and 1994 found that despite initial TB screening by U.S.-authorized physicians in India prior to immigration to the U.S., 51% of the chest radiographs taken in Minneapolis were abnormal (Truong, *et al.*, 1997). A comparison with the results from the chest radiograph evaluations conducted in India indicated that 79% of the Tibetans had unchanged readings and 21% showed evidence of potentially progressive disease. A study of all tuberculosis cases occurring in Broward, Dade, and Palm Beach Counties in Florida during calendar year 1995 found that 49% of the 629 individuals with reported tuberculosis had been born in 40 countries. Of those individuals with a known date of arrival in the U.S., 68% had been in the U.S. for more than five years; overseas immigrant screening for tuberculosis had identified only three cases (Granich, *et al.*, 1998).

A large number of persons entering the U.S., including most nonimmigrants, such as tourists and students, are not subject to screening procedures. A recent study of culture-positive tuberculosis patients in the Fort Worth-Dallas, Texas metroplex, the ninth largest metropolitan area in the U.S., found that a greater proportion of nonimmigrants had multi-drug resistant TB and were HIV-positive, compared to those with permanent residence and those who were undocumented (Weis, *et al.*, 2001). Although individuals seeking permanent resident status in the U.S. must be screened for tuberculosis and be found noninfectious to others in order to obtain their visas, data indicate that the screening procedures utilized currently are less effective than is desired and the requisite follow-up of immigrants entering the U.S. who are known to be infected with TB is less than adequate. These deficiencies in screening and follow-up procedures are particularly worrisome in view of the likelihood that immigrants may delay seeking care following entry to the U.S. absent troublesome symptoms and the possibility of disease transmission to others, particularly in crowded, urban living and working situations.

The delay in seeking care for tuberculosis may result from a number of factors including a fear of immigration authorities and misconceptions about the disease and its treatment. It has been found, for instance, that legislation that increases the fear of detection by immigration authorities may exacerbate delays in seeking care (Asch, *et al.*, 1994). Misconceptions about the nature of the disease and its treatment may also play a role. In absolute numbers, immigrants from Mexico and the Philippines are the two largest immigrant groups in the U.S. to develop TB (Zuber, *et al.*, 1997). A focus group study conducted with Filipino immigrants at California and Hawaii community health centers to explore beliefs about TB found that the participants viewed TB as being highly contagious and caused by environmental exposures, such as cigarettes and alcohol, unsanitary conditions, wet clothing, and bacteria and viruses, imbalances of the body occasioned by overwork, poor nutrition, respiratory illness, worrying and family problems, and family inheritance, and contagion from an infected person through touch, the sharing of utensils, or airborne spread (Yamada, *et al.*, 1999). It was believed that the disease could be treated through modern medical attention, traditional medicines, improved sanitation and air, smoking cessation, and the correction of imbalances of the body through proper rest, exercise, discipline, diet, and a positive outlook. Participants also noted the highly stigmatizing nature of the disease and the resulting isolation, shame, and loneliness, leading sufferers to delay or avoid medical diagnosis entirely. Focus groups conducted with foreign-born Vietnamese participants in Orange County, California revealed a belief in two forms of TB, the psychological and the physical (Houston, *et al.*, 2002). The conceptualization of physical TB converged with Western biomedical knowledge of TB as a communicable disease.

However, psychological TB, which was said to be characterized by fatigue, lethargy, and a loss of appetite that could lead to an impairment of immune system functioning and the onset of physical TB, was not believed by participants to be transmissible to others.

These findings underscore the need for prompt screening for TB following arrival in the U.S., a consideration of extrapulmonary TB, and the development of outreach programs and informational messages that address the transmission, symptoms, and treatment for TB in a linguistically and culturally appropriate manner. This may be particularly critical in urban areas due to the insular nature of some immigrant communities and the possibility of disease transmission as a result of close contact with others that is associated with urban living, such as the use of crowded public transportation and residence in high-rise apartment buildings with ventilation systems of varying effectiveness.

From the health care provider perspective, heightened sensitivity to detection of infectious diseases in this population, especially the more rare tropical diseases, is needed. It is critical that care providers at urban area emergency centers and inner city hospitals be familiar with the symptoms of other communicable diseases of high prevalence in other countries, and that they be trained to obtain and consider a patient's travel or migration history. A failure to do so can result in misdiagnosis and failure to provide appropriate and timely care. A retrospective case series conducted at a large, inner city medical center in Los Angeles identified 20 cases of falciparum malaria with initial medical evaluation in the emergency department during the period from 1979 through 1993, but found that malaria had been considered as a diagnosis in only 12 of these cases. Nineteen of these 20 individuals were recent immigrants or immigrants returning to the U.S. after visiting relatives abroad (Kyiacou, *et al.*, 1996).

Temporary visitors to the U.S. and, until recently, individuals immigrating permanently to the U.S. have not been required to have many vaccinations that are common in the U.S. As a result, they have been at greater risk of contracting diseases that had become relatively less common in the U.S., such as rubella. Because the vaccination requirements apply primarily to those seeking permanent resident status and were incorporated into immigration laws relatively recently, it cannot be assumed that immigrants will have had immunizations common in the U.S. A retrospective case series of tetanus cases presenting at the emergency department of a large inner-city medical center between the years 1986 and 1997 found that many of them had occurred in recent immigrants who had not received childhood immunizations (Henderson, *et al.*, 1998).

There is substantial evidence to suggest that immigrant children may also have higher rates of childhood diseases for which vaccinations are available in comparison to U.S.-born children. As an example, an investigation of a rubella outbreak in North Carolina found that the majority of the 83 cases occurred among latino immigrants and that the children had not received rubella vaccination in the countries from which they had migrate because of differing vaccination policies (Rangel, *et al.*, 1999). An assessment of vaccination coverage in a survey of 314 children under 2 years of age in New York City found that foreign-born children had vaccination coverage similar to that of U.S.-born children for diphtheria-pertussis-tetanus, oral polio vaccine, and measles-mumps-rubella, but had been underimmunized for *Haemophilus influenzae* type b and hepatitis B (Findley, *et al.*, 1999) Even children processing for adoption by U.S. parents may lack necessary immunizations or experience incomplete immune responses to vaccines (Schulte, *et al.*, 2002). The lack of adequate immunization may be of particular concern with respect to those immigrant children living in urban areas due to the increased likelihood of their exposure to infectious individuals in these more densely populated environments (Strine, *et al.*, 2002).

Increased attention has been paid to the occurrence of sexually transmitted infections among immigrant populations, due in large part to controversies surrounding the admission to the U.S. of HIV-infected immigrants and criteria excluding immigrants with sexually transmitted disease from entry into this country (Editorial Desk, 1993). Relatively little information is available about the risk for or rates of sexually transmitted infections among urban immigrants. An analysis of health care utilization patterns at one Houston clinic found that Central American immigrants accounted for 4% of the 30,000 annual clinic visits and a large proportion of care was devoted to the treatment of sexually transmitted diseases (Eichenberger and Shandera, 1999). A study of 274 TB culture-positive individuals with varying immigration statuses in the Fort Worth-Dallas metropolitan area found a higher prevalence of HIV infection among individuals traveling to the U.S. as non-immigrants, in comparison with those who were permanent residents and those who were undocumented (Weis, *et al.*, 2001). Although a number of studies have examined the incidence and prevalence of STDs among rural immigrant migrant workers (Bertolli, 1993; Brammeier, *et al.*, 2002; Centers for Disease Control and Prevention, 1992; Ruiz *et al.*, 1997; Organista and Balls Organista, 1997; Organista, *et al.*, 1996; Paz-Bailey, *et al.*, 2004), little research has been conducted with urban immigrant migrant workers. A relatively recent screening for syphilis of 235 male immigrants from Latin America living in San Francisco found that 0.4% had secondary syphilis; among the 198 persons screened for gonorrhea and Chlamydia, it was found that 3.5% had Chlamydia and 0.5% had gonorrhea (Wong, *et al.*, 2003). Data were unavailable to identify contextual or social factors that may have increased the risk of transmission. As with tuberculosis, fear of immigration authorities, stigma associated with the disease itself, and misconceptions about the disease may result in delay in the receipt of diagnosis and care (Kang, *et al.*, 2003).

Behavioral studies including immigrant populations also indicate the need for health care providers to screen patients for risk behaviors in order to determine the need for additional counseling and/or testing and treatment. A survey study of 1,789 students at two high schools in northern California during 1988 and 1989 found that the mean number of risk behaviors was highest among latino immigrant students, as compared with native-born latinos and native non-latino white students (Brindis, *et al.*, 1995). Eight different risk behaviors had been included in the assessment: the use of alcohol, marijuana, cigarette, and other illicit substances; self-violence; drunk driving; unintended pregnancy; and violence. Rates of sexual activity were particularly high among the immigrant students as compared to the others. The authors hypothesized that the level of risk was related to the duration of residence in the U.S., with those residing longer engaging in increasing sexual activity.

A 1990 survey of 3,049 Boston public middle and high school students surveyed in their own languages yielded similar findings. Thirty-five percent of the students had been born outside of the U.S. (Hingson, *et al.*, 1991). Immigrant students were more likely to worry about getting AIDS, but were less likely than U.S.-born students to be familiar with HIV/AIDS prevention strategies or where to obtain information or HIV testing. A similar proportion of the immigrant students reported having had sexual intercourse as compared with the U.S.-born students, but a larger proportion of those foreign-born students having sexual intercourse reported intercourse with injection drug users and without condoms. The authors suggested the need to provide HIV education in students' native languages and reliance on student peer educators to deliver the information. It is important to note, though not emphasized by the study investigators, that these relatively low rates of HIV knowledge and relatively high risk behaviors occurred among students in a public school setting located in a large, urban area, where multiple sources of information outside of the school system were not accessible or not accessed by the students. This underscores the need for clinicians and other health professionals to convey health information and screen for risk behavior when opportunities present themselves, such as when students present for an annual physical examination for school or for participation in team sports.

2.2. Chronic Disease

2.2.1. Cancer

Studies of various forms of cancer, including breast, colorectal, and stomach cancers, have found that the incidence of these cancers in immigrant populations to the U.S. tends to converge towards the rates seen in the U.S. and away from those in their countries of origin even within the first generation. For instance, Ziegler and colleagues (1993) reported from their study of breast cancer incidence rates from 1983 through 1987 among Chinese, Filipino, and Japanese women under the age of 55 that the incidence rates in the immigrating generation were higher than in their native countries and converged towards the even higher rates of similarly aged women in the San Francisco, Oakland, Los Angeles, and Oahu areas. A study of cancer mortality in Chinese immigrants to New York City, U.S.-born whites, and Chinese in Tianjin during the years 1986 through 1990 found that the standardized breast ratio for cancer mortality among the New York City Chinese was intermediate between the lower ratio among Chinese in Tianjin and the higher ratio among U.S.-born whites (Stellman and Wang, 1994).

Risk factors for colon cancer, which is the third most common cancer for both men and women worldwide (Coleman, *et al.*, 1993), may include diet, occupational exposures (Garabrant, *et al.*, 1984), and reduced physical activity (Tomatis, *et al.*, 1990). It is of note that although the rates of colon cancer are relatively low in Africa, Asia, and Latin America, they are increasing in places of rapid urbanization (Tomatis, *et al.*, 1990). A study of rates of colorectal cancer among Puerto Rican immigrants to Connecticut found that the rates among the immigrants were higher than those found in Connecticut, but lower than the rates observed in Puerto Rico (Polednak, 1992).

Rates of prostate cancer have been found to be higher in developed and developing countries, as compared to undeveloped countries (Tomatis, *et al.*, 1990). Incidence rates of prostate cancer among immigrants have often been found to be intermediate between those of the immigrants' native country and those of the U.S., like the rates for breast and colorectal cancer. Dunn (1975) reported from his study of the incidence rates of prostate cancer among Chinese and Japanese immigrants to the San Francisco Bay area that the rates were higher than U.S. rates, but lower than the rates in the countries of nativity.

While these migration studies have been used for hypotheses relating to the influence of genes and environment, one must question whether the apparently elevated risk of various forms of cancer among immigrants groups may be attributable, at least in part, to the significant gaps in health screening utilization by immigrants, including those living in urban areas. It was reported from an analysis of the 2000 National Health Interview Survey that women who had immigrated to the U.S. during the previous 10 years were among those least likely to have had a mammogram within the previous two years or a Pap test within the previous three years (Swan, *et al.*, 2003). Among men and women, recent immigrants were among those least likely to have had a fecal occult blood test or endoscopy within the recommended screening interval. A greater proportion of those surveyed who lived in Metropolitan Statistical Areas (MSAs) had had a mammogram in the two previous years compared to non-MSA residents. (An MSA is defined by the U.S. Office of Management and Budget (OMB) as a county or group of counties with at least one city of 50,000 or by the Census Bureau as an urbanized area of at least 50,000 with a metropolitan population of at least 100,000.)

Other studies similarly indicate less than optimal utilization of cancer screening procedures. In a study of 148 foreign-born women of latino ethnicities living in or around Washington, D.C., it was found that although 93% of the women reported ever having had a Pap smear, only 42% had had one in the year prior to the study and 71% had had one in the three years immediately preceding the study; 24% had not followed screening recommendations for cervical cancer (Fernandez, *et al.*, 1998). Among women over the age of 40, 62% had ever had a mammogram, but only 33% had followed the screening recommendations for their age (a mammogram once every year or two years for women ages 40 to 49, and once a year for women 50 years of age or older). Knowledge about screening recommendations was extremely low. The women offered various explanations for why they had not obtained a Pap smear or mammogram including embarrassment about the exam, fear of the test itself, fear of detecting cancer, cost, and the absence of any symptoms that they believed would indicate the existence of cancer. Women living in the U.S. for five to nine years were found to be more likely than recent immigrants to have complied with screening recommendations. It was hypothesized that this difference may have been related to additional barriers experienced by recent immigrants, including language, ineligibility for federal programs due to undocumented status, and competing priorities (Fernandez, *et al.*, 1998).

A study of 533 latina immigrants, 270 U.S.-born latinas, and 422 white women in Orange County, California reported similar findings. A smaller proportion of the immigrant women, compared to the U.S.-born latina and white women, had received a Pap test during the preceding three years. Those lacking health insurance and those of lower acculturation levels were least likely to have obtained Pap tests. The study additionally found that latina immigrants were more likely than members of the other groups to believe that early sexual intercourse, multiple sexual partners, and having a spouse with multiple sexual partners were risk factors for cervical cancer (Hubbell, *et al.*, 1996). However, they were also more likely to believe that the risk of cervical cancer was increased as a result of poor hygiene, having an abortion, fate, vaginal trauma, antibiotics, and having sex while menstruating.

Utilization of cancer screening tests has also been found to be low among Korean immigrants. A survey of 438 Korean-American women in Maryland found that English language proficiency was associated with ever having had a mammogram and the proportion of lifetime spent in the U.S. was associated with having a Pap test (Juan, *et al.*, 2000).

Relatively little attention has been devoted to an examination of the urban environment on the development of cancer and cancer mortality risk among immigrants. One cancer researcher explained the need for and difficulty of such investigations as follows:

> [I]nvestigation into differential exposures to fat-soluble environmental chemicals may reveal etiologies of breast and prostate cancers. In addition to diet and alcohol consumption, the environment is encountered through contact with skin and lungs. Numerous chemical compounds, such as hair dressings, skin lotions, and contaminated water come into contact with the skin. Determination of the possible relationship of a specific pollutant with incidence of cancer is difficult as pollution is usually a mix of chemicals. For example, ambient air content of benzene, which is associated with mammary cancer in animal models, is frequently higher than U.S. Environmental Protection Agency guidelines in urban areas; however, the effort to separate the putative effect from effects of other chemicals also found in the environment is daunting (Gordon, 1998).

2.2.2. *Childhood Chronic Disease*

Immigrant children may suffer from chronic disease existing prior to their arrival that may not have been diagnosed. A retrospective medical records review in Portland, Maine of 132 refugees aged 2 months through 18 years arriving from diverse countries to the U.S. found that, although the overall health status of many children appeared good, almost one-fifth of the children had hepatitis B surface antibody, anemia was detected in almost one-fifth of the children, and almost one-fifth of the children under the age of 6 had elevated blood lead levels (Hayes, *et al.*, 1998). The oral health of inner-city immigrant children from Central American countries has been found to be related to the recency of the mothers' arrival in the U.S. (Watson, *et al.*, 1999).

Other conditions among immigrants are not carried into the U.S. but may be associated with circumstances in the U.S. A study of asthma prevalence among Asian American school children in Boston found that rates of diagnosed and undiagnosed asthma among immigrant children in Boston found a lower rate of asthma among the children in Chinatown (Lee, *et al.*, 2003). It was hypothesized that the lower rate may have been a function of recent immigration and shorter duration to environmental exposures in the U.S. and/or reliance on traditional remedies to treat symptoms. A study of acute appendicitis cases over a one-year period in California and New York found that latino and Asian children had a higher likelihood of appendiceal rupture in California, while black children had a higher risk of rupture in New York (Guagliardo, *et al.*, 2003). The authors concluded that immigration and acculturation level may be risk factors for delayed emergency care, resulting in appendicitis rupture. The underlying reasons for the delay in emergency care were not explored.

2.2.3. *Mental Health*

A significant body of literature exists that addresses mental health issues among immigrant populations. This section presents findings relating to mental illness diagnoses among immigrants living in urban areas. However, published research often fails to indicate whether the immigrant-participants of a study are living in urban areas. In addition, the impact of migration to and/or residence in an urban area on immigrants' mental health or services utilization has not been well-explored and significant additional research is warranted. Unfortunately, basic questions remain unanswered: Does residence in urban areas, compared to suburban or rural living, increase the incidence of mental illness among immigrants due to the stresses of urban living? Is prognosis from a diagnosed mental illness worse due to difficulties associated with the complexities of accessing care in large urban areas, or improved because of access to a greater number of services? Does residence in urban ethnic enclaves serve to protect severely mentally ill persons from victimization or does it serve to isolate mentally ill immigrants still further due to stigmatization, alternative models to explain and/or treat behaviors, and a distrust of the western medical system?

2.2.3.a. Posttraumatic Stress Disorder. A number of studies have examined the occurrence of posttraumatic stress disorder and/or depression among immigrants residing in urban areas. However, these studies did not consider separately the impact of urban living on individuals' experience of symptoms. A study of 460 Vietnamese immigrants in Orange County, California found that 35% were experiencing symptoms of posttraumatic stress disorder (Yamamoto, *et al.*, 1989, cited in Shapiro, *et al.*, 1999). In comparison, the National Comorbidity Survey, based on a stratified, multi-stage, area probability sample of noninstitutionalized civilian individuals ages 15 to 54 in the U.S., reported a 12-month prevalence of 3.9% for PTSD (Kessler, *et al.*, 1999).

2.2.3.b. Depression. A recent study of 215 Vietnamese immigrants, also conducted in Orange County, California, found that the younger adults in the study were more likely to be highly acculturated and employed, but were more likely to be depressed and reported significantly more family conflict and greater dissatisfaction with life in the U.S. than were the older respondents (Shapiro, *et al.*, 1999). The relationship between acculturation level and depression, however, remains unclear. Yet another study conducted with 1,789 latinos in rural and urban counties in the Sacramento area of California found that the prevalence of depression was highest among immigrants and higher still among those who were least acculturated (Gonzalez, *et al.*, 2001). It would be helpful to the development of intervention programs to understand, for instance, if exposure to urban violence appeared to trigger the manifestations of PTSD or exacerbate depression.

2.2.3.c. Suicide. A study of suicides from 1970 through 1992 among persons aged 15 to 34 in California found that immigrants were underrepresented among the 32,928 deaths (Sorenson and Shen, 1996b). Firearms were the most common method of suicide among both immigrants and U.S.-born individuals, and the home was the most common site for suicide among both groups. Foreign-born latinos, who came primarily from Mexico, appeared to account for the apparent lower risk of suicide. They appeared to be at higher risk of suicide than their counterparts in Mexico, but at lower risk than their counterparts born in the U.S. (Sorenson and Shen, 1996b). It has been hypothesized that the tendency of immigrants to settle in ethnic enclaves in large cities, close to other immigrants as well as family and friends, may serve as a preventive factor for suicide by reducing social isolation and promoting contact with those with similar circumstances and a common language (Shen and Sorenson, 1998).

2.2.3.d. Mental Health Services. In general, reports indicate that mental health services are greatly underutilized by immigrant groups, including immigrants in urban areas. A study of 3,012 randomly sampled Mexican Americans in urban, small town, and rural areas of Fresno County, California reported that only 15.4% of the immigrant respondents found through study screening to have a mental disorder had utilized mental health services, compared to 37.5% of the U.S.-born study participants with such a diagnosis (Vega, *et al.*, 1999). Proportionately more mental health services were utilized by immigrants living in urban areas as compared to rural areas. The authors of the study hypothesized that the low utilization of mental services could be explained by reference to one or more factors requiring further investigation: cultural beliefs about mental health problems, ineffective and inappropriate therapies, a relative scarcity of Spanish-speaking therapists, difficulties accessing services, and/or the protective effects of family members and social network supports.

Urban areas, however, cannot be assumed to have the necessary services or networks to provide immigrants with the support that is needed. A study of loneliness in 110 elderly Korean immigrants in a large metropolitan area in the U.S. found that, despite long periods of residence in the U.S., the majority indicated a high level of identification with their ethnic group (Kim, 1999). Most continued to speak little English. The majority of respondents relied upon adult children, spouses, and Korean neighbors and church members for support and, importantly, did not identify any non-Korean individual as providing support. The women reported high levels of loneliness. Most of those individuals who respondents identified as providing support lived in the same housing complex, suggesting that the type of housing may influence social support and the degree of loneliness that is experienced (Kim, 1999).

2.2.4. *Substance Use*

A number of studies indicate that substance use may be a particular problem among immigrant latinos residing in urban areas. A study conducted in northern California found that compared to non-latino white students, latino students were both more likely to use alcohol, tobacco, marijuana, and other substances and to engage in various forms of violence and drunken driving (Brindis, *et al.*, 1995). Young Central American immigrants have been found to have higher alcohol and illegal substance use, particularly hallucinogens, marijuana, cocaine, and PCP, in comparison with other latinos (Tomasello, *et al.*, 1993). Kurtines and Szapocznik (1995) found from their work with immigrants in the Miami area that drug use may be related to difficulties with assimilation and the effects of immigration on family cohesiveness. Their research indicates that young people in immigrant families acculturate more rapidly and completely than older family members, resulting in the exacerbation of struggles by adolescent members for increasing independence, parental loss of traditional leadership roles, and reduced emotional support for the youths. These findings are consistent with those of several other studies that have similarly reported an association between acculturation and/or duration of U.S. residence and increased risk of substance use or dependence. It was found in a study of 3,012 participants of Mexican origin residing in rural and urban areas of Fresno

County, California that longer residence in the U.S. and acculturation as measured by language preference were significantly associated with a higher risk of drug abuse or dependence (Alderete, *et al.*, 2000). Another study found that increased duration of residence in New York City by Puerto Rican youth was associated with increased levels of substance use (Velez and Ungemack, 1989).

Although previous research indicated that latino girls often initiated their substance use through their relationships with men (Bullington, 1977), Moore (1994) found from her study of female adolescents from street-oriented families in barrio neighborhoods of Los Angeles female heroin-using gang members often are born into a "bad girl" label, to parents who have a history of gang membership and drug use. Moore hypothesized that traditionally conservative values generally protect girls from substance use, but girls born into a "bad-girl" label are disadvantaged by these same values, which result in their isolation from more positive social contact. Additionally, these traditional values may serve to increase the risk of substance use and gang membership among males, who are often allowed significant freedom to be on the streets.

These studies taken together suggest that longer residence in the U.S., higher levels of immigrant youth acculturation to U.S. culture, and parental ascription to traditional gender roles for their children may increase the risk of substance use among immigrant youth. Accordingly, it may be advisable to incorporate into prevention programs for immigrant youth components that address the stress associated with the immigration process, adjustment to U.S. society, changing family dynamics and family member roles resulting from immigration, the positive and negative aspects of traditional and nontraditional gender roles, and positive strategies for addressing these changes and accompanying stress.

2.3. Intentional and Unintentional Injury

A study by Sorenson and Shen (1996a) found that immigrants were overrepresented among the homicide deaths of 64,510 Californians during the years 1970 through 1992. Although immigrants comprised an estimated 17.4% of California's population during these years, they accounted for almost one-quarter of the state's homicide victims. The researchers found that non-latino white immigrants were 1.66 times as likely to die due to homicide as non-latino whites born in the U.S., while black immigrants were less likely than U.S.-born blacks to die due to homicide. Shen and Sorenson (1998) hypothesized that the increased risk of homicide among non-latino whites may be attributable to an increase in exposure, since many come from European countries that regulate access to firearms more strictly than does the U.S.

3.0. STRUCTURAL BARRIERS TO CARE

An analysis of data from the 1989 and 1990 National Health Interview Surveys and the 1989 Insurance and 1990 Family Resource Supplements found that, compared to native-born residents, foreign-born residents of the U.S. were more likely to be uninsured, less likely to have private insurance or Medicare, and somewhat more likely to have Medicaid (Thamer and Rinehart, 1998). Subsequent legal reforms at both the state and federal levels may have impacted even further immigrants' ability to obtain medical care due to a lack of health care coverage.

As an example of state-level legal changes, the ballot initiative known as Proposition 187 was passed by California voters in 1994. If implemented, this initiative would have barred undocumented individuals from using public benefits, including Medicaid. (Palinkas and Arciniega, 1999; Ziv and Talo, 1995). Following the passage of Proposition 187, the California Department of Health Services (California Department of Health Services, 1996) developed a special program in collaboration with the then-Immigration and Naturalization Service (INS) to demand that foreign-born noncitizen women returning to the U.S. through California ports of entry and airports repay Medicaid for any benefits they had used. [The INS was disestablished and its functions incorporated into the Bureau of Immigration and Customs Enforcement (BICE) of the Department of Homeland Security (DHS). For ease of reference, this chapter will continue to refer to the agency as the INS.] The women were advised that failure to repay these sums could result in a denial of their re-entry into the country. (California State Auditor, 1999; Wiles, *et al.*, 1997). However, no such requirement for repayment existed under either Medicaid law or immigration law. (Schlosberg and Wiley, 1998) These efforts to garner payments from the women exacerbated fears among even legal immigrants that their legitimate reliance on Medicaid benefits could lead to their characterization by INS as "public charges" and result in their exclusion or expulsion from the U.S. (Berk, *et al.*, 2000; Sun-Hee Park, *et al.*, 2000; Schlosberg and Wiley, 1998).

The implementation of various provisions of Proposition 187, including the cessation of prenatal care to undocumented mothers, was ultimately enjoined by various California courts. However, subsequent to voter passage in California of Proposition 187, the U.S. Congress passed the Personal Responsibility and Work Opportunity Reform Act (PRWORA) and the Illegal Immigration Reform and Immigrant Responsibility Act (IIRAIRA), which became effective on August 22, 1996. PRWORA created two classes of immigrants for the purpose of determining potential eligibility for specified publicly funded benefits, including nonemergency medical services, such as prenatal care. Immigrants who obtained their legal permanent resident status prior to August 22, 1996, the date of the law's enactment, were to be known as "qualified aliens." Individuals who obtained their legal permanent resident status after the date of enactment were to be classified as "nonqualified aliens." Pursuant to provisions in the legislation, most such individuals would be ineligible to receive publicly funded benefits, including Medicaid-funded services, for a period of five years following their receipt of their legal status.

Exceptions were created for certain classes of immigrants, including refugees, asylum seekers, immigrants with 40 quarters of qualifying work history, and noncitizens who had served in the U.S. military. Somewhat later, an exception was created for specified noncitizens whose need for publicly funded medical care was attributable to domestic violence. Nonqualified aliens would be subject to a deeming requirement, whereby the income of the U.S. citizen or permanent resident individual(s) who sponsored them for immigration would be considered in calculating eligibility for the benefit. In addition to the restrictions that were imposed on the receipt of benefits by certain legally immigrated individuals, the federal legislation provides that states may not provide nonemergency services to nonqualified aliens, including undocumented persons, without first passing new state legislation providing for the use of state funding for this coverage.

Findings relating to the effect of immigration and welfare reforms on immigrants' ability to access care have been inconsistent. Asch and colleagues (1998) reported that the passage of Proposition 187 in California may have discouraged immigrants in Los Angeles County from seeking screening and/or early treatment for tuberculosis infection. The passage of Proposition 187 was also found to be associated with a decrease in new walk-in patients at an ophthalmology clinic at a major public inner-city hospital in Los Angeles County (Marx et al.. 1996) and a decrease in patients at an STD clinic (Hu, *et al.*, 1995). However, Loue and colleagues (in press) found no statistically significant difference in time between onset of gynecological illness and seeking of care, or length of time between seeking care and receipt of care among women of Mexican ethnicity of varying immigration statuses in San Diego County. Another study of immigrants of various nationalities, languages, and immigration statuses in Cuyahoga County, Ohio similarly found no effect of the reform laws on immigrants' ability to access care (Loue, *et al.*, 2000). A high proportion of respondents in this latter study, however, had entered the U.S. as refugees and, as such, were not subject to the restrictions on their receipt of publicly funded health care.

4.0. PROMOTING HEALTH AND PREVENTING DISEASE

4.1. Creative Clinical Programs

A number of programs have been developed to deliver health care services to immigrants in urban areas that are particularly creative and responsive to the needs of their patient communities. Two of these will be highlighted here.

A new clinical service was developed in Washington State to permit pharmacists for an urban ambulatory pediatric clinic serving a large immigrant population to evaluate and treat children and adolescents aged 6 months to 19 years who were suffering from minor acute illnesses and to provide patients with bilingual education materials (Kalister, *et al.*, 1999). The program developed protocols and encounter forms for the evaluation of coughs and colds, fever, diaper rash, vomiting and diarrhea, and head lice. In addition, patient education materials addressing these topics were prepared and published in 8 different languages. Safety was assessed by reviewing the records of all patients who returned within one week of an encounter with the pharmacy, and through a telephone survey of the parents. Almost three-quarters of the 191 patients treated during the first year of the pharmacy service were immigrants. A retrospective review of 48 records found that the majority of the errors were attributable to failures of documentation; 7 reflected a failure to refer to a physician as mandated by the protocols that were in place. Parents were extremely satisfied with the quality and promptness of attention received through the pharmacy service.

The Indochinese Psychiatry Clinic (IPC) was founded in Boston in 1981 to meet the needs of Cambodian, Vietnamese, and Lao refugees suffering from trauma and trauma-related mental disorders (Allden, 1998). IPC strives to provide culturally sensitive mental health services in a framework that is acceptable to the patient families. As such, it has been cited as a model for refugee clinics in various other countries and has been lauded for its pioneering, bicultural work with traumatized refugees. Available services include intake and assessment, psychopharmacology, the coordination of medical, neurological, and neuropsychological evaluations and care, individual and group psychotherapy, family and patient psychoeducation, home-based care, crisis intervention, inpatient and partial hospital care; case management, community outreach, and a Cambodian shadow puppet project. Notably, the evaluation team includes a Western-trained social worker or nurse clinician, a bicultural mental health specialist who serves as the cultural and linguistic facilitator-cotherapist-case manager, and a psychiatrist. In addition, the facility provides 24-hour coverage in conjunction with a medical center emergency department.

4.2. Community-Based Health Programs

A number of successful community health education programs have been developed that specifically target urban immigrants. Only a few will be reviewed here, and readers are urged to consult other resources for additional examples.

Many programs that have specifically targeted immigrant communities have relied upon community health workers, or CHAs. CHAs are also referred to in the literature as "lay health advisors," "natural helpers," "village health workers," and "community health advocates." Health promotion and health delivery programs in many countries from which immigrants come have a tradition of reliance on CHAs. In much of Latin America, for instance, health information is delivered door-to-door by community *promotoras.* Like the CHAs in the U.S., they are community residents who receive special training to deliver health services and health education to members of their communities (Swider and McElmurry, 1990).

The Urban Immigrant Outreach Health Program in Chicago sought to identify underserved and immigrant families, assess their health needs, and link them to necessary health, social, and human services (McElmurry, *et al.*, 2003). Additional program objectives included the enhancement of immigrants' social networks and the strengthening of their capacity to influence the health-related environment in their communities. The bilingual CHAs worked closely with a community health nurse. Program data indicated that the project was successful in (1) reducing immigrant families' barriers to care by strengthening social networks within the communities through the establishment of immigrant support groups and volunteer efforts; and (2) in reducing the burden on local clinics by referring families to appropriate alternative services (McElmurry, *et al.*, 2003).

Urban latino immigrants were also the focus of Compañeros en Salud (Partners in Health), a church-based health promotion project that sought to reduce the risk of breast, cervical, and diet-related cancers (Candelaria, *et al.*, 1998). Like Project Salsa, Compañeros en Salud recruited and trained women to serve as CHAs, to hold a series of 11 classes on diet-related cancers, including breast cancer, and to provide referrals to community health services (Castro, *et al.*, 1995).

A San Diego County survey of 282 Asian Pacific Islander individuals from 11 different ethnic communities, many of whom were immigrants, found that more than half of the respondents could not identify even one medically accepted cause of HIV transmission (Loue, *et al.*, 1996). A community-based project, initially known as Project HAPI (Health for Asians and Pacific Islanders), utilized various culturally sensitive approaches to HIV education and outreach, including the dissemination of HIV-related information through community leaders and the development of decorated gift boxes to disguise condoms for public distribution. The project continues to exist beyond its initial funding and is now known as the Asian Pacific Islander Community AIDS Project (APICAP).

One of the most visible projects addressing the health of urban immigrants has been Project Salsa, which was constituted as a community-based nutritional health promotion project for the latino community on the U.S-Mexico border, just south of San Diego, California. This project, which was premised on components of social learning theory, consisted of chronic disease risk factor screening, cooking classes, a newspaper column, nutritional shopping instruction, school interventions for teachers, students, cafeteria staff, and parents; and community health advisor (CHA) training on breast feeding (Candelaria, *et al.*, 1998; Elder, *et al.*, 1998).

The Center for Immigrant Health in New York City, first established in 1989 as the New York Task Force on Immigrant Health, consists of a partnership between community members, practitioners, researchers, social scientists, policy makers, and health advocates. The Center trains community members to provide outreach, education, and screening relating to various topics, such as cancer and tuberculosis; conducts provider education in caring for immigrant and refugee populations, provides technical assistance to institutions; and conducts research related to immigrant and refugee populations (Center for Immigrant Health, n.d.).

These programs possess several common features that may have contributed to their success. First, as indicated above, each of these programs utilized the skills of community health advisors to disseminate information to the relevant communities. These CHAs knew the both the people and the geography of the communities and were known and trusted by members of the relevant communities. Each of the programs was founded on a theory to guide its development. For example, Project Salsa was premised on social learning theory, while Project HAPI relied on the health belief model. In addition to relying on trained CHAs for the delivery of services, these programs developed and worked closely with community advisory boards, consisting of representatives from the target communities. Each of these projects also attempted to leave something with the communities after the cessation of the initial funding, demonstrating a longer-term commitment to the communities.

5.0. CONCLUSION

The majority of individuals coming to the U.S. from other countries, whether temporarily or permanently, settle in urban areas. Many of these individuals may bring with them health conditions or health related issues that are not familiar to U.S. physicians due to their inexperience in these areas and/or the rarity of these conditions in the U.S., such as diagnosis of falciparum malaria, for instance. It is critical that appropriate screening programs be developed to detect disease at its earliest stage in order to maximize treatment opportunities and to minimize both the possibility of transmission to others and the development of preventable disease sequelae. Additionally, urban physicians and institutions must maximize training in order to detect the signs and symptoms of disease and conditions that may be more rare in U.S. populations.

Many urban immigrants, like non-urban immigrants, may confront difficulties in accessing care due to language differences, lack of physician training, and lack of health insurance, among other factors. These difficulties may be exacerbated by laws that require or threaten the reporting of individuals' immigration status to authorities or that specifically prohibit the provision of care to those without specific forms of documentation. Such provisions have been found to result in delays in seeking care. The potential for disastrous consequences through further disease transmission, such as in the case of tuberculosis, is enhanced in urban venues due to the circumstances of urban living, such as contact with large numbers of persons in relatively confined areas.

Despite the fact that most immigrants reside in urban areas, relatively little is known about their health status as compared with non-urban immigrants or non-immigrant urban residents, the effect of urban living on their health status and health access, and the interaction of urban life with the effects of immigrant status. A study of the physical activity of latina immigrants in North Carolina provides a good example of the kind of research that could be conducted to address such issues. This study found that only 37% of the 671 participants met vigorous or moderate recommendations for physical activity (Evenson, *et al.*, 2003). Urban conditions, such as traffic, street lighting, unattended dogs, and the presence or absence of sidewalks, were found to be unrelated to whether women exercised. However, knowing people who exercised, seeing people exercise in the neighborhood, and having lived in a community with places to exercise were associated with increased physical activity.

Future research should similarly consider the effect of urban conditions on specific health, illness, and disease utilization in immigrant populations. Urban conditions to be examined include, but are not limited to, community characteristics that may affect utilization of health services, such as the availability of a transportation services and the location of health services; the availability and affordability of ancillary health care services, such as interpreter and translation services; and the availability and location of health care services sensitive to particular cultural and linguistic populations. Local laws and governmental or institutional policies must also be examined to determine their effects, if any, on access to and utilization of care. For instance, cooperation between local law enforcement and federal immigration authorities in the detection of undocumented individuals may deter immigrants from utilizing public transportation, potentially resulting in a decrease in utilization of clinic services. The provision of local government-funded care to immigrants may increase service utilization despite restrictive federal legislation seeking to limit its availability through the use of federal funds. Urban conditions, such as crime rates, population density, pollution, and working conditions also require examination for their impact on the incidence of specific diseases, health status, and disease progression and prognosis.

REFERENCES

Adair, R., and Nwaneri, O. (1999). Communicable disease in African immigrants in Minneapolis. *Arch. Intern. Med.* 159(1): 83–85.

Alderete, E., Vega, W.A., Kolody, B., and Aguilar-Gaxiola, S. (2000). Effects of time in the United States and Indian Ethnicity on DSM-III-R psychiatric disorders among Mexican Americans in California. *J. Nervous Mental Disease* 188: 90–100.

Allden, K. (1998). The Indochinese Psychiatry Clinic: Trauma and refugee mental health treatment in the 1990s. *Journal of Ambulatory Care Management* 21(2): 30–38.

Anon. (2002). Increase in African immigrants and refugees with tuberculosis—Seattle-King County, Washington, 1998-2001. *MMWR.* 51(39): 882–883.

Asch, S., Leake, B., Abderson, R., and Gelberg, L. (1998). Why do symptomatic patients delay obtaining care for tuberculosis? *American Journal of Respiratory and Critical Care Medicine* 157: 1244–1248.

Asch, S., Leake, B., and Genlberg, L. (1994). Does fear of immigration authorities deter tuberculosis patients from seeking care? *Western Journal of Medicine* 161(4): 373–376.

Berk, M.L., Schur, C.L., Chavez, L.R., and Frankel, M. (2000). Health care use among undocumented Latino immigrants. *Health Affairs* 19: 51–64.

Bertolli, J. (1993). Prevention and control of sexually transmitted diseases among migrant farmworkers. *Public Health Rep.* 108: 177–178.

Billeaud, J. (2004). Illegal immigrants face hardships in houses run by smugglers. The San Diego Union-Tribune, March 16. (May 14, 2004.); http://signonsandiego.com.

Bodnar, J. (1987). *The Transplanted: A History of Immigrants in Urban America.* Indiana University Press, Bloomington, Indiana.

Brammeier, M., Gould, G., Miller, J., Chow, J., Lighthall, D., and Bolan, G. (2002). Sexually transmitted disease risk among California agricultural workers: results from a population-based survey (abstract no. 131). Presented at the National STD Prevention Conference, San Diego, California.

Brindis, C., Wolfe, A.L., McCarter, V., Ball, S., and Starbuck-Morales, S. (1995). The associations between immigrant status and risk-behavior in Latino adolescents. *J. Adolescent Health* 17:99–105.

Bullington, B. (1997). *Heroin Use in the Barrio.* Lexington Books, Lexington, Massachusetts.

California Department of Health Services. (1996). Adequacy of Prenatal Care Utilization—California 1989–1994. *MMWR.* 45: 655.

California State Auditor. (1999). *Department of Health Services: Use of Its Port of Entry Fraud Detection Program Is No Longer Justified.* California Bureau of State Audits, Sacramento, California.

Candelaria, J., Campbell, N., Lyon, G., Elder, J.P., and Villaseñor, A. (1988). Strategies for health education: Community-based methods. In: Loue, S. (Ed.). *Handbook of Immigrant Health.* pp. 587–606. New York: Plenum Press.

Cantwell, M.F., Snider, D.E., Cauthen, G.M., and Onorato, I.M. (1994). Epidemiology of tuberculosis in the United States, 1985 through 1992. *JAMA.* 272: 535–539.

Castro, F.G., Elder, J., Coe, K., Tafoya-Barraza, H.M., Moratto, S., Campbell, N., and Talavera, G. (1995). Mobilizing churches for health promotion in Latino communities: Compañeros en Salud. *Journal of National Cancer Monographs* 18: 127–135.

Center for Immigrant Health. (n.d.) About Us. (August 17, 2004); http://www.med.nyu.edu/cih/about/index.html.

Center for Disease Control and Prevention. (1998). 1997 Surveillance Slides. Center for Disease Control and Prevention, October 11, 2004; http://www.cdc.gov/nchstp/tb/pubs/slidesets/surv/surv1997/html/surv_slides.htm

Centers for Disease Control and Prevention. (1992). HIV infection, syphilis, and tuberculosis screening among migrant farm workers Florida, 1992. *MMWR.* 41: 723–724.

Coleman, M.P., Esteve, J., Damieck, P., Arslan, A., and Renard, H. (1993). *Trends in Cancer Incidence and Mortality* (IARC Scientific Publications No. 121, 1-806). World Health Organization and the International Agency for Research on Cancer, Lyons, France.

Daniels, R. (1990). *Coming to America: A History of Immigration and Ethnicity in American Life.* Harper, New York.

Dunn, J.E. (1975). Cancer epidemiology in populations of the United States—with emphasis on Hawaii and California—and Japan. *Cancer Research* 35(11, Pt. 2): 3240–3245.

Editorial. (1997). The abuse of illegal immigrants. *New York Times,* July 22, (May 14, 2004); http://www.eco.utexas.edu/~archive/chiapas95/1997. 07/msg00332.html.

Editorial Desk. (1993). Immigrants infected with HIV, New York Times, February 20, sec. 1, p. 18, col. 1. (June 18, 2004); http://web.lexis-nexis.com/universe.

Eichenberger, R.K., and Shandera, W.X. (1999). The public health care of Central Americans in Houston. *Texas Medicine* 95(6): 55–62.

Elder, J.P., Campbel, N., Candelaria, J.I., Talavera, G.A., Mayer, J.A., Mreno, C., Medel, Y.R., and Lyons, G.K. (1998). Project Salsa: Development and institutionalization of a nutritional health promotion project in a Latino community. *Am. J. Health Promotion* 12(6): 391.

Enchautegui, M.E. (1993). Immigration impact on local employment and ethnic minorities. In N. Carmon. (ed.), *Immigrants: Liability or Asset.* Haifa: The Center for Urban and Regional Studies, Technion—Israel Institute of Technology.

Evenson, K.R., Sarmiento, O.L., Tawney, K.W., Macon, L., and Ammerman, A.S. (2003). Personal, social, and environmental correlates of physical activity in North Carolina Latina immigrants. *Am. J. Prev. Med.* 25(3Si): 77–85.

Fernandez, M.E., Tortolero-Luna, G., and Gold, R.S. (1998). Mammography and Pap test screening among low-income foreign-born Hispanic women in the USA. *Cad. Saude Publica Rio de Janeiro.* 14(Sup 3): 133–147.

Findley, S.E., Irigoyen, M., and Schulman, A. (1999).Children on the move and vaccination coverage in a low-income, urban Latino population. *Am. J. Public Health* 89(11): 1728–1731.

Garabrant, D.H., Peters, J.M., Mack, T.M., and Bernstein, L. (1984). Job activity and colon cancer risk. *Am. J. Epid.* 119 (6):1005–1014.

Gonzalez, H.M., Haan, M.N., and Hinton, L. (2001). Acculturation and the prevalence of depression in older Mexican Americans: Baseline results of the Sacramento area Latino study on aging. *J. Am. Geriatr. Soc.* 49: 948–953.

Gordon, N. (1998). Cancer. In: Loue, S. (ed.). *Handbook of Immigrant Health.* Plenum Press, New York, pp. 389-406.

Granich, R.M., Zuber, P.L.F., McMillan, M., Cobb, J.D., Burr, J., Sfakianaki, E.D., Fussell, M., and Binkin, N.J. (1998). Tuberculosis among foreign-born residents of southern Florida, 1995. *Public Health Rep.* 113: 552–113.

Greenhouse, S. (2002). Migrant-camp operators face forced labor charges, *New York Times,* June 21, (May 14, 2004); http://www.flsny.org.

Guagliardo, M.F., Teach, S.J., Huang, Z.J., Chamberlain, J.M., and Joseph, J.G. (2003). Racial and ethnic disparities in pediatric appendicitis rupture rate. *Academic Emergency medicine: Official Journal of the Society for Academic Emergency Medicine* 10(11): 1218–1227.

Hayes, E.B., Talbot, S.B., Matheson, E.S., Pressler, H.M., Hanna, A.B., and McCarthy, C.A. (1998). Health status of pediatric refugees in Portland, Maine. *Archives of Pediatric and Adolescent Medicine* 152: 564–568.

Henderson, S.O., Mody, T., Groth, D.E., Moore, J.J., and Newton, E. (1998). The presentation of tetanus in an emergency department. *J. Emerg. Med.* 16(5): 705–708.

Hingson, R.W., Strunin, L., Grady, M., Strunk, N., Carr, R., Berlin, B., and Craven D.E. (1991). Knowledge about HIV and behavioral risks of foreign-born Boston public school students. *Am. J. Public Health* 81(12): 1638–1641.

Houston, R.K., Harada, N., and Makinodan, T. (2002). Development of a culturally sensitive educational intervention program to reduce the high incidence of tuberculosis among foreign-born Vietnamese. *Ethn. Dis.* 7(4): 255–265.

Hu, Y., Donovan, S., Ford, W., Courtney, K., Rulnick, S., and Richwald, S. (1995). The impact of Proposition 187 on the use of public health services by undocumented immigrants in Los Angeles County [abstract 1008]. *123rd Meeting of the American Public Health Association Meeting.*

Hubbell, F.A., Chavez, L.R., Mishra, S.I., and Burciaga Valdez, R. (1996). Beliefs about sexual behavior and other predictors of Papanicolaou smear screening among Latinas and Anglo women. *Arch. Int. Med.* 156: 2353–2358.

Immigration and Naturalization Service. (2000). *INS Statistical Yearbook.* Washington, D.C.

Juan, H.S., Choi, Y., and Kim, M.T. (2000). Cancer screening among Korean-American women. *Cancer Detection and Prevention* 24(6): 589–601.

Kalister, H., Newman, R.D., Read, L., Walters, C., Hrachovec, J., and Graham, E.A. (1999). Pharmacy-based evaluation and treatment of minor illnesses in a culturally diverse pediatric clinic. *Archives of Pediatric and Adolescent Medicine* 153: 73–735.

Kang, E., Rapkin, B.D., Springer, C., and Kim, J.H. (2003). The "demon plague" and access to care among Asian undocumented immigrants living with HIV disease in New York City. *Journal of Immigrant Health* 5(2): 49–58.

Kessler, R.C., Zhao, S., Katz, S.J., Kouzis, A.C., Frabk, RG., Edlund, M., and Leaf, P. (1999). Past-year use of outpatient services for psychiatric problems in the National Comorbidity Survey. *Am. J. Psychiatry* 156(1): 115–123.

Kim, O. (1999). Predictors of loneliness in elderly Korean immigrant women living in the United States of America. *J. Adv. Nurs.* 29: 1082–1088.

Kurtines, W.M., and Szapocznik, J. (1995). Cultural competence in assessing Hispanic youths and families: Challenges in the assessment of treatment needs and treatment evaluation for Hispanic drug-abusing adolescents. In: Rahdert, E., and Czechowicz, D. (Eds.), *Adolescent Drug Abuse: Clinical Assessment and Therapeutic Interventions.* National Institute on Drug Abuse Research Monograph 156. Rockville, Maryland: National Institutes of Health, U.S. Department of Health and Human Services, pp. 172–189.

Kyiacou, D.N., Spira, A.M., Talan, D.A., and Mabey, D.C.W. (1996). Emergency department presentation and misdiagnosis of imported falciparum malaria. *Ann. Emer. Med.* 27(6):696– 699.

Lee. T., Brugge. D., Francis. C., and Fisher, O. (2003). Asthma prevalence among inner-city Asian American schoolchildren. *Public Health Rep.* 118: 215–220.

Lifson, A.R., Thai, D., O'Fallon, A., Mills, W.A., and Hang, K. (2002). Prevalence of tuberculosis, hepatitis B virus, and intestinal parasitic infections among refugees to Minnesota. *Public Health Rep.* 117: 69–77.

Lipson, J.G., Omidian, P.A., and Paul, S.M. (1995). Afghan health education project: A community survey. *Public Health Nurs.* 12: 143–150.

Lou, S., Cooper, M., Lloyd, L.S. (2004). Welfare and Immigration Reform and Use of Prenatal Care among Women of Mexican Ethnicity in San Diego, California. *Journal of Immigrant Health* In Press.

Loue, S., Faust, M., and Bunce, A. (2000). The effect of immigration and welfare reform legislation on immigrants' access to health care, Cuyahoga and Lorain Counties. *Journal of Immigrant Health* 2: 23-30.

Loue, S., Lloyd, L.S., and Loh, L. (1996). HIV prevention in U.S. Asian Pacific islander communities: An innovative approach. *Journal of Health Care for the Poor and Underserved* 7(4): 364–376.

Luna, C., and Tran, M. (2004). Arrest in sex slave case. *Los Angeles Times*, Feb. 13 (May 14, 2004); http://www.iabolish. com/news/press-coverage/2004/lat02-13-04.htm.

Makinodan, T., Liu, J., Yuno, E., Knowles, L.K., Davidson, P.T., and Harada, N. (1999). Profile of tuberculosis among foreign-born Asians residing in Los Angeles County, California, 1985-1994. *Asian American Pacific Islander Journal of Health* 7(1): 38–46.

Maltoni, C., Cilibarti, A., Cotti, G., Conti, B., and Belpoggi, F. (1989). Benzene, an experimental multi potential carcinogen: Results of a long-term bioassays performed at the Bologna Institute of Oncology. *Environmental Health Perspectives* 82: 109–124.

Marcuse, P. (1996). Of walls and immigrant enclaves. In: Carmon, N. (ed.), *Immigration and Integration in Post-Industrial Societies: Theoretical Analysis and Policy-Related Research*. St. Martin's Press, Inc, New York, pp. 86–186.

Marx, J.L., Thach, A.B., Grayson, G., Lowry, L.P., Lopez, P.F., and Lee, P.P. (1996). The effects of California Proposition 187 on an ophthalmology clinic utilization at an inner-city urban hospital. *Ophthalmology* 103: 847–851.

McCormick, E., and Zamora, J.H. (2000). Slave trade still alive in US: Exploited women, children trafficked from poorest nations. *San Francisco Examiner*, Feb. 13, (May 14, 2004); http://www.siptn.org/Kentucky/slavetrade2.html.

McElmurry, B.J., Park, C.G., and Buseh, A.G. (2003). The nurse-community health advocate team for urban immigrant primary health care. *Journal of Nursing Scholarship* 35(3): 275–281.

McFadden, R.D. (1993). Smuggled to New York: The overview—7 die as crowded immigrant ship grounds off Queens. *New York Times*. June 7, 142: 1.

Metropolitan Desk. (1993). Fear and intimidation slow identification of six bodies. *New York Times*. September 5, 142: 51.

Moore, J. (1994). The chola life course: Chicana heroin users and the barrio gang. *International Journal of the Addictions* 29:1115–1126.

Office of Immigration Statistics. (2003). *Fiscal Year 2002 Yearbook of Immigration Statistics*, (May 14, 2004); http://uscis.gov.

Office of immigration Statistics. (2002). *Fiscal Year 2002 yearbook of Immigration Statistics* October 11, 2004; http://uscis.gov/graphics/shared/aboutus/ statistics/IMM02yrbk/IMMExcel/table8.xls

Organista, K.C., and Balls Organista, P. (1997). Migrant laborers and AIDS in the United States: A review. *AIDS Education and Prevention* 9: 83–93.

Organista, K.C., Balls Organista, P., Garcia de Alba, G.J.E., Castillo Moran, M.A., and Carillo, H. (1996). AIDS and condom-related knowledge, beliefs, and behaviors in Mexican migrant laborers. *Hispanic Journal Behavioral Science* 18: 392–406.

Pacenti, J. (1998). Enslaved women in Florida ring. *Laredo Morning Times* February 25, 1998: 2A, col 3.

Palinkas, L.A., and Arciniega, J.L. (1999). Immigration reform and the health of Latino immigrants in California. *J. Immigr. Health* 1:19–30.

Paz-Bailey, G., Teran, S., Levine, W., and Markowitz, L.E. (2004). Syphilis outbreak among Hispanic immigrants in Decatur, Alabama. *Sex. Transm. Dis.* 31(1): 20–25.

Polednak, A.P. (1992). Cancer incidence in the Puerto Rican-born population of Connecticut. *Cancer* 70(5): 1172–1176.

Rangel, M.C., Sales, R.M., and Valeriano, E.N. (1999). Rubella outbreaks among Hispanics in North Carolina: Lessons learned from a field investigation. *Ethn. Dis.* 9(2): 230–236.

Rodriguez, B. (2002). 6 accused in migrant slavery operation: Suspects deny charges involving workers sent to NY farms. *Dallas Morning News*, June 26, (May 14, 2004); http://www.flsny.org.

Ruiz, J.D., Da Valle, L., Junghkei, M., Mobed, K., and Lopez, R. (1997). *Seroprevalence of HIV and syphilis and assessment of risk behaviors among migrant and seasonal farmworkers in Northern California*. Office of AIDS, California Department of Health Services, Sacramento, California.

Rumbaut, R.G., Chavez, L.R., Moser, R.J., Pickwell, S.M., and Wishnik, S.M. (1988). The politics of migrant health care: A comparative study of Mexican immigrants and Indochinese refugees. *Research in the Sociology of Health Care* 7: 143–202.

Schlosberg, C., and Wiley, D. (1998). *The Impact of INS Public Charge Determinations on Immigrant Access to Health Care*. Washington, D.C.: National Health Law Program and National Immigration Law Center, May. (April 25, 2002); http://healthlaw.org/pubs/19980522publiccharge.html.

Schulte, J.M., Maloney, S., Aronson, J., San Gabriel, P., Zhou, J., and Saiman, L. (2002). Evaluating acceptability and completeness of overseas immunization records of internationally adopted children. *Pediatrics* 109(2).

Sennett, R. (1992). The origins of the modern ghetto. Paper delivered at Arden House Urban Forum on Place and Right. Quoted in P. Marcuse, Of walls and immigrant enclaves. In: Carmon, N. (Ed.). *Immigration and Integration in Post-Industrial Societies: Theoretical Analysis and Policy-Related Research.* St. Martin's Press, Inc., New York, pp. 86—186.

Shapiro, J., Douglas, K., de la Rocha, O., Radecki, S., Vu, C., and Dinh, T. (1999). Generational differences in psychosocial adaptation and predictors of psychological distress in a population of recent Vietnamese immigrants. *J. Community Health* 24(2): 95–113.

Shen, H., and Sorenson, S.B. (1998). Violence and injury among immigrants: An epidemiological review. In S. Loue (Ed.). *Handbook of Immigrant Health.* Plenum Press, New York, pp. 545—565.

Solitar, B.M., Lozada, C.J., Tseng, C.E., Lowe, A.M., Krajewski, W.M., Blanchard, K., Pillinger, M., and Weissman, G. (1998). Reiter's syndrome among Asian shipboard immigrants: The case of the *Golden Venture. Seminars in Arthritis and Rheumatism* 27: 293–300.

Sorenson, S.B., and Shen, H. (1996a). Homicide risk among immigrants in California, 1970 through 1992. *Am. J. Public Health* 86: 97–100.

Sorenson, S.B., and Shen, H. (1996b). Youth suicide trends in California: An examination of immigrant and ethnic group risk. *Suicide and Life-Threatening Behavior* 26: 143–154.

Stellman, S.D., and Wang, Q.S. (1994). Cancer mortality in Chinese immigrants to New York City: Comparison with Chinese in Tianjin and with United States-born Whites. *Cancer* 73(4): 1270–1275.

Strine, T.W., Barker, L.E., Mokdad, A.H., Luman, E.T., Sutter, R.W., and Chu, S.Y. (2002). Vaccination coverage of foreign-born children 19 to 35 months of age: Findings from the National Immunization Survey, 1999-2000. *Pediatrics* 110(2).

Sun-Hee Park, L., Sarnoff, R., Bender, C., and Korenbrot, C. (2000). Impact of recent welfare and immigration reform on use of Medicaid for prenatal care by immigrants in California. *J. Immigr. Health* 2:5–22.

Swan, J., Breen, N., Coates, R.J., Rimer, B.K., and Lee, N.C. (2003). Progress in cancer screening practices in the United States: Results from the 2000 National Health Interview Survey. *Cancer* 97: 1528–1540.

Swider, S.M., and McElmurry, B.J. (1990). A women's health perspective in primary health care: A nursing and community health worker demonstration project in urban America. *Family and Community Health* 13(3): 1–17.

Thamer, M., and Rinehart, C. (1998). Public and private insurance of US foreign-born residents: Implications of the 1996 welfare reform law. *Ethn. Health* 3(1,2): 19–29.

Tomasello, A., Tyler, F.B., Tyler, S.L., and Zhang, Y. (1993). Psychosocial correlates of drug use among Latino youth leading autonomous lives. *Int. J. Addictions* 28: 435–450.

Tomatis, L., Aitio, A., Day, NE., Heseltine, E., Kaldo, J., Miller, A.B., Parkin, D.M., and Riboli, E. (1990). *Cancer: Causes, Occurrence, and Control.* (IARC Scientific Publication No. 100). Lyons, France: World Health Organization and International Agency for Research on Cancer.

Truong, D.H., Hedemark, L.L., Mickman, J.K., Mosher, L.B, Dietrich, S.E., and Lowry, P.W. (1997). Tuberculosis among Tibetan immigrants from India and Nepal in Minnesota, 1992-1995. *JAMA.* 277(9): 735–738.

United States Census Bureau. (2002). News Release, February.

United States Department of Justice. (2003). Leader of Ukrainian alien smuggling operation sentenced to 17-1/2 years in federal prison. Press release, March 10, (May 14. 2004); http://www.usdoj.gov/usao/cac/pr2003/041.htm.

Vega, W.A., Kolody, B., Aguilar-Gaxiola, S., and Catalano, R. (1999). Gaps in service utilization by Mexican Americans with mental health problems. *Am. J. Psychiatry* 156: 928–934.

Velez, C.N., and Ungemack, J.A. (1989). Drug use among Puerto Rican youth: An exploration of generational status differences. *Soc. Sci. Med.* 29: 779–789.

Watson, M.R., Horowitz, A.M., Garcia, I., and Canto, M.T. (1999). Caries conditions among 2-5-year old immigrant Latino children related to parents' oral health knowledge, opinions and practices. *Community Dent. Oral Epidemiol.* 27: 8–15.

Weis, S.E., Moonan, P.K., Pogoda, J.M., Turk, L., King, B., Freeman-Thompson, S., and Burgess, G. (2001). Tuberculosis in the foreign-born population of Tarrant County, Texas by immigration status. *American Journal of Respiratory Critical Care Medicine* 164: 953–957.

Wiles, M.H., Wright, D.F., Parks, M, and Clayton, J. (1997). Abuse by officials at the border. *Los Angeles Times.* Dec. 23; B6 (editorial).

Wong, W., Tambis, J.A., Hernandez, M.T., Chaw, J.K., and Klausner, J.D. (2003). Prevalence of sexually transmitted diseases among Latino immigrant day laborers in an urban setting—San Francisco. *Sex. Transm. Dis.* 30(8): 661– 663.

Yamada, S., Caballero, J., Matsunaga, D.S., Agustin, G., and Magana, M. (1999). Attitudes towards tuberculosis in immigrants from the Philippines to the United States. *Fam. Med.* 31(7):477-482.

Yamamoto, J., Niem, T.T., Nguyen, D., and Snodgrass, L. (1989). Post traumatic stress disorder in Vietnamese refugees. Unpublished manuscript, University of California Los Angeles, School of Medicine, Neuropsychiatric Institute.

Ziegler, R.G., Hoove, R.N., Pike, M.C., Hildesheim, A., Nomura, A.M.Y., Wes, D.W., Wu-Williams, A.H., Kolonel, L.N., Horn-Ross, P.L., Rosenthal, J.F., and Hyer, M.B. (1993). Migration patterns and breast cancer risk in Asian-American women. *J. Natl. Cancer Inst.* 85: 1819-1827.

Ziv, A., and Talo, B. (1995). Denial of care to illegal immigrants. *N. Engl. J. Med.* 332: 1095–1098.

Zuber, P.L.F., McKenna, M.T., Binkin, N.J., Onorato, I. M., and Castro, K. (1997). Long-term risk of tuberculosis among foreign-born people in the United States. *JAMA.* 278: 304-307.

Chapter 7

The Urban Environment, Drug Use, and Health

Danielle Ompad and Crystal Fuller

"The heroin habit is essentially a matter of city life . . ."
Pierce Bailey in "The Heroin Habit." *The New Republic,* 1916

1.0. INTRODUCTION

Drug use incorporates a wide variety of drugs, including licit (i.e. tobacco and alcohol) and illicit drugs (e.g. marijuana, hallucinogens, cocaine, heroin, etc.). Both licit and illicit drugs result in substantial morbidity and mortality despite concerted efforts aimed at minimizing or preventing the use of these drugs. Drug use results in significant societal economic costs; addiction costs the U.S. approximately $400 billion in health care costs, lost worker productivity, and crime (McGinnis and Foege, 1999).

In 2000, most (80.3%) U.S. residents lived in metropolitan areas (U.S. Census Bureau, 2000) and most studies of drug abuse have been conducted in urban areas. Thus, our current understanding of drug abuse reflects primarily an urban perspective and historically, drug use has been conceptualized as an urban problem (Bailey, 1916; Hunt and Chambers, 1976; Kleber, 1994; Storr, *et al.*, 2004). While there has been some focus in the literature on illicit drug use in rural areas (National Institute on Drug Abuse, 1997; Sarkar, *et al.*, 1997), in this chapter we will focus on use of illicit drugs and its contextual determinants in urban settings. We will work from the theoretical framework proposed by Galea, Ahern and Vlahov (Galea, *et al.*, 2003) where the social and physical environment, along with structural considerations such as availability of social services, municipal structures and national and international policies (e.g. the "War on Drugs"), will be considered. We will examine the occurrence of drug use and its associated morbidity and mortality within the context of multiple levels of influence including individual, network, and neighborhood influences. This chapter begins with a review of the epidemiology of drug use in which we focus on the prevalence and incidence of drug use within and between cities. We will then discuss key characteristics of the urban environment that are associated with drug use in urban settings, and consider the medical consequences of drug use and the extent to which the urban environment can affect these outcomes. Finally, we will highlight effective prevention and treatment programs that have been implemented in urban areas.

2.0. DRUG USE EPIDEMIOLOGY

Before examining the role of the urban environment in the occurrence and consequences of drug use, we begin with a brief overview of the epidemiology of drug use. In the U.S., there are a number of surveillance and survey efforts to estimate prevalence of drug use. Two important sources include the National Survey on Drug Use and Health (NSDUH) and Monitoring the Future (MTF); both are based on probability samples of U.S. residents outside of institutions (including correctional facilities) and thus likely represent conservative estimates. Furthermore, as the majority of Americans live in urban areas, findings from these studies may approximate the current situation in U.S. urban areas.

2.1. Prevalence

According to the 2002 NSDUH, approximately 108 million persons over age 12 had used an illicit drug in their lifetime and in the U.S. 35.1 million had used an illicit drug in the past year (Substance Abuse and Mental Health Services Administration and Office of Applied Studies, 2003b). The most frequently reported illicit drug used was marijuana (40.4% reported lifetime use, 11.0% past year use). In terms of lifetime use, cocaine and hallucinogens were also quite prevalent (14.4% and 14.6%, respectively), while amphetamines (9.0%) and heroin (1.6%) were less so.

In 2003, drug use was especially prevalent among adolescents. According to 2003 estimates from the MTF Study, a study of public and private high school and middle school students in the U.S., 51.1% of high school seniors had used an illicit drug in their lifetime and 39.3% had used an illicit drug in the last year (Johnston, *et al.*, 2004). In terms of lifetime use, the most commonly reported illicit drug was marijuana (46.1%), followed by amphetamines (14.4%), narcotics other than heroin (13.2%; i.e., oxycontin, percocet, vicodin, etc.), inhalants (11.2%) and hallucinogens (10.6%).

Drug use is a global phenomenon. The United Nations Office on Drugs and Crime provides estimates of annual prevalence of drug use among individuals aged 15 and older in countries that have estimates available (United Nations and Office on Drugs and Crime, 2003). For example, the annual prevalence of marijuana use in Central and South America ranges between 0.1% in Belize to 9.2% in El Salvador as compared to 9.3% in the U.S. Marijuana prevalence in African countries range from 0.01% in Cote d'Ivoire to 21.5% in Ghana; and the highest prevalence estimates are from Papua New Guinea and the Federated States of Micronesia (29.5% and 29.1%, respectively). These estimates illustrate both the enormous variability in drug use from country to country and the global burden of drug use.

2.2. Incidence

The 2002 NSDUH also provided estimates of drug use incidence, or the number of new users of illicit drugs during a given year in the U.S. (Figure 1) (Substance Abuse and Mental Health Services Administration and Office of Applied Studies, 2003b). Incidence of marijuana has ebbed and flowed over the past four decades. Between 1965 and 1973, the estimated number of marijuana initiates rose from 0.8 million to 3.6 million. After approximately five years of stable initiation rates, the number of initiates declined from almost 3.5 million in 1978 to 1.6 million in 1990, then again rose to 2.8 million in 1995. Estimates of the number of initiates ranged between 2.5 and 3.0 million per year between 1995 and 2001.

Trends in incidence within the U.S. vary over time for different drugs. Cocaine hit a peak of 1.7 million new users in 1981 and slowly declined through the 1980s and early 1990s. In the mid-1990s, incidence again began to rise resulting in a recent estimate of almost 1.2 million new users in 2001. The number of new hallucinogen users was stable throughout the 1970s and 1980s, but increased throughout 1990s growing from approximately 713,000 new users in 1989 to 1.6 million new users in 2001. In contrast, methamphetamine and heroin incidence has remained relatively stable during the past decade.

2.3. Polydrug Use

Polydrug use is a common occurrence that is generally not assessed in national datasets which instead tend to report on drugs separately. Compared to using specific drugs by themselves, polydrug use has been associated with more traffic accidents (Bo, *et al.*, 1975), increased toxicity (Hearn, *et al.*, 1991), and higher risk of death from overdose (Coffin, *et al.*, 2002a). Data are consistent in showing that polydrug use in general contributes substantially to overdose mortality. Up to 90% of overdoses presenting to an emergency department in Switzerland were shown to be positive for multiple drugs (Cook, *et al.*, 1998) and 84% of cocaine overdose deaths in Spain also involved heroin (Lora-Tamayo, *et al.*, 1994). Among injection drug users (IDUs), benzodiazepine use was associated with increased risk of both death from all causes and death preceding AIDS diagnosis (Van Haastrecht, *et al.*, 1996). In a study of the relative contributions of different drug combinations of opiates, cocaine and alcohol to overdose deaths from 1990-1998 in New York City, the majority of the variation in overdose death rates observed during the 1990s was attributed to drug combinations (Coffin, *et al.*, 2002).

2.4. Age of Onset

There is a substantial literature characterizing the initiation of drug use. Most studies have examined tobacco and alcohol initiation, while a growing number of studies have addressed initiation of illicit drugs, including injection drug use. Over the last several decades, individuals from younger age cohorts have initiated drug use at younger ages, noted both in Australia and the U.S. The Australian National Drug Strategy Household Survey, a representative study of Australians over the age of 14 (Figure 2) (Degenhardt, *et al.*, 2000) noted that for marijuana, LSD and heroin in particular, the age of initiation dramatically decreased for each successive age cohort. The mean age of initiation of marijuana went from 30 years for those born between 1940 and 1944 to 16 years for those

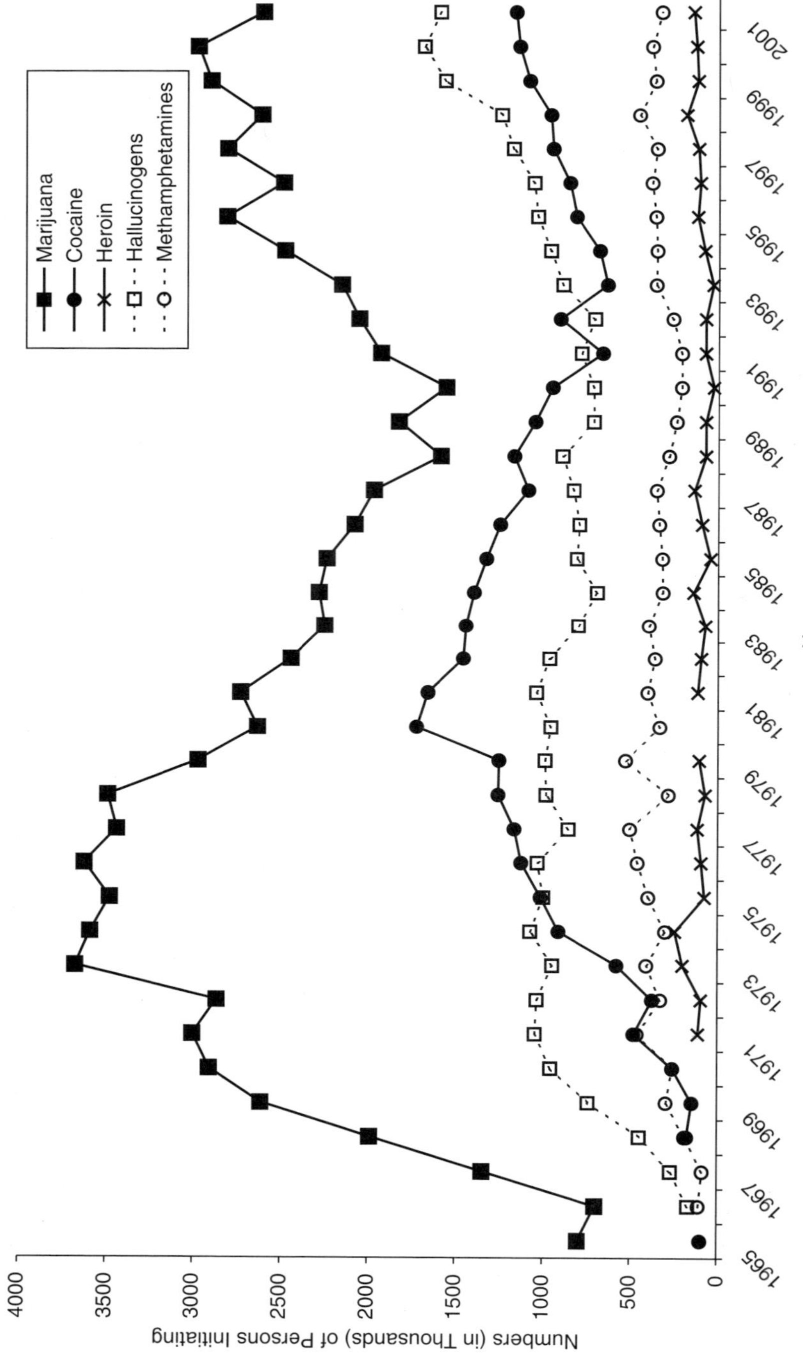

Figure 1. Illicit Drug Use Incidence in the U.S., 1965–2001 (Adapted from NSDUH 2002)

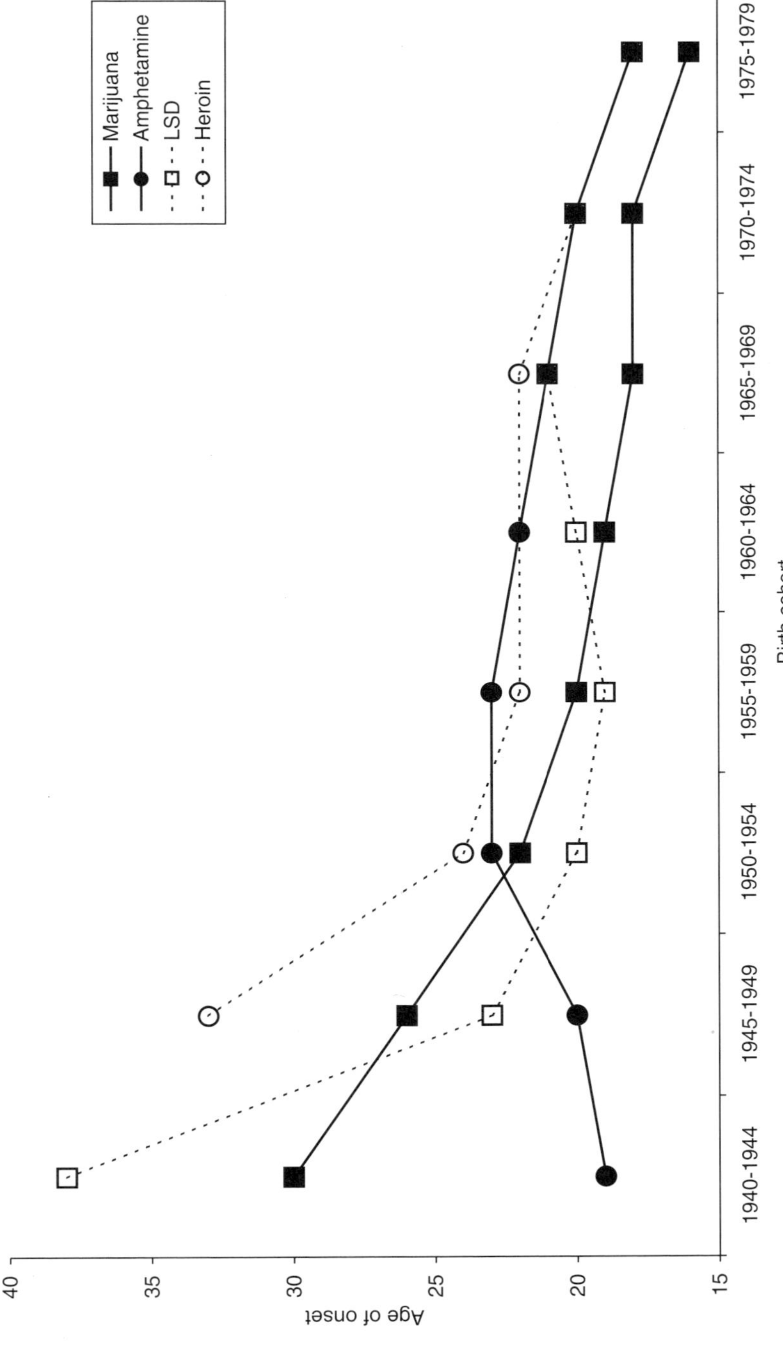

Figure 2. Cohort Trends in the Age of Initiation of Drug Use in Australia (Adapted from Degenhardt, *et al*, 2004)

born between 1975 and 1979, from 38 years to 18 years for LSD and from 33 years to 18 years for heroin.

Data from the NSDUH show recent trends in the age at initiation of drug use in the U.S. (Figure 3) (Substance Abuse and Mental Health Services Administration, 2001; Substance Abuse and Mental Health Services Administration and Office of Applied Studies, 2003a). Between 1988 and 2002, the age at marijuana initiation dropped from approximately 19 to 18 years. The age at initiation of hallucinogens and heroin increased, from 18.2 to 18.9 years and 20.2 to 22.1 years, respectively.

Figure 3 also highlights the differences in initiation ages for different drugs. Cigarette initiation occurs the earliest, followed by alcohol, marijuana and hallucinogens and finally heroin and cocaine. Such patterns in drug use initiation have served as evidence for supporting the gateway theory of drug use. The gateway theory describes a sequential pattern of drug use that often begins with licit drugs such as alcohol and tobacco which can progress to illicit drugs including marijuana, cocaine, and heroin (Kandel, 1975; Kandel, *et al.*, 1992). Morral and colleagues (Morral, *et al.*, 2002a; Morral, *et al.*, 2002b) have argued that while the marijuana gateway theory may exist, drug use propensity can explain that the same phenomenon observed in the gateway theory, namely that use of a softer drug can lead to use of a harder drug. Others have argued that it is the *opportunity* to use a given drug, rather than use of a less serious drug, that determines whether an

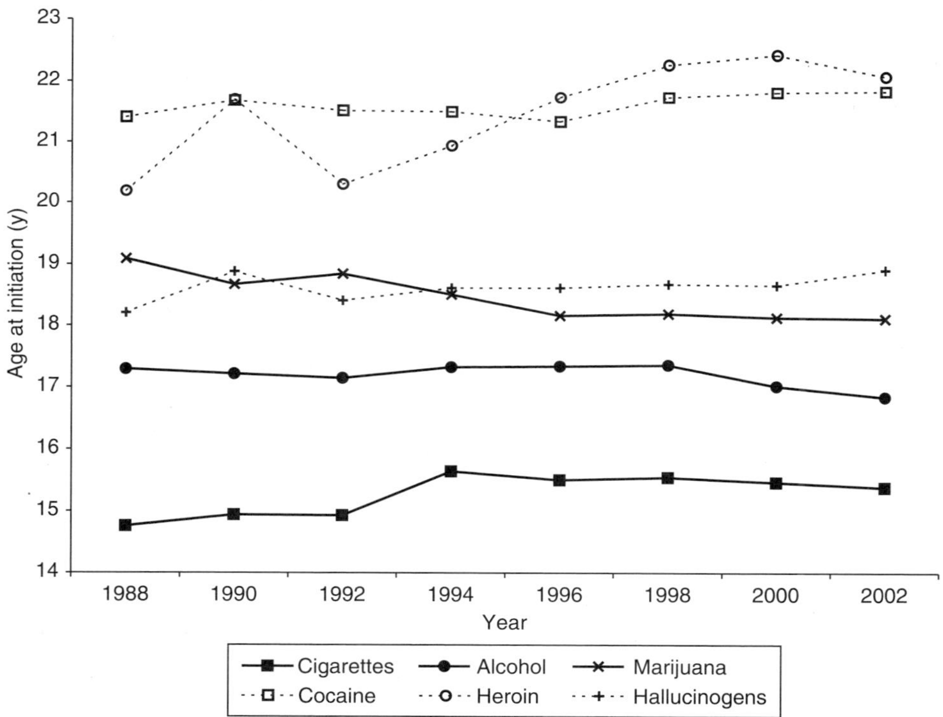

Figure 3. Age at Initiation for Selected Drugs of Abuse (Adapted from NSUDH 2002 and NHSDA 1988-2000).

individual transitions from one drug to another (Crum, *et al.*, 1996; Storr, *et al.*, 2004; Van Etten and Anthony, 2001; Van Etten, *et al.*, 1997; Wagner and Anthony, 2002; Wilcox, *et al.*, 2002).

2.5. Gender Differences

Generally, women have lower overall rates of drug use as compared to men (Substance Abuse and Mental Health Services Administration and Office of Applied Studies, 2003b; Johnston, *et al.*, 2004; Warner, *et al.*, 1995). In the 2002 NSDUH, men were more likely to report illicit drug use (10.3% vs. 6.4%) (Substance Abuse and Mental Health Services Administration and Office of Applied Studies, 2003b). However, in recent years the differences between men and women have not been as straightforward. For example, in the 2003 MTF data (Johnston, *et al.*, 2004), 12th grade boys had higher annual prevalence rates for most illicit drugs. Compared to 12th grade girls, 12th grade boys were more likely to have used marijuana (37.8% vs. 31.6%), inhalants (5.2% vs. 2.9%), hallucinogens (7.8% vs. 3.8%), cocaine (5.9% vs. 3.7%) and most other drugs in the last year. However, for 8th and 10th graders there are few gender differences. In fact, in 8th grade, girls had higher annual prevalence rates as compared to boys for several drugs including inhalants (9.6% vs. 7.7%), cocaine (2.3% vs. 1.9%), heroin (0.9% vs. 0.8%) and methamphetamines (3.0% vs. 2.0%). Women have also been shown to have a lower likelihood of being an injection drug user (Gossop, *et al.*, 1994).

Although men are generally more likely than women to use specific drugs, women have been shown to have higher rates of problems related to their drug use. Among heroin users, women are more likely to be addicted and become addicted sooner as compared to men (Anglin, *et al.*, 1987), as well as consume more heroin as compared to men (Bretteville-Jensen, 1999). However, other studies have shown that women consume less heroin than men (Powis, *et al.*, 1996). Despite the indications that women may have more problems related to their drug use, the Treatment Episode Data Set (TEDS) – a study of national admissions to drug abuse treatment services, reports that between 1992 and 2002 approximately 70% of individuals in treatment were men (Substance Abuse and Mental Health Service Administration and Office of Applied Studies, 2004). Whether this reflects gender difference in prevalence or that women feel more stigmatized and reluctant to appear in these programs is not entirely clear.

2.6. Racial/Ethnic Differences

The relation between race/ethnicity and use of drugs is complex. National surveys have failed to demonstrate consistently different drug use consumption between racial/ethnic groups (Office of Applied Studies, SAMHSA, 2002), yet other studies have demonstrated significant differences in terms of patterns of use. The MTF Study examined tobacco, alcohol, and illicit drug use among high school seniors between 1976 and 2000 (Wallace, Jr., *et al.*, 2002). On average, American Indian seniors had the highest rates of marijuana, inhalant, stimulant, and tranquilizer use in the past year compared to other racial/ethnic groups. Among latinos, Mexican Americans had the highest rates of marijuana use in the last year (40.4% compared to 36.2% among Cuban Americans, 37.6% among Puerto Rican Americans and 29.7% among other Latin Americans). However, Cuban Americans had the highest rates of inhalant, hallucinogen, cocaine, heroin and stimulant use. The lowest rates of drug use were reported by Asian Americans, blacks and Latin Americans other than those of Cuban, Mexican, and Puerto Rican ethnicity.

Research has shown race/ethnicity to play an important role in initiation of illicit drug use. For example, initiation of illicit non-injection and injection drug use at a younger age is more common in white as compared to black injection drug users(IDUs) (Fuller, *et al.*, 2002; Fuller, *et al.*, 2001; Golub and Johnson, 2001; Kral, *et al.*, 2000; Ellickson and Morton, 1999). In addition, whites are more likely to be polydrug users (Epstein, *et al.*, 1999). A similar trend is observed when comparing non-injection drug users (NIDUs) to IDUs, where reports have shown white drug users are more likely to be an IDU than black drug users (Fuller, *et al.*, 2002; Golub and Johnson, 2001). Most reports suggest that differences observed in the prevalence of drug abuse between racial/ethnic groups likely reflect socio-economic differences between groups (Lillie-Blanton, *et al.*, 1996; Ensminger, *et al.*, 1997).

In addition to drug use, racial/ethnic differences in the medical consequences of drug use have also been observed. Minority IDUs have higher rates of HIV than white IDUs, and this difference cannot be attributed entirely to risk behavior (Centers for Disease Control and Prevention, 2002; Chaisson, *et al.*, 1987; Kral, *et al.*, 1998; Kottiri, *et al.*, 2002; Schoenbaum, *et al.*, 1989; Watters, *et al.*, 1994). This racial/ethnic difference in risk of HIV infection has not been fully explained. It has been suggested that behavioral factors play a role in these differences: among blacks, 56% of incident HIV infections are attributed to injection drug use as compared to 20% among latinos (Centers for Disease Control and Prevention, 2002). However, these differences cannot be attributed solely to behavioral differences (Schoenbaum, *et al.*, 1989; Vlahov, *et al.*, 1990) nor can they be attributed to HIV entering minority communities earlier than white communities (Novick, *et al.*, 1989).

Racial/ethnic differences have also been observed in overdose mortality. In New York City, black and latino drug users have a higher rate of overdose mortality compared to whites (Galea, *et al.*, 2003). However, racial/ethnic differences in overdose morality differ between cities (Harlow, 1990; Lerner and Nurco, 1970). In San Francisco, latino drug users had a lower mortality rate as compared to whites and blacks (Davidson, *et al.*, 2003). Again, it has been suggested that behavioral factors play a role in these differences in terms of the drugs being used, the context of use (e.g. alone vs. with others) and the responses of witnesses to overdose events (Galea, *et al.*, 2003).

2.7. Medical Consequences

Drug users, and particularly injection drug users, experience increased death rates as compared to the general population even when HIV-related mortality is excluded (Vlahov, *et al.*, 2004; Perucci, *et al.*, 1991). A well-established body of research has demonstrated that drug users are disproportionately affected by a number of health problems, including HIV, other blood-borne diseases (e.g., hepatitis), and overdose. This literature has been well summarized elsewhere (Cherubin, 1967; Cherubin, *et al.*, 1972; Cherubin and Sapira, 1993; Galea, *et al.*, 2004), and a comprehensive review of these issues is beyond the scope of this chapter. Knowledge and understanding of these health issues, which are certainly more concentrated in cities with large drug using populations, are critical for planning effective urban health strategies and interventions. Some drug user health problems are the result of unique exposures to risks related to drug use and sexual behavior (e.g. overdose, HIV acquisition, etc.). However, it is important to note that many of these health problems also appear to be related to social conditions (Marzuk, *et al.*, 1997a). Here, we summarize several key health problems that affect drug users. In the following section we will examine how the urban environment can affect these outcomes.

2.7.1. *Overdose*

Drug overdose is a common occurrence among habitual drug users; approximately 30 to 68% of drug users report a nonfatal overdose in their lifetime (Darke, *et al.*, 1996a; Tobin and Latkin, 2003; Seal, *et al.*, 2001). According to estimates from the Drug Abuse Warning Network, there were 258, 931 emergency room visits for overdoses in 2002 (Substance Abuse and Mental Health Service Administration and Office of Applied Studies, 2003).

Factors in the immediate drug using environment (the immediate "context") are likely related to fatal drug overdose; specifically, use of drugs in an unfamiliar environment, alone, or with persons who are afraid to call for help (Darke and Zador, 1996; Manning and Ingraham, 1983) have all been associated with a higher likelihood of fatal overdose risk. Larger contextual factors that may be implicated in determining fatal overdose mortality and will be discussed in the next section include poverty, neighborhood-level income distribution, and availability of treatment resources, drug availability, and policing efforts.

2.7.2. *HIV*

Injection drug use remains an important and well-established risk factor for HIV and other blood-borne infections. There have been several studies conducted across North and South America as well as Europe, Asia, and Australia that have estimated the prevalence of HIV infection among adult IDUs dating as early as 1977. For example, Holmberg conducted a study of HIV in 96 metropolitan statistical areas in the U.S. (Holmberg, 1996). He estimated that approximately half of all estimated new infections were occurring among injection drug users, most of them in northeastern cities, Miami, and San Juan, Puerto Rico. HIV prevalence rates among IDUs in North America remained highest in the northeast area of the U.S. ranging from 61% in New York City to 43% in Asbury Park during the late 1980s (Lange, *et al.*, 1988; Battjes, *et al.*, 1991). More recently, the prevalence of HIV among injection drug users has decreased in some areas like New York City (Des Jarlais, *et al.*, 1998; Des, *et al.*, 2003; Rockwell, *et al.*, 2002).

In addition to IDUs, non-injection drug users (NIDUs) who use intranasal (sniffing or snorting) and inhaled (smoking) routes of drug administration are also at increased risk for HIV infection (Neaigus, *et al.*, 1996; Gyarmathy, *et al.*, 2002; Booth, *et al.*, 1993). Much of the increased risk for HIV infection among NIDUs is thought to occur through sexual risk behavior like trading sex for drugs (Montoya and Atkinson, 1996; Kral, *et al.*, 2001), inconsistent condom use (Kral *et al.*, 1998b; Woody, *et al.*, 1999b), and having multiple sex partners (Montoya and Atkinson, 1996). These associations have been well-documented among crack and cocaine users (Hser, *et al.*, 1999; Edlin, *et al.*, 1994; Fullilove, *et al.*, 1990; Booth, *et al.*, 1993; Logan and Leukefeld, 2000b; Kral, *et al.*, 1998b; Woody, *et al.*, 1999a; Ross, *et al.*, 2002; Flom, *et al.*, 2001). Among crack users, the exchange of sex for drugs or money, having multiple sex partners, and the infrequent use of condoms place many at increased risk of HIV infection (Edlin, *et al.*, 1994; Fullilove, *et al.*, 1990;

Booth, *et al.*, 1993; Kral, *et al.*, 1998d; Logan and Leukefeld, 2000a). Heroin (Sanchez, *et al.*, 2002; Gyarmathy, *et al.*, 2002; Neaigus, *et al.*, 2001) and methamphetamine NIDUs (Molitor, *et al.*, 1998) have also been shown to engage is risky sexual behavior, although these sub-groups have not been well studied.

2.7.3. *Hepatitis*

Drug users often engage in a variety of behaviors that place them at risk for Hepatitis B virus (HBV) and Hepatitis C virus (HCV) infection. Both infections are responsible for considerable morbidity and mortality both nationally and internationally. HBV infection continues to be a major public health concern, with an estimated 2 billion people with serologic evidence of current or past infection and 350 million people chronically infected worldwide (Kane, 1995). It has been estimated that 170 million people are infected with HCV globally (1999). Approximately 3.9 million Americans are infected with the hepatitis C virus, which corresponds to a prevalence rate of 1.8%, according to estimates from the Third National Health and Nutrition Examination Study (Alter, *et al.*, 1999b).

The prevalence of HBV infection is high among injection drug users, ranging between 20 and 81% (Murrill, *et al.*, 2002; 2001; Hwang, *et al.*, 2000; Edeh and Spalding, 2000; Karapetyan, *et al.*, 2002; Renwick, *et al.*, 2002). In the U.S., approximately 13.8% of cases are attributable to parenteral transmission through injection drug use practices (Goldstein, *et al.*, 2002). Non-injection drug users (NIDUs) also have been shown to have higher rates of HBV infection as compared to the general population (Gyarmathy, *et al.*, 2002; Hwang, *et al.*, 2000).

Previous studies have shown strong associations between acquisition of HCV infection and "direct" sharing of needles and syringes, as well as "indirect" sharing of injection paraphernalia, including cookers and cotton filters (Alter, *et al.*, 1999; Diaz, *et al.*, 2001; Stark, *et al.*, 1997; Thorpe, *et al.*, 2000; Villano, *et al.*, 1997). HCV transmission is also closely associated with duration of drug injection. Among persons newly initiated into illicit drug injection in Baltimore, 65% had acquired HCV infection within one year (Garfein, *et al.*, 1996). In a large cohort of IDUs, researchers estimated rates of HCV infection relative to HBV and HIV. By the tenth month of injection drug use, 78% of IDUs were HCV seropositive, compared to 58% having HBV and 16% having HIV (Garfein, *et al.*, 1996).

In addition to IDUs, NIDUs have been observed to have an HCV prevalence between 5-12% compared to the general population prevalence of approximately 2% (Koblin, *et al.*, 2003). The source of this increased risk has yet to be fully explained although it is hypothesized that drug use behaviors (i.e., sharing non-injecting drug equipment), personal hygiene practices (i.e., sharing razors or clippers), non-commercial tattooing, and/or high risk sexual behaviors may play a role (Koblin, *et al.*, 2003; Gyarmathy, *et al.*, 2002; Conry-Cantilena, *et al.*, 1996; McMahon and Tortu, 2003; McMahon, *et al.*, 2004; Tortu, *et al.*, 2004; Tortu, *et al.*, 2001; Quaglio, *et al.*, 2003).

3.0. DRUG USE AND URBAN ENVIRONMENTS

Thus far we have discussed the epidemiology of drug use from a national perspective, with a focus on the trends in the U.S., where approximately 80% of the population is categorized as living in metropolitan areas. As noted previously, drug use is generally conceived as an urban problem. In this next section, we will focus specifically on urban areas and factors associated with drug use in these areas. We will begin by highlighting urban-rural, inter-urban, and intra-urban similarities and differences to provide perspective. We will then work from the theoretical framework proposed by Galea, and colleagues, (Galea, *et al.*, 2003) to explore the urban context through the social environment, the physical environment, and structural considerations such as availability of social services, municipal structures and national and international policies.

3.1. Urban comparisons

3.1.1. Urban vs. rural

Differences in drug use between urban and rural areas vary over time and by geographical area. Some studies have demonstrated higher rates of drug use among urban populations as compared to rural populations (Mueser, *et al.*, 2001), while others have shown the opposite (Othieno, *et al.*, 2000; Leukefeld, *et al.*, 2002). Data from the Monitoring the Future Study suggest that lifetime and annual drug use rates among adolescents are relatively similar across communities (table 1), and that in some cases use in rural areas exceeds that in urban areas (e.g. lifetime methamphetamine prevalence) (Johnston, *et al.*, 2004).

Another analysis of the MTF data suggested temporal changes in urban versus rural differences between 1976 and 1992 (Cronk and Sarvela, 1997). During the late 1970s and 1980s, rates of marijuana and cocaine use were higher among urban than rural adolescents. However, by the early 1990s use of these drugs among rural adolescents matched or exceeded those of their urban counterparts.

Data from the National Survey on Drug Use and Health (table 2) reveals different trends for persons over the age of 18 (Substance Abuse and Mental Health Services Administration and Office of Applied Studies, 2004). Large metropolitan counties (defined as having one million or more residents) had higher lifetime and annual rates of marijuana, inhalant, hallucinogen, and cocaine use as compared to small metropolitan counties (defined as having less than one million residents) and non-metropolitan counties (defined as urbanized, less urbanized and rural counties). With the findings from the MTF study, this suggests that urban-rural differences in drug use differ by age.

Table 1. Lifetime and Annual Prevalence of Use of Selected Drugs among 12th Graders by Population Density (Adapted from MTF, 2003)

	Large Metropolitan Statistical Areas		Other Metropolitan Statistical Areas		Non-Metropolitan Statistical Areas	
	Lifetime	Annual	Lifetime	Annual	Lifetime	Annual
Marijuana	43.4	32.3	49.5	38.1	43.5	32.2
Inhalants	10.6	3.5	11.4	4.4	11.7	3.7
Hallucinogens	8.9	4.4	12.3	7.2	9.6	5.5
Cocaine	6.2	3.8	8.6	5.7	7.9	4.6
Heroin	1.1	0.7	1.6	0.8	1.9	0.9
Methamphetamines	3.4	0.2	6.2	1.0	9.8	0.7

Table 2. Lifetime and Annual Prevalence of Use of Selected Drugs among Persons Aged 18 and Older by Geographic Characteristics (Adapted from NSDUH, 2003)

	Large Metropolitan County		Small Metropolitan County		Non-Metropolitan County	
	Lifetime	Annual	Lifetime	Annual	Lifetime	Annual
Marijuana	45.0	10.4	43.4	10.6	36.8	8.1
Inhalants	10.3	0.5	9.2	0.5	7.9	0.3
Hallucinogens	16.5	1.7	15.8	1.4	12.1	1.0
Cocaine	17.8	2.8	15.5	2.4	12.0	2.1

Beyond national estimates of drug use, researchers have also examined urban-rural differences in the natural history of drug use. For example, a study of incarcerated drug users in Kentucky revealed significant differences in the age of onset of drug use between urban and rural inmates. Urban inmates initiated alcohol (13.5 vs. 13.7 years), marijuana (13.9 vs. 14.5 years), and cocaine use (20.6 vs. 22.0 years) at significantly younger ages as compared to rural inmates (Leukefeld, *et al.*, 2002). In Australia, the primary drug use by injection drug users differed in the urban and rural settings (Aitken, *et al.*, 1999). Urban injection drug users were more likely to use heroin (73.6% for urban IDUs vs. 20.5% for rural IDUs) as compared to rural injection drug, who were more likely to be amphetamines users (79.5% for rural IDUs vs. 25.5% for urban IDUs).

Urban-rural differences have been noted in drug treatment experiences. Urban drug users were significantly more likely to have a history of drug treatment as compared to their rural counterparts (Warner and Leukefeld, 2001). This association has also been shown in a sample of drug users from Miami and rural Georgia, where urban drug users were approximately 2.5 times more likely to have been in drug treatment as compared to rural drug users (Metsch and McCoy, 1999).

Urban-rural differences in drug use behaviors and blood-borne infections have also been an area of interest. A Scottish study found few differences between rural and urban injection drug users in terms of recent injection and treatment access (Haw and Higgins, 1998). However, urban IDUs were significantly more likely to be HIV infected as compared to rural IDUs. This difference was attributed to higher levels of risky injection behaviors, limited migration from urban to rural areas, and reluctance on the part of rural IDUs to share with IDUs outside their social and kinship networks. Rural Australian IDUs also had significantly lower injection (2.8 vs. 5.3 injections per week) and needle sharing frequencies (0.3 vs. 1.2 shared injections per week) and were less likely to have HCV (41.2% vs. 67.9%) as compared to their urban counterparts (Aitken, *et al.*, 1999).

Collectively, these studies highlight the inconsistency of drug use trends when comparing urban areas to rural areas. Urban versus rural differences in drug use vary by geographical area and sub-populations.

3.1.2. Inter- and Intra-urban Comparisons

Inter-urban comparisons are useful in highlighting regional and geographical variance in drug use, as well as investigating possible mechanisms for observed differences and similarities. In particular, comparisons of similar populations in different areas have provided some insight into inter-urban differences in drug use. For example, a well-described cohort of Puerto Rican drug injectors in New York City and Bayamón, Puerto Rico has revealed several differences between the two ethnically similar populations. IDUs in Puerto Rico injected more frequently (5.4 vs. 2.8 mean injections per day) (Colon, *et al.*, 2001) and had higher rates of needle sharing as compared to their New York counterparts (Deren, *et al.*, 2001).

Intra-urban comparisons are probably one of the more widely used methods for investigating the urban context. By looking for differences between neighborhoods researchers have examined the impact of income inequality, a feature of the social environment, on drug use outcomes (Fuller, *et al.*, 2002; Galea, *et al.*, 2003). Other studies have shown that behaviors are not always similar between neighborhoods. In a study in two New York neighborhoods there were significant differences in terms of risk for blood-borne pathogens and their correlates. IDUs in the Lower East Side of Manhattan were significantly more likely to be infected with HBV and HCV as compared to IDUs in Harlem (Des Jarlais, *et al.*, 2003). Among IDUs on the Lower East Side, HCV infection was associated with older age, injecting with someone who had hepatitis, longer duration of injection drug use, and drug treatment (Diaz, *et al.*, 2001). In Harlem, HCV infection was associated with longer duration of injection drug use, cocaine injection, sharing filter cottons during injection preparation and drug treatment (Diaz, *et al.*, 2001). As we will see in section 4.2, intra-urban studies contributed much to our understanding of the role of the urban environment in shaping the occurrence and natural history of drug use.

3.2. The Urban Context

As illustrated previously, drug use is not exclusively an urban phenomenon although it is often thought of as such (Bailey, 1916; Storr, *et al.*, 2004). Indeed, much of the current drug abuse research had been conducted in urban settings (Abraham, 1999; Boardman, *et al.*, 2001; Ensminger, *et al.*, 1997; Kral, *et al.*, 2003; Latkin, *et al.*, 2003; Roy, *et al.*, 2003). However, surprisingly little research has been conducted to examine the role of the urban environment in the occurrence of drug use. In this section we seek to summarize the literature addressing these relations.

Urban areas have often suffered from large-scale drug use epidemics (Hughes, *et al.*, 1972; Bailey, 1916; Hunt and Chambers, 1976). In particular, it has been suggested that urban environments can serve as a crossroad, and final destination, in the drug distribution network (Furst, *et al.*, 2004; Frischer, *et al.*, 2002; Hunt and Chambers, 1976).

During the past decade, a growing body of research has begun to consider the role that the urban context (e.g. the social and physical environment and structural considerations) plays in shaping risk behavior and health (Syme and Balfour, 1998). However, there has been relatively less research about how these factors are related both to the natural history of drug use and to the negative consequences of drug abuse. In this next section, we will explore the urban context of drug use drawing on much of the inter- and intra-urban literature alluded to previously

3.2.1. Social Environment

The urban environment is comprised of contextual factors that include social norms and attitudes, disadvantage (e.g., neighborhood socioeconomic status), and social capital (e.g., social trust, social institutions, etc.) (Galea and Vlahov, 2005). The literature pertaining to the social environment and drug use has been reviewed in detail elsewhere (Galea, *et al.*, 2004), and a comprehensive review of these issues is beyond the scope of this chapter. However, some points are worth noting as they relate to the urban social environment.

There is limited information about the influence of the social environment of drug use behaviors in most areas. Features of the social environment may have an impact on both the prevalence and patterns of drug use (Bachman, *et al.*, 1984; Bachman, *et al.*, 1999) as well as modify well-recognized correlates of drug abuse including violence and ill-health (Scribner, *et al.*, 1999; Wallace, *et al.*, 1992; Marczynski, *et al.*, 1999). We summarize research on the relation between the social environment and the occurrence of drug use paying particular attention to the multiple levels of influence (e.g. network, neighborhood, and societal) that are at work in these complex relationships. When possible, we have moved beyond simply looking at prevalence rates and focused on more specialized areas such as opportunity to use and initiation of use.

3.2.1.a. Social Norms and Attitudes. Social norms and attitudes play an important role in drug use and related behaviors. Norms are societal such as those transmitted through schools and churches, but the influence of norms can be expressed at the network level of family and peers. Beginning with the family network, we can see that parental norms play an important role in adolescent drug use. Specifically, family members' use of cigarettes and alcohol was related to illicit drug use in a study of Greek youth (Madianos, *et al.*, 1995). Similarly, parental drug use has been associated with illicit drug use in adults in several studies (Newcomb and Bentler, 1986; von, *et al.*, 2002; Lindenberg, *et al.*, 1999).

Peer norms have also been shown to influence drug use. In a study of adolescents in Sydney, Australia, those who reported marijuana use among friends and siblings were more likely to use marijuana (Levy and Pierce, 1990). Similar associations have been observed in other international studies of adolescents, where positive attitudes towards hashish (Madianos, *et al.*, 1995; Newcomb and Bentler, 1986) and drug use (Madianos, *et al.*, 1995; Newcomb and Bentler, 1986) or the perception of drug use by close friends (Schmid, 2001) was associated with illicit drug use. In one Canadian study of street youth, girls with an IDU friend were 4.6 times more likely to initiate injection drug use than girls without an IDU friend (Roy, *et al.*, 2002).

Beyond the social norms characterized by the behavior and perceived behavior of peers and families, the larger social constructs of school and society impact drug use. For example, in the Monitoring the Future study, school-level disapproval of marijuana use was associated with a lower probability of students' use of marijuana, even after controlling for their own disapproval and demographic characteristics (Kumar, *et al.*, 2002). Research has shown that increases in the perceived risks and disapproval of drug use are associated with declines in drug use on a population level (Bachman, *et al.*, 1990; Beyers, *et al.*, 2004). In the U.S., societal tolerance or support for drug use began to wane during the 1970s and 1980s. These changes in social norms were associated with reduced incidence of drug use (Johnson and Gerstein, 2000).

3.2.1.b. Neighborhood Disadvantage. Another aspect of the social environment is neighborhood disadvantage or low neighborhood-level socio-economic status. Although many studies of drug use have been conducted within disadvantaged neighborhoods, only a handful of studies have investigated a broader array of communities to examine the association between drug use and neighborhood disadvantage.

Beginning with opportunity to try drugs, we can see consistent associations between drug use and neighborhood disadvantage. In a study of high school students in Guam, Storr and colleagues (2004) reported an association between neighborhood disadvantage and the opportunity to try drugs. Guamanian youth with higher levels of neighborhood disadvantage were significantly more likely to have had the opportunity to try marijuana (Storr, *et al.*, 2004).

Neighborhood disadvantage has also been shown to be associated with drug use initiation. A prospective cohort study of 1,416 Baltimore middle school students found that neighborhood disadvantage was associated with initiation of drug use, where children from most disadvantaged neighborhoods were more likely to have been offered cocaine, inhalants, and marijuana (Crum, *et al.*, 1996). Similarly, Fuller and colleagues reported that neighborhood disadvantage was related to initiation of injection drug use (Fuller, *et al.*, 2002). IDUs from high poverty/high minority neighborhoods were significantly more likely to initiate injection drug use during adolescence as compared to IDUs from low poverty/low minority neighborhoods.

Researchers have just begun to evaluate the relations between the urban social environment and the medical consequences of drug use. One study demonstrated a significant association between poverty and fatal accidental drug overdoses of cocaine and opiates in New York City (Marzuk, *et al.*, 1997b). Recently, the role of income distribution in shaping consequences of drug use such as drug overdose had been examined (Galea, *et al.*, 2003b). Overdose deaths were more likely in neighborhoods with higher levels of drug use and with more unequal income distribution. Circumstantial evidence suggests that levels of policing in the community affects drug use patterns (Karlsson and Romelsjo, 1997) and that policing activity may play a role in the causal links between use of drugs and fatal drug overdose (Darke, *et al.*, 1996b).

In these examples, as with most studies of neighborhood disadvantage, there is no way to tell whether these associations are causal as most studies are cross-sectional in nature. Despite this limitation, these studies suggest that neighborhood disadvantage is associated with an increased opportunity to use drugs as well as increased drug use prevalence and mortality.

3.2.1.d. Social Capital. Social cohesion/capital, as expressed by trust and willingness to participate in community's activities, can provide shared social resources that facilitate collective action (Kawachi and Berkman, 2000). There is evidence that erosion of social cohesion/capital is associated with negative health outcomes such as increases in mortality, poor self-rated perception of health, higher crime rates and violence (Kawachi, *et al.*, 1997; Kennedy, *et al.*, 1998).

Studies of social cohesion and drug use are sparse. Some research suggests that racialized practices and ideologies may influence drug use through the structure and process of interpersonal relationships (Wallace, Jr., 1999), subsequently reducing trust in society and systems. Similarly, a recent study found that experiencing social stressors (defined as experiencing unfair treatment, e.g. compared to other people treated with less courtesy, less respect or poorer service) at the neighborhood level were associated with drug use (Boardman, *et al.*, 2001). Thus, lack of social capital in this case is associated with increased drug use. In a study in rural Mexico, communities with little or no drug use demonstrate more social cohesion (Wagner, *et al.*, 2002). Social cohesion is also associated with greater perceived neighborhood problems with youth alcohol and drug use (Duncan, *et al.*, 2002).

3.2.1.e. Summary. Some modest evidence suggests that the social environment, through social norms and attitudes, neighborhood disadvantage, and social capital might impact the occurrence and initiation of drug use. However, this area of inquiry is in its infancy. Future studies will further elucidate the roles of the various aspects of the urban social environment on the full spectrum of drug use, from initiation to cessation.

3.2.2. Physical Environment

According to Galea and Vlahov (2005) the urban physical environment refers to the built environment, urban infrastructure (e.g. sanitation), pollution, access to green space, transportation systems and the geological and climate conditions of the area the city occupies. Examination of the association of built environment and health overall is a relatively recent area of inquiry (see the September 2003 issues of the *Journal of Urban Health* and the *American Journal of Public Health* that examined health and the built environment), and few studies have been conducted to examine relations between the urban physical environment and drug use.

While studies of the physical environment and drug use are scant, there is a growing literature looking at a variety of other diseases. For example, researchers have noted the relationship between the physical environment and STDs. Using a "broken windows" index that measured housing quality, abandoned cars, graffiti, trash, and public school deterioration, Cohen and colleagues found an association between the deteriorated physical conditions of local neighborhoods with gonorrhea rates, which was independent of poverty (Cohen, *et al.*, 2000). In a study of syphilis in North Carolina, an increase in drug activity in the counties along the Interstate 95 corridor preceded a rise in syphilis cases (Cook, *et al.*, 1999).

Although few studies have investigated the role of the physical environment as it relates to drug use, there is preliminary evidence for an association between the use of drugs and airport noise (Knipschild and Oudshoorn, 1977; Grandjean, *et al.*, 1976), but this association has not been examined further. Thus, studies examining the relationship between the physical environment and drug use or its consequences are almost nonexistent and conceptualization of possible associations is still in the early stages (Galea and Vlahov, 2004; Freudenberg, *et al.*, 2005).

3.2.3. Structural Considerations

Structural considerations such as availability of health and social services (e.g., drug treatment), municipal structures (e.g. law enforcement) and national and international policies (e.g. legislation and trade policies) can be both positively and negatively associated with drug use.

3.2.3.a. Health and Social Services. The availability of health and social services remains a key determinant of good health. In this section, we will focus specifically on drug treatment. It should be noted that the structural considerations detailed here do not apply exclusively to urban areas. Between 1920 and 1964, while not illegal, physicians faced possible prosecution and conviction for treating opiate abusing patients with opiates (Jaffe and O'Keeffe, 2003). The development of drug abuse treatment options, especially pharmacotherapy, has not been a high priority in the U.S., given the restrictive atmosphere for treatment. Until recently, the treatment of opiate abuse has been limited because pharmacotherapy has not been a part of the medical mainstream (Ling and Smith, 2002).

Currently, treatment options include inpatient and outpatient counseling, detoxification with methadone or clonidine, methadone maintenance therapy and more recently LAAM (levacetylmethadol), buprenorphine and naloxone (Warner, *et al.*, 1997; Federal Registry, 2003; FDA Consumer, 2003). The limited pharmacopoeia for opiate abuse is tightly regulated in the U.S. for both patients and doctors by the Department of Health and Human Services and the Drug Enforcement Agency (DEA) (Molinari, *et al.*, 1994), resulting in a drug treatment system characterized by restricted access, strict rules about discharging patients who do not comply with treatment guidelines, and treatment clinicians who are cautious about treatment flexibility for fear of running into trouble with regulators. For cocaine and methamphetamine, there are few treatment options, since there is virtually no approved pharmacotherapy (Cretzmeyer, *et al.*, 2003; Warner, *et al.*, 1997). In contrast, there is a vast pharmacopoeia for other mental health disorders like depression and anxiety. Clinicians treating patients with these conditions can exercise discretion in adjusting medications to fit the symptoms.

Effective drug treatment remains an issue of legislation, regulation, and enforcement in the U.S. Policy and regulations continue to walk a thin line by avoiding "sending the wrong message." Unfortunately, the implication of such policies is that drug users are not provided treatment in a way that is acceptable to the patient, so treatment is often delayed until individuals "hit rock bottom."

3.2.3.b. Law Enforcement. Law enforcement practices and initiatives can have a significant effect on drug use. A large scale drug enforcement operation in Vancouver, Canada resulted in displacement of injection drug use from neighborhoods in the city to adjacent ones (Wood, *et al.*, 2004). Not only can policing efforts move drug markets, but they can also have an impact of risk and protective behaviors. A study of Russian drug users suggests that IDUs are reluctant to carry needles due to fears of being arrested, which was subsequently associated with an increased risk of sharing needles and syringes (Rhodes, *et al.*, 2003; Rhodes, *et al.*, 2004).

In the U.S., in places like Connecticut where syringe and paraphernalia laws were deregulated, decreases in self-reported syringe-sharing and increases in purchasing by IDUs of sterile syringes from reliable sources have been reported (Groseclose, *et al.*, 1995). Policing can also affect overdose outcomes, where police attendance or potential for police involvement at overdoses had been reported to be a deterrent for heroin users to call for medical assistance (Darke, *et al.*, 1996a; Sergeev, *et al.*, 2003).

3.2.3.c. Legislation. State, national and international policies and regulations can have considerable impact on drug users and their families. We have already mentioned legislation as it applies to drug treatment in the U.S. Here we will highlight other state, national and international policies and their impact on drug users.

State laws have a significant impact on drug users and their families. A powerful example of such laws is in New York State. In 1973 the New York State Legislature, with the encouragement of the Governor Nelson Rockefeller (Rockefeller, 1973), enacted some of the most stringent state drug laws in the U.S. (2000). Characterized by mandatory minimums and harsh sentences, the Rockefeller Drug Laws (RDLs) have led to the incarceration of over 100,000 drug users since there implementation (Drucker, 2002). Those incarcerated under the RDLs are overwhelming New York

City residents (78%) and black or latino (94%). Drucker estimated the potential years of life lost as a result of the RDLs to be equivalent to 8,667 deaths.

From a national perspective, three policy areas that have had significant impacts on the lives of drug users are policies regarding the provision of pharmacotherapy, the ban on federal funding of needle exchange programs and the "War on Drugs." We have briefly discussed the issues surrounding pharmacotherapy. The issues surrounding NEPs and the federal response to drug use are often controversial.

Needle exchange programs (NEPs) have been shown to be effective in reducing the transmission of HIV among IDUs (Vlahov and Junge, 1998; Paone, *et al.*, 1995). Access to clean needles through NEPs or pharmacy sales has been associated with decreased syringe sharing (Groseclose, *et al.*, 1995; Calsyn, *et al.*, 1991). Needle stick injuries to the general public (Buning, 1991) and police have not increased with the implementation of such programs (Macalino, *et al.*, 1998). In addition, the incidence of HIV infection among NEP participants has decreased in a number of settings (Kaplan and Heimer, 1995; Hurley, *et al.*, 1997; Des Jarlais, *et al.*, 1996). In fact, increases in HIV risk behavior have been observed in a city where the needle exchange program was forced to close (Broadhead, *et al.*, 1999). Despite the overwhelming evidence in support of NEPs, the U.S. government has maintained a ban of federal funding of NEPs. Currently needle exchange programs rely on local, state and private funding (Des Jarlais, *et al.*, 2004).

The U.S. "War on Drugs" was declared by President Richard Nixon in 1971 (2000). The war on drugs included allocations of funds for prevention and treatment. A major program of the war was the Drug Abuse Resistance Education (DARE) program. Project DARE was a school-based drug prevention program. Recent evaluations of the program indicate that it had little or no effect on drug use (Ennett, *et al.*, 1994; Lynam, *et al.*, 1999).

The War on Drugs has resulted in a concentration of police activity in lower-income neighborhoods in cities (Gordon, 1994; Goetz, 1996). Law enforcement activities have included crime reduction programs in housing projects, which have had a significant impact on residents. For example, 46% of the 1,200 households evicted in New York City in 1989 were due to anti-drug activities (Keyes, 1992). Family members of drug dealers evicted from public housing are not always protected from removal (Goetz, 1996).

4.0. FUTURE DIRECTIONS

Several innovative yet controversial interventions have been identified for further exploration, including heroin maintenance programs, safer injection rooms and Naloxone provision to drug users. In some communities, these interventions have been piloted and/or implemented.

Naloxone is a specific opiate antagonist (Chamberlain and Klein, 1994) that is often used to revive individuals during an opiate overdose. The provision of Naloxone to drug users for the prevention of overdose fatalities has been examined in Europe (Dettmer, *et al.*, 2001) and is currently being studied in the U.S. (Russell, 2002). Preliminary studies suggest that the provision of take home naloxone has prevented deaths due to overdose (Dettmer, *et al.*, 2001).

Heroin maintenance programs have been active in Europe for decades (Kintz, *et al.*, 1997; Logan, 1973; Perneger, *et al.*, 1998) while the debate in the U.S. has raged for at least as long (Logan, 1973; Parry, 1992). Safer injection rooms, places where IDUs can inject their drugs in a safe and clean environment, now operate in Europe (Dolan and Wodak, 1996; Fischer, 1995) and Australia (Dolan, *et al.*, 2000) and are being piloted in Canada (Read, 2003). The reported benefits of these facilities include improved health and social functioning of participants and reductions in drug injection, intoxication, overdoses and risk behaviors for disease transmission. In the meantime, such programs remain clinically and politically controversial.

5.0. CONCLUSION

Drug use continues to be a major concern in urban centers and significantly affects the health of cities at the beginning of the new millennium. Drug users still face considerable challenges to their health and well-being. The extent to which the urban environment affects the occurrence of drug use and its consequences is an area of growing research. Early investigations suggest that specific features of the urban environment are related to not only the occurrence of drug use, but also its course and consequences. Many questions remain unanswered with respect to the impact of the urban social and physical environment, along with larger societal structures, on illicit drug use. Because of the large number of drug users in urban areas, cities provide a unique opportunity for public health practitioners, urban planners, and policy makers to develop and test creative programs and interventions to improve the health outcomes for this population.

REFERENCES

Abraham, M. D. (1999). Illicit drug use, urbanization, and lifestyle in the Netherlands. *J. Drug Issues* 29:565–586.

Aitken, C., Brough, R., and Crofts, N. (1999). Injecting drug use and blood-borne viruses: a comparison of rural and urban Victoria, 1990-95. *Drug Alcohol Rev.* 18:47–52.

Alter, M. J., Kruszon-Moran, D., Nainan, O. V., McQuillan, G. M., Gao, F., Moyer, L. A., Kaslow, R.A., and Margolis, H.S. (1999). The prevalence of hepatitis C virus infection in the United States, 1988 through 1994. *N. Engl. J. Med.* 341:556– 562.

Anglin, M. D., Hser, Y. I., and McGlothlin, W. H. (1987). Sex differences in addict careers. 2. Becoming addicted. *Am. J. Drug Alcohol Abuse* 13:59–71.

Bachman, J. G., Freedman-Doan, P., O'Malley, P. M., Johnston, L. D., and Segal, D. R. (1999). Changing patterns of drug use among US military recruits before and after enlistment. *Am.J. Public Health* 89:672–677.

Bachman, J. G., Johnston, L. D., and O'Malley, P. M. (1990). Explaining the recent decline in cocaine use among young adults: further evidence that perceived risks and disapproval lead to reduced drug use. *J. Health Soc. Behav.* 31:173–184.

Bachman, J. G., O'Malley, P. M., and Johnston, L. D. (1984). Drug use among young adults: the impacts of role status and social environment. *J. Pers. Soc. Psychol.* 47:629–645.

Bailey, P. (1916). The heroin habit. *The New Republic. April 22, 1916.* 6:314–316.

Battjes, R. J., Pickens, R. W., and Amsel, Z. (1991). HIV infection and AIDS risk behaviors among intravenous drug users entering methadone treatment in selected U.S. cities. *J. Acquir. Immune. Defic. Syndr.* 4:1148–1154.

Belenko, S.R. (ed.). (2000). *Drugs and drug policy in America: A documentary history.* Westport, CT: Greedwood Press.

Berkman, L. F. and Kawachi, I. (2000). *Social Epidemiology.* Oxford University Press, New York.

Beyers, J. M., Toumbourou, J. W., Catalano, R. F., Arthur, M. W., and Hawkins, J. D. (2004). A cross-national comparison of risk and protective factors for adolescent substance use: the United States and Australia. *J. Adolesc. Health* 35:3–16.

Bo, O., Haftner, J. F., Langard, O., Trumpy, J. H., Bredesen, J. E., and Lunden, P. K. M. (1975). Ethanol and diazepam as causative agents in road traffic accidents. In: Israelstan, S., and Lambert S. (eds.), *Alcohol, drugs, and traffic safety*. Addiction Research Foundation, Toronto, pp 62–81.

Boardman, J. D., Finch, B. K., Ellison, C. G., Williams, D. R., and Jackson, J. S. (2001). Neighborhood disadvantage, stress, and drug use among adults. *J. Health Soc. Behav.* 42:151–165.

Booth, R. E., Watters, J. K., and Chitwood, D. D. (1993). HIV risk-related sex behaviors among injection drug users, crack smokers, and injection drug users who smoke crack. *Am. J. Public Health* 83:1144–1148.

Bretteville-Jensen, A. L. (1999). Gender, heroin consumption and economic behavior. *Health Econ.* 8:379–389.

Broadhead, R. S., van Hulst, Y., and Heckathorn, D. D. (1999). The impact of a needle exchange's closure. *Public Health Rep.* 114:439–447.

Buning, E. C. (1991). Effects of Amsterdam needle and syringe exchange. *Int. J. Addict.* 26:1303–1311.

Calsyn, D. A., Saxon, A. J., Freeman, G., and Whittaker, S. (1991). Needle-use practices among intravenous drug users in an area where needle purchase is legal. *AIDS* 5:187–193.

Centers for Disease Control and Prevention, (2002), Division of HIV/AIDS Prevention, Washington, D.C., (September 28, 2004); http://www.cdc.gov/hiv/pubs/facts.htm.

Chaisson, R. E., Moss, A. R., Onishi, R., Osmond, D., and Carlson, J. R. (1987). Human immunodeficiency virus infection in heterosexual intravenous drug users in San Francisco. *Am. J. Public Health* 77:169–172.

Chamberlain, J. M., and Klein, B. L. (1994). A comprehensive review of naloxone for the emergency physician. *Am.J. Emerg. Med.* 12:650–660.

Cherubin, C., McCusker, J., Baden, M., Kavaler, F., and Amsel, Z. (1972). Epidemiology of death in narcotic addicts. *Am. J. Epidemiol.* 96:11–22.

Cherubin, C. E. (1967). The medical sequelae of narcotic addiction. *Ann. Intern. Med.* 67:23–33.

Cherubin, C. E., and Sapira, J. D. (1993). The medical complications of drug addiction and the medical assessment of the intravenous drug user: 25 years later. *Ann. Intern. Med.* 119: 1017-1028.

Coffin, P. O., Galea, S., Ahern, J., Leon, A. C., Vlahov, D., and Tardiff, K. (2002a). Opiates, cocaine and alcohol combinations in accidental drug overdose deaths in New York City, 1990-1998. *Addiction* 98(6):711.

Cohen, D., Spear, S., Scribner, R., Kissinger, P., Mason, K., and Wildgen, J. (2000). "Broken windows" and the risk of gonorrhea. *Am. J. Public Health* 90:230–236.

Colon, H.M., Robles, R.R., Deren, S., Sahai, H., Finlinson, H.A., Andia, J., Cruz, M.A., Kang, S.Y., and Oliver-Velez, D.(2001). Between-city variation in frequency of injection among Puerto Rican injection drug users: East Harlem, New York, and Bayamon, Puerto Rico. *J. Acquir. Immune Defic. Syndr.* 27:405–413.

Conry-Cantilena, C., Van Raden, M., Gibble, J., Melpolder, J., Shakil, A. O., Viladomiu, L.,Cheung, L., DiBisceglie, A., Hoofnagle, J., Shih, J.W., Kaslow, R., Ness, P., and Alter, H.J. (1996). Routes of infection, viremia, and liver disease in blood donors found to have hepatitis C virus infection. *N. Engl. J. Med.* 334:1691–1696.

Cook, R. L., Royce, R. A., Thomas, J. C., and Hanusa, B. H. (1999). What's driving an epidemic? The spread of syphilis along an interstate highway in rural North Carolina. *Am. J. Public Health* 89:369–373.

Cook, S., Moeschler, O., Michaud, K., and Yersin, B. (1998). Acute opiate overdose: characteristics of 190 consecutive cases. *Addiction* 93:1559–1565.

Cretzmeyer, M., Sarrazin, M. V., Huber, D. L., Block, R. I., and Hall, J. A. (2003). Treatment of methamphetamine abuse: research findings and clinical directions. *J. Subst. Abuse Treat.* 24:267–277.

Cronk, C. E., and Sarvela, P. D. (1997). Alcohol, tobacco, and other drug use among rural/small town and urban youth: a secondary analysis of the monitoring the future data set. *Am. J. Public Health* 87:760–764.

Crum, R. M., Lillie-Blanton, M., and Anthony, J. C. (1996). Neighborhood environment and opportunity to use cocaine and other drugs in late childhood and early adolescence. *Drug Alcohol Depend.* 43:155–161.

Darke, S., Ross, J., and Hall, W. (1996a). Overdose among heroin users in Sydney, Australia: I. Prevalence and correlates of non-fatal overdose. *Addiction* 91:405–411.

Darke, S., Ross, J., and Hall, W. (1996b). Overdose among heroin users in Sydney, Australia: II. responses to overdose. *Addiction* 91:413–417.

Darke, S., and Zador, D. (1996). Fatal heroin 'overdose': a review. *Addiction* 91:1765–1772.

Davidson, P. J., McLean, R. L., Kral, A. H., Gleghorn, A. A., Edlin, B. R., and Moss, A. R. (2003). Fatal heroin-related overdose in San Francisco, 1997-2000: a case for targeted intervention. *J. Urban Health* 80:261–273.

Degenhardt, L., Lynskey, M., and Hall, W. (2000). Cohort trends in the age of initiation of drug use in Australia. *Aust. N. Z. J. Public Health* 24:421–426.

Deren, S., Robles, R., Andia, J., Colon, H. M., Kang, S. Y., and Perlis, T. (2001). Trends in HIV seroprevalence and needle sharing among Puerto Rican drug injectors in Puerto Rico and New York: 1992-1999. *J. Acquir. Immune Defic. Syndr.* 26:164–169.

Des Jarlais, D.C., Diaz, T., Perlis, T., Vlahov, D., Maslow, C., Latka, M., Rockwell, R., Edwards, V., Friedman, S.R., Monterroso, E., Williams, I., and Garfein, R.S. (2003). Variability in the incidence of human immunodeficiency virus, hepatitis B virus, and hepatitis C virus infection among young injecting drug users in New York City. *Am. J. Epidemiol.* 157:467–471.

Des Jarlais, D.C., Marmor, M., Paone, D., Titus, S., Shi, Q., Perlis, T., Jose, B., and Friedman, S.R. (1996). HIV incidence among injecting drug users in New York City syringe-exchange programmes. *Lancet* 348:987–991.

Des Jarlais, D. C., McKnight, C., and Milliken, J. (2004). Public funding of US syringe exchange programs. *J. Urban Health* 81:118–121.

Des Jarlais, D.C., Perlis, T., Friedman, S.R., Deren, S., Chapman, T., Sotheran, J.L., Tortu, S., Beardsley, M., Paone, D., Torian, L.V., Beatrice, S.T., DeBernardo, E., Monterroso, E., and Marmor, M. (1998). Declining seroprevalence in a very large HIV epidemic: injecting drug users in New York City, 1991 to 1996. *Am. J. Public Health* 88:1801–1806.

Des Jarlais, D.C., Diaz, T., Perlis, T., Vlahov, D., Maslow, C., Latka, M., Rockwell, R., Edwards, V., Friedman, S.R., Monterroso, E., Williams, I., and Garfein, R.S. (2003). Variability in the incidence of human immunodeficiency virus, hepatitis B virus, and hepatitis C virus infection among young injecting drug users in New York City. *Am. J. Epidemiol.* 157:467–471.

Dettmer, K., Saunders, B., and Strang, J. (2001). Take home naloxone and the prevention of deaths from opiate overdose: two pilot schemes. *BMJ.* 322:895–896.

Diaz, T., Des Jarlais, D.C., Vlahov, D., Perlis, T.E., Edwards, V., Friedman, S.R, Rockwell, R., Hoover, D., Williams, I.T., and Monterroso, E.R. (2001). Factors associated with prevalence hepatitis C: Differences among young adult injection drug users in lower and upper Manhattan, New York City. *Am. J. Public Health* 91:23–30.

Dolan, K., Kimber, J., Fry, C., Fitzgerald, J., McDonald, D., and Trautmann, F. (2000). Drug consumption facilities in Europe and the establishment of supervised injecting centres in Australia. *Drug Alcohol Rev.* 19:337–346.

Dolan, K., and Wodak, A. (1996), Switzerland, (September 28, 2004); http://www.lindesmith.org/library/dolan2.cfm

Drucker, E. (2002). Population impact of mass incarceration under New York's Rockefeller drug laws: an analysis of years of life lost. *J. Urban Health* 79:434–435.

Drugs approved for opiate dependence (2003). *FDA Consum.* 37:6.

Duncan, S. C., Duncan, T. E., and Strycker, L. A. (2002). A multilevel analysis of neighborhood context and youth alcohol and drug problems. *Prev. Sci.* 3:125–133.

Edeh, J., and Spalding, P. (2000). Screening for HIV, HBV and HCV markers among drug users in treatment in rural south-east England. *J. Public Health Med.* 22:531–539.

Edlin, B.R., Irwin, K.L., Faruque, S., McCoy, C.B., Word, C., Serrano, Y., Inciardi, J.A., Bowser, B.P., Schilling, R.F., and Holmberg, S.D. (1994a). Intersecting epidemics–crack cocaine use and HIV infection among inner-city young adults. Multicenter Crack Cocaine and HIV Infection Study Team. *N. Engl. J. Med.* 331:1422–1427.

Ellickson, P. L., and Morton, S. C. (1999). Identifying adolescents at risk for hard drug use: racial/ethnic variations. *J. Adolesc. Health* 25: 82–395.

Ennett, S. T., Tobler, N. S., Ringwalt, C. L., and Flewelling, R. L. (1994). How effective is drug abuse resistance education? A meta-analysis of Project DARE outcome evaluations. *Am. J. Public Health* 84:1394–1401.

Ensminger, M. E., Anthony, J. C., and McCord, J. (1997b). The inner city and drug use: initial findings from an epidemiological study. *Drug Alcohol Depend.* 48:175–184.

Epstein, J. A., Botvin, G. J., Griffin, K. W., and Diaz, T. (1999). Role of ethnicity and gender in polydrug use among a longitudinal sample of inner-city adolescents. *J. Alcohol Drug Education* 45:1–12.

FDA Consumer. (2003). Drugs approved for opiate dependence. *FDA Consumer* 37(1):6.

Federal Registry. (2003). Opioid drugs in maintenance and detoxification treatment of opiate addiction; addition of buprenorphine and buprenorphine combination to list of approved opioid treatment medication. Interim final rule. *Federal Registry* 68(99):27937-27939.

Fischer, B. (1995). Drugs, communities, and "harm reduction" in Germany: the new relevance of "public health" principles in local responses. *J. Public Health Policy* 16:389–411.

Flom, P.L., Friedman, S.R., Kottiri, B.J., Neaigus, A., Curtis, R., Des Jarlais, D.C., Sandoval, M., and Zenilman, J.M. (2001). Stigmatized drug use, sexual partner concurrency, and other sex risk network and behavior characteristics of 18- to 24-year-old youth in a high-risk neighborhood. *Sex. Transm. Dis.* 28:598–607.

Freudenberg, N., Vlahov, D., and Galea, S. (2005). Beyond urban penalty and urban sprawl: Back to living conditions as the focus of urban health. *J. Communinty Health* 30(1): 1-11.

Frischer, M., Anderson, S., Hickman, M., and Heatlie, H. (2002). Diffusion of drug misuse in Scotland: Findings from the 1993 and 1996 Scottish Crime Surveys. *Addiction Research & Theory* 10:83–95.

Fuller, C. M., Borrell, L. N., Galea, S., and Vlahov D. (2002). The effect of race, neighborhood, and social network on adolescent initiation of injection drug use among recont-onset injection drug users in Baltimore, Maryland. Paper presented at the *2002 AIDS Conference,* Barcelona Spain, 7-12 July 2002.

Fuller, C. M., Vlahov, D., Arria, A. M., Ompad, D. C., Garfein, R. S., and Strathdee, S. A. (2001). Factors associated with adolescent initiation of injection drug use. *Public Health Rep.* 116:136–145.

Fuller, C. M., Vlahov, D., Ompad, D. C., Shah, N., Arria, A., and Strathdee, S. A. (2002). High-risk behaviors associated with transition from illicit non-injection to injection drug use among adolescent and young adult drug users: a case-control study. *Drug Alcohol Depend.* 66:189-198.

Fullilove, R. E., Fullilove, M. T., Bowser, B. P., and Gross, S. A. (1990). Risk of sexually transmitted disease among black adolescent crack users in Oakland and San Francisco, Calif. *JAMA.* 263:851–855.

Furst, R. T., Herrmann, C., Leung, R., Galea, J., and Hunt, K. (2004). Heroin diffusion in the mid-Hudson region of New York State. *Addiction* 99:431–441.

Galea, S., Ahern, J., Tardiff, K., Leon, A. C., Coffin, P. O., Derr, K., and Vlahov, D. (2003). Racial/ethnic disparities in overdose mortality trends in New York City, 1990-1998. *J. Urban Health* 80:201–211.

Galea, S., Ahern, J., and Vlahov, D. (2003). Contextual determinants of drug use risk behavior: a theoretic framework. *J. Urban Health* 80:iii50-iii58.

Galea, S., Ahern, J., Vlahov, D., Coffin, P. O., Fuller, C., Leon, A. C., and Tardiff, K. (2003). Income distribution and risk of fatal drug overdose in New York City neighborhoods. *Drug Alcohol Depend.* 70:139–148.

Galea, S., Ahern, J., Vlahov, D., Coffin, P. O., Leon, A. C., and Tardiff, K. (2003b). Income distribution and risk of fatal drug overdose in New York City neighborhoods. *Drug Alcohol Depend.* 70(2):139–48.

Galea, S., Nandi, A., and Vlahov, D. (2004). The social epidemiology of substance use. *Epidemiol Rev.* 26:36–52.

Galea, S., and Vlahov, D. (2005). Urban Health: Evidence, Challenges, and Directions. *Annu. Rev. Public Health* 26; 341-365.

Garfein, R. S., Vlahov, D., Galai, N., Doherty, M. C., and Nelson, K. E. (1996). Viral infections in short-term injection drug users: the prevalence of the hepatitis C, hepatitis B, human immunodeficiency, and human T-lymphotropic viruses. *Am. J. Public Health* 86:655–661.

Global surveillance and control of hepatitis C. Report of a WHO Consultation organized in collaboration with the Viral Hepatitis Prevention Board, Antwerp, Belgium (1999). *J. Viral Hepat.* 6:35–47.

Goetz, E. G. (1996). The US war on drugs as urban policy. *J. Urban Regional Res.* 20:539–549.

Goldstein, S. T., Alter, M. J., Williams, I. T., Moyer, L. A., Judson, F. N., Mottram, K. Fleenor, M., Ryder, P.L., and Margolis, H.S. (2002). Incidence and risk factors for acute hepatitis B in the United States, 1982-1998: implications for vaccination programs. *J. Infect. Dis.* 185:713–719.

Golub, A. and Johnson, B. D. (2001). Variation in youthful risks of progression from alcohol and tobacco to marijuana and to hard drugs across generations. *Am. J. Public Health* 91:225–232.

Gordon, D. R. (1994). *The return of the dangerous classes: Drug prohibition and policy politics.* W.W. Norton & Co., New York.

Gossop, M., Griffiths, P., and Strang, J. (1994). Sex differences in patterns of drug taking behaviour. A study at a London community drug team. *Br. J. Psychiatry* 164:101–104.

Grandjean, E., Graf, P., Lauber, A., Meier, H., and Muller, R. (1976). Survey on the effects of noise around three civil airports in Switzerland. In: Kerlin, R. (ed.), *Internoise '76.* Institute of Noise Control Engineers, Washington D.C., pp 85–90.

Groseclose, S. L., Weinstein, B., Jones, T. S., Valleroy, L. A., Fehrs, L. J., and Kassler, W. J. (1995). Impact of increased legal access to needles and syringes on practices of injecting-drug users and police officers–Connecticut, 1992-1993. *J Acquir. Immune. Defic. Syndr. Hum. Retrovirol.* 10:82–89.

Gyarmathy, V. A., Neaigus, A., Miller, M., Friedman, S. R., and Des, J. (2002b). Risk correlates of prevalent HIV, hepatitis B virus, and hepatitis C virus infections among noninjecting heroin users. *J Acquir. Immune. Defic. Syndr.* 30:448–456.

Harlow, K. C. (1990). Patterns of rates of mortality from narcotics and cocaine overdose in Texas, 1976-87. *Public Health Rep.* 105:455–462.

Haw, S., and Higgins, K. (1998). A comparison of the prevalence of HIV infection and injecting risk behaviour in urban and rural samples in Scotland. *Addiction* 93: 855–863.

Hearn, W. L., Rose, S., Wagner, J., Ciarleglio, A., and Mash, D. C. (1991). Cocaethylene is more potent than cocaine in mediating lethality. *Pharmacol. Biochem. Behav.* 39:531–533.

Hepatitis B vaccination for injection drug users–Pierce County, Washington, 2000 (2001). *MMWR. 50,* 388–90, 399.

Holmberg, S. D. (1996). The estimated prevalence and incidence of HIV in 96 large US metropolitan areas. *Am. J. Public Health* 86:642-654.

Hser, Y. I., Chou, C. P., Hoffman, V., and Anglin, M. D. (1999). Cocaine use and high-risk sexual behavior among STD clinic patients. *Sex. Transm. Dis.* 26:82–86.

Hughes, P. H., Barker, N. W., Crawford, G. A., and Jaffe, J. H. (1972). The natural history of a heroin epidemic. *Am. J. Public Health* 62:995–1001.

Hunt, L. G., and Chambers, C. D. (1976). *The heroin epidemics : a study of heroin use in the United States, 1965-1975.* Spectrum Publications, New York, New York.

Hurley, S. F., Jolley, D. J., and Kaldor, J. M. (1997). Effectiveness of needle-exchange programmes for prevention of HIV infection. *Lancet* 349:1797–1800.

Hwang, L. Y., Ross, M. W., Zack, C., Bull, L., Rickman, K., and Holleman, M. (2000a). Prevalence of sexually transmitted infections and associated risk factors among populations of drug abusers. *Clin. Infect. Dis.* 31:920–926.

Jaffe, J. H., and O'Keeffe, C. (2003). From morphine clinics to buprenorphine: regulating opioid agonist treatment of addiction in the United States. *Drug Alcohol Depend.* 70:S3-S11.

Johnson, R. A., and Gerstein, D. R. (2000). Age, period, and cohort effects in marijuana and alcohol incidence: United States females and males, 1961-1990. *Subst. Use Misuse.* 35:925–948.

Johnston, L. D., O'Malley, P. M., Bachman, J. G., and Schulenberg, J. E. (2004). Monitoring the Future national survey results on drug use, 1975-2003. Volume I: Secondary school students Rep. No. NIH Publication No. 04-5507. National Institute on Drug Abuse, Bethesda, MD.

Kandel, D. (1975). Stages in adolescent involvement in drug abuse. *Science* 190:912–914.

Kandel, D. B., Yamaguchi, K., and Chen, K. (1992). Stages of progression in drug involvement from adolescence to adulthood: Further evidence for the gateway theory. *J. Stud. Alcohol* 53:447–457.

Kane, M. (1995). Global programme for control of hepatitis B infection. *Vaccine* 1:S47–9.

Kaplan, E. H., and Heimer, R. (1995). HIV incidence among New Haven needle exchange participants: updated estimates from syringe tracking and testing data. *J. Acquir. Immune. Defic. Syndr. Hum. Retrovirol.* 10:175–176.

Kaplan, G. A., Everson, S. A., and Lynch, J. W. (2000). The contribution of social and behavioral research to an understanding of the distribution of disease: A multi-level approach. In: Smedley B.D., and Syme., S.L. (eds.), *Promoting health: Intervention strategies from social and behavioral research.* National Academy Press, Washington D.C., pp 37–80.

Kaplan, G. A., Pamuk, E. R., Lynch, J. W., Cohen, R. D., and Balfour, J. L. (1996). Inequality in income and mortality in the United States: analysis of mortality and potential pathways. *BMJ.* 312:999–1003.

Karapetyan, A. F., Sokolovsky, Y. V., Araviyskaya, E. R., Zvartau, E. E., Ostrovsky, D. V., and Hagan, H. (2002). Syphilis among intravenous drug-using population: epidemiological situation in St Petersburg, Russia. *Int. J. STD AIDS.* 13: 618–623.

Karlsson, G., and Romelsjo, A. (1997). A longitudinal study of social, psychological and behavioural factors associated with drunken driving and public drunkenness. *Addiction* 92:447–457.

Kawachi, I., and Berkman, L. (2000). Social cohesion, social capital and health. In: Berkman L., and I. Kawachi, I. (eds.), *Social epidemiology.* Oxford Unviersity Press, New York, pp 174–190.

Kawachi, I., and Kennedy, B. P. (1997). Health and social cohesion: why care about income inequality? *BMJ.* 314:1037–1040.

Kawachi, I., Kennedy, B. P., Lochner, K., and Prothrow-Stith, D. (1997). Social capital, income inequality, and mortality. *Am. J. Public Health* 87:1491–1498.

Kennedy, B. P., Kawachi, I., Prothrow-Stith, D., Lochner, K., and Gupta, V. (1998). Social capital, income inequality, and firearm violent crime. *Soc. Sci. Med.* 47:7-17.

Keyes, L. C. (1992). *Strategies and saints: Fighting drugs in subsidized housing.* The Urban Institute Press, Washington, D.C.

Kintz, P., Brenneisen, R., Bundeli, P., and Mangin, P. (1997). Sweat testing for heroin and metabolites in a heroin maintenance program. *Clin. Chem.* 43:736–739.

Kleber, H. D. (1994). Our current approach to drug abuse–progress, problems, proposals. *N. Engl. J. Med.* 330:361–365.

Knipschild, P., and Oudshoorn, N. (1977). VII. Medical effects of aircraft noise: drug survey. *Int. Arch. Occup. Environ. Health* 40:197–200.

Koblin, B. A., Factor, S. H., Wu, Y., and Vlahov, D. (2003). Hepatitis C virus infection among non-injecting drug users in New York City. *J. Med. Virol.* 70:387–390.

Kottiri, B. J., Friedman, S. R., Neaigus, A., Curtis, R., and Des, J. (2002). Risk networks and racial/ethnic differences in the prevalence of HIV infection among injection drug users. *J. Acquir. Immune. Defic. Syndr.* 30:95–104.

Kral, A. H., Bluthenthal, R. N., Booth, R. E., and Watters, J. K. (1998b). HIV seroprevalence among street-recruited injection drug and crack cocaine users in 16 US municipalities. *Am. J Public Health* 88:108–113.

Kral, A.H., Bluthenthal, R.N., Booth, R.E., and Watters, J.K. (1998a) HIV seroprevalence among street-recruited injection drug and crack cocaine users in 16 US municipalities. *Am. J. Public Health* 88(1):108-113.

Kral, A. H., Bluthenthal, R. N., Lorvick, J., Gee, L., Bacchetti, P., and Edlin, B. R. (2001). Sexual transmission of HIV-1 among injection drug users in San Francisco, USA: risk-factor analysis. *Lancet* 357:1397–1401.

Kral, A. H., Lorvick, J., and Edlin, B. R. (2000). Sex- and drug-related risk among populations of younger and older injection drug users in adjacent neighborhoods in San Francisco. *J. Acquir. Immune. Defic. Syndr.* 24:162–167.

Kral, A. H., Lorvick, J., Gee, L., Bacchetti, P., Rawal, B., Busch, M., and Edlin, B.R. (2003). Trends in human immunodeficiency virus seroincidence among street-recruited injection drug users in San Francisco, 1987-1998. *Am. J. Epidemiol.* 157:915–922.

Kumar, R., O'Malley, P. M., Johnston, L. D., Schulenberg, J. E., and Bachman, J. G. (2002). Effects of school-level norms on student substance use. *Prev. Sci.* 3:105–124.

Lange, W. R., Snyder, F. R., Lozovsky, D., Kaistha, V., Kaczaniuk, M. A., and Jaffe, J. H. (1988). Geographic distribution of human immunodeficiency virus markers in parenteral drug abusers. *Am. J. Public Health* 78:443–446.

Latkin, C. A., Forman, V., Knowlton, A., and Sherman, S. (2003). Norms, social networks, and HIV-related risk behaviors among urban disadvantaged drug users. *Soc. Sci. Med.* 56:465–476.

Lerner, M., and Nurco, D. N. (1970). Drug abuse deaths in Baltimore, 1951-1966. *Int. J. Addict.*. 5:693–716.

Leukefeld, C. G., Narevic, E., Hiller, M. L., Staton, M., Logan, T. K., Gillespie, W., Webster, J.M., Garrity, T.F., and Purvis, R. (2002). Alcohol and drug use among rural and urban incarcerated substance abusers. *Int. J. Offender. Ther. Comp. Criminol.* 46: 715–728.

Levy, S. J., and Pierce, J. P. (1990). Predictors of marijuana use and uptake among teenagers in Sydney, Australia. *Int. J. Addict.* 25:1179–1193.

Lillie-Blanton, M., Parsons, P. E., Gayle, H., and Dievler, A. (1996). Racial differences in health: not just black and white, but shades of gray. *Annu. Rev. Public Health* 17:411–48.

Lindenberg, C. S., Strickland, O., Solorzano, R., Galvis, C., Dreher, M., and Darrow, V. C. (1999). Correlates of alcohol and drug use among low-income Hispanic immigrant childbearing women living in the USA. *Int. J. Nurs. Stud.* 36:3–11.

Ling, W., and Smith, D. (2002). Buprenorphine: blending practice and research. *J. Subst. Abuse Treat.* 23:87–92.

Logan, D. G. (1973). Heroin maintenance clinics: does the "British System" have answers for U.S. addiction treatment shortcomings? *Proc. Natl. Conf. Methadone. Treat.* 1:579–585.

Logan, T. K., and Leukefeld, C. (2000a). Sexual and drug use behaviors among female crack users: a multi-site sample. *Drug Alcohol Depend.* 58:237–245.

Logan, T. K., and Leukefeld, C. (2000b). Sexual and drug use behaviors among female crack users: a multi-site sample. *Drug Alcohol Depend.* 58:237–245.

Lora-Tamayo, C., Tena, T., and Rodriguez, A. (1994). Cocaine-related deaths. *J. Chromatogr. A.* 674:217–224.

Lynam, D. R., Milich, R., Zimmerman, R., Novak, S. P., Logan, T. K., Martin, C., Leukefeld, C., and Clayton R. (1999). Project DARE: no effects at 10-year follow-up. *J. Consult. Clin. Psychol.* 67:590–593.

Macalino, G.E., Springer, K.W., Rahman, Z.S., Vlahov, D., and Jones, T.S. (1998). Community-based programs for safe disposal and used needles and syringes. *J. Acquir. Immune, Defic. Syndr. Hum. Retrovirol.* 18(Suppl 1):S111-9.

Madianos, M. G., Gefou-Madianou, D., Richardson, C., and Stefanis, C. N. (1995). Factors affecting illicit and licit drug use among adolescents and young adults in Greece. *Acta. Psychiatr. Scand.* 91:258–264.

Manning, F. J., and Ingraham, L. H. (1983). Drug "overdoses" among U.S. soldiers in Europe, 1978-1979. I. Demographics and toxicology. *Int. J. Addict.* 18:89–98.

Marczynski, K. S., Welte, J. W., Marshall, J. R., and Ferby, E. N. (1999). Prevalence and determinants of alcohol-related problems. *Am. J. Drug Alcohol Abuse* 25:715–730.

Marzuk, P. M., Tardiff, K., Leon, A. C., Hirsch, C. S., Stajic, M., Portera, L., and Hartwell, N. (1997a). Poverty and fatal accidental drug overdoses of cocaine and opiates in New York City: an ecological study. *Am. J. Drug Alcohol Abuse* 23:221–228.

McGinnis, J. M., and Foege, W. H. (1999). Mortality and morbidity attributable to use of addictive substances in the United States. *Proc. Assoc. Am. Physicians* 111:109–118.

McMahon, J. M., Simm, M., Milano, D., and Clatts, M. (2004). Detection of hepatitis C virus in the nasal secretions of an intranasal drug-user. *Ann. Clin. Microbiol. Antimicrob.* 3:6.

McMahon, J. M., and Tortu, S. (2003). A potential hidden source of hepatitis C infection among noninjecting drug users. *J. Psychoactive Drugs* 35:455–460.

Metsch, L. R., and McCoy, C. B. (1999). Drug treatment experiences: rural and urban comparisons. *Subst. Use. Misuse.* 34:763–784.

Molinari, S. P., Cooper, J. R., and Czechowicz, D. J. (1994). Federal regulation of clinical practice in narcotic addiction treatment: purpose, status, and alternatives. *J. Law Med. Ethics* 22:231–239.

Molitor, F., Truax, S. R., Ruiz, J. D., and Sun, R. K. (1998). Association of methamphetamine use during sex with risky sexual behaviors and HIV infection among non-injection drug users. *West J. Med.* 168:93–97.

Montoya, I. D., and Atkinson, J. S. (1996). Determinants of HIV seroprevalence rates among sites participating in a community-based study of drug users. *J. Acquir. Immune. Defic. Syndr. Hum. Retrovirol.* 13:169–176.

Morral, A. R., McCaffrey, D. F., and Paddock, S. M. (2002). Reassessing the marijuana gateway effect. *Addiction* 97:1493–1504.

Morral, A. R., McCafrey, D. F., and Paddock, S. M. (2002). Evidence does not favor marijuana gateway effects over a common-factor interpretation of drug use initiation: responses to Anthony, Kenkel & Mathios and Lynskey. *Addiction* 97:1509–1510.

Mueser, K. T., Essock, S. M., Drake, R. E., Wolfe, R. S., and Frisman, L. (2001). Rural and urban differences in patients with a dual diagnosis. *Schizophr. Res.* 48:93–107.

Murrill, C. S., Weeks, H., Castrucci, B. C., Weinstock, H. S., Bell, B. P., Spruill, C., and Gwinn, M. (2002). Age-specific seroprevalence of HIV, hepatitis B virus, and hepatitis C virus infection among injection drug users admitted to drug treatment in 6 US cities. *Am. J. Public Health* 92:385–387.

Murrill, C.S., Prevots, D.R., Miller, M.S., Linley, L.A., Royalty J.E., and Gwinn, M. (2001). Incidence of HIV among injection drug users entering drug treatment programs in four U.S. cities. *J. Urban Health* 78(1):152-61.

National Household Survey on Drug Abuse, 1997. (11-28-2002). Substance Abuse and Mental Health Service Administration.

National Institute on Drug Abuse. (1997). Rural substance abuse: State of knowledge and Issues. vols. 168. National Institutes of Health, Rockville, MD.

Neaigus, A., Friedman, S. R., Jose, B., Goldstein, M. F., Curtis, R., Ildefonso, G., and Des Jarlais, D.C. (1996). High-risk personal networks and syringe sharing as risk factors for HIV infection among new drug injectors. *J. Acquir. Immune. Defic. Syndr. Hum. Retrovirol.* 11:499–509.

Neaigus, A., Miller, M., Friedman, S. R., and Des, J. (2001). Sexual transmission risk among noninjecting heroin users infected with human immunodeficiency virus or hepatitis C virus. *J. Infect. Dis.* 184:359–363.

Newcomb, M. D., and Bentler, P. M. (1986). Cocaine use among young adults. *Adv. Alcohol. Subst. Abuse* 6:73–96.

Novick, D. M., Trigg, H. L., Des, J., Friedman, S. R., Vlahov, D., and Kreek, M. J. (1989). Cocaine injection and ethnicity in parenteral drug users during the early years of the human immunodeficiency virus (HIV) epidemic in New York City. *J. Med. Virol.* 29:181–185.

Office of Applied Studies, Substance Abuse and Mental Health Services Administration. (1998). *Preliminary results from the 1997 National Household Survey on Drug Abuse,* DHHS Publication No. SMA 98-3251. Department of Health and Human Services, Rockville, MD.

Opioid drugs in maintenance and detoxification treatment of opiate addiction; addition of buprenorphine and buprenorphine combination to list of approved opioid treatment medications. (2003b). Interim final rule. F*ed. Regist.* 68:27937–27939.

Othieno, C. J., Kathuku, D. M., and Ndetei, D. M. (2000). Substance abuse in outpatients attending rural and urban health centres in Kenya. *East Afr. Med. J.* 77:592-595.

Paone, D., Des, J., Gangloff, R., Milliken, J., and Friedman, S. R. (1995). Syringe exchange: HIV prevention, key findings, and future directions. *Int. J. Addict.* 30:1647–1683.

Parry, A. (1992). Taking heroin maintenance seriously: the politics of tolerance. *Lancet* 339:350-351.

Perneger, T. V., Giner, F., del, R. M., and Mino, A. (1998). Randomised trial of heroin maintenance programme for addicts who fail in conventional drug treatments. *BMJ.* 317:13–18.

Perucci, C. A., Davoli, M., Rapiti, E., Abeni, D. D., and Forastiere, F. (1991). Mortality of intravenous drug users in Rome: a cohort study. *Am. J. Public Health* 81:1307-1310.

Powis, B., Griffiths, P., Gossop, M., and Strang, J. (1996). The differences between male and female drug users: community samples of heroin and cocaine users compared. *Subst. Use Misuse.* 31:529–543.

Quaglio, G., Lugoboni, F., Pajusco, B., Sarti, M., Talamini, G., Lechi, A., Mezzelani, P., and Des Jarlais, D.C. (2003). Factors associated with hepatitis C virus infection in injection and noninjection drug users in Italy. *Clin. Infect. Dis.* 37:33–40.

Read, N. (2003). Canada's first safe-injection site opens: Mirrored booths, 'chill out' room featured in controversial, taxpayer-funded centre. *Ottawa Citizen* September 16, 2003.

Renwick, N., Dukers, N. H., Weverling, G. J., Sheldon, J. A., Schulz, T. F., Prins, M. Coutinho, R.A., and Goudsmit, J. (2002). Risk factors for human herpesvirus 8 infection in a cohort of drug users in the Netherlands, 1985-1996. *J. Infect. Dis.* 185:1808–1812.

Rhodes, T., Judd, A., Mikhailova, L., Sarang, A., Khutorskoy, M., Platt, L., Lowndes, C.M., and Renton, A. (2004). Injecting equipment sharing among injecting drug users in Togliatti City, Russian Federation: maximizing the protective effects of syringe distribution. *J. Acquir. Immune. Defic. Syndr.* 35:293–300.

Rhodes, T., Mikhailova, L., Sarang, A., Lowndes, C. M., Rylkov, A., Khutorskoy, M., and Renton A. (2003). Situational factors influencing drug injecting, risk reduction and syringe exchange in Togliatti City, Russian Federation: a qualitative study of micro risk environment. *Soc. Sci. Med.* 57:39-54.

Rockefeller, N. G. (1973). Annual message to the New York State legislature. Ref Type: Unpublished Work.

Rockwell, R., Deren, S., Goldstein, M. F., Friedman, S. R., and Des, J. (2002). Trends in the AIDS epidemic among New York City's injection drug users: localized or citywide? *J. Urban Health* 79:136–146.

Ross, M. W., Hwang, L. Y., Zack, C., Bull, L., and Williams, M. L. (2002). Sexual risk behaviours and STIs in drug abuse treatment populations whose drug of choice is crack cocaine. *Int. J. STD AIDS* 13:769–774.

Roy, E., Haley, N., Leclerc, P., Cédras, L., Blais, L., and Boivin, J. (2002). Drug injection among street youth: Predictors of initiation. *J. Urban Health* 80:92–105.

Roy, E., Haley, N., Leclerc, P., Cedras, L., Blais, L., and Boivin, J. F. (2003). Drug injection among street youths in Montreal: predictors of initiation. *J. Urban Health* 80:92–105.

Russell, S. (2002). Pilot program for heroin addicts saved lives, doctors say; Emergency antidote given for overdoses. *San Francisco Chronicle* December 3, 2002.

Sanchez, J., Comerford, M., Chitwood, D. D., Fernandez, M. I., and McCoy, C. B. (2002). High risk sexual behaviours among heroin sniffers who have no history of injection drug use: implications for HIV risk reduction. *AIDS Care* 14:391–398.

Sarkar, K., Panda, S., Das, N., and Sarkar, S. (1997). Relationship of national highway with injecting drug abuse and HIV in rural Manipur, India. *Indian J. Public Health* 41:49–51.

Schmid, H. (2001). Cannabis use in Switzerland: The role of attribution of drug use to friends, urbanization and repression. *Swiss J. Psychol.* 60:99–107.

Schoenbaum, E. E., Hartel, D., Selwyn, P. A., Klein, R. S., Davenny, K., Rogers, M., and Feiner, C., and Friedland, G. (1989). Risk factors for human immunodeficiency virus infection in intravenous drug users. *N. Engl. J. Med.* 321:874-879.

Scribner, R., Cohen, D., Kaplan, S., and Allen, S. H. (1999). Alcohol availability and homicide in New Orleans: conceptual considerations for small area analysis of the effect of alcohol outlet density. *J. Stud. Alcohol.* 60:310–316.

Seal, K. H., Kral, A. H., Gee, L., Moore, L. D., Bluthenthal, R. N., Lorvick, J., and Edlin, B.R. (2001). Predictors and prevention of nonfatal overdose among street-recruited injection heroin users in the San Francisco Bay Area, 1998-1999. *Am. J. Public Health* 91:1842–1846.

Sergeev, B., Karpets, A., Sarang, A., and Tikhonov, M. (2003). Prevalence and circumstances of opiate overdose among injection drug users in the Russian Federation. *J. Urban Health* 80:212–219.

Stark, K., Bienzle, U., Vonk, R., and Guggenmoos-Holzmann, I. (1997). History of syringe sharing in prison and risk of hepatitis B virus, hepatitis C virus, and human immunodeficiency virus infection among injecting drug users in Berlin. *Int. J. Epidemiol.* 26:1359-1366.

Storr, C. L., Arria, A. M., Workman, Z. R., and Anthony, J. C. (2004). Neighborhood environment and opportunity to try methamphetamine ("ice") and marijuana: evidence from Guam in the Western Pacific region of Micronesia. *Subst. Use. Misuse.* 39:253–276.

Substance Abuse and Mental Health Service Administration & Office of Applied Studies (2004). Treatment Episode Data Set (TEDS) 1992-2002: National admissions to substance abuse treatment services Report No. DHHS Publication No. SMA 04-3965. Department of Health and Human Services, Rockville, MD.

Substance Abuse and Mental Health Service Administration & Office of Applied Studies (2003). Emergency Department Trends From DAWN: Final Estimates 1995 – 2002. Report No. DAWN Series D-24, DHHS Publication No. SMA 03-3780. Rockville, MD.

Substance Abuse and Mental Health Services Administration, 2001, National Household Survey on Drug Abuse, 1988-2000, (September 28, 2004); http://www.oas.samhsa.gov/nhsda/2k1nhsda/vol1/toc.htm

Substance Abuse and Mental Health Services Administration & Office of Applied Studies (2003a). National Survey on Drug Use and Health, 2002 Rockville, MD.

Substance Abuse and Mental Health Services Administration & Office of Applied Studies (2003b). Results from the 2002 National Survey on Drug Use and Health: National Findings Report No. NHSDA Series H-22, DHHS Publication No. SMA 03–3836. Rockville, MD.

Substance Abuse and Mental Health Services Administration & Office of Applied Studies (2004). Results from the 2003 National Survey on Drug Use and Health: National Findings Report No. NHSDA Series H-25, DHHS Publication No. SMA 04-3964. Rockville, MD.

Syme, L. S., and Balfour, J. L. (1998). Social determinants of disease. In: R.B.Wallace, R.B., and Doebbeling, B.H. (eds.), Public Health and Preventive Medicine (12 ed.). Appleton and Lange, Stanford, CT.

Thorpe, L. E., Ouellet, L. J., Levy, J. R., Williams, I. T., and Monterroso, E. R. (2000). Hepatitis C virus infection: prevalence, risk factors, and prevention opportunities among young injection drug users in Chicago, 1997-1999. *J. Infect. Dis.* 182:1588–1594.

Tobin, K. E., and Latkin, C. A. (2003). The relationship between depressive symptoms and nonfatal overdose among a sample of drug users in Baltimore, Maryland. *J. Urban Health* 80: 220–229.

Tortu, S., McMahon, J. M., Pouget, E. R., and Hamid, R. (2004). Sharing of noninjection drug-use implements as a risk factor for hepatitis C. *Subst. Use Misuse.* 39:211–224.

Tortu, S., Neaigus, A., McMahon, J., and Hagen, D. (2001). Hepatitis C among noninjecting drug users: a report. *Subst. Use Misuse.* 36:523–534.

U.S. Census Bureau. (2000). U.S. Census 2000. U.S. Department of Commerce, Economic and Statistics Administration, Washington D.C.

United Nations & Office on Drugs and Crime (2003). *Global illicit drug trends 2003.* United Nations, New York.

Van Etten, M. L., and Anthony, J. C. (2001). Male-female differences in transitions from first drug opportunity to first use: searching for subgroup variation by age, race, region, and urban status. *J. Womens Health Gend. Based. Med.* 10:797–804.

Van Etten, M. L., Neumark, Y. D., and Anthony, J. C. (1997). Initial opportunity to use marijuana and the transition to first use: United States, 1979-1994. *Drug Alcohol Depend.* 49:1–7.

Van Haastrecht, H. J., van Ameijden, E. J., Van den Hoek, J. A., Mientjes, G. H., Bax, J. S., and Coutinho, R. A. (1996). Predictors of mortality in the Amsterdam cohort of human immunodeficiency virus (HIV)-positive and HIV-negative drug users. *Am. J. Epidemiol.* 143: 380–391.

Villano, S. A., Vlahov, D., Nelson, K. E., Lyles, C. M., Cohn, S., and Thomas, D. L. (1997). Incidence and risk factors for hepatitis C among injection drug users in Baltimore, Maryland. *J. Clin. Microbiol.* 35:3274–3277.

Vlahov, D., Anthony, J. C., Munoz, A., Margolick, J., Nelson, K. E., Celentano, D. D. Solomon, L., and Polk, B.F. (1991). The ALIVE study, a longitudinal study of HIV-1 infection in intravenous drug users: description of methods and characteristics of participants. *NIDA Res. Monogr.* 109: 75–100.

Vlahov, D., and Junge, B. (1998). The role of needle exchange programs in HIV prevention. *Public Health Rep.* 113 Suppl 1:75–80.

Vlahov, D., Munoz, A., Anthony, J. C., Cohn, S., Celentano, D. D., and Nelson, K. E. (1990). Association of drug injection patterns with antibody to human immunodeficiency virus type 1 among intravenous drug users in Baltimore, Maryland. *Am. J. Epidemiol.* 132:847–856.

Vlahov, D., Wang, C. L., Galai, N., Bareta, J., Mehta, S. H., Strathdee, S. A., and Nelson, K.E. (2004). Mortality risk among new onset injection drug users. *Addiction* 99:946–954.

von, S. K., Lieb, R., Pfister, H., Hofler, M., and Wittchen, H. U. (2002). What predicts incident use of cannabis and progression to abuse and dependence? A 4- year prospective examination of risk factors in a community sample of adolescents and young adults. *Drug Alcohol Depend.* 68:49–64.

Wagner, F., Diaz, D. B., Lopez, A. L., Collado, M. E., and Aldaz, E. (2002). Social cohesion, cultural identity, and drug use in Mexican rural communities. *Subst. Use Misuse.* 37:715-747.

Wagner, F. A., and Anthony, J. C. (2002). Into the world of illegal drug use: exposure opportunity and other mechanisms linking the use of alcohol, tobacco, marijuana, and cocaine. *Am. J. Epidemiol.* 155:918–925.

Wallace, J. M., Jr. (1999). The social ecology of addiction: race, risk, and resilience. *Pediatrics* 103:1122–1127.

Wallace, J. M., Jr., Bachman, J. G., O'Malley, P. M., Johnston, L. D., Schulenberg, J. E., and Cooper, S. M. (2002). Tobacco, alcohol, and illicit drug use: racial and ethnic differences among U.S. high school seniors, 1976-2000. *Public Health Rep.* 117(Suppl 1):S67–S75.

Wallace, R., Fullilove, M. T., and Wallace, D. (1992). Family systems and deurbanization: Implications for substance abuse. In: Lowinson, J.H., Ruiz, P., and Millman, R.B. (eds.), *Substance abuse: A comprehensvie textbook* (2nd ed.). Williams and Wilkins, Baltimore, MD, pp 944-955.

Warner, B. D., and Leukefeld, C. G. (2001). Rural-urban differences in substance use and treatment utilization among prisoners. *Am. J. Drug Alcohol Abuse 27*:265–280.

Warner, E. A., Kosten, T. R., and O'Connor, P. G. (1997). Pharmacotherapy for opioid and cocaine abuse. *Med. Clin. North Am.* 81:909–925.

Warner, L. A., Kessler, R. C., Hughes, M., Anthony, J. C., and Nelson, C. B. (1995). Prevalence and correlates of drug use and dependence in the United States. Results from the National Comorbidity Survey. *Arch. Gen. Psychiatry* 52:219–229.

Watters, J. K., Estilo, M. J., Kral, A. H., and Lorvick, J. J. (1994). HIV infection among female injection-drug users recruited in community settings. *Sex. Transm. Dis.* 21:321–328.

Wilcox, H. C., Wagner, F. A., and Anthony, J. C. (2002). Exposure opportunity as a mechanism linking youth marijuana use to hallucinogen use. *Drug Alcohol Depend.* 66:127–135.

Wood, E., Spittal, P. M., Small, W., Kerr, T., Li, K., Hogg, R. S., Tyndall, M.W., Montaner, J.S.G., and Schechter, M.T. (2004). Displacement of Canada's largest public illicit drug market in response to a police crackdown. *CMAJ.* 170:1551–1556.

Woody, G. E., Donnell, D., Seage, G. R., Metzger, D., Marmor, M., Koblin, B. A., Buchbinder, S., Gross, M., Stone, B., and Judson, F.N. (1999). Non-injection substance use correlates with risky sex among men having sex with men: data from HIVNET. *Drug Alcohol Depend.* 53:197–205.

Chapter 8

The Health of Children in Cities

M. Chris Gibbons, Vijay Singh, Kisha Braithwaite, and Bernard Guyer

1.0. INTRODUCTION

According to the 2000 census, 72.6 million children aged 0–18 live in the U.S., accounting for approximately one fourth of the total population (Federal Interagency Forum on Child and Family Statistics, 2003). Nearly one-third of these children live in central cities and one-half live in the suburbs (Sawhill and Chadwick, 1999). The number of children under 5 years of age has increased by 0.5% since 1990, while the number of children ages 5–19 years increased by 12.4% during the same time period (Maternal and Child Health Bureau, 2004). Over the next 50 years the proportion of children in the U.S. population will fall, as the population ages and birth rates plateau. By 2050, it is estimated that children will constitute 24% of the population, down from 26% in 1995 (Guyer, *et al.*, 1996). On the other hand, the ethnic diversity of this child population will be even greater than that of the overall population; in 2050, only 22% of U.S. children will be non-latino white, compared to 50.1% of the total population (U.S. Department of Commerce, 1996). These changing U.S. child population demographics suggest that more children will live in cities and that these urban children will be more ethnically and racially diverse than the child population as a whole.

While many similarities exist, the health of children and adolescents living in urban centers differs in several important ways when compared to that of children and adolescents not living in urban centers. Children living in urban centers are more likely to, 1) lack health insurance, 2) be living with a family with an income below the poverty line and receiving cash welfare benefits, 3) be living with a parent who does not possess a high school education, and 4) be more likely to be living in a single parent home (Wertheimer, *et al.*, 2002). All of these unique features have implications for the health of urban children.

Clearly within every city unique characteristics can be found that distinguish it from other cities. Yet, large urban centers also share many social, cultural, physical, and public infrastructure characteristics (Vlahov and Galea, 2002). Examination of the 100 largest urban areas in the U.S. reveals that they are increasingly populated by racial, ethnic, and immigrant minorities (Vlahov and Galea, 2002). This is due to both immigration of foreign nationals to the city and emigration of middle-class white U.S. citizens to the suburbs. The term "urban health penalty" describes the conditions that exist when healthier, more affluent persons leave the city and the remaining, often immigrant, residents experience health problems that interact with the city's physical and economic deterioration (Prewitt, 1997). The poverty zones created by this deterioration become epicenters for economic decline, job loss, and major health problems (Greenberg, 1991).

Increased population density, insufficient incomes, inadequate housing, and outdoor air pollution are all characteristic of urban centers (Galea, *et al.*, 2005; Hinrichsen, *et al.*, 2004). Health status and outcomes of children living under these conditions generally lag behind that of those living in non-urban areas. Understanding the causes and developing efficacious solutions is complicated by the issues of health care costs, quality, and access. While both rural and urban communities struggle with these issues, often urban communities exhibit a much higher degree of variability, intensity, and scope of the problem than rural communities. Fortunately, the picture is not all bad in regards to the urban environment. As will be discussed later in this chapter, among urban centers child survival rates are on average better than those for children living in rural areas (Hinrichsen, *et al.*, 2004). Cities offer youths a rich institutional environment with museums, theaters, libraries, schools, parks, zoos, movie theaters, music halls, stadiums, shops, houses of worship, restaurants, and other facilities. Racial and social diversity introduce children to a multicultural environment of languages, traditions, festivals, and foods. These, and a wide variety of other factors common to the urban environment, are undoubtedly a positive influence on the psychological and physical health of the children living in the urban environment.

This chapter will highlight some of the broad themes and major determinants of the health of children living in the inner city. The purpose of this chapter is to address three areas: 1) the urban characteristics that may affect the health of children; 2) how children contribute to the overall population health of cities; and 3) discuss gaps in knowledge and needed areas of research.

2.0. URBAN CHARACTERISTICS THAT MAY AFFECT THE HEALTH OF CHILDREN

2.1 Health Insurance Status

The Institute of Medicine's Committee on Children, Health Insurance, and Access to Care, concluded that health insurance coverage was the major determinant of access to care during childhood (IOM Committee on Children, 1998). While several child health insurance products are currently available, the largest source of coverage for children is via parental employers (Rolett, *et al.*, 2001). In 2002, 64.5% of children were insured through private insurance products, almost all provided by their parents' insurers. Still almost 14% or 11 million children were uninsured (Elixhauser, *et al.*, 2002). Even among working families, children are less well insured than their working parents. This is because many employers do not offer health insurance benefits for dependents, or many employees, particularly lower wage and part time employees, cannot afford to purchase these dependent health benefits (Rolett, *et al.*, 2001). Urban children, in particular, are at increased risk for uninsurance because they are more likely to be from single parent families, less likely to be from two parent families in which both parents are working and more likely to be from a racial or ethnic minority group (Coburn, *et al.*, 2002).

Although these differences in insurance status appear to have significant negative consequences for the health of urban children, the relationship between parental employment, childhood health insurance status, and child health in the urban environment is not completely clear. For example, while lack of health insurance is associated with lack of a regular source of care and an increased use of publicly funded clinics and emergency rooms (IOM Committee on Children, 1998), poor child health status and the likelihood of chronic health problems are more directly associated with lower parental employment (Kuhlthau and Perrin, 2001) and increased barriers to employment (Smith, *et al.*, 2002). Thus the lack of parental employment appears to be more strongly associated with negative health consequences than lack of health insurance.

2.2. Socio-Economic Status (SES) and Social Capital

A gradient in outcomes is consistently seen between people of lower and higher socioeconomic status along many diseases and health outcomes (Berkman and Kawachi, 2000; Marmot, *et al.*, 1991; Hemingway, *et al.*, 1997; Fuller, *et al.*, 1980; Poundstone, *et al.*, 2004; Galea, *et al.*, 2005; Brown, *et al.*, 2004; Galobardes, *et al.*, 2004; Muntaner, *et al.*, 2004). For example, low socio-economic status has been associated with poor mental health (Muntaner, *et al.*, 2004; Kalff, *et al.*, 2001), poor school achievement, (Duncan, *et al.*, 1994), increased infant mortality (Waldmann, 1999), HIV infection (Poundstone *et al.*, 2004), and Diabetes Mellitus (Brown, *et al.*, 2004). This relationship has been demonstrated among children and adolescents (Drukker, *et al.*, 2003). In addition, when a life course perspective is employed it appears that socioeconomic circumstances occurring at different stages of the life course may subsequently influence specific adulthood health outcomes including adult mortality (Galobardes, *et al.*, 2004). These relationships are of particular importance in the urban environment where concentrated pockets of low SES children and adults live.

Social cohesion has also been associated with health outcomes among adults and children (Berkman and Kawachi, 2000). Social cohesion refers to the extent of connectedness and solidarity among groups in a society. Social capital has also been associated with health outcomes in children (Aneshensel and Sucoff, 1996; Gold, *et al.*, 2002). Social capital is defined as those features of social organizations which act as resources for individuals and facilitate collective action (Berkman and Kawachi, 2000). These would include neighborhood trust and the existence of robust social networks (Kawachi, *et al.*, 1997). Socially cohesive communities then, are ones in which there exists greater stocks of social capital (Berkman and Kawachi, 2000). In terms of health outcomes, lower levels of social capital are associated with poorer mental health, increased school delinquency, inhibition of successful child development, increased teen pregnancy rate, increased child abuse, and increased infant mortality rates (Berkman and Kawachi, 2000; Waterston, *et al.*, 2004). Many of these child health outcomes have been linked to the urban environment.

The urban school system may be an important factor influencing both health and intellectual development of children (Mansour, *et al.*, 2003). There is evidence that school connectedness, defined as a child's perception of experiences of caring or closeness to school personnel and the school environment, is associated with child health (Mansour, *et al.*, 2003; Bonny, *et al.*, 2000). Resnick and colleagues found that higher levels of school connectedness were more protective against adolescent pregnancy than any other factor including family connectedness, unintentional injury, poly drug use, school delinquency, or absenteeism (Resnick, *et al.*, 1993). Higher levels of school connectedness are also positively associated with parental level of education (Bonny, *et al.*, 2000), and negatively associated with minority race, urban school type, cigarette use, alcohol utilization, and increasing school nurse visits (Bonny, *et al.*, 2000). Finally, evidence suggests that children's perceptions of school connectedness are malleable and positive improvements in school connectedness are associated with improved health outcomes (Hawkins, *et al.*, 1999).

2.3. Food and Urban Child Health

Several food and dietary characteristics of the urban environment have been associated with the health of inner city residents. For example, grocery store location, cost of food, and quality of supermarkets have all been linked to dietary choices and nutrient availability in the inner city (Morland, *et al.*, 2002a, 2002b). Specifically, urban centers tend to have smaller family owned food stores largely stocked with calorie dense, fatty, and refined foods, and with limited availability of fresh fruits and vegetables; these items are often sold at higher prices than similar items at suburban food stores. Suburban grocery stores are more often larger chain-type grocery stores, with a better supply of nutritious foods including an array of fresh fruits and vegetables that are offered at lower prices than in the inner city. This is important because the consumption of foods in a given community has been shown to correlate with the availability of foods in the community. (Cullen, *et al.*, 2001; Morland, *et al.*, 2002a; 2002b).

This association of retail outlet proximity and diet is also true for the consumption of tobacco and alcoholic beverages. Increased density of tobacco outlets and liquor establishments is associated with the urban inner city (Hyland, *et al.*, 2003; LaVeist and Wallace, 2000), the amount of alcohol ingested per capita, altered dietary nutrient intake, and with excess health risk among residents living in these communities (LaVeist and Wallace, 2000; Hyland, *et al.*, 2003). It is not widely recognized (with the exception of tobacco) that regulatory policies, such as business zoning and liquor licensing laws, that enable these situations to exist, have the unintended and perhaps unrecognized consequences of influencing disease risk of residents living in the urban environment.

2.4. Urbanization and Industrialization

As urban areas grow in population, they expand both vertically and horizontally, often overwhelming the natural environment and destroying ecosystems thereby imposing much larger ecological footprints and more significant health consequences for the involved populace (Hinrichsen, *et al.*, 2004). Urbanization and industrialization inevitably bring the continuing challenge of how to dispose of refuse and waste materials. Historically, incineration, burial, or dumping has been used most often, usually with little concern for potential long-term health effects (Powell and Stewart, 2001).

Growing awareness of a potential problem led to the development of the EPA in 1970 and the passage of legislation including the Comprehensive Environmental

Response, Compensation and Liability Act (CERCLA), also known as the *Superfund Act.* Superfund sites are generally the most serious and hazardous waste sites. To date, more than 1327 Superfund sites are in existence, with a disproportionate number located in poor or minority communities. Low-income and minority groups are more likely than are affluent and non-minority groups to live near landfills, incinerators, hazardous waste treatment facilities, and other toxic sites (Morello-Frosch, *et al.*, 2002; Powell and Stewart, 2001; Faber and Krieg, 2002).

Children are often the victims of environmental injustices, and poor and minority children, just as their parents, are affected disproportionately. In the U.S. almost 4 million children or approximately 25% of children live within 1 mile of a hazardous waste site (Powell and Stewart, 2001). Urban poor and minority children comprise the bulk of exposed children. The effects of childhood exposure to toxic agents are many and include neurodevelopment abnormalities, developmental, learning, and behavioral disabilities. Exposure sources have been documented in urban homes, schools, and industrial sites in close proximity to residential neighborhoods. Agents most commonly implicated are lead, Dioxins, and Polychlorinated Biphenyls (Powell and Stewart, 2001).

Despite the creation of federal and state agencies and a series of laws, regulations, policies, and a recent Institute of Medicine report calling attention to the issue, improving and eliminating environmental justice problems have proven to be intellectually daunting and highly resistant to positive change (Lee, 2002).

3.0. HOW CHILDREN CONTRIBUTE TO THE OVERALL HEALTH OF CITIES

3.1. Infant Mortality Rate (IMR)

In the U.S., the infant mortality rate (the number of deaths of infants under one year of age per 1,000 live births) has declined rather steadily throughout the twentieth century, largely due to improvements in control of infectious diseases, health care (particularly neonatal intensive care), and nutrition. In 1900, the rate was about 162 deaths per 1,000 births (Linder and Grove, 1947); by the year 2000 it had declined to 6.9 (Iyasu, *et al.*, 2002). Although marked improvements in infant survival have occurred among all racial and ethnic groups, higher infant mortality rates are seen among many minority groups and the magnitude of the disparity has in some cases increased (Arias, *et al.*, 2003). For example, between 1980 and 2000, infant mortality among whites declined 47.7% (from 10.9 to 5.7), while infant mortality among blacks declined only 36.9% (from 22.2 to 14.0). Consequently, the black-white ratio of infant mortality increased 25% (from 2.0 to 2.5) over this time period (Iyasu, *et al.*, 2002).

Cities have high infant mortality rates (IMR) because their residents share certain high-risk characteristics. The variability in IMR among the nation's 60 largest cities tends to segregate by race, ethnicity, and other characteristics common to the urban environment. For example, those cities with the highest infant mortality rates tend to have a larger proportion of black births and a smaller proportion of latino births. Conversely, cities with the lowest infant mortality rates tend to have a smaller proportion of black births and a larger proportion of latino births. Additionally, cities with higher IMRs were more commonly in the more urbanized Midwest, Southeast, and Northeast, and those with lower IMRs were clustered in the less urban Pacific West and West Central regions (Haynatzka, *et al.*, 2002). Several factors including low birth weight (Iyasu, *et al.*, 2002), low socioeconomic status, teen motherhood, single motherhood (Forssas, *et al,*. 1999), low maternal educational attainment, poor access to prenatal care (Barros, *et al.*, 2001), maternal tobacco use (Matthews, *et al.*, 2002), and biologic or genetic factors have been suggested as important causes of these unequal urban disparities in infant mortality.

Biologic and genetic factors do not appear to exert significant independent effects on infant mortality rates in the U.S. population (Ekwo and Moawad, 2000). While the primary reason for infant mortality disparities appears to be attributable to a higher proportion of low birth weight deliveries among minority and particularly black women, the etiology of black-white disparities in low birth weight is complex and not explained entirely by demographic risk factors such as maternal age, education, or income (Schoendorf, *et al.*, 1992; Buka, *et al.*, 2003). Other factors that might contribute to the disparity include racial differences in maternal medical conditions, stress, lack of social support, bacterial vaginosis, other co-morbidities, previous preterm delivery, and maternal health experiences that might be unique to black women (Hogan, *et al.*, 2001; Milligan, *et al.*, 2002; Buka, *et al.*, 2003).

In 1991, the U.S. Department of Health and Human Services began the national Healthy Start Initiative. This was a five year, $170 million infant mortality prevention demonstration program for communities with very high infant mortality rates (Boroff and O'Campo, 1996). This program funded 15 sites (mostly urban) in communities with infant mortality rates that were 1.5 – 2.5 times the national average. The program began with a five-year demonstration phase to identify and develop community-based system-level approaches to reducing infant mortality by 50% over the five-year period and to improve the health and well-being of women, infants, children, and their families. Healthy Start projects address multiple issues, including: providing adequate prenatal care, promoting positive prenatal health behaviors, meeting basic health needs (nutrition, housing, psychosocial support), reducing barriers to access, and enabling client empowerment.

While a formal national evaluation of the program showed mixed results, analyses of data from specific sites are promising (Devaney, *et al.*, 2000). One such evaluation detailed the Baltimore City Healthy Start's impact on medical reform, a component of the healthy start program, which works in conjunction with prenatal clinics, pediatric clinics, and family planning clinics in an effort to improve community access to services. Although obtaining long-term funding remains a challenge, preliminary data indicate that Healthy Start has begun to increase the utilization of prenatal and pediatric care, improve linkages between providers, and increase male involvement in perinatal care. In turn, these activities are helping to improve birth outcomes among very high risk inner city Baltimore women.

3.2. Asthma

The observation that urban air pollution is a potential cause of asthma and respiratory disease dates back to Greek and Roman antiquity (Holgate, *et al.*, 1999). In the early to mid twentieth century acute exacerbations of air pollution in urban centers of Belgium, London, Germany, and the Netherlands were all associated with increases in coughing, wheezing, shortness of breath, hospitalizations, and cardiopulmonary mortality among children and adults (Alberg and Samet, 2003). Towards the later half of the twentieth century, during the last three decades, the prevalence of asthma has increased significantly in all age and race/ethnicity groups across the world, with disproportional increases among impoverished, minority children living in urban inner cities (Shapiro and Stout, 2002; Mannino, *et al.*, 1998; 2002; Eggleston, *et al.*, 1999). The prevalence of asthma in children under the age of 18 is approximately seven percent in the U.S. However the rates may be as high as 20–25% among certain inner city census tracts in the northeast and Midwest (Graham, 2004; Aligne, *et al.*, 2000; Webber, *et al.*, 2002).

Many interrelated factors contribute to the epidemiology of urban childhood asthma. Individual and community level factors including exposure and sensitization to cockroach, rat and mouse allergens, dust mites, environmental tobacco smoke, cat dander, ozone, particulate matter, outdoor air pollution, lead, deteriorated urban housing stock and diesel exhaust, and poor access to care are all important (Eggleston, *et al.*, 1999; Shapiro and Stout, 2002; Holgate, *et al.*, 1999; Litonjua, *et al.*, 2001; Rosenstreich, *et al.*, 1997; Rauh, *et al.*, 2002; Kattan, *et al.*, 1997; Phipatanakul, *et al.*, 2000; Perry, *et al.*, 2003; Stevenson, *et al.*, 2001). These asthma determinants may operate via direct and indirect mechanisms. For example ambient air toxicants may act as direct irritants of bronchial mucosa. Alternatively an indirect pathway is also being increasingly recognized where toxicants act as immunmodulators via affecting the production of IgE and TH2 (Thymus-derived helper), thereby modulating the inflammatory response to alveolar antigens in genetically predisposed children (Shapiro and Stout, 2002; Eggleston, *et al.*, 1999).

Along with these individual and community level factors certain more global associations have been demonstrated between asthma and the urban environment. For example, rising levels of carbon dioxide (CO_2) trap atmospheric heat, promote plant pollen production, and alter species composition by favoring growth of ragweed, opportunistic weeds and molds. The combination of air pollutants, aeroallergens, heat waves and unhealthy air masses are increasingly associated with a changing climate and are collectively thought to contribute to global warming, in addition to causing damage to the respiratory systems, particularly for growing children and minority groups living in the inner cities (Epstein and Rogers, 2004).

Childhood morbidity and mortality associated with asthma and the urban environment have generally been on the increase for at least the last two to three decades. Over this time period the number of physician office and outpatient visits, emergency department visits, and hospitalizations have steadily increased, with children under the age of 18 consistently having the highest rates (Mannino, *et al.*, 1998; 2002; Webber, *et al.*, 2002).

The ultimate prevention and control of urban childhood asthma will require a comprehensive multifaceted approach. While appropriate medical management is important, its ultimate effectiveness is limited to the degree of success achieved at improving asthma determinants found in the urban environment (Clark, *et al.*, 1999).

School-based asthma education and prevention programs are an area of active research. According to the 2002 State Survey of School-Based Health Center Initiatives, there are 1,498 school-based health centers in the U.S. 61% of these centers are in schools located in urban areas. Most of them (63%) being in urban high schools (Lear, 2004). The potential efficacy of this strategy is supported by studies that suggest providing asthma self management education during school time can reduce symptoms and improve school performance (Webber, *et al.*, 2003; Lurie, *et al.*, 1998; Evans, *et al.*, 1997). Unfortunately the utilization of these sites as asthma education, prevention and control sites appears to be low. In a recent survey, none of nearly 1,500 school-based health centers listed asthma as a top priority (Lear, 2004).

3.3. Injury

National injury mortality data are not readily available by level of urbanization (Frattaroli, *et al.,* 2002). However, injury rates are greatest in those areas with low socioeconomic status residents, especially urban black children (Centers for Disease Control and Prevention, 2004). In the literature, two of the most commonly described forms of injury outcomes for children in urban areas are pedestrian accidents and youth violence.

Overall, motor vehicle traffic injuries occur more often among rural than urban children (National Center for Health Statistics, 1997). These rural children are usually injured as passengers (Lapidus, *et al.*, 1998; King, *et al.*, 1994), reflecting the fact that rural children spend more time in cars and drive longer distances. Urban children, however, are injured by motor vehicles more often as pedestrians than as occupants (Laraque, *et al.*, 1995). Nationally 18,000 children under age 15 were injured as pedestrians, and 434 died in 2002 (National Highway Traffic Safety Administration, 2002).

Environmental factors associated with childhood motor vehicle pedestrian injuries include two types of factors; 1) social, societal, systems and cultural factors and 2) physical characteristics like the home, streets, and playground (Grossman and Rivara, 1992). The concentration of poverty in inner cities, along with recent increases in residential segregation by income and race in U.S. metropolitan areas, create circumstances that lead to worse motor vehicle related injury outcomes for children in poor neighborhoods (Katz, *et al.*, 2001). Specifically, poverty in the urban child's social environment can create conditions that promote pedestrian injuries. For example, higher average and posted speed limits are likely to occur in areas of low socioeconomic status (Rivara, 1990). These higher speeds inevitably lead to more significant pedestrian motor vehicle injury.

Poverty also influences the physical environment in pedestrian accidents. Children from regions of concentrated poverty generally experience greater traffic exposure. This is because lower rates of parental home and car ownership are associated with more streets to cross on foot per day per child, and less likelihood of being driven home from school (Rao, *et al.*, 1997). Higher traffic volumes and increased traffic density are also associated with low SES neighborhoods (Rivara, 1990). Children from poor families are fivefold less likely to live in private houses or have adequate play space in their yards (Grossman and Rivara, 1992). Thus, urban children have fewer alternatives to street and sidewalk play (Posner, *et al.*, 2002). Finally, fewer pedestrian control devices occur in impoverished areas, and a recent review demonstrated that many sites of pediatric pedestrian trauma in Miami were located in long intervals between marked intersections (Hameed, *et al.*, 2004). These larger distances allow greater vehicle acceleration and more random pedestrian crossing patterns, which in turn predispose children to injury when they "dart-out" mid-block, between areas of obstructed view (DiMaggio and Durkin, 2002).

One strategy being investigated to lessen pedestrian injuries among urban children is based on community behavioral education. Unfortunately the scientific evidence suggests that community-based education alone is insufficient to improve traffic safety behavior among young children (Klassen, *et al.*, 2000). Recently the urban physical environment has emerged as a potentially more effective interventional target to prevent pedestrian injury. Creating safe playgrounds was one aspect of the Safe Kids/Healthy Neighborhood Coalition program, which brought together city agencies, volunteer organizations, and citizen groups in Central Harlem to try to improve child health outcomes (Davidson, *et al.*, 1994; Laraque, *et al.*, 1994). After two years of the intervention, injuries such as trauma from motor vehicles decreased 23% from baseline, and this was attributable to the increased availability of safe play areas for the urban children (Laraque, *et al.*, 1995). Other aspects of the urban physical environment can be manipulated through "traffic calming" engineering strategies. These include speed bumps, which by design are passive prevention strategies that work without any direct action on the part of the individual. A recent matched case-control study discovered that speed humps in Oakland, CA were associated with a 53% to 60% reduction in the odds of pediatric pedestrian injury or death within a child's neighborhood (Tester *et al.*, 2004). Intentional, or violence-related injuries include assault by firearms, blunt trauma and cutting or piercing (Centers for Disease Control and Prevention, 1997). Analysis of data from 88 cities across 33 states reveals 645 homicides reported in 2000 for children under age 18 (Department of Justice, 2003). In the past, numerous studies have shown that homicide rates are higher in urban centers than in rural areas (National Center for Health Statistics, 1997; Czerwinski and Moloney-Harmon, 1997; Zavoski, *et al.*, 1995; Weesner, *et al.*, 1994). Trend data from Boston, however, are encouraging and suggest a 12% annual decline in pediatric violence-related injuries, over a four year period (Sege, *et al.*, 2002).

Among childhood violence-related injuries, firearms are most commonly used. Fifty-seven percent of homicides nationwide in 2001 among children 10–14 years of age involved firearms (National Center for Health, 2001). Firearms are widely available in cities and may be unsafely stored (Weesner, *et al.*, 1994). Concentrated poverty in the urban environments can create fear for safety and promote weapon carrying. A survey in 1993 of ten inner city high school students showed that 22% of respondents reported possession of any type of firearm (Smith, 1996). The urban environment also generates child exposure to community and family violence, where violence can become a learned behavior (Czerwinski and Moloney-Harmon, 1997).

Strategies to intervene in violence-related injuries among children in cities including school-based education programs and peer mentoring have been able to change childhood attitudes towards violence (Sheehan, *et al.*, 1999). However, evaluations of other violence outcomes are needed for these interventions.

Policy and regulatory interventions represent another approach to firearm injury control among urban children. Available options include required designs that limit access of unauthorized, high-risk users (Frattaroli, *et al.*, 2002), like urban children. Intervention legislation and programs, such as tracing crime guns, strengthening the regulation of licensed firearm retailers, and screening prospective gun buyers (Wintemute, 2002), can decrease firearm availability, especially for urban youth. Community coalitions may even improve the urban environment as evidenced by the Safe Kids/Healthy Neighborhoods program, which showed a 44% decrease in injury risk for all targeted injuries, including physical assault and firearm mechanisms (Davidson *et al.*, 1994). Finally, the Moving to Opportunity Demonstration Program is a federal initiative that chose poor inner city participants, at random, to receive moving assistance to enable them to relocate to wealthier neighborhoods. Early results document a 56% decrease in violent crime perpetrated by juvenile's aged 11–16 in Baltimore, MD (Ludwig, *et al.*, 2001) and a 42% decrease in behavior problems among boys, as well as a 74% reduction in child injuries requiring medical attention, in Boston, MA (Katz, *et al.*, 2001). These studies suggest that the seemingly intractable problems of urban violence may indeed be amenable to improvement among urban youths.

3.4. Obesity

Across the world the incidence and prevalence of childhood obesity is on the rise (Wang, *et al.*, 2002; Wang, 2001). In the U.S., the percentage of school-age children six through eleven that are overweight more than doubled between the late 1970s and the year 2000, rising from 6.5% to 15.3%. The percent of overweight adolescents aged 12 – 19 tripled from 5.0% to 15.5% during the same time period (National Center for Heath Statistics, 2003). The increase in overweight prevalence is highest among non-latino black and Mexican-origin adolescents (Strauss and Pollack, 2001), where more than 23% of non-latino black and Mexican-origin adolescents were overweight in 1999–2000 (Ogden, *et al.*, 2002). In a population of urban kindergarten school children in Chicago, IL, approximately 25% of the predominately Mexican-American children were already overweight (Ariza, *et al.*, 2004). Among urban populations as a whole, as many as 40% of children may be overweight or obese (Nelson, *et al.*, 2004; Johnson-Down, *et al.*, 1997).

Childhood obesity can lead to adult obesity and all its complications (Satcher, 2001). It may also negatively impact the pathogenesis or epidemiology of other childhood chronic diseases such as asthma. Several studies now point to childhood obesity as a risk factor for asthma prevalence and increased asthma morbidity among urban youths (Gennuso, *et al.*, 1998; Luder, *et al.*, 1998; 2004).

From an economic standpoint childhood obesity is related to the large increase in the percentage of hospital discharges with obesity related diseases. These include hypertension, diabetes gallbladder disease, sleep apnea, and asthma. Obesity associated hospital costs increased by threefold from $35 million in the late 1970s and early 1980s to $127 million in the late 1990s (Wang and Dietz, 2002).

The determinants of childhood obesity are complex and involve multiple factors including over-nutrition, inadequate physical activity, and other socio-environmental and physical characteristics associated with the urban inner city (Goran and Treuth, 2001; Strauss and Knight, 1999; O'Loughlin, *et al.*, 2000; 1998; Gordon-Larsen, 2001; Stettler *et al.*, 2000). It has been suggested that limited access to safe outdoor play and recreational facilities in the urban environment might be associated with obesity levels particularly among low income urban children (Cummins and Jackson, 2001; Burdette and Whitaker, 2004). The excess consumption and access to fast food restaurants located within the urban environment has also been hypothesized to contribute to the obesity problem among urban children and youths. However much more work is needed to fully characterize and confirm this potential association (Burdette and Whitaker, 2004).

Several public health approaches to childhood obesity reduction especially among those living in the urban environment are under investigation. Preliminary data suggest that such strategies as behavior modification (Moon, *et al.*, 2004), reduction in TV and movie watching, and decreased video gaming (Robinson, 1999), and early initiation of breast feeding (Armstrong and Reilly, 2002) may be beneficial in reducing overweight and obesity levels in children (Campbell, *et al.*, 2001). Experience with obesity prevention is limited, and the need for more research remains a priority.

Finally, interest and investigation in the association of community and neighborhood design (the built environment) and obesity is rapidly emerging. It is hypothesized that design strategies such as community sidewalks, walk-to-school programs, and reducing traffic speeds could facilitate physical activity, and thus reduce child obesity particularly in the urban environment (Cummins and Jackson, 2001). Currently there is insufficient data to draw valid evidence-based conclusions regarding these hypotheses.

3.5. Mental Health and Urban Youth

Recently several lines of evidence have converged to kindle growing public concern about the mental health of children and adolescents in the U.S. In 1999, the Surgeon General's Report on Mental Health suggested that the prevalence of psychological disorders might be significantly higher in the U.S. than is generally appreciated. The report indicates that 20% of children suffer from a psychiatric or substance abuse disorder (NIH, 1999). Additionally, the American Psychiatric Association estimated that 15 to 25% of children evaluated in primary care settings have significant psychosocial disorders requiring some type of intervention (American Psychiatric Association, 2004).

Because childhood and adolescence are inherently characterized by biological, psychological, and socio-emotional developmental changes, it is often challenging to uncover mental health issues and accurately determine a youth's psychological well-being. This problem is further complicated because of environmental factors including family, peers, community, schools, impoverished conditions, violence, drug abuse, crime, and gang-related activities, which can profoundly influence teen psychological well-being. Over two decades ago Rutter first suggested an association between child mental health and the urban environment (Rutter and Quinton, 1977). In the years that followed several other studies (Raine, *et al.*, 1998; 1997; 1996) documented associations between a child's individual health status, social/environmental risk factors, and the development of mental disorders, particularly in the areas of depression, suicide substance abuse, and addiction.

Depression affects up to 2.5% of children and 8.3% of adolescents in the U.S. at any given time. Lifetime prevalence for adolescents has been estimated at 15% to 20%, mirroring the rate seen in adults. Although in childhood the rates of depression are approximately the same for girls and boys, by adolescence girls are twice as likely as boys to develop depression (Lagges and Dunn, 2003). Children with depression are at risk for several other psychiatric disorders. Before the onset of depression, children may develop ADHD, oppositional defiant disorder, or conduct disorder, while adolescents are at increased risk for developing anxiety disorders after the onset of depression (Lagges and Dunn, 2003). Depressed adolescents are also at an increased risk for suicidal behavior and substance abuse (Birmaher, *et al.*, 1998; Weissman, *et al.*, 1999). More than 90% of children and adolescents who committed suicide had a history of a psychological disorder before their death. The most common disorder observed was depression (Gould, *et al.*, 2003).

While the actual numbers of youths who successfully kill themselves are relatively small (1.5 per 100,000 among 10- to 14-year-olds and 8.2 per 100,000 among 15- to 19-year-olds), data from several sources document a much larger problem. The Youth Risk Behavior Survey conducted by the CDC indicated that during the past year, 19% of high school students "seriously considered attempting suicide," nearly 15% made a specific plan to attempt suicide, 8.8% reported any suicide attempt, and 2.6% made a medically serious suicide attempt that required medical attention (Gould, *et al.*, 2003).

These data suggests a significant increase in the youth/adolescent suicide problem over the course of the last 30 years. Typically the highest rates are seen among American Indians and the lowest among Asians. In addition, the gap between those at high risk and low risk is narrowing particularly between low risk blacks and high risk whites. The reasons for the increase overall or among blacks is not entirely clear however the increased exposure to drugs and alcohol as well as the increased availability of firearms, both of which are common to the urban environment, have been postulated as causative (Gould, *et al.*, 2003).

Current treatment for depression in children and adolescents begins with either behavioral therapy or medications. Several forms of behavioral psychotherapy administered individually or in group settings have been shown to be effective as a clinical intervention (Shaffer and Craft, 1999). For suicide, much of the preventive studies have evaluated interventions in school and community-based settings. School-based interventions tend to employ the utilization of suicide awareness curricula with children and adolescents. Despite the widespread use of these materials the efficacy has not been validated (Guo and Hartsall, 2002).

A positive relationship has been said to exist between youth and adolescent substance abuse or addiction and the residence in an urban environment (Gracey, 2002; Freudenberg, 2001). Several studies however have called this notion into question asserting that urban populations are no more likely than rural populations to engage in high risk behaviors or even that rural populations are at highest risk for these activities (Judd, *et al.*, 2002; Levine and Coupey, 2003). Although the policy implications of determining "who's worse" will ensure that this debate is likely to continue for the foreseeable future, one aspect of this debate may be a bit more straightforward.

Local, state, and federal crime data indicate that the incidence of substance abuse and addiction is related to incarceration rates among users. In fact, the burgeoning of the U.S. correctional facility population over the last 2 decades has largely been the result of mandatory sentencing for substance abuse offenses (Glaser and Greifinger, 1993; Zanis, *et al.*, 2003). Among youths and adolescents, those entering the correctional system may be at higher risk than un-incarcerated youths for sexually transmitted diseases, drug abuse, issues regarding pregnancy and parenting, human immunodeficiency virus (HIV) infection, and preexisting mental health disorders (AAP Committee on Adolescence, 2001).

In this country, jails and prisons are disproportionately located in urban communities. Because the average length of stay at U.S. jails is a few weeks (Freudenberg, 2001; Glaser and Greifinger, 1993), the turnover rates are very high. Thus significant numbers of adults and adolescents cycle through the correctional system each year. Some estimates put the number as high as ten million individuals including three quarters of a million juveniles every year (Glaser and Greifinger, 1993; AAP Committee on Adolescence, 2001). As such, the existence of a jail or prison in a given community can significantly impact the health of incarcerated and ultimately non-incarcerated residents living in that community (Freudenberg, 2001).

The availability of treatment and intervention services for incarcerated, detained, and recently released adolescents and juveniles is inadequate. Over two decades ago Knitzer concluded that children and adolescents in the juvenile justice system were largely neglected and ignored (Soler, 2002). Today questions still linger regarding an adolescents "right" to treatment, the proper interventional treatment to use and who should fund such treatments (Soler, 2002). These issues only serve to complicate the fact that many juveniles involved with the correctional system lack a regular source of medical care or private physician and many with a preexisting medical problem come from families that seem to be unable or unwilling to assist in ensuring that the adolescent receive proper medical care after release (AAP Committee on Adolescence, 2001).

The science of intervention and treatment of youth and adolescent mental health issues is under flux and continually developing. In fact, it has been estimated that even under the best of circumstances, where the number of people seeking treatment is maximized, clinician competence and patient compliance were also all maximized. Moreover, approximately half the burden of substance abuse, depression, and anxiety disorders among youth could not be averted with current interventions and knowledge, irrespective of the funding availability (Andrews and Wilkinson, 2002). For this reason, preventive interventional approaches among the youngest possible cohorts of children has been advocated (Andrews and Wilkinson, 2002), and the efficacy of such preventive, school-based cognitive behavior therapy administered by teachers or clinicians has been demonstrated (Andrews and Wilkinson, 2002). However, while efficacy can be demonstrated under controlled settings, similar levels of effectiveness in population-based environment have yet to be achieved (Andrews and Wilkinson, 2002).

School-based therapeutic programs have generally targeted certain maladaptive behaviors most prominent in the school setting (disruptive behavior, violence, substance abuse etc) rather than treating distinct identifiable clinical syndromes like anxiety, ADHD, and depression (Rones and Hoagwood, 2000). Programs show a wide variability in scope, intensity and duration with some programs requiring parental involvement over the school year and others being brief student interventions (Rones and Hoagwood, 2000). Despite this programmatic heterogeneity, a significant literature exists documenting the efficacy of therapeutic approaches administered in the school based-setting (Rones and Hoagwood, 2000).

Even though clinicians have efficacious interventions at their disposal, the practical and widespread administration of these mental health services remain fragmented and uncoordinated for most youth living in the urban environment (Pratt, *et al.*, 2000). To improve this situation, the American Psychiatric Association recently suggested that child and adolescent mental health services should be community-based and family-centered with access to services facilitated through school-based and primary care settings (APA Taskforce for the vision for the mental health system, 2003). While this approach may be desirable, living in the urban environment presents significant challenges to the realization of this vision. Urban public school systems are generally under funded and under staffed. Many have only part-time health personnel or no health personnel at all on site. It is difficult to see how, under current fiscal constraints, schools or many urban public school systems could dedicate resources or staff to gain the skills and resources needed to be adequately equipped to handle these health issues. While teachers may perform mental health interventions in the setting of a trial or research study, many are reluctant to integrate these services into the daily activities of the classroom (Rones and Hoagwood., 2000). Thus advocates of family centered, school-clinic coordinated services must overcome several social, financial, and practical barriers before this is likely to occur. In the end, significant impact on the mental health of children living in urban environments will likely require much more policy and interventional research, increased funding of current programs, and the creation of new and innovative treatment programs at schools and other community based sites.

4.0. CHILD HEALTH BENEFITS OF LIVING IN THE URBAN ENVIRONMENT

There's no reason to believe that children living in cities are inherently or biologically different than those living in suburban or rural settings; that is, there is no "urban genotype." Since children have little choice as to where they live, their residence in urban environments is determined inadvertently by the circumstances of their parents' lives. Yet, cities have profound influences on children, and children, in turn, shape the urban landscape. Much of this chapter has focused on the negative aspects of the urban environment on the health of children. Because we reviewed the medical and public health literature, where most epidemiological and health services studies have been carried out in urban populations, and because the research on health problems is dominated by a deficit model, the picture of the children in cities that emerges is one of exposures to hazards, high-risk behaviors, and serious health problems.

We recognize that this picture of children's health in cities is biased. Cities are complex, rich environments that bring to children an array of influences, both positive and negative. The job of childhood is progressive growth and development, ongoing learning, and constant change. Children are at the same time vulnerable and resilient. They learn from what we might consider the most negative of environments. They search, explore, mimic, and react to all stimuli in their lives. Bronfenbrenner, among others, has described the complex and multi-leveled ecological environment in which children grow and develop. It is not always clear which forces are positive, and which are negative (1992).

We must acknowledge that there are positive aspects to growing up in cities that reflect the unique assets of the urban landscape. Cities offer a rich institutional environment with museums, theaters, libraries, schools, parks, zoos, movie theaters, music halls, stadiums, shops, houses of worship, restaurants, and other facilities. Cities bring to children a large and dense peer group that participates in teams, choirs, classrooms, and clubs, among other groupings. Most cities are ethnically, racially, and socially diverse introducing children to a multicultural environment of languages, traditions, festivals, and foods. Cities are made up of collections of neighborhoods-center city business districts, industrial estates, parks and vacant lots, dense poor residential areas as well as middle-class and affluent housing-each of which is of interests and instructs children. Urban children are exposed to a rich ecology of traffic, crowds, noises, diverse architecture, and all variations of humankind. Finally, as we are concerned here about health, it must be noted that cities are home to the best and worst of health care facilities-sophisticated academic medical centers, medical institutions of various sizes, multiple health care facilities, and doctors' offices. Geographic access to such facilities is not likely to be a barrier to receipt of care.

Similarly, we acknowledge the negative aspects of growing up in cities that play a part in determining the health problems of children. The concentration of poverty in cities can be extreme, and it is particularly these poor children with whom we are most concerned. Cities face enormous burdens of crime, drugs, and violence. But cities also show us the extremes of wealth and it may be this exaggerated inequality that also shapes the health of urban children. Cities are congested with human populations that are ever shifting and migrating. Housing quality can be poor. Air quality may be poor. Food may be poor in quality and quantity. In such a congested, complex ecology, childhood diseases flourish.

Unfortunately, the literature on the health of children in cities does not provide enough evidence to weigh and evaluate the influences of these positive and negative forces. The challenge to improving the health of urban children is not just designing and delivering health care programs to them, but of redesigning and shaping their urban environments to bring them the richest assets of city life while minimizing the negative consequences. At the end of the 19th century in the U.S., the clearest disparity that existed in the health of populations was between the healthy country folk and the sick and dying city dwellers (Preston and Haines, 1991). That disparity largely disappeared by the end of the 20th century, but we continue to face the challenge of making city life the healthiest it can be for growing children. It's also worth concluding this chapter by saying something about the influence of children on cities.

5.0. RESEARCH GAPS

As documented in the preceding discussion, a significant amount of research and scientific discourse is being conducted regarding the health of urban children. While much has been done, even more remains to be done. More work is needed to complete our understanding of the unique health impacting characteristics of the urban environment both positive and negative. Most of the factors usually discussed as critical urban factors (e.g. poverty, healthcare access) are also important determinants among rural communities as well. Are urban centers then only qualitatively unique? One factor common to urban environments, but perhaps not to rural environments is noise and its relationship to child health and development. While there may indeed be noise associated with rural environments (heavy agricultural machinery), qualitative and quantitative differences undoubtedly exist among rural and urban noise exposures. What is the nature of these differences and what, if any, are the associated health impacts on child growth and development? Are these impacts reversible or treatable? What are the cost implications of these exposures? Should this knowledge be incorporated into the design, engineering, and development of the machines and engines of the future?

There is a great need to identify biologic markers of urban factors and the cellular and molecular biologic mechanisms through which urban socio-behaviorally mediated outcomes operate. The question of qualitative versus quantitative difference in urban living must be evaluated. So too must the question of a hypothesized dose-response relationship to health outcomes associated with living in cities. If these relationships exist, are they static and fixed or dynamic and change over time? What factors influence this dynamism? Are child biological and psychosocial development or socio-environmental forces the most important factors influencing this dose-response relationship?

The health effects of school connectedness, unintended health consequences of business and zoning laws and the relationship of the built environment on child health outcomes and child obesity prevention each need further study and analysis. Conversely, our understanding of the benefits of urban living on child health is virtually non-existent in the health literature. Work in this area has the very real possibility of yielding currently inconceivable insights and valuable new knowledge that will ultimately benefit the health and improve the care all the worlds' children. As we move forward, as the number and size of the worlds' urban centers continues to grow, the challenge for scientists, researchers, and practitioners is to not only determine what makes urban living different, but also what can make it better.

REFERENCES

AAP Committee on Adolescence. (2001). American Academy of Pediatrics: Health care for children and adolescents in the juvenile correctional care system. *Pediatrics* 107:799-803.

Alberg, A.J., and Samet, J.M. (2003). Epidemiology of lung cancer. *Chest* 123:21S-49S.

Aligne, C.A., Auinger, P., Byrd, R.S., and Weitzman, M. (2000). Risk factors for pediatric asthma. Contributions of poverty, race, and urban residence. *Am. J. Respir. Crit. Care Med.* 162:873-877.

American Psychiatric Association. (2004). Addressing the Mental Health needs of America's children; http://www.psych.org/advocacy_policy/leg_issues/fac-children.cfm.

Andrews, G., and Wilkinson, D.D. (2002). The prevention of mental disorders in young people. *Med. J. Aust.* 177:S97-S100.

Aneshensel, C.S., and Sucoff, C.A. (1996). The neighborhood context of adolescent mental health. *J. Health Soc. Behav.* 37:293-310.

APA Taskforce for the vision for the mental health system. (2003). *A vision for the mental health system.* American Psychiatric Association, Virginia.

Arias, E., MacDorman, M.F., Strobino, D.M., and Guyer, B. (2003). Annual summary of vital statistics—2002. *Pediatrics* 112:1215-1230.

Ariza, A.J., Chen, E.H., Binns, H.J., and Christoffel, K.K. (2004). Risk factors for overweight in five- to six-year-old Hispanic-American children: a pilot study. *J. Urban Health* 81:150-161.

Armstrong, J., and Reilly, J.J. (2002). Breastfeeding and lowering the risk of childhood obesity. *Lancet* 359:2003-2004.

Barros, F.C., Victora, C.G., and Horta, B.L. (2001). Ethnicity and infant health in Southern Brazil. A birth cohort study. *Int. J. Epidemiol.* 30:1001-1008.

Berkman, L.F., and Kawachi, I. (2000). *Social Epidemiology.* Oxford University Press, New York.

Birmaher, B., Brent, D.A., and Benson, R.S. (1998). Summary of the practice parameters for the assessment and treatment of children and adolescents with depressive disorders. *J. Am. Acad. Child Adolesc. Psychiatry* 37:1234-1238.

Bonny, A.E., Britto, M.T., Klostermann, B.K., Hornung, R.W., and Slap, G.B. (2000). School disconnectedness: identifying adolescents at risk. *Pediatrics* 106:1017-1021.

Boroff, M., and O'Campo, P. (1996). Baltimore City Healthy Start Medical Reform for reducing infant mortality. *Patient Educ. Couns.* 27:41-52.

Bronfenbrenner, U. (1992). Ecologic Systems Theory. In: Vasta, R, (ed.), *Six theories of child development: Revised formulations and current issues.* Jessica Kingsley Publishers, Ltd., Pennsylvania, pp. 187-249.

Brown, A.F., Ettner, S.L., Piette, J., Weinberger, M., Gregg, E., Shapiro, M.F., Karter, A.J., Safford, M., Waitzfelder, B., Prata, P.A., and Beckles, G.L. (2004). Socioeconomic position and health among persons with diabetes mellitus: a conceptual framework and review of the literature. *Epidemiol. Rev.* 26:63-77.

Buka, S.L., Brennan, R.T., Rich-Edwards, J.W., Raudenbush, S.W., and Earls, F. (2003). Neighborhood support and the birth weight of urban infants. *Am. J. Epidemiol.* 157:1-8.

Burdette, H.L., and Whitaker, R.C. (2004). Neighborhood playgrounds, fast food restaurants, and crime: relationships to overweight in low-income preschool children. *Prev. Med.* 38:57-63.

Campbell, K., Waters, E., O'Meara, S., and Summerbell, C. (2001). Interventions for preventing obesity in childhood. A systematic review. *Obes. Rev.* 2:149-157.

Centers for Disease Control and Prevention (1997). Recommended framework for presenting injury mortality data. *MMWR. Recomm. Rep.* 46:1-30.

Centers for Disease Control and Prevention. (2004). Childhood injury fact sheet; www.cdc.gov/ncipc/factsheets/childh.htm.

Clark, N.M., Brown, R.W., Parker, E., Robins, T.G., Remick, D.G., Jr., Philbert, M.A., Keeler, G.J., and Israel, B.A. (1999). Childhood asthma. *Environ. Health Perspect.* 107(Suppl 3): 421-429.

Coburn, A.F., McBride, T.D., and Ziller, E.C. (2002). Patterns of health insurance coverage among rural and urban children. *Med. Care. Res. Rev.* 59:272-292.

Cullen, K.W., Baranowski, T., Rittenberry, L., Cosart, C., Hebert, D., and de Moor, C. (2001). Child-reported family and peer influences on fruit, juice and vegetable consumption: reliability and validity of measures. *Health Educ. Res.* 16:187-200.

Cummins, S.K., and Jackson, R.J. (2001). The built environment and children's health. *Pediatr. Clin. North Am.* 48:1241-1252.

Czerwinski, S.J., and Moloney-Harmon, P.A. (1997). Caught in the crossfire. Children, guns, and trauma: an update. *Crit. Care Nurs. Clin. North Am.* 9:201-210.

Davidson, L.L., Durkin, M.S., Kuhn, L., O'Connor, P., Barlow, B., and Heagarty, M.C. (1994). The impact of the Safe Kids/Healthy Neighborhoods Injury Prevention Program in Harlem, 1988 through 1991. *Am. J. Public Health* 84:580-586.

Department of Justice. (2003). Bureau of Justice Statistics data online; http://bjsdata.ojp.usdoj.gov/dataonline/ Search/Homocide/Local/OneYearOfData.cfm

Devaney, B., Howell, E., McCormick, M., and Moreno, L. (2000). *Reducing infant mortality; lessons learned from healthy start.* Mathematica Policy Reserch, Final Report No. MPR Ref # 8166-113. Princeton, NJ.

DiMaggio, C., and Durkin, M. (2002). Child pedestrian injury in an urban setting: descriptive epidemiology. *Acad. Emerg. Med.* 9:54-62.

Drukker, M., Kaplan, C., Feron, F., and van Os, J. (2003). Children's health-related quality of life, neighborhood socio-economic deprivation and social capital. A contextual analysis. *Soc. Sci. Med.* 57:825-841.

Duncan, G.J., Brooks-Gunn, J., and Klebanov, P.K. (1994). Economic deprivation and early childhood development. *Child Dev.* 65:296-318.

Eggleston, P.A., Buckley, T.J., Breysse, P.N., Wills-Karp, M., Kleeberger, S.R., and Jaakkola, J.K. (2004). The environment and asthma in US inner-cities. *Health Perspect.* 107:439-459.

Ekwo, E.E., and Moawad, A. (2000). Maternal age and preterm births in a black population. *Paediatr. Perinat. Epidemiol.* 14:145-151.

Elixhauser, A., Machlin, S.R., Zodet, M.W., Chevarley, F.M., Patel, N., McCormick, M.C., and Simpson, L. (2002). Health care for children and youth in the United States: 2001 annual report on access, utilization, quality, and expenditures. *Ambul. Pediatr.* 2:419-437.

Epstein, P.R., and Rogers, C. (2004). *Inside the Greenhouse: The Impacts of CO2 and Climate Change on Public Health in the Inner City.* Harvard Medical School, Massachusetts.

Evans, D., Mellins, R., Lobach, K., Ramos-Bonoan, C., Pinkett-Heller, M., Wiesemann, S, Klein, I., Donahue, C., Burke, D., Levinson, M., Levin, B., Zimmerman, B., and Clark, N. (1997). Improving care for minority children with asthma: professional education in public health clinics. *Pediatrics* 99:157-164.

Faber, D.R., and Krieg, E.J. (2002). Unequal exposure to ecological hazards: environmental injustices in the Commonwealth of Massachusetts. *Environ. Health Perspect.* 110(Suppl 2):277-288.

Federal Interagency Forum on Child and Family Statistics. (2003). *America's Children: Key National Indicators of Well-being 2003.* Government Printing Office, Washington, DC.

Forssas, E., Gissler, M., Sihvonen, M., and Hemminki, E. (1999). Maternal predictors of perinatal mortality: the role of birthweight. *Int. J. Epidemiol.* 28:475-478.

Frattaroli, S., Webster, D.W., and Teret, S.P. (2002). Unintentional gun injuries, firearm design, and prevention: what we know, what we need to know, and what can be done. *J. Urban Health* 79:49-59.

Freudenberg, N. (2001). Jails, prisons, and the health of urban populations: a review of the impact of the correctional system on community health. *J. Urban Health* 78:214-235.

Fuller, J.H., Shipley, M.J., Rose, G., Jarrett, R.J., and Keen, H. (1980). Coronary-heart-disease risk and impaired glucose tolerance. The Whitehall study. *Lancet* 1:1373-1376.

Galea, S., Freudenberg, N., and Vlahov, D. (2005). Cities and Population Health. *Soc. Sci. Med.* 60(5): 1017-1033.

Galea, S., Nandi, A., and Vlahov, D. (2004). The social epidemiology of substance use. *Epidemiol. Rev.* 26:36-52.

Galobardes, B., Lynch, J.W., and Davey, S.G. (2004). Childhood socioeconomic circumstances and cause-specific mortality in adulthood: systematic review and interpretation. *Epidemiol. Rev.* 26:7-21.

Gennuso, J., Epstein, L.H., Paluch, R.A., and Cerny, F. (1998). The relationship between asthma and obesity in urban minority children and adolescents. *Arch. Pediatr. Adolesc. Med.* 152:1197-1200.

Glaser, J.B., and Greifinger, R.B. (1993). Correctional health care: a public health opportunity. *Ann. Intern. Med.* 118:139-145.

Gold, R., Kennedy, B., Connell, F., and Kawachi, I. (2002). Teen births, income inequality, and social capital: developing an understanding of the causal pathway. *Health Place* 8:77-83.

Goran, M. I., and Treuth, M.S. (2001). Energy expenditure, physical activity, and obesitin children. *Pediatr. Clin. North Am.* 48:931-953.

Gordon-Larsen, P. (2001). Obesity-related knowledge, attitudes, and behaviors in obese and non-obese urban Philadelphia female adolescents. *Obes. Res.* 9:112-118.

Gould, M.S., Greenberg, T., Velting, D.M., and Shaffer, D. (2003). Youth suicide risk and preventive interventions: a review of the past 10 years. *J. Am. Acad. Child Adolesc. Psychiatry* 42:386-405.

Gracey, M. (2002). Child health in an urbanizing world. *Acta Paediatr.* 91:1-8.

Graham, L.M. (2004). All I need is the air that I breath: outdoor air quality and asthma. *Paediatr. Respir. Rev.* 5(Suppl A):S59-S64.

Greenberg, M. (1991). American cities: good and bad news about public health. *Bull. N.Y Acad. Med.* 67:17-21.

Grossman, D.C., and Rivara, F.P. (1992). Injury control in childhood. *Pediatr. Clin. North Am.* 39: 471-485.

Guo, G., and Hartsall, C. (2002). *Efficacy of suicide prevention programs for children and youth* Report No. HTA 26. Alberta Heritage Foundation for Medical Research, Canada.

Guyer, B., Strobino, D.M., Ventura, S.J., MacDorman, M., and Martin, J.A. (1996). Annual summary of vital statistics–1995. *Pediatrics* 98:1007-1019.

Hameed, S.M., Popkin, C.A., Cohn, S.M., and Johnson, E.W. (2004). The epidemic of pediatric traffic injuries in South Florida: a review of the problem and initial results of a prospective surveillance strategy. *Am. J. Public Health* 94:554-556.

Hawkins, J.D., Catalano, R.F., Kosterman, R., Abbott, R., and Hill, K.G. (1999). Preventing adolescent health-risk behaviors by strengthening protection during childhood. *Arch. Pediatr. Adolesc. Med.* 153:226-234.

Haynatzka, V., Peck, M., Santibanez, S., Iyasu, S., and Scoendorf, K. (2002). Racial and ethnic disparities in infant mortality rates—60 Largest U.S. Cities, 1995—1998. *MMWR.* 51:329-332.

Hemingway, H., Nicholson, A., Stafford, M., Roberts, R., and Marmot, M. (1997). The impact of socioeconomic status on health functioning as assessed by the SF-36 questionnaire: the Whitehall II Study. *Am. J. Public Health* 87:1484-1490.

Hinrichsen, D., Salem, R., and Blackburn, R. (2004). *Meeting the urban challenge: Population reports*, Report No. Series M # 16. Johns Hopkins Bloomberg School of Public Health.

Hogan, V.K., Richardson, J.L., Ferre, C.D., Durant, T., and Boisseau, M. (2001). A public health framework for addressing black and white disparities in preterm delivery. *J. Am. Med. Womens Assoc.* 56:177-80, 205.

Holgate, S., Samet, J., Koren, H., and Maynard, R. (1999). *Air Pollution and Health.* Academic Press, New York.

Hyland, A., Travers, M.J., Cummings, K.M., Bauer, J., Alford, T., and Wieczorek, W.F. (2003). Tobacco outlet density and demographics in Erie County, New York. *Am. J. Public Health* 93:1075-1076.

IOM Committee on Children, H. I. a. A. t. C. (1998). *America's Children: Healthcare Insurance and Access to Care.* National Academy Press, Washington, DC.

Iyasu, S., Tomashek, K., and Barfield, W. (2002). Infant mortality and low birth weight among black and white infants; US 1980-2000. *MMWR.* 51:589-592.

Johnson-Down, L., O'Loughlin, J., Koski, K.G., and Gray-Donald, K. (1997). High prevalence of obesity in low income and multiethnic schoolchildren: a diet and physical activity assessment. *J. Nutr.* 127:2310-2315.

Judd, F.K., Jackson, H.J., Komiti, A., Murray, G., Hodgins, G., and Fraser, C. (2002). High prevalence disorders in urban and rural communities. *Aust. N. Z. J. Psychiatry* 36:104-113.

Kalff, A.C., Kroes, M., Vles, J.S., Hendriksen, J.G., Feron, F.J., Steyaert, J., van Zeben, T.M., Jolles, J., and van Os, J. (2001). Neighbourhood level and individual level SES effects on child problem behaviour: a multilevel analysis. *J. Epidemiol. Community Health* 55:246-250.

Kattan, M., Mitchell, H., Eggleston, P., Gergen, P., Crain, E., Redline, S., Weiss, K., Evans, R.3rd., Kaslow, R., Kercsmar, C., Leickly, F., Malveaux, F., and Wedner, H.J. (1997). Characteristics of inner-city children with asthma: the National Cooperative Inner-City Asthma Study. *Pediatr. Pulmonol.* 24:253-262.

Katz, L.F., Kling, J.R., and Liebman, J.B. (2001). Moving to opportunity in Boston: Early results f a randomized mobility experiment. *Q. J. Econ.* 116:607-654.

Kawachi, I., Kennedy, B.P., Lochner, K., and Prothrow-Stith, D. (1997). Social capital, income inequality, and mortality. *Am. J. Public Health.* 87:1491-1498.

King, W. D., Nichols, M.H., Hardwick, W.E., and Palmisano, P.A. (1994). Urban/rural differences in child passenger deaths. *Pediatr. Emerg. Care* 10:34-36.

Klassen, T.P., MacKay, J.M., Moher, D., Walker, A., and Jones, A.L. (2000). Community-based injury prevention interventions. *Future Child* 10:83-110.

Kuhlthau, K.A., and Perrin, J.M. (2001). Child health status and parental employment. *Arch. Pediatr. Adolesc. Med.* 155:1346-1350.

Lagges, A.M., and Dunn, D.W. (2003). Depression in children and adolescents. *Neurol. Clin.* 21:953-960.

Lapidus, G., Lerer, T., Zavoski, R., and Banco, L. (1998). Childhood injury in Connecticut. *Conn. Med.* 62:323-331.

Laraque, D., Barlow, B., Davidson, L., and Welborn, C. (1994). The Central Harlem playground injury prevention project: a model for change. *Am. J. Public Health* 84:1691-1692.

Laraque, D., Barlow, B., Durkin, M., and Heagarty, M. (1995). Injury prevention in an urban setting: challenges and successes. *Bull. N.Y. Acad. Med.* 72:16-30.

LaVeist, T.A., and Wallace, J.M., Jr. (2000). Health risk and inequitable distribution of liquor stores in African American neighborhood. *Soc. Sci. Med.* 51:613-617.

Lear, J.G. (2004). 2002 Survey of school-based health center initiatives. The George Washington University School of Public Health Center for health and healthcare in schools; http://www.health inschools.org/sbhcs/method.asp.

Lee, C. (2002). Environmental justice: building a unified vision of health and the environment. *Environ. Health Perspect.* 110(Suppl 2):141-144.

Levine, S.B., and Coupey, S.M. (2003). Adolescent substance use, sexual behavior, and metropolitan status: is "urban" a risk factor? *J. Adolesc. Health* 32:350-355.

Linder, F.E., and Grove, R.D. (1947). *Vital statistics rates in the United States 1900-1940.* US Government Printing Office, Washington, DC.

Litonjua, A.A., Carey, V.J., Burge, H.A., Weiss, S.T., and Gold, D.R. (2001). Exposure to cockroach allergen in the home is associated with incident doctor-diagnosed asthma and recurrent wheezing. *J. Allergy Clin. Immunol.* 107:41-47.

Luder, E., Ehrlich, R.I., Lou, W.Y., Melnik, T.A., and Kattan, M. (2004). Body mass index and the risk of asthma in adults. *Respir. Med.* 98:29-37.

Luder, E., Melnik, T.A., and DiMaio, M. (1998). Association of being overweight witgreater asthma symptoms in inner city black and Hispanic children. *J. Pediatr.* 132:699-703.

Ludwig, J., Duncan, G., and Hirschfield, P. (2001). Urban poverty and juvenile crime: evidence from a randomized housing-mobility experiment. *Q. J. Econ.* 116:655-680.

Lurie, N., Straub, M.J., Goodman, N., and Bauer, E. J. (1998). Incorporating asthma education into a traditional school curriculum. *Am. J. Public Health* 88:822-823.

Mannino, D.M., Homa, D.M., Akinbami, L.J., Moorman, J.E., Gwynn, C., and Redd, S.C. (2002). Surveillance for asthma–United States, 1980-1999. *MMWR. Surveill. Summ.* 51:1-13.

Mannino, D. M., Homa, D.M., Pertowski, C.A., Ashizawa, A., Nixon, L.L., Johnson, C.A., Ball, L.B., Jack, E., and Kang, D.S. (1998). Surveillance for asthma–United States, 1960-1995. *MMWR. CDC. Surveill. Summ.* 47:1-27.

Mansour, M.E., Kotagal, U., Rose, B., Ho, M., Brewer, D., Roy-Chaudhury, A., Hornung, R.W., Wade, T.J., and DeWitt, T.G. (2003). Health-related quality of life in urban elementary schoolchildren. *Pediatrics* 111:1372-1381.

Marmot, M.G., Smith, G.D., Stansfeld, S., Patel, C., North, F., Head, J., White, I., Brunner, E., and Feeney, A. (1991). Health inequalities among British civil servants: the Whitehall II study. *Lancet* 337:1387-1393.

Maternal and Child Health Bureau. (2004). *Child Health USA 2002* DHHS, HealthResources and Services Administration.

Matthews, T., Menacker, F., and MacDorman, M. (2002). *Infant mortality statistics from the 2000 period linked birth/infant death data set.* Centers for Disease Control and Prevention, Georgia.

Milligan, R., Wingrove, B.K., Richards, L., Rodan, M., Monroe-Lord, L., Jackson, V., Hatcher, B., Harris, C., Henderson, C., and Johnson, A.A. (2002). Perceptions about prenatal care: views of urban vulnerable groups. *BMC. Public Health* 2:25.

Moon, Y.I., Park, H.R., Koo, H.Y., and Kim, H.S. (2004). Effects of behavior modification on body image, depression and body fat in obese Korean elementary school children. *Yonsei Med. J.* 45:61-67.

Morello-Frosch, R., Pastor, M., Porras, C., and Sadd, J. (2002b). Environmental justice and regional inequality in southern California: Implications for future research. *Env. Health. Per.* 110(supp 2): 149-154.

Morland, K., Wing, S., and Diez, R.A. (2002a). The contextual effect of the local food environment on residents' diets: the atherosclerosis risk in communities study. *Am.J. Public Health* 92:1761-1767.

Morland, K., Wing, S., Diez, R.A., and Poole, C. (2002). Neighborhood characteristics associated with the location of food stores and food service places. *Am. J. Prev. Med.* 22:23-29.

Muntaner, C., Eaton, W.W., Miech, R., and O'Campo, P. (2004). Socioeconomic position and major mental disorders. *Epidemiol. Rev.* 26:53-62.

National Center for Health Statistics. (1997). *1996-1997 Injury Chartbook* Hyattsville, MD.

National Center for Health (2001). *Ten leading causes of injury and death by age group – 2001.* Center for Disease Control. Statistics; http://www.cdc.gov/nchs/fastats/lcod.htm

National Center for Health Statistics. (2003). *Health US 2003,* Center for Disease Control; http://www.cdc.gov/nchs/hus.htm

National Highway Traffic Safety Administration. (2002). *Traffic safety facts 2002.*

Nelson, J.A., Chiasson, M.A., and Ford, V. (2004). Childhood overweight in a New York City WIC population. *Am. J. Public Health* 94:458-462.

NIH. (1999). *Mental Health: A Report of the surgeon general.* Government Printing Office, Rockville, MD.

O'Loughlin, J., Gray-Donald, K., Paradis, G., and Meshefedjian, G. (2000). One- and two-year predictors of excess weight gain among elementary schoolchildren in multiethnic, low-income, inner-city neighborhoods. *Am. J. Epidemiol.* 152:739-746.

O'Loughlin, J., Paradis, G., Renaud, L., Meshefedjian, G., and Gray-Donald, K. (1998). Prevalence and correlates of overweight among elementary schoolchildren in multiethnic, low income, inner-city neighbourhoods in Montreal, Canada. *Ann. Epidemiol.* 8:422-432.

Ogden, C.L., Flegal, K.M., Carroll, M.D., and Johnson, C.L. (2002). Prevalence and trends in overweight among US children and adolescents, 1999-2000. *JAMA.* 288:1728-1732.

Perry, T., Matsui, E., Merriman, B., Duong, T., and Eggleston, P. (2003). The prevalence of rat allergen in inner-city homes and its relationship to sensitization and asthma morbidity. *J. Allergy Clin. Immunol.* 112:346-352.

Phipatanakul, W., Eggleston, P.A., Wright, E.C., and Wood, R.A. (2000). Mouse allergen. I. The prevalence of mouse allergen in inner-city homes. The National Cooperative Inner-City Asthma Study. *J. Allergy Clin. Immunol.* 106:1070-1074.

Posner, J.C., Liao, E., Winston, F.K., Cnaan, A., Shaw, K.N., and Durbin, D.R. (2002). Exposure to traffic among urban children injured as pedestrians. *Inj. Prev.* 8:231-235.

Poundstone, K.E., Strathdee, S.A., and Celentano, D.D. (2004). The social epidemiology of human immunodeficiency virus/acquired immunodeficiency syndrome. *Epidemiol. Rev.* 26:22-35.

Powell, D.L., and Stewart, V. (2001). Children. The unwitting target of environmental injustices. *Pediatr. Clin. North Am.* 48:1291-1305.

Pratt, M.K., Davidson, L., and McMahon, T.J. (2000). Comprehensive services for at risk urban youth: applying lessons from the community mental health unit. *Children's services: social policy, research and practice* 3:63-83.

Preston, S.H., and Haines, M.R (1991). *Fatal Years; Child Mortality in Late Nineteenth Century America.* Princeton University Press, New Jersey.

Prewitt, E. (1997). Inner City Health Care. *Ann. Int. Med.* 26:485-490.

Raine, A., Brennan, P., Mednick, B., and Mednick, S. A. (1996). High rates of violence, crime, academic problems, and behavioral problems in males with both early neuromotor deficits and unstable family environments. *Arch. Gen. Psychiatry* 53:544-549.

Raine, A., Brennan, P., and Mednick, S. A. (1997). Interaction between birth complications and early maternal rejection in predisposing individuals to adult violence: specificity to serious, early-onset violence. *Am. J. Psychiatry* 154:1265-1271.

Raine, A., Reynolds, C., Venables, P. H., Mednick, S. A., and Farrington, D. P. (1998). Fearlessness, stimulation-seeking, and large body size at age 3 years as early predispositions to childhood aggression at age 11 years. *Arch. Gen. Psychiatry* 55:745-751.

Rao, R., Hawkins, M., and Guyer, B. (1997). Children's exposure to traffic and risk of pedestrian injury in an urban setting. *Bull. N.Y. Acad. Med.* 74:65-80.

Rauh, V. A., Chew, G. R., and Garfinkel, R. S. (2002). Deteriorated housing contributes to high cockroach allergen levels in inner-city households. *Environ. Health Perspect.* 110(Suppl 2):323-327.

Resnick, M. D., Harris, L. J., and Blum, R. W. (1993). The impact of caring and connectedness on adolescent health and well-being. *J. Paediatr. Child Health* 29(Suppl 1):S3-S9.

Rivara, F. P. (1990). Child pedestrian injuries in the United States. Current status of the problem, potential interventions, and future research needs. *Am. J. Dis. Child* 144:692-696.

Robinson, T. N. (1999). Reducing children's television viewing to prevent obesity: a randomized controlled trial. *JAMA.* 282:1561-1567.

Rolett, A., Parker, J. D., Heck, K. E., and Makuc, D. M. (2001). Parental employment, family structure, and child's health insurance. *Ambul. Pediatr.* 1:306-313.

Rones, M., and Hoagwood, K. (2000). School-based mental health services: a research review. *Clin. Child Fam. Psychol. Rev.* 3:223-241.

Rosenstreich, D. L., Eggleston, P., Kattan, M., Baker, D., Slavin, R. G., Gergen, P., Mitchell, H., McNiff-Mortimer, K., Lynn, H., Ownby, D., and Malveaux, F. (1997). The role of cockroach allergy and exposure to cockroach allergen in causing morbidity among inner-city children with asthma. *N. Engl. J. Med.* 336:1356-1363.

Rutter, M., and Quinton, D. (1977). Psychiatric disorders: Ecological factors and conceptsof causation. In: McGurk, H. (ed.), *Ecologic factors in human development* Amsterdam, Holland, pp. 173-187.

Satcher, D. (2001). *The surgeon general's call to action to prevent and decrease overweight and obesity.* DHHS, Washington, DC.

Sawhill, I., and Chadwick, L. (1999). *Children in cities: Uncertain futures.* The Brookings Institute, Washington, DC.

Schoendorf, K.C., Hogue, C. J., Kleinman, J. C., and Rowley, D. (1992). Mortality among infants of black as compared with white college-educated parents. *N. Engl. J. Med.* 326:1522-1526.

Sege, R. D., Kharasch, S., Perron, C., Supran, S., O'Malley, P., Li, W., and Stone, D. (2002). Pediatric violence-related injuries in Boston: results of a city-wide emergency department surveillance program. *Arch. Pediatr. Adolesc. Med.* 156:73-76.

Shaffer, D., and Craft, L. (1999). Methods of adolescent suicide prevention. *J. Clin. Psychiatry* 60(Suppl 2):70-74.

Shapiro, G.G., and Stout, J.W. (2002). Childhood asthma in the United States: urban issues. *Pediatr. Pulmonol.* 33:47-55.

Sheehan, K., DiCara, J.A., LeBailly, S., and Christoffel, K.K. (1999). Adapting the gang model: peer mentoring for violence prevention. *Pediatrics* 104:50-54.

Smith, M.D. (1996). Source of firearm acquisition among a sample of inner-city youths: research results and policy implications. *J. Crim. Justice* 24:361-367.

Smith, L.A., Romero, D., Wood, P.R., Wampler, N.S., Chavkin, W., and Wise, P.H. (2002). Employment barriers among welfare recipients and applicants with chronically ill children. *Am. J. Public Health* 92:1453-1457.

Soler, M. (2002). Health issues for adolescents in the justice system. *J. Adolesc. Health* 31:321-333.

Stettler, N., Tershakovec, A.M., Zemel, B.S., Leonard, M.B., Boston, R.C., Katz, S.H. and Stallings, V.A. (2000). Early risk factors for increased adiposity: a cohort study of African American subjects followed from birth to young adulthood. *Am. J. Clin. Nutr.* 72:378-383.

Stevenson, L.A., Gergen, P.J., Hoover, D.R., Rosenstreich, D., Mannino, D.M., and Matte, T.D. (2001). Sociodemographic correlates of indoor allergen sensitivity among United States children. *J. Allergy Clin. Immunol.* 108:747-752.

Strauss, R.S., and Knight, J. (1999). Influence of the home environment on the development of obesity in children. *Pediatrics* 103:e85.

Strauss, R.S., and Pollack, H.A. (2001). Epidemic increase in childhood overweight, 1986-1998. *JAMA* 286:2845-2848.

Tester, J.M., Rutherford, G.W., Wald, Z., and Rutherford, M.W. (2004). A matched case-control study evaluating the effectiveness of speed humps in reducing child pedestrian injuries. *Am. J. Public Health* 94:646-650.

US Department of Commerce, B. o. t. c. (1996). *Current population reports: Population projections of the United States by age, sex, race and hispanic origin: 1995 to 2050.* US Census Bureau; http://www.census.gov/prod/1/pop/p25-1130/

Vlahov, D., and Galea, S. (2002). Urbanization, urbanicity, and health. *J. Urban Health* 79:S1-S12.

Waldmann, R.J. (1999). Income distribution and infant mortality. In: Kawachi I, Kennedy BP, and Wilkinson R.G. (eds.), *The society and population health reader.* The New York Press, New York, pp. 14-27.

Wang, G., and Dietz, W.H. (2002). Economic burden of obesity in youths aged 6 to 17 years: 1979-1999. *Pediatrics* 109:E81.

Wang, Y. (2001). Cross-national comparison of childhood obesity: the epidemic and the relationship between obesity and socioeconomic status. *Int. J. Epidemiol.* 30:1129-1136.

Wang, Y., Monteiro, C., and Popkin, B.M. (2002). Trends of obesity and underweight in older children and adolescents in the United States, Brazil, China, and Russia. *Am. J. Clin. Nutr.* 75:971-977.

Waterston, T., Alperstein, G., and Stewart, B.S. (2004). Social capital: a key factor in child health inequalities. *Arch. Dis. Child* 89:456-459.

Webber, M.P., Carpiniello, K.E., Oruwariye, T., and Appel, D.K. (2002). Prevalence of asthma and asthma-like symptoms in inner-city elementary schoolchildren. *Pediatr. Pulmonol.* 34:105-111.

Webber, M.P., Carpiniello, K.E., Oruwariye, T., Lo, Y., Burton, W.B., and Appel, D.K. (2003). Burden of asthma in inner-city elementary schoolchildren: do school-based health centers make a difference? *Arch. Pediatr. Adolesc. Med.* 157:125-129.

Weesner, C.L., Hargarten, S.W., Aprahamian, C., and Nelson, D.R. (1994). Fatal childhood injury patterns in an urban setting. *Ann. Emerg. Med.* 23:231-236.

Weissman, M.M., Wolk, S., Goldstein, R.B., Moreau, D., Adams, P., Greenwald, S., Klier, C.M., Ryan, N.D., Dahl, R.E., and Wickramaratne, P. (1999). Depressed adolescents grown up. *JAMA.* 281:1707-1713.

Wertheimer, R., O'Hare, W., Croan, T., Jager, J., Long, M., and Reynolds, M. (2002). *The right start for america's newborns: A decade of city and state trends (1990-1999).* National Crime Prevention Control; http://www.ncpc.org/ncpc/ncpc/?pg=2088-7236.

Wintemute, G.J. (2002). Where the guns come from: the gun industry and gun commerce. *The Future of Children* 12: 55-71.

Zanis, D.A., Mulvaney, F., and Coviello, D. (2003). Health issues in prisons and jails: implications for urban health. *J. Drug Issues* 33:223-236.

Zavoski, R.W., Lapidus, G.D., Lerer, T.J., and Banco, L.I. (1995). A population-based study of severe firearm injury among children and youth. *Pediatrics* 96:278-282.

Chapter 9

Older Adults

Guardians of Our Cities

Linda Fried and Jeremy Barron

1.0. THE HEALTH STATUS OF OLDER ADULTS IN URBAN AREAS: ISSUES AND CHALLENGES

1.1. Demography

The American population is aging. The percentage of America's population that is age 65 or older will rise from 12% currently to 20% by 2030. Urban populations are similarly aging and will continue to do so in the coming decades. These trends are due to the increasing life expectancy both at younger ages and once people reach 65. Primary, secondary, and tertiary prevention along with medical advances are all contributors to the improved survivorship resulting in the now 76 million strong Baby Boom cohort.

In 1990, the U.S. Census found that 73% of older men and 77% of older women live in metropolitan areas (cities and suburbs). Out of 56 million families in metropolitan areas (cities and suburbs) in the U.S., 10 million families (i.e. 18%) include at least one member over age 65, according to March 1998 census data (CPS, 1998). Consistent with U.S. averages, 11.2% of the urban U.S. central city population is at least 65 years old, and 5.5% of the urban population is at least 75 years old (Eberhart, *et al.*, 2001). The age distribution of cities and suburbs is similar. Rural counties have even higher proportions of older adults than urban counties; 14.7% of the non-metropolitan U.S. population is at least 65 years old.

Cities and inner suburbs have generally experienced population losses in recent decades, as individuals have migrated to outer suburbs. The number of older Americans residing in suburbs has increased 19% from 1990 to 2000. However, the number of older Americans in central cities has remained stable from 1990 to 2000 (Frey, 2003). In 2002, 25.9% of all older heads of households lived in a central city, while 51.3% live in a metropolitan area outside of a central city, and 22.7% live in nonmetropolitan areas (CPS, 2002) (Figure 1). The percentage of all older adults who live in central cities has declined from 29% in 1992 to

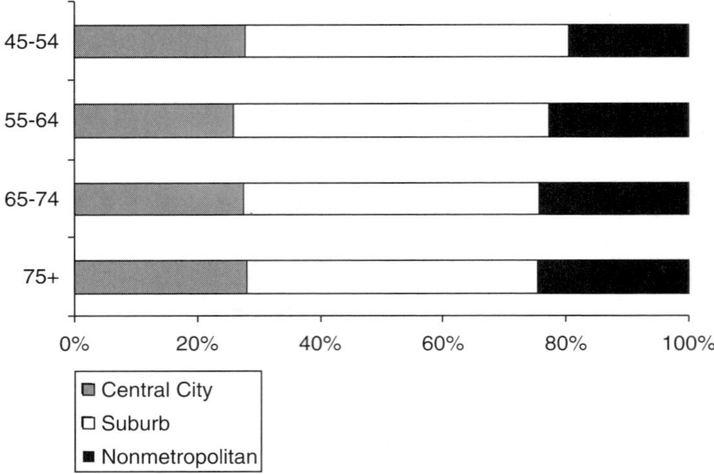

Figure 1. Metropolitan Location by Age of Older American Adults, 2001 (*Source*: U.S. Census Bureau, 2001 American Housing Survey).

26% in 2003, while the absolute number has remained the same. The percentage of older adults who live in suburbs has increased from 41% to 47% in this period. However, urban residence is more common among the oldest old (>85 years old), possibly representing reverse migration to the cities so as to live closer to family as disability develops.

The poverty rate among older Americans has declined in recent decades. However, over 15% of older adults have household incomes under $10,000 per year (Figure 2). The urban elderly poverty rate is 14%, much higher than the 7% rate in suburban older residents (Frey, 1999). However, urban poverty is not more concentrated among the old than the young. In Baltimore City, 10% of persons living below the poverty level are at least 65 years old, comparable to national figures (U.S. Census Bureau, 2000). Overall, although cities have a higher percentage of poor older adults than suburban communities, cities typically have a heterogeneous population that also includes many wealthy older residents (Figure 2).

Older adults from minority populations and foreign-born populations are particularly overrepresented in urban communities. In 2002, 51.5% of blacks lived in a central city, compared to 21.1% of non-latino whites (McKinnon, 2003). However, the black population tends to be younger: 11% of metropolitan-dwelling black adults are at least age 65, compared to 15% of metropolitan-dwelling white (Saluter, 1994). Older blacks have a 21.9% poverty rate, compared to an 8.1% rate for older non-latino whites in 2001. In high-poverty urban areas in the U.S, approximately 80% of the population is comprised of racial or ethnic minorities (Geronimus, 2000).

Foreign-born older adults disproportionately live in the Western U.S. and typically live with family. Poverty rates are higher for older immigrants than for older native-born Americans. Similarly, older immigrants are much more likely to lack health insurance than native-born Americans (6% v. 0.8%) (He, 2002). Although most foreign-born older Americans are European, in the future, older foreign-born

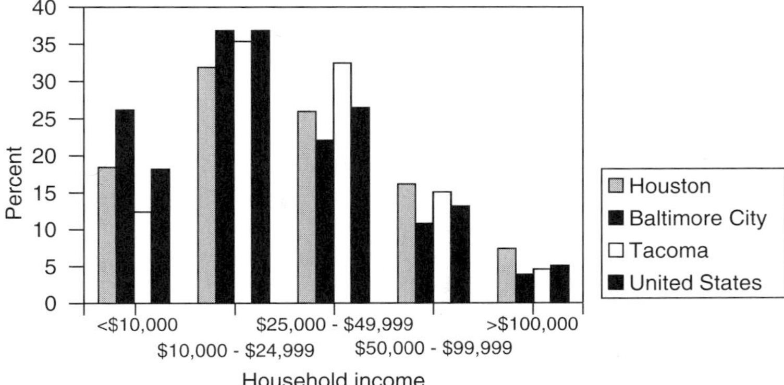

Figure 2. Income distribution among Householders Age 75 Years and Over in Three cities and in the United States (*Source*: U.S. Census 2000: Summary File, self-analysis).

populations will be primarily Latin American and Asian (United Way of Tri-State, 1999).

Women represent both a majority of older Americans and a majority of older urban adults. In the U.S., the Census Bureau in 1990 calculated 64 men per 100 women age 65 and over in urban communities (Kinsella and Velkoff, 2001). Overall, 56.1% of older adults living in metropolitan areas are married, while 33.3% are widowed, and 5.8% are divorced. This distribution mirrors the marital status distribution of the total older population. A higher percentage of older men are married than older women (76.5% v. 42.0%) (Saluter, 1994) (See Figure 3). According to the 2000 Census, 9.3% of central city households are comprised of older adults living alone, compared to 8.4% of suburban households. Rates of living alone modestly rise with advancing age above 65. A much higher proportion of older women than older men live alone. In 1998, 40.8% of women 65 years of age or older in the U.S. lived alone, compared to 17.3% of older men (FIFA, 2000).

In 1997, 64% of urban older adults were high school graduates, compared to 71% of suburban older adults. Notably, three-quarters (72%) of urban older Americans are homeowners (Frey, 1999); in some urban communities, older adults are the primary homeowners. Public health efforts which enable older people to maintain enough vigor and independence to remain in their homes have the potential for broad community benefits, including stability of many urban communities.

In 2001, 61.2% of older Americans in metropolitan areas had private health insurance over and above Medicare, whereas 68.1% of older adults in nonmetropolitan areas had this type of insurance. Approximately 8% of older adults in both urban and rural communities had Medicaid coverage. In 2001, 15.8% of metropolitan-dwelling Medicare beneficiaries were covered by Medicare managed care programs, compared to only 3.1% in rural areas (National Center for Health Statistics, 2003).

Although migration by older adults between countries is rare, migration within the U.S. is fairly common. However, older adults move less frequently than younger

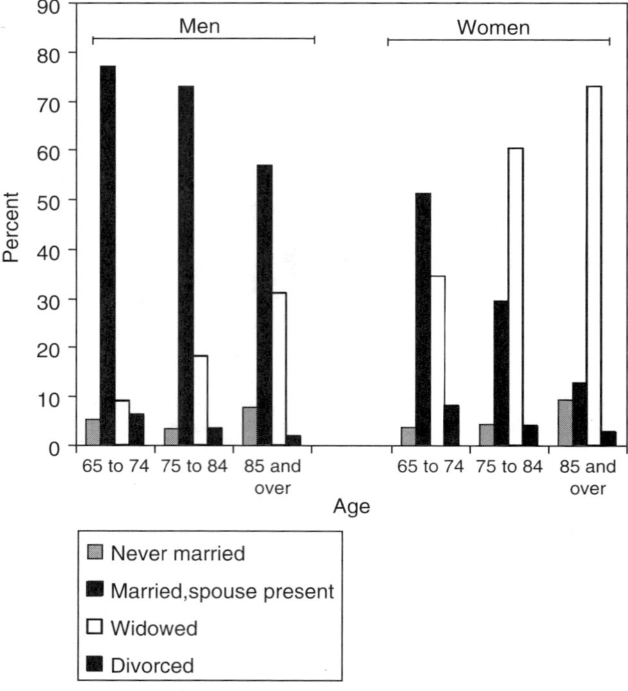

Figure 3. Marital Status of Metropolitan-Dwelling Persons 65 Years and Over by Age and Sex (*Source*: Saluter, US Census, 1994. *Data from Current Population Reports: Population Characteristics*, March 1994).

adults. In recent decades, fit retirees would often move to migration centers like Florida and Arizona. Some of these individuals eventually move back to their home communities if they become ill or disabled. In recent years, regional migration centers (closer to home) and naturally-occurring retirement communities (streets and neighborhoods with populations aging in place) are also becoming common.

Florida continues to have cities with the highest percentage of adults over age 65 and over age 85 (U.S. Census Bureau, 2000a). For example, in Clearwater City, Florida, 21.5% of the population is at least 65 years old and 3.6% of the population is at least 85 years old, compared to 6.5% and 1.5% respectively in the U.S. as a whole (U.S. Census Bureau, 2000a). Florida's Charlotte County, where 34.7% of residents are at least 65 years old, has the highest percentage of older adults of any large county in the U.S.

Overall, the older population in urban communities can expect to grow in the coming decades. Within several decades, many urban areas will have similar proportions of older adults to that now found in Florida. At present, minority, immigrant, and poor populations are disproportionately represented in cities and have special health needs. However, as affluent and well-educated Baby Boomers age and increasingly remain in or return to cities, the socioeconomic status of older adults in cities will evolve, with increasing heterogeneity of resources and needs of urban older adults.

1.2. Key Health Issues

Older adults in our rapidly aging society are a highly heterogeneous group. Some individuals remain active and vigorous into extremely advanced age, while others become frail or ill much earlier. Some older individuals age in place (possibly with home services), others seek assisted living settings, and others require institutionalization. This heterogeneity leads to different prevention, care, and access needs at different stages of health. Due to differential resources and environment, attention is required to understand the characteristics and needs of a variety of population subsets.

1.2.1. Mortality

The most frequently recognized indices of health status are mortality rates and causes. The top five causes of death, in rank order, among adults over age 65 are heart disease, cancer, stroke, chronic obstructive pulmonary disease, and pneumonia (Eberhart, *et al.*, 2001). Mortality rates are lowest for older adults in large metropolitan counties and highest in nonmetropolitan counties (Eberhart, *et al.*, 2001) (See Figure 4). Although inner cities such as Central Harlem have particularly high death rates, excessive mortality is seen primarily among children and young adults rather than older adults (McCord and Freeman, 1990). Death rates from heart disease and stroke have been falling for 40 and 60 years respectively, due to improved control of modifiable risk factors and improved treatment (Hunink, *et al.*, 1997). Among blacks in Southern states, heart disease death rates have declined more substantially in urban areas than in rural areas (Barnett, *et al.*, 1996).

Although age is considered a strong predictor of mortality, age becomes less central below age 85 after adjusting for health conditions, health habits, and sociodemographic characteristics (Fried, *et al.*, 1998). Rather, subclinical and clinical diseases, physical activity, smoking, alcohol use, disability, compromised cognition, income less than $50,000/year, and male gender are the major independent predictors of mortality in old age; they confer additive risk. Notably, education levels of

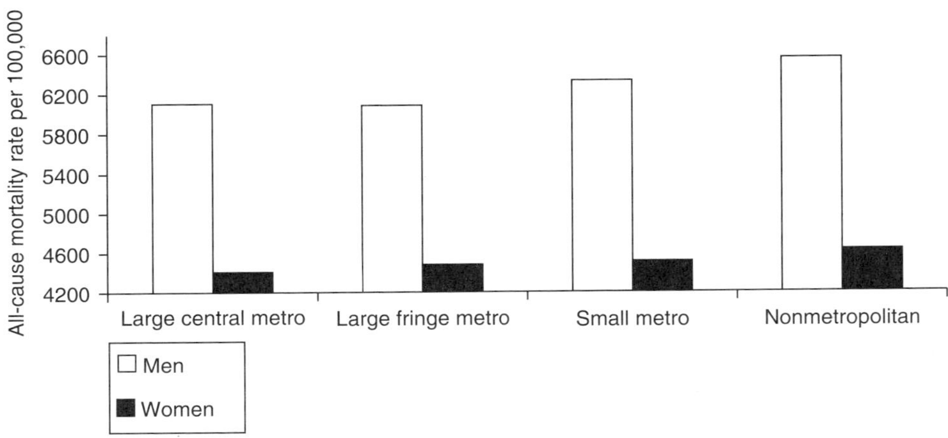

Figure 4. All-Cause Mortality Rate among Men and Women Age 65 and Older, 1996–1998, by Residence (*Source*: Eberhardt *et al.*, 2001).

high school or greater are associated with 40% decreased mortality rates even to the oldest ages, however, this association loses significance after adjusting for income. Adjusting for all of the above factors including age, male gender is associated with 2.3-fold increased risk of mortality among people at least 65 years old. This finding is consistent with the evidence that older men are more likely to die from chronic disease earlier than women, while women are more likely to live with these diseases and their resultant disability.

All of the leading causes of death among older Americans, except for pneumonia and influenza, are chronic conditions. In fact, the prevalence of chronic conditions that people live with, i.e. morbidity, is increasing. Eighty percent of people 65 years and older have one or more chronic diseases, 50% have two or more, and 48% have three or more, among community-dwelling older adults.

1.2.2. Morbidity

This underestimates the overall prevalence of serious chronic illnesses, as 5% of older adults reside in nursing homes due to these diseases and their resulting disability. The major chronic conditions associated with aging include both chronic diseases and geriatric conditions such as falls, frailty and incontinence. The prevalence of chronic disease increases substantially with age, so that by age 65 and older over 50% of older adults report arthritis, 30% report heart disease, 14% have a cancer diagnosis, 10% report diabetes, and 7% have prevalent stroke histories. The prevalence of these chronic diseases increases after age 65. The prevalence of moderate or severe memory impairment also rises with age with estimates for those 85 and older ranging approximately 35% for women and 37% for men (Fried, 2004). Between 20 and 50% of all persons with these chronic diseases are 65 and older, depending on the disease, so that screening for risk of these diseases and intervention to prevent their consequences is an important issue for this older age group and for improving health associated with aging. Screening approaches also need to change with age for a variety of reasons: First, risk factors may change with age and dictate altered approaches. Thus, evidence from the Cardiovascular Health Study indicates that the most effective way to identify people 65 and older who are at risk of cardiovascular disease is by identifying those with subclinical disease; in this group, risk factor modification is likely to be beneficial. Those without subclinical disease by this age appear to be at very low risk. Second, because many older adults have multiple diseases and health problems, positive findings on screening may need to be considered in light of prognosis from other diseases and patient priorities in deciding how to balance potentially competing therapies for multiple conditions in order to arrive at a therapeutic regimen that is feasible for the individual.

Geriatric conditions also become increasingly prevalent with increasing age. These conditions are multifactorial in etiology, and generally are not distinct pathologic entities in the way that diseases are defined. They include falls, which occur in one-third of older adults annually; frailty, a wasting syndrome which is clinically prevalent in 7% of those 65 and older; and incontinence, prevalent in 8-9%; all of these rates are described for community-dwelling older adults. Falls are problematic in themselves, leading to serious injuries and conferring a high risk of mortality (Tinetti, *et al.*, 1988). Frailty has been shown to identify a group at very high risk of mortality, falls, disability, and hospitalization (Fried, *et al.*, 2001). Incontinence, along with falls and frailty, are all risk factors for need for long-term care. All are identifiable by new screening methods, and appear responsive to interventions.

Syndromes such as incontinence and falls are common in frail older adults. Urinary incontinence is very common, particularly in disabled individuals. For example, in a sample of the one-third most disabled community-dwelling older women in eastern Baltimore City, the prevalence of urinary incontinence in the past month was 54% (Guralnik, *et al.*, 1995). One-third of older adults fall each year. Falls are associated with serious injuries as well as with institutionalization and mortality. The U.S. Preventive Services Task Force recommends screening for fall risk in adults 75 years and older; screening and risk factor modifications have been shown to have substantial impact in decreasing risk of falls and serious injuries (Tinetti, *et al.*, 1988).

The prevalence of dementia also rises with advanced age from 5% at ages 75-79 to 20-30% in adults over age 85. These rates may be higher among blacks than among whites, perhaps due to educational differences. Alzheimer's disease is the most common cause for dementia in older adults. However, new data from the Cardiovascular Health Study indicates that vascular disease is a much more common cause of dementia than previously thought. Almost one-third of older adults without a history of stroke had evidence for infarct-like lesions on brain MRI. In blacks, stroke is a particularly prominent cause for dementia (Froelich, *et al.*, 2001). Depression is also extremely common among older adults. Although women are diagnosed with depression more often than men, the prevalence becomes similar between genders among the oldest old (FIFA, 2000).

Common conditions vary in prevalence according to race and ethnicity. For example, in 1995, blacks over age 70 reported a 67% prevalence of arthritis, while 58% of non-latino whites and 50% latinos reported arthritis (FIFA, 2000). Blacks also display higher rates of hypertension, which likely contributes to a higher risk of stroke. Older latinos and blacks have comparably high rates of diabetes mellitus.

Given the high rates of comorbidity among the older population, many older adults are prescribed a large number of medications. These complicated medical regimens are difficult for older patients to take correctly and also difficult for many to afford. As a result, adherence to prescribed medication regimens declines with increasing numbers of medications.

The health consequences of comorbidity are only beginning to be understood. In particular, the number of diseases present, and particular pairs of diseases, such as osteoarthritis and heart disease, confer greatly increased risk of disability (Fried, 2004). Chronic diseases individually and the high rates of comorbidity are major risk factors for disability and loss of independence with age.

1.2.3. Disability

Disability refers to physical or cognitive limitations to an individual's ability to perform essential or socially defined roles. Disability occurs when a person's capabilities are unable to match either the tasks or environmental demands, and the individual has difficulty performing necessary or desired tasks and activities. Disability is a feared condition in late life and a risk factor for loss of independence, institutionalization, social isolation, and financial devastation. In 2001, 6.1% of metropolitan older adults reported limitations in activities of daily living, i.e. basic self-care tasks including bathing, dressing, and toileting, compared to 7.3% of older adults outside of metropolitan areas. Similarly, 12.2% of older adults in metropolitan areas reported limitations in instrumental activities of daily living, such as meal preparation, shopping, or using the telephone, while 13.7% of non-metropolitan older adults described these limitations (National Center for Health Statistics, 2003).

A higher percentage of blacks than whites over age 70 reported inability to perform at least one of nine physical activities such as walking or stooping (32.6% v. 24.6%) in 1995 (FIFA, 2000) (See Figure 5). Furthermore, in a comparison of inner city St. Louis and the U.S. population, inner city older blacks are more likely to live alone, be disabled, and describe poor health than other older blacks (Miller, *et al.*, 1996). Rates of disability appear to be a major component in the growing disparity as in health between older blacks and whites (Clark, 1997).

Disability in older adults is primarily an outcome of chronic diseases and geriatric conditions, exacerbated by environmental conditions, such as the presence of stairs for a person who has difficulty climbing stairs, and access to resources – from social support to transportation to prescription medicines and effective secondary and tertiary prevention. Approximately one-third of community-dwelling older adults report difficulty walking, one aspect of disability, while almost 20% report difficulty doing the tasks of household management, such as shopping, meal preparation, and financial management, essential to living independently in one's home. Almost 20% report difficulty with basic self care tasks such as bathing or dressing. Difficulty in these tasks is a risk factor for becoming dependent, i.e. being unable to perform these tasks without assistance. On the other hand, environmental or personal modifications can permit the individual to compensate for limitations and be able to continue to live independently. Many aspects of urban living, such as apartment buildings with elevators, facilitate preservation of independence.

1.2.4. Prevention Strategies

Primary, secondary, and tertiary prevention and health promotion strategies are cornerstones of management for older adults with chronic disease and geriatric conditions, with or without resulting disability. This includes the recommendations of the U.S. Preventive Services Task Force for asymptomatic older adults, and a range of public health and clinical approaches to improved management of chronic conditions. Interventions like these are important to ameliorate the risk factors

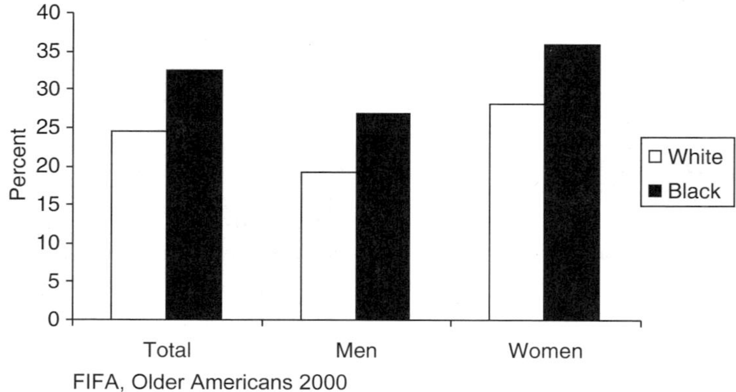

Note: Physical functioning activities are walking a quarter of a mile, walking up ten steps, standing for two hours, sitting for two hours, crouching/kneeling, reaching over the head, reaching out, using fingers to grasp, lifting ten pounds. Unable indicates unable to perform alone and without aids.

Figure 5. Percentage of Persons Age 70 and Over Who Are Unable to Perform Any One of Nine Physical Functions, by Sex and Race, 1995 (*Sources*: Federal Interagency Forum on Age-Related statistics 2000; Civilian noninstitutionalized population data from Supplement on Aging).

for loss of independence and the need for long-term care, and for improving quality of life.

Prevention is also important for acute illnesses such as influenza or pneumococcal pneumonia. Influenza causes 20,000-40,000 deaths each year, and 90% occur in adults over age 65. Pneumococcal disease continues to be a major infectious disease in the U.S., causing 40,000 deaths per year. The case fatality rate for severe pneumococcal infections with bacteremia is 25-35%. Older adults are disproportionately affected by this serious illness (Robison, *et al.*, 2001) and have higher mortality rates; this risk increases in congregate housing facilities, such as nursing homes. Unfortunately, because antibiotic resistance is high in large hospitals, urban adults may have a higher incidence of resistant infections than rural adults (Panlilio *et al.*, 1992). However, suburban residents seem to have high rates of resistant pneumococcal infection, possibly due to access to care and physician prescribing practices (Hofmann, *et al.*, 1995). The U.S. Preventive Services Task Force recommends that all older adults receive the influenza vaccine annually and the pneumococcal vaccine once after reaching age 65.

Meanwhile, as a result of improved treatment regimens, HIV will become more prevalent among older adults in coming decades, and will continue to affect urban communities disproportionately. This emerging cohort will have unique medical and social needs. Already, 11% of Americans diagnosed with HIV are at least age 50 (CDC, 2001). Forty-nine percent of men over age 50 with AIDS and 70% of women over age 50 with AIDS are black or latino.

Controlling disease risk factors can prevent the onset of disease and prevent disease complications. For example, primary and secondary prevention have substantial potential to reduce vascular dementia through blood pressure and cardiovascular disease prevention and management. Multifactorial interventions to address risk factors can also prevent incontinence and falls and there is mounting evidence that strengthening exercise is important to the prevention and treatment of frailty. In order to achieve maximal benefit from disease prevention interventions, it is necessary to screen high risk populations, including those at risk of progression or recurrence of existing health conditions.

Older adults are disproportionately large users of health care, universally and also in cities. Although only 13% of the American population is at least 65 years old, this group accounts for almost half of inpatient hospital days. Health care utilization is similar in rural and metropolitan communities. For example, older adults in metropolitan areas had 286.8 discharges from short-stay hospitals per 1,000 people while older adults in nonmetropolitan areas had 295.8 discharges per 1,000 people. Older adults in rural communities experienced slightly shorter length of hospital stays than did urban older adults (5.2 days v. 5.5 days) (National Center for Health Statistics, 2003). The proportion of older adults living in nursing homes in major cities is comparable to national rates.

2.0. HOW URBAN LIVING MAY AFFECT THE HEALTH OF OLDER ADULTS

Characteristics of urban communities can both positively and negatively influence the health and independent functioning of older adults. Most obviously, the urban environment can present a variety of challenges for maintaining and promoting the health of older adults. Air pollution, substandard housing, street crime, traffic, and weakened neighborhood institutions form a legion of health and social challenges for all citizens, particularly the most vulnerable. On the other hand, urban environments can provide greater mobility due to public transportation, buildings with elevators, community transport vans, and increased density and access to cultural stimulation and health care access. Urban environments also provide greater access to community services and support intergenerational interaction as well as opportunities for social engagement and stimulation. We review some of the salient issues below.

2.1. Physical Environment

Older adults as well as children are more sensitive to urban environmental threats like air pollution than are middle-aged adults. High levels of ground level ozone (Delfino, *et al.*, 1998) and particulate matter have been associated with morbidity (such as from respiratory disease) and mortality among the urban elderly (Schwartz, 1994). Ground level ozone is generated by car exhaust, while particulate matter is released from factories and energy plants. Asthma and other respiratory illnesses cause severe morbidity and mortality among urban older adults and are exacerbated by air pollution. An example of this impact is that asthma hospitalization rates in 1996 in Chicago were twice as high as in the surrounding suburbs (Thomas and Williams, 1999). Exposure to particulate matter is associated with overall increases in both hospitalizations and outpatient care among older urban adults. In a comparison of most polluted and least polluted metropolitan areas, the most polluted areas have 18% higher outpatient costs for whites age 65-84 and 7% higher inpatient care costs (Fuchs and Frank, 2002). Code red air days are a health threat for vulnerable older people.

Another risk of the physical environment is overcrowding (Howden-Chapman, 2004). Crowding is particularly a concern among immigrant populations. Overcrowding increases transmission of infectious diseases and often increases noise and stress. Noise pollution from traffic or crowding which interrupts sleep can be an important problem for older adults who are awakened easily due to reduced stage IV sleep.

Urban residents living in impoverished areas often have excellent neighborhood access to liquor stores and pawn shops but poor access to markets selling affordable healthy food. Notably, few older urban adults meet dietary recommendations (Tangney, 2000) for grains, vegetables, and dairy products. Approximately 40-50% of older adults are undernourished. Possibly due to high poverty rates, older adults in cities, particularly in Southern states, have higher rates of hunger and food insecurity than other older adults (Nord, 2002).

Older adults have a great fear of street crime, although young people are victimized more often. Fear of violence or intimidation has been reported to limit physical activity and promote social isolation. Factors such as loneliness are associated with fear of crime in the neighborhood as well as in the home (Bazargan, 1994). Older adults living in cities are also frequent targets for fraud, from telemarketers and others. Twenty-seven percent of 200 Houston senior center participants reported being victimized by fraud (Otiniano, *et al.*, 2002). Such victimization increases feelings of fear, guilt, and self-doubt. Finally, the terrorist attack of September 11, 2001 traumatized the nation's populace, including older adults, and reminds us of a new threat to urban communities. The different ways that older adults, and children, are particularly vulnerable to threats of bioterrorism and as well as targeted methods to safeguard these groups, remain to be addressed.

2.2. Housing

Housing conditions affect the health of older urban adults. Older adults have the highest rates of being homeowners. In New York City, 27% of homeowners are at least 65 years old (U.S. Census Bureau, 2002), approximately twice as high as the percentage of older residents. The proportion of female homeowners who are at least 65 years old in this survey is slightly greater than the proportion of older male homeowners (14.4 versus 12.7%). Older blacks have lower rates of home ownership than whites (U.S. Census Bureau, 1995). Older adults who are homeowners in urban communities often have homes that are old and possess outdated plumbing and electrical systems (See Figure 6). Effective heating and air conditioning is critical for older adults who lack the physiologic and social mechanisms to compensate for threatening climates. Hundreds of older urban adults died during recent heat waves in Chicago and in Paris (e.g., Naughton *et al.*, 2002). Physical housing problems are most common among old minority seniors. One of every six older blacks lives in inadequate housing (defined as moderate to severe physical problems), compared to one of every 23 older whites, according to a 1995 U.S. government survey (U.S HUD, 1999), and certainly the black population is more concentrated in central cities. Due to the frequency of inadequate electrical and heating systems, poor (Mierley and Baker, 1983), older (Istre, *et al.*, 2001) urban adults are disproportionately injured and killed in house fires (See Figure 7). Many urban residences have unhealthy characteristics, according to a study of six U.S. cities (Muller, *et al.*, 2002).

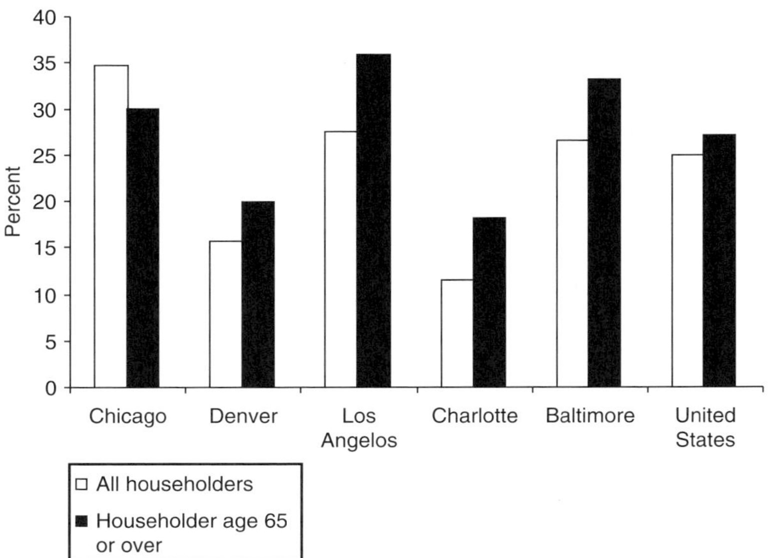

Note: Metropolitan areas include city as well as surrounding suburbs according to US Census definition.

Figure 6. Percentage of Structures Built in 1949 or Earlier by Age of Householder: Five Metropolitan Areas and Total United States (*Source*: American Housing Survey, 1995-2002).

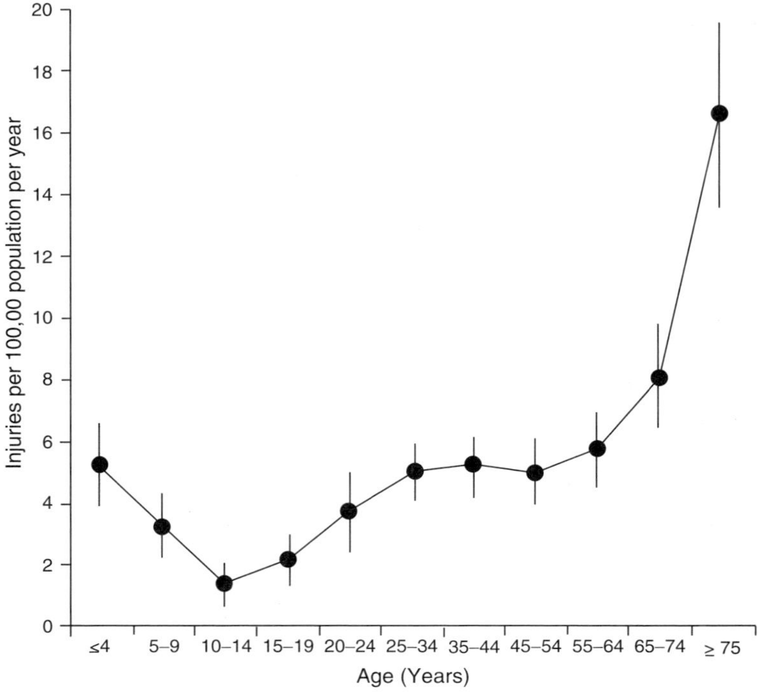

Note: Fire injuries in Dallas, Texas from 1991 to 1997 reported by Emergency Medical Services, local burn center, and medical examiner.

Figure 7. Fire Injuries by Age Group (*Source*: Istre, 2001).

There is evidence that many older homeowners have difficulty maintaining housing stock, due both to financial considerations and physical limitations. This can result in poorly maintained and unhealthful homes with increasing risk of accidents, fires, and injuries. These poorly maintained homes are a threat to the neighborhood's security and value. Also, older homes are typically not designed for access by disabled individuals. These homes often have narrow doorways and lack first floor bathrooms. A health event such as a stroke may trigger institutionalization unless the home can be modified for wheelchair use, etc. Often, healthy home buyers do not plan for future mobility disability or difficulties with activities of daily living when comparing homes. Finally, because a home with a paid mortgage is a major component of household wealth for many older adults, a deteriorating home or neighborhood substantially diminishes a person's total assets.

2.3. Transportation

Residents of cities with public transportation have less need to drive, a benefit for many older adults. In addition, cities often offer access to services within walking distance. Although older adults rely on personal vehicles as frequently as younger adults, older drivers take fewer and shorter trips (Collia, *et al.*, 2003).

Aging is associated with decreased peripheral vision, slowed reaction times, and sometimes other sensory, physical, or cognitive impairments, which make driving hazardous. These physiologic alterations can add to the challenge of driving in central cities such as navigating difficult traffic patterns, sitting in traffic jams with frequent stops and starts, and fighting for parking close to the home. Motor vehicle collisions involving older drivers are more likely to occur at intersections than collisions involving younger drivers. Overall, the number of older Americans killed in traffic accidents increased 27% from 1991 to 2001 (TRIP, 2003).

A study of urban older adults who have recently stopped driving found that all of them had motor vehicle collisions before forfeiting a driver's license and most described immobility and loneliness (Johnson, 1999). For these individuals, family and friends were often not available to provide transportation. Fortunately, many cities provide excellent mass transit options, compared to suburban and nonmetropolitan settings. These transportation alternatives can prevent isolation or dependency of older adults who have curtailed or eliminated driving. Unfortunately, however, older adults are walking and using public transportation less frequently than twenty years ago, even in urban communities (Glasgow, 2000). Many transit systems have noted ridership declines (Mason, 1998). Suburban sprawl and lack of persistent public investment in transit probably contribute to this decline. Although common in Europe, walking and bicycling are very rare among older Americans (See Figure 8). Moreover, many cities in the West and Southwest that have recently seen a dramatic rise in numbers of older citizens have poor transit systems. When vigorous older individuals stop driving in these settings, they face significant isolation unless they relocate or unless new services are provided (Frey, 1999).

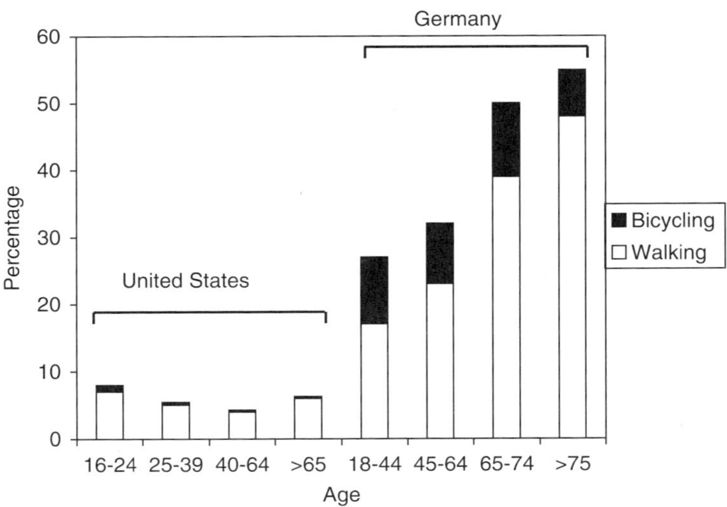

Note: Data from the US Department of Transportation, Federal Highway Administration surveys,and German Ministry of Transport

Figure 8. Percentage of Trips in Urban Areas Made by Walking and Bicycling in the United States and Germany, by Age Group, 1995 (*Source*: Pucher 2003).

Heavy traffic is a danger to pedestrians, particularly to older people. Although they spend less time as pedestrians than younger adults, in 2000, older adults accounted for 21% of pedestrian deaths (NHTSA, 2001). Older adults have the highest pedestrian-motor vehicle collision mortality rate. Although older adults are more cautious pedestrians, slowed walking speed contributes strongly to their high risk (Oxley, *et al.*, 1997). Traffic signals are helpful in preventing motor vehicle collisions involving older pedestrians (Koepsell, *et al.*, 2002). Unfortunately, electronic walk signs often do not provide the time needed by older adults with slower walking speeds so that they can cross the street safely.

2.4. Activities of Older Adults

There is increasing evidence that, for urban older adults, high frequency of participation in leisure and productive activities is associated with improved health and reduced depression due to a positive sense of agency (Herzog, *et al.*, 1998). Older urban adults have more opportunities than those in the suburbs for socializing with neighbors and participation in group activities (Felton, *et al.*, 1981). However, fears of crime, increased prevalence of abandoned homes, and decreased neighborhood social capital have diminished the communication and interaction between neighbors in many urban communities. Cities often have a cadre of senior centers offering social activities as well as health screenings. National survey data suggests that participation in senior center activities is most common among older, poorly educated, nonwhite, and socially active seniors (Sabin, 1993). Many senior centers are focused on activities for frail older adults, with few options for the vast majority of community-dwelling older adults who are not frail. In the last decade, slot machine gambling has become an increasingly accessible and desirable social activity for older adults in cities. Liberalization of state gambling laws has triggered an increase in the number of older adults who gamble (Petry, 2002), as well as an increase in numbers seeking treatment for problem gambling.

The percentage of men who continue to do paid work at age 65 has declined steadily for 50 years, but recently has plateaued. In 1999, the labor force participation rate for men at least 65 years old was 16.9%, a figure slightly higher than in 1985. The 1999 labor force participation rate for older women was 8.9% (Purcell, 2000). Older adults who continue in the workforce beyond usual retirement age typically either cannot financially afford to retire or are self-employed.

Many older adults have caregiving responsibilities. An increasing percentage of children in cities are being raised by grandparents with neither of the parents in the home (Bryson and Casper, 1999). Although caregiving is associated with stress, depression, and neglect of medical needs, it can also provide a sense of purpose and value (Kramer, 1997).

There is also evidence that 30% of older adults would like to be engaged in volunteer activities or other productive activities, but are not. There is a substantial structural lag (Riley, *et al.*, 1994) between the needs and desires to remain productively engaged in society and the dearth of such meaningful roles available for older adults. For many adults, post-retirement years are a time to "give back." According to Erik and JoAnn Erikson's theories of late life development, (Erickson, *et al.*, 1986) fulfillment of this need, being generative and leaving one's legacy, are important to a sense of meaning in one's life and "successful" aging. This suggests tremendous potential for contributions of our aging population to the well-being of our cities, which is, as yet, unrealized.

2.5. Access to Health Care

Vulnerable older urban adults disproportionately receive medical care from academic medical centers, typically located in urban centers (Kahn, *et al.*, 1994). These academic medical centers are often sources of high-quality care (Ayanian and Weissman, 2002), and improved outcomes, potentially due to greater expertise, volume, or more technology. Also, urban density means better access to a more diverse set of health care institutions than in rural settings.

However, older adults with inadequate or no health insurance are less likely to receive consistent primary care, where preventive services and meaningful chronic disease care are typically delivered. Older blacks receive fewer preventive services than older whites, and the least affluent receive fewer preventive services than the more affluent (Gornick, *et al.*, 1996). For example, older blacks are less likely to be vaccinated against influenza than whites. Thus, some older urban adults may be at risk for a variety of preventable adverse health outcomes due to limitations of the urban health delivery system. The U.S. health care system is organized primarily for provision of acute medical care, rather than the chronic care of older adults' health conditions. Acute care often does not include attention to, or reimbursement of providers for the prevention, chronic disease management, and care coordination that improve health outcomes, for older adults with chronic diseases.

3.0. HOW OLDER ADULTS CONTRIBUTE TO THE HEALTH OF THEIR COMMUNITIES

In successful communities, older adults are often the glue that dynamically binds together a family and a neighborhood. The varied contributions of older adults to a community reflect the heterogeneity of this population. A substantial proportion of homeowners in urban communities are older adults. As homeowners, these older adults have a stake in preserving the quality of the neighborhood and the value of their property. They therefore often provide necessary social capital by serving as guardians and observers in neighborhoods. Because social cohesion in a community is associated with lower rates of violence (Sampson *et al.*, 1997), older adults can be important contributors to increased neighborhood safety.

Similarly, because they are less likely to migrate than younger adults, seniors provide stability in a family and neighborhood. These stabilizing forces provide moral leadership and mentoring for younger family members as well as others in the neighborhood. Households led by a person at least 65 years old have a lower risk of being victims of property crime than households headed by someone under age 65 (FIFA, 2000). Conversely, when these citizens become too frail to maintain their homes, communities suffer. Declines in health, declines in physical function, and home deterioration can lead to migration out of the community to institutional care or to a family member's home. Investments in disease and disability prevention as well as investments in home maintenance are likely to keep people in their homes and preserve housing stock and neighborhood stability.

While many young adults leave the city, healthy affluent retired adults often return in order to take advantage of cultural attractions (Mulrine, 1999). For example, the Upper West Side of Manhattan and Friendship Heights in Washington DC have large populations of older adults. These vigorous and affluent retirees bring resources into the city through property taxes, discretionary spending, and charitable contributions including support of cultural activities.

As noted above, older adults, particularly women, are frequent volunteers in urban communities, bringing services and support to many others. Older people who do not do paid work or formal volunteering often serve as informal caregivers, providing important care to spouses or to grandchildren. Thus, older adults bring substantial social and financial capital, as well as neighborhood stability, to urban communities.

4.0. BUILDING NEW URBAN COMMUNITIES THAT WILL IMPROVE THE HEALTH OF OLDER ADULTS

Structural lag refers to the time delay between the onset of a change in population needs and the political and social mobilization to address these needs (Riley *et al.*, 1994). There is a profound challenge ahead for our aging society due to structural lag in the development and support of institutions, services, and infrastructure to promote the health, well-being, and engagement of older adults. Prevention strategies can guide policies to address the structural lag in our response to the aging of our society. Exploiting the strengths of urban communities, such as public transportation, population density, and the presence of academic medical centers, can overcome barriers to optimum health and health care for an aging population (See Table 1).

4.1. Environmental Engineering

Given a variety of residential options, many people would like to live in a home in a small town or a community with a small town's characteristics: people are friendly and most destinations are in walking distance. To support older adults' ability to reside in cities, cities would do well to adopt zoning strategies that encourage homes being near supermarkets and shopping opportunities, as well as libraries, schools, senior centers, and other opportunities for engagement. Such zoning policies empower all citizens to participate easily in the life of the community. The ideal city reflects civic virtues and encourages each person to achieve full growth and potential (Jennings, 2001).

A healthy urban environment needs to contain sufficient green space to provide opportunities for pleasurable and social leisure-time physical activity. Such

Table 1. Urban Opportunities and Challenges

Opportunities	Challenges
Population density	Poverty
Mass transit	Low opportunities to harness social capital
Academic medical centers	Crime
Density of community services	Old homes
Arts/Culture	Pollution
Industry/Jobs	Lack of green space
Universities	Access to grocery stores in poorer neighborhoods
Access to opportunities to remain productive and engaged	

green spaces would promote the health of older adults (Takano, *et al.*, 2002) as long as they are safe.

Mixed use zoning, permitting proximity of commercial and residential properties, would reduce the need for automobiles and promote physical activity. Adequate urban public transportation and paratransit services also enable more people to stay integrated in the community and increase incentives for unsafe drivers to surrender their car keys. Increasing transit ridership among older adults requires frequently serviced and useful routes and comfortable vehicles.

To protect older pedestrians, ensuring long enough walk signs to allow people to cross the street or reach a median safe area is important. Also, widening sidewalks and placing more benches on sidewalks would make walking easier for frail or disabled older people, providing stopping points as needed.

Modern homes should be accessible for the individual, with first floor bathrooms, wide doorways and, potentially, ramps to the outdoors. Prospective home buyers should be informed of the accessibility of a home to disabled individuals. In older homes where adults wish to "age in place," home modifications will likely be needed in the event of temporary or permanent disability. These older homeowners may need financial or physical assistance to maintain a home in good condition. Public-private partnerships may be the most practical and sustainable mechanism to facilitate home repairs and modifications.

4.2. Social Mobilization

As a society, we are confronted by the new phenomenon of the "third age": the one-third of life that people will be living after retirement. Roles and responsibilities in this third age are in need of development. It is critical to recognize, from a public health point of view, that older adults' health is positively affected by remaining active and engaged in meaningful activities that have an impact and "give back" to society (for example, see Erikson *et al.*). At the same time, we have profound unmet social needs to which older adults could bring social capital in a mutually beneficial relationship. In fact, for cities, older adults could be the "only increasing natural resource" (Fried *et al.*, 2000). Recognizing the needs and desires of older adults to remain active and generative and developing institutions that facilitate this will serve to promote the health of our aging population (Fried, *et al*, 1997).

There are a number of examples of new models of volunteerism as well as phased retirement that are being developed in response to these challenges. One model for a volunteer program that was intentionally developed as a health promotion program for the older volunteers while creating roles with high impact for society is the Experience Corps (Fried, 2004; Freedman and Fried, 1999). This program places a critical mass of older adult volunteers in public elementary schools in a high intensity model (15 hours per week) in roles designed to significantly improve academic outcomes for children. At the same time, the program is intentionally designed to increase physical, social, and cognitive activity for the older volunteers as well as provide opportunities for regular, structured activities and to leave a legacy. There is early evidence from this program that this multi-risk factor modification approach may be effective in prevention of disability and loss of independence with aging (Fried, 2004). This type of intervention provides a vehicle for health promotion to many older adults who would not otherwise participate in long-term health promotion activities.

4.3. Chronic Care Reform and Disease Prevention

Maintaining the health of older urban adults with chronic illness requires effective chronic disease management, as well as care that is well-coordinated between health care providers in health facilities and health care providers at home. Effective chronic disease management and prevention or minimization of disability requires a spectrum of approaches. For example, individuals with chronic illness benefit from education in managing their own diseases. Such disease management approaches have demonstrated the ability to improve health status without increasing health costs (Phelan, *et al.*, 2002). Physicians, nurses, educators, and community health workers all can contribute to disease management programs designed to prevent disability, institutionalization, and death. The urban environment, with a high density of providers, can facilitate communication and effective coordination of care, including case management and discharge planning. One example of successful coordination is a discharge planning and home visit intervention for hospitalized older adults in Philadelphia which reduced rehospitalization rates as well as health care costs (Naylor, *et al.*, 1999).

In older adults, prevention has demonstrated to be effective in reducing death from conditions including cardiovascular disease, colon cancer, and influenza. Prevention strategies such as physical activity have also improved quality of life in older adults of varying health status and appear to be important in prevention of frailty and loss of independence with aging, improving both physical function and well-being and cognitive function. The U.S. Preventive Services Task Force recommends a variety of screening and counseling interventions for older adults. Although individual-level prevention is often practiced effectively by clinicians, these strategies are not sufficient to benefit all urban seniors. The reason that these strategies are designed for periodic screenings of asymptomatic older adults, and some case findings. These need to be coupled with "community-based" health education and screening and secondary and tertiary prevention of progression of disease and of disability. Home-level prevention strategies such as effective air conditioning and accessible bathrooms and kitchens are a critical component of the prevention continuum important to supporting maintenance of ability to function independently in one's home with aging.

4.4. Health System Reform

American health systems will need to be reinvented to provide optimum care for older urban adults, as well as effective chronic disease care broadly. New models of care delivery for frail older adults feature interdisciplinary teams that coordinate care between providers and between care settings. The Program of All-inclusive Care for the Elderly (PACE) is an example of a care model that serves frail, chronically ill, older urban adults well (Eng, *et al.*, 1997). PACE programs, centered on an adult day center, serve as medical provider and insurer and coordinate community services to maintain functioning and independence. Meanwhile, adult day centers themselves are increasingly utilized, with nearly 75% being located in urban areas. These day centers typically are private, not for profit, and sponsored by a church, nursing home, or other organization (Wacker, *et al.*, 1998). These day care centers provide both social services and limited medical services for community-dwelling older adults. Day centers offer frail older adults a chance for social interaction as well as an opportunity to be evaluated by trained staff who can screen for problems and hopefully prevent progression of illness and disability, and hospitalizations. The respite and support provided by day centers and PACE programs serves to prevent unnecessary institutionalization and, in many instances, offer models for long term care at home.

Programs which support people remaining in the home and community rather than being institutionalized when long term care is needed are increasingly favored for social as well as economic reasons. Cities are potentially well-positioned to develop assisted living and life care communities for non-driving older adults due to proximity to necessary health and social services as well as to cultural attractions. Land acquisition and zoning are current barriers to building such communities in cities. New York State has been investing (with federal funds) in maintaining the health and quality of life of older adults in naturally occurring retirement communities, particularly in New York City (Pine and Pine, 2002). Low-income individuals aging in a subsidized building not designated as senior housing receive heath and care management services as well as social and educational opportunities.

4.5. End of Life Care

The support of family and close friends can help to maintain dignity at the end of life. 40% of baby boomers will require at least a brief nursing home stay during their lives. Urban long-term care facilities tend to be large, and Medicaid is the dominant payer for nursing home care. Dementia patients who reside in urban nursing homes are 14% more likely than similar patients in non-urban areas to have a feeding tube, either due to greater access to care or due to other factors (Mitchell, *et al.*, 2003). Although such institutional care may well be depersonalized, communal living in proximity to family and friends with opportunities for outside excursions could make urban nursing homes preferred. Additionally, the highest rate of hospice use is in large urban areas (Virnig, *et al.*, 2004). At the end of life, urban hospice programs can provide attentive, compassionate care. Because most hospice care is provided in the home rather than in inpatient settings, a dense population is most conducive to a successful and responsive hospice program.

5.0. CONCLUSION

Individuals as well as society can take important steps to influence health and well-being later in life. Robust aging requires either good health and good functioning or the ability to manage chronic health conditions and compensate for functional difficulties. As they age, people can remain engaged with family, community, and society – and this is important to well-being with aging. Cities of the future will need to develop innovative environments that enhance autonomy and support the function, engagement and well-being of older people at different levels of health status. Urban communities can create networks of health and social programs that provide the optimum continuum of care and opportunities for older adults.

There are numerous models of innovative health and social programs which, if scaled up, could beneficially affect older adults in urban settings, and potentially prevent out-migration after retirement. Programs which improve the health of older urban adults may benefit from public-private partnerships to shoulder the burdens of leadership and financing. Government, the non-profit sector, and private industry all have an interest in strengthening the health of older urban adults.

Public health education interventions can promote healthy behaviors and self-management of disease, as well as the appropriate use of medical care. Cities offer distinct opportunities for providing integration of clinical care with community services that can provide meals, transportation, home repairs, and opportunities for social engagement for older adults at different levels of health status. Because of the location of academic health centers along with the public health system in urban settings, there is great potential for collaboration in development of more effective and novel integrated health care delivery systems that span the home, community, and health care delivery sites. Thoughtful, creative research will improve our ability to determine best practices for improving the lives of older adults in urban settings. Community-based participatory research allows investigators to evaluate strategies for translating clinical and public health knowledge into improved community care. This research can answer important questions and can be sustained with community commitment and leadership.

REFERENCES

Ayanian, J.Z., and Weissman, J.S. (2002). Teaching hospitals and quality of care: A review of the literature. *Milbank Q.* 80:569-585.

Barnett, E., Strogatz, D., Armstrong, D., and Wing, S. (1996). Urbanization and Coronary Heart Disease Mortality among African-Americans in the U.S. South. *J. Epidemiol. Community Health* 50:252-257.

Bazargan, M. (1994). The Effects of health, environmental, and socio-psychological variables on fear of crime and its consequences among urban black elderly individuals. *Int. J. Aging Hum. Dev.* 38: 99-115.

Bryson, K., and Casper, L.M. (1998). Coresident grandparents and grandchildren. *Current Population Reports, Special Studies.* U.S. Census Bureau Report No. 26, pp. 23-198; http://www.census.gov/population/www/documentation/twps0026/twps0026.html

Budson, A.E., Simons, J.S., Sullivan, A.L., Beier, J.S., Solomon, P.R., Scinto, L.F., Daffner, K.R., and Schacter, D.L. (2004). Memory and emotions for the September 11, 2001, terrorist attacks in patients with Alzheimer's disease, patients with mild cognitive impairment, and healthy older adults. *Neuropsychology* 18(2):315-27.

Centers for Disease Control and Prevention. (2001). *HIV/AIDS surveillance report.* (2001). Centers for Disease Control and Prevention, Atlanta, GA: 13(2): 5-6; http://www.cdc.gov/hiv/stats/hasr1302.htm

Clark, D.O. (1997). U.S. trends in disability and institutionalization among older blacks and whites. *Am. J. Public Health* 87:438-440.

Collia, D.V., Sharp, J., and Giesbrecht, L. (2003). The 2001 National Household Travel Survey: A Look into the travel patterns of older Americans. *J. Safety Res.* 34:461-470.

Current Population Survey, March 1998 Supplement. US Census Bureau

Current Population Survey, March 2002 Supplement. US Census Bureau

Current Population Survey, March 2003 Supplement. US Census Bureau

Delfino, R.J., Murphy-Moulton, A.M., and Becklake, M.R. (1998). Emergency room visits for respiratory illnesses among the elderly in Montreal: Association with low level ozone exposure. *Environ. Res.* 76:67-77.

Eberhardt, M.S., Ingram, D.D., Makuc, D.M., Pamuk, E.R., Freid, V.M., Harper, S.B., Schoenborn, C.A., and Xia, H. (2001). *Urban and Rural Health Chartbook. Health, United States, 2001.* National Center for Health Statistics, Hyattsville MD:

Eng, C., Pedulla, J., Eleazer, G.P., McCann, R., and Fox, N. (1997). Program of all-inclusive care for the elderly (PACE): An innovative model of integrated geriatric care and financing. *J. Am. Geriatr. Soc.* 45:223-232.

Erikson, E.H., Erikson, J.M., and Kivnick, H.Q. (1986). *Vital Involvement in Old Age.* W.W. Norton and Company, New York.

Federal Interagency Forum on Aging-Related Statistics (FIFA). (2000). *Older Americans 2000: Key Indicators of Well-Being.* U.S. Government Printing Office, Washington DC.

Felton, B.J., Hinrichsen, G.A., and Tsemberis, S. (1981). Urban-suburban differences in the predictors of morale among the aged. *J. Gerontol.* 36:214-222.

Freedman, M., and Fried, L.P. (1999). Launching Experience Corps: Findings from a 2-year Pilot Project Mobilizing Older Americans to Help Inner-City Elementary Schools. (January, 1999) Civic Ventures, Oakland, CA.

Freedman, M. (1999). *Prime Time: How Baby Boomers Will Revolutionize Retirement and Transform America.* Public Affairs, New York, pp. 292.

Frey, W.H. (1999). *Beyond Social Security: The Local Aspects of an Aging America.* Brookings Institution, Washington DC.

Frey, W.H. (2003). Boomers and seniors in the suburbs: Aging patterns in census 2000. *The Living Cities Census Series,* 2003 (May 3 2004); www.brookings.edu/es/urban/publications/freyboomers.pdf.

Fried, L.P. (2004). Epidemiology of Aging: Implications of the Aging of Society. In: Goldman, L., and Ausieollo, D., (eds.), *Cecil Textbook of Medicine,* 22nd *ed,* Chapter 21. Elsevier Science, United States, pp. 100-105.

Fried, L.P., Carlson, M.C., Freedman, M., Frick, K.D., Glass, T.A., Hill, J., McGill S., Rebok, G.W., Seeman, T., Tielsch, J., Wasik, B.A., and Zeger, S. (2004). A Social model for health promotion for an aging population: Initial evidence on the Experience Corps model. *J. Urban Health* 81:64-78.

Fried, L.P., Freedman, M., Endres, T.E., and Wasik, B. (1997). Building communities that promote successful aging. *WJM.* 167:216-219.

Fried, L.P., Kronmal, R.A., Newman, A.B., Bild, D.E., Mittelmark, M.B., Polak, J.F., Robbins, J.A., and Gardin, J.M. (1998). Risk factors for 5-year mortality in older adults: The Cardiovascular Health Study. *JAMA.* 279:585-592.

Fried, L.P., Tangen, C.M., Walston, J., Newman, A.B., Hirsch, C., Gottdiener, J., Seeman, T., Tracey, R., Kop, W., Burke, G., and McBurnie, M.A. (2001). Frailty in older adults: Evidence for a phenotype. *J. Gerontol. Med. Sci.*56:M146-56.

Froehlich, T.E., Bogardus, S.T. Jr, and Inouye S.K. (2001). Dementia and race: are there differences between African Americans and Caucasians? *J. Am. Geriatr. Soc.* 49:477-84.

Fuchs, V.R., and Frank, S.R. (2002). Air pollution and medical care use by older Americans: A Cross area analysis. *Health Aff.* 21:207-14.

Geronimus, A.T. (2000). To Mitigate, resist, or undo: Addressing structural influences on the health of urban populations. *Am. J. Public Health* 90:867-872.

Glasgow, N. (2000). Older Adults Patterns of Driving and Using Other Transportation. *Rural America* 15:26-31, 2000; http://www.ers.usda.gov/publications/ruralamerica/sep2000/sep2000f.pdf.

Gornick, M.E., Eggers, P.W., Reilly, T.W., Mentnech, R.M., Fitterman, L.K., Kucken, L.E., and Vladeck, B.C. (1996). Effects of race and income on mortality and use of services among Medicare beneficiaries. *N. Engl. J. Med.* 335:791-9.

Guralnik J.M., Fried L.P., Simonsick E.M., Kasper J.D., and Lafferty M.E., (eds.). (1995). *The Women's Health and Aging Study: Health and Social Characteristics of Older Women with Disability.* National Institute on Aging, National Institute of Health, Publication Bethesda, MD; http://www.nia.nih.gov/health/pubs/whasbook/chap5/chap5.htm.

He, W. (2002). The Older foreign-born population in the United States. Current Population Reports, Series P23-211. U.S. Census Bureau. U.S. G.P.O., Wahington, DC.

Herzog, A.R., Franks, M.M., Markus, H.R., and Holmberg, D. (1998). Activities and well-being in older age: Effects of self-concept and educational attainment. *Psychol. Aging* 13:179-85.

Hofmann, J., Ctron, M.S., Farley, M.M., Baughman, W.S., Facklam, R.R., Elliott, J.A., Deaver, K.A., and Breiman, R.F. (1995). The Prevalence of drug-resistant *Streptococcus pneumoniae* in Atlanta. *N. Engl. J. Med.* 333:481-486.

Howden-Chapman, P. (2004). Housing standards: A Glossary of housing and health. *J. Epidemiol. Community Health* 58:162-168.

Hunink, M.G., Goldman, L., Tosteson, A.N., Mittleman, M.A., Goldman, P.A., Williams, L.W., Tsevat, J., and Weinstein, M.C. (1997). The recent decline in mortality from coronary heart disease, 1980-1990: The effect of secular trends in risk factors and treatment. *JAMA.* 277:535-542.

Istre, G.R., McCoy, M.A., Osborn, L., Barnard, J.J., and Boton, A. (2001). Deaths and injuries from house fires. *N. Engl. J. Med.* 344:1911-6.

Jennings, B. (2001). From the urban to the civic: The moral possibilities of the city. *J. Urban Health.* 78: 88-97.

Johnson, J.E. (1999). Urban older adults and the forfeiture of a driver's license. *J. Gerontol. Nurs.* 25:12-18.

Kahn, K.L., Pearson, M.L., Harrison, E.R., Desmond, K.A., Rogers, W.H., Rubenstein, L.V., Brook, R.H., and Keeler, E.B. (1994). Health care for black and poor hospitalized Medicare patients. *JAMA.* 271:1169-74.

Kinsella, K. and Velkoff, V. (2001). *An Aging World: 2001.* U.S. Census Bureau, Series 95101-1, U.S. GPO, Washington DC.

Koepsell, T., McCoskey, L., Wolf, L. Moudon, A.V., Buchner, D., Kraus, J., and Patterson, M. (2002). Crosswalk markings and the risk of pedestrian-motor vehicle collisions in older pedestrians. *JAMA*. 288:2136-143.

Kramer, B.J. (1997). Gains in the caregiver experience: Where are we? What next? *Gerontologist* 37: 218-232.

Mason, J.W. (1998). The buses don't stop here anymore. *The American Prospect*; www.prospect.org/print/ V9/37/mason-j.html.

McCord, C., and Freeman, H.P. (1990). Excess mortality in Harlem. *N. Engl. J. Med.* 322:173-177.

McKinnon, J. (2003). The Black Population in the United States: March 2002. *Current Population Reports*, U.S. Census Bureau, US GPO, Washington DC, pp. 20-541.

Mierley, M.C., and Baker, S.P. (1983). Fatal House Fires in an Urban Population. *JAMA*. 249:1466-1468.

Miller, D.K., Carter, M.E., Miller, J.P., Fornoff, J.E., Bentley, J.A., Boyd, S.D., Rogers, J.H., Cox, M.N., Morley, J.E., Lui, L.Y., and Coe, R.M. (1996). Inner city older blacks have high levels of functional disability. *J. Am. Geriatr. Soc.* 44:1166-1173.

Mitchell, S.L., Teno, J.M., Roy, J., Kabumoto, G., and Mor, V. (2003). Clinical and organizational factors associated with feeding tube use among nursing home residents with advanced cognitive impairment. *JAMA*. 290:73-80.

Muller, C., Gnanasekaran, K., Knapp, K., and Dushi, I. (2002). Older homeowners and renters in six U.S. cities: Housing and economic resources. *International Longevity Center Working Paper*. ILC-USA, New York; http://www.ilcusa.org/_lib/pdf/rpt_oldpeoplehousing.pdf

Mulrine, A. (1999). Retire to the suburbs: Over my dead body. *U.S. News World Rep.* 126(25):81.

National Center for Health Statistics. (2003). *Health, United States. Trend Tables on 65 and Older Population.* U.S. Department of Health and Human Services; http://www.cdc.gov/nchs/products/pubs/pubd/ hus/trendtables.htm

National Highway Traffic Safety Administration. (2001). *Traffic Safety Facts 2000: Pedestrians*. US Department of Transportation, Washington, DC, Report DOT HS 809331.

Naughton, M.P., Henderson, A., Mirabelli, M.C., Kaiser, R., Wilhelm, J.L., Kieszak, S.M., Rubin, C.H., and McGeehin, M.A. (2002). Heat-related mortality during a 1999 heat wave in Chicago. *Am. J. Prev. Med.* 22(4):221-7.

Naylor, M.D., Brooten, D., Campbell, R., Jacobsen, B.S., Mezey, M.D., Pauly, M.V., and Schwartz, J.S. (2002). Comprehensive discharge planning and home follow-up of hospitalized elders. *JAMA*. 281:613-620.

Nord, M. (2002). Food security rates are high for elderly households. Food Review. Economic Research Service, United States Department of Agriculture; www.ers.usda.gov/publications/FoodReview/ Sep2002/ frvol25i2d.pdf.

Oxley, J., Fildes, B., Ihsen, E., Charlton, J., and Day, R. (1997). Differences in traffic judgments between young and old adult pedestrians. *Accid. Anal. Prev.* 29:839-847.

Otiniano, M.E., Lorimor, R., MacDonald, E., and Du, X.L. (2002). Common fraud experienced by the elderly: Findings from a 1998 survey in Houston Texas. *Tex. Med.* 98:46-50.

Panlilio, A.L., Culver, D.H., Gaynes, R.P., Banerjee, S., Henderson, T.S., Tolson, J.S., and Martone, W.J. (1992). Methicillin-resistant *Staphylococcus aureus* in U.S. hospitals, 1975-1991. *Infect. Control Hosp. Epidemiol.* 13:582-6.

Petry, N.M. (2002). A comparison of young, middle-aged, and older treatment-seeking pathological gamblers. *Gerontologist* 42:92-99.

Phelan, E.A., Williams, B., Leveille, S., Snyder, S., Wagner, E.H., and LoGerfo, J.P. (2002). Outcomes of a community-based dissemination of the health enhancement program. *J. Am. Geriatr. Soc.* 50:1519-1524.

Pine, P.P., and Pine, V.R. (2002). Naturally occurring retirement community-supportive service program: An example of devolution. *J. Aging. Soc. Policy* 14:181-193.

Pucher, J., and Dijkstra, L. (2003). Promoting safe walking and cycling to improve public health: Lessons from the Netherlands and Germany. *Am. J. Public Health* 93:1509-1516.

Purcell, P.J. (2000). Older workers: Employment and retirement trends. U.S. Department of Labor; http://rider.wharton.upenn.edu/~prc/PRC/WP/WP2004-11.pdf

Riley, M.W., Kahn, R.L., and Foner, A. (eds.). (1994). *Age and Structural Lag: Societies' Failure to Provide Meaningful Opportunities in Work, Family, and Leisure.* John Wiley and Sons, New York.

Robinson, K.A., Baughman, W., Rothrock, G., Barrett, N.L., Pass, M., Lexau, C., Damaske, B., Stefonek, K., Barnes, B., Patterson, J., Zell, E.R., Schuchat, A., and Whitney, C.G. (2001). Epidemiology of invasive Streptococcus pneumoniae infections in the United States, 1995-1998. *JAMA*. 285:1729-1735.

Sabin, E.P. (1993). Frequency of senior center use: A preliminary test of two models of senior center participation. *J. Gerontol. Soc. Work.* 20:97-114.

Saluter, A. (1994). *Marital Status and Living Arrangements: March 1994.* Current Population Reports: Population Characteristics, U.S. Census Bureau, Washington DC, pp.20-484

Sampson, R.J., Raudenbush, S.W., and Earls, F. (1997). Neighborhoods and violent crime: a multilevel study of collective efficacy. *Science* 277(5328):918-24.

Schwartz, J. (1994). Air pollution and hospital admissions for the elderly in Detroit, Michigan. *Am. J. Respir. Crit. Care Med.* 150:648-55.

Takano, T., Nakamura, K., and Watanabe, M. (2002). Urban residential environments and senior citizens' longevity in megacity areas: The importance of walkable green spaces. *J. Epidemiol. Community Health* 56: 913-918.

Tangney, C. (2000). Dietary intake in an older urban population. *J. Nutr.* 130:2393.

The Road Information Program (TRIP). (2003). Designing Roadways to Safely Accommodate the Increasingly Mobile Older Driver; http://www.tripnet.org/OlderDrivers2003Study.PDF.

Thomas, S.D., and Whitman, S. (1999). Asthma hospitalizations and mortality in Chicago: An epidemiologic overview. *Chest* 116:135S-141S.

Tinetti, M.E., Speechley, M., and Ginter, S.F. (1988). Risk factors for falls among elderly persons living in the community. *N. Engl. J. Med.* 319(26):1701-7.

U.S. Census Bureau. (2000a) Summary File tables, U.S. Census Bureau; www.census.gov/population/cen2000/phc-t13/tab05.pdf

U.S. Census Bureau. (1995). *Housing in metropolitan areas: Black households.* Statistical Brief. SB/95-5; www.census.gov/apsd/www/statbrief/sb95_5.pdf.

U.S. HUD Publication. (1999). *Housing our Elders;* www.hud.gov/pressrel/elderlyfull.pdf

United Way of Tri-State. (1999). Twenty Million Neighbors: Update on the Older Elderly; www.uwts.org/scs3.pdf.

United States Preventive Services Task Force. (1996) *Guide to Clinical Preventive Services.* 2nd ed. Washington DC; http://www.ncbi.nlm.nih.gov/books/bv.fcgi?rid=hstat3.chapter.10062

Virnig, B.A., Moscovice, I.S., Durham, S.B., and Casey, M.M. (2004). Do rural elders have limited access to Medicare hospice services? *J. Am. Geriatr. Soc.* 52:731-735.

Wacker, R.R., Roberto, K.A., and Piper, L.E. (1998). *Community Resources for Older Adults: Programs and Services in an Era of Change.* Pine Forge Press, Thousand Oaks.

Wolinsky, F.D., Wyrwich, K.W., Kroenke, K., Babu, A.N., and Tierney, W.M. (2003). 9-11, Personal stress, mental health, and sense of control among older adults. *J. Gerontol.* 58B:S146-150.

Chapter 10

The Health of Urban Populations in Developing Countries

An Overview

Mark R. Montgomery and Alex C. Ezeh

1.0. INTRODUCTION

In the next thirty years, the developing countries of Africa and Asia are likely to cross an historic threshold, becoming, for the first time, more urban than rural (United Nations, 2003). In so doing, they will join the great majority of countries in Latin America, a region that is already as urbanized as North America and Europe. As the developing world converges to the developed world in its urban percentages, one might expect to see an accompanying transition in the dominant concepts, methods, and central concerns of health research. Surely, one would think, the upsurge of interest in social epidemiology that has so marked the developed-country literature over the past decade must also have been evident in the developing-country literature. The implications for health of socioeconomic inequality, relative deprivation, neighborhood effects, segregation, and poverty would seem, if anything, even more likely to be vividly expressed in the cities of poor countries than in the cities of the West. It is therefore somewhat disconcerting to find comparatively little research underway for poor countries in which these perspectives and concepts figure centrally in empirical studies of urban health. At least where these themes are concerned, the health literature remains oddly compartmentalized.

Chapter 17 explores the potential for the concepts and methodological tools of urban social epidemiology to be applied in the cities of poor countries. In the current chapter we sketch the health context in which such concepts may be explored. Urban health in poor countries is a very large topic, of course, and no single chapter can begin to do it justice. To focus our efforts, we refer the reader seeking more on the big picture to a recent National Research Council report (Panel on Urban Population Dynamics, 2003), which gives a lengthy review of urban health in poor countries. In what follows, we first describe the urban demographic transition in more detail, indicating how, in company with other new currents in economic development, this transition may bring attention to bear on the health of city-dwellers in poor countries. We proceed to describe, in very broad strokes, the nature of urban health conditions in these countries, and then give attention to specific features of health environments and behavior that might be profitably studied with social epidemiological tools.

2.0. THREE TRANSFORMATIONS

Three transformations are underway that have the potential to bring research and policy attention to bear on developing-country urban health. The first of these is the demographic transition mentioned above; the second is the consequence of new currents of thought in economic development; and the third has to do with the profound reorganization of political economy now taking place across the developing world. We begin with the demographic considerations.

Over the next thirty years, the world's population is expected to grow by nearly one-third, but this growth will be highly concentrated in the cities and towns of poor, developing countries (United Nations, 2003). Of the anticipated 2 billion persons to be added to the world's total by the year 2030, fully 1.9 billion are expected to reside in the cities and towns of Africa, Asia, and Latin America. Rural population totals, by contrast, are likely to undergo little net change over the period (see Figure 1) and relatively small changes are also expected for the urban populations of rich countries. This urban transformation is also evident in national percentages. Whereas in 1950 less than 20% of the population of poor countries lived in cities and towns, by 2030 the figure will have risen to nearly 60%. Within a few years, according to these forecasts, it will no longer be possible to speak of the developing world as if it were mainly composed of rural villages.

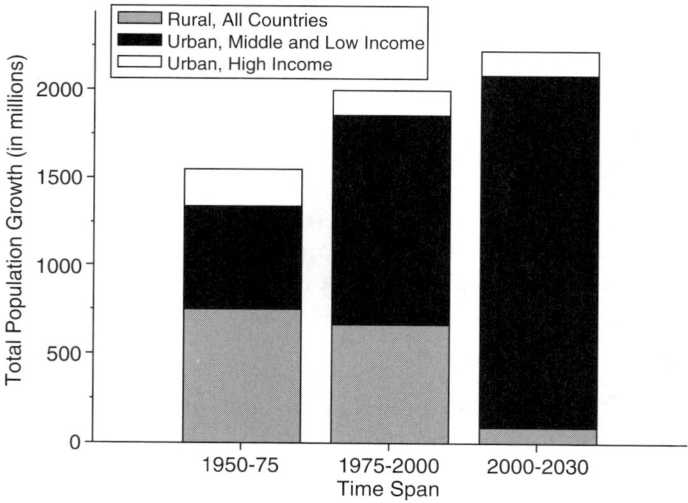

Figure 1. Distribution of World Population Growth by Urban/Rural and National Income Level Estimates and Projections for 1950–2030 (*Sources*: United Nations [2003]; World Bank [2001]).

Today the world as a whole contains 40 cities with populations of 5 million or more, and 30 of them are found in poor countries. United Nations projections indicate that between 2000 and 2015, a further 19 cities of this size will be added to the world's total, and 18 of these will be located in poor countries. In the decades ahead, the governments of these countries will face daunting challenges in managing such large cities and improving the health of their residents.

All this may suggest an urban future dominated by very large cities. Yet the majority of developing-country urban residents will probably reside in much smaller settlements. Figure 2 shows the number of urban residents who will likely be added to cities of different sizes over the period 2000 to 2015. As can be seen, the largest share of the increase will be absorbed by urban areas with fewer than 1 million inhabitants. In 2015 these towns and cities are expected to account for about 60% of the developing-country urban total (not shown in the figure). Cities from 1 to 5 million in size will house another 26%, leaving just 14% of all urban dwellers in the largest cities.

As the Panel on Urban Population Dynamics (2003) has shown, smaller urban places—especially those under 100,000 in population—are notably underserved by their governments, often lacking electricity, piped water, and adequate waste disposal. Small cities can exhibit environmental and health conditions not unlike those of rural villages. The sheer scale of the challenge presented by the largest cities should not cause the health problems of these small cities to be overlooked.

The second transformation that is drawing attention to urban contexts has to do with the Millennium Development Goals around which the United Nations, the World Bank, and other major multilaterals have been organizing their efforts. The theme that unites this enterprise is the need to reduce poverty in the developing world; its novel feature is the insistence on quantification of development targets

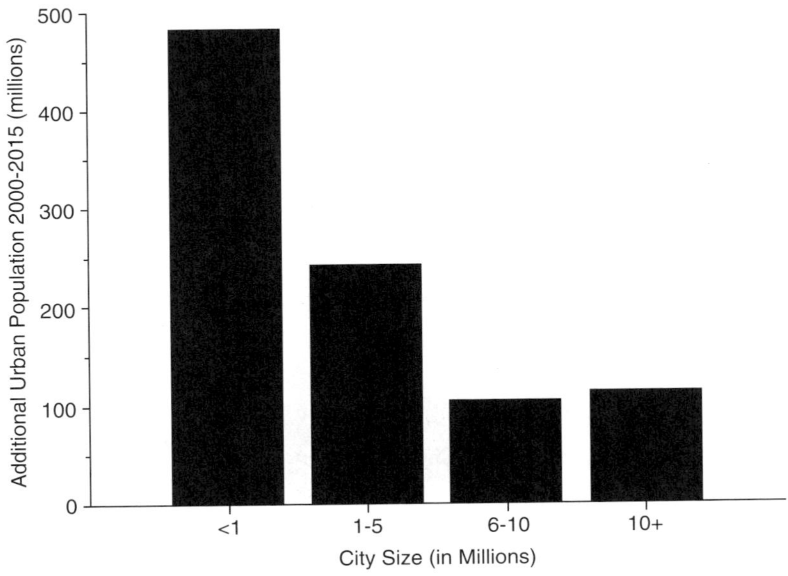

Figure 2. Net Additions to Urban Population in Developing Countries Over the Period 2000–2015, by City Size (*Source*: United Nations [2003]).

and measures of progress. (See www.un.org/millenniumgoals for further information on the Millennium Declaration and its associated goals, specific targets, and research programs). A number of the targets refer to health but make no explicit mention of urban health as a distinct area of interest). From an urban perspective, the most pertinent of the targets is Target 11: to achieve by 2020 "significant improvements in the lives of at least 100 million slum dwellers". According to the most recent estimates (UN-Habitat, 2003a), which are shown by region in Figure 3, there are some 870 million slum dwellers in the developing world, accounting for 43% of its urban residents. Set against the 870 million total, the ambitions of Target 11 would appear modest indeed. Yet because development agencies and researchers have long put their emphasis on rural poverty, Target 11 serves as a pointed reminder of the fact that poor people are also to be found in cities. Whatever the prospects may be of actually meeting Target 11, substantial payoffs are already evident from the efforts of the United Nations and its research partners to quantify the urban component of national poverty.

The third transformation is the result of sweeping changes underway in the nature of governance in developing countries. We refer to the phenomenon of decentralization, whereby national governments are transferring to lower-level governments many political, fiscal, and administrative responsibilities. Across the developing world, new local governmental forms and units are proliferating at an astonishing rate (Chapter 9, Panel on Urban Population Dynamics, 2003). Of course, in many countries health services are still being delivered through vertically organized national ministries of health, much as they have been for decades. But in many others, the decentralization of health services is being actively contemplated and in some it is already well underway.

Decentralization is often welcomed, but it implies that for some time to come, health programs will be overseen by new units of municipal, state, and regional

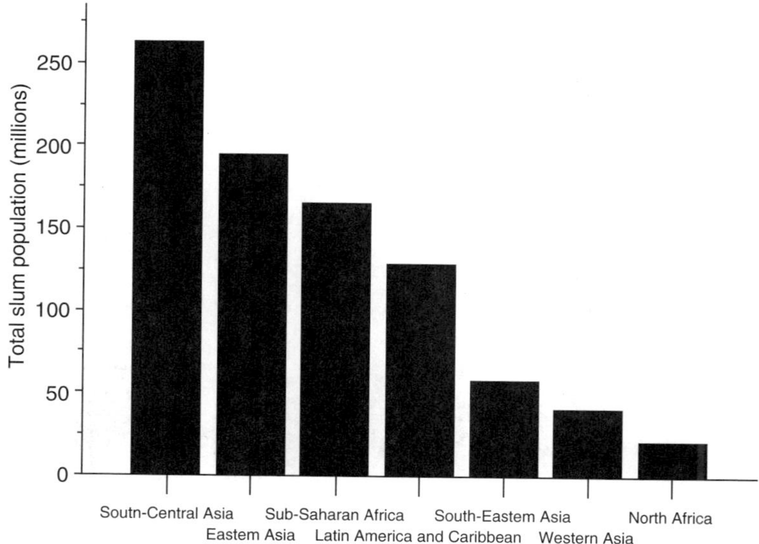

Figure 3. Total Populations Living in Slums, by Region of the Developing World (*Source*: UN-Habitat [2003a]).

governments with little-to-no prior experience in health. Local authorities will need much more by way of spatially disaggregated data to understand the health needs of their constituents, and ways will have to be found for local governments to pass information back to the national level to guide the allocation of national health budgets. One benefit of decentralization may be expected: As it proceeds, the shift of responsibilities to the local level may at last force recognition of the health inequities that exist within cities.

3.0. LOOKING BENEATH THE URBAN AVERAGES

On average, as the Panel on Urban Population Dynamics (2003) has shown, city populations in developing countries exhibit lower levels of child mortality than are found in rural populations, and similar urban–rural differences are evident across a range of health indicators. But urban averages can obscure striking within-city differentials in health—the urban poor often face health risks that are nearly as bad as those seen in the countryside, and sometimes the risks are decidedly worse. Figure 4 illustrates this. In the slums of Nairobi, rates of child mortality substantially exceed those found elsewhere in the city; they are high enough even to exceed rural Kenyan mortality. If urban populations do have an advantage in health relative to rural populations, then it seems that this advantage must be very unequally shared.

The Nairobi example suggests that the spatial concentration of poverty may well exact health penalties beyond those of household poverty alone. As Chapter 17 will discuss, however, not enough research has been conducted in the cities of developing countries to identify with any confidence the health implications of concentrated poverty and neighborhood disadvantage. Moreover, there is a growing

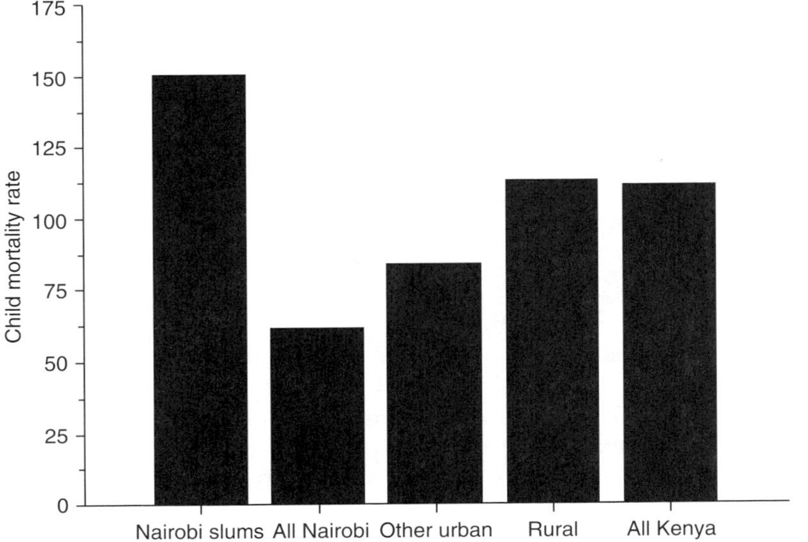

Figure 4. Comparison of Child Mortality Rates in the Nairobi Slums Sample with Rates for Nairobi, Other Cities, Rural Areas, and Kenya (*Source*: African Population and Health Research Center [2002]).

awareness that the term "slum" is itself far from an adequate description of the social and economic heterogeneity that marks the neighborhoods of many urban poor. Careful scholars have generally taken pains to distinguish the population of the urban poor from the population of slum-dwellers, and they tend to employ the term "slum" only as convenient shorthand (UN-Habitat, 2003a). Still, the continuing shortage of rigorous quantitative research on neighborhood heterogeneity is remarkable in view of the emphasis on slums seen in so much of the literature.

4.0. A BRIEF PORTRAIT OF URBAN HEALTH

It is difficult to give any comprehensive account of urban health in the developing world that considers the full range of risks facing infants, children, adolescents, prime-age adults, and the elderly. Few developing countries possess reliable vital statistics systems, and much of what is known and statistically generalizable about health must therefore be drawn from sample surveys. Surveys are useful vehicles for the collection of all-cause data on infant and child mortality, to be sure, but they are less helpful in assessing the risks of adult death. Even for children, survey-based data on cause of death are generally of doubtful reliability. Some health morbidities—those with clearly identifiable symptoms—can be effectively investigated through household surveys of adults and children. (Only recently have systematic measurement efforts been mounted across the developing world. The World Health Survey program of the World Health Organization (WHO) has fielded a number of surveys in a wide range of developing countries, but the data from these surveys have not yet appeared in the public domain. The Demographic and Health Surveys, to be described below, are restricted to women of reproductive age and their spouses or partners; hence, they do not gather information on all adults.) Data gathering on other diseases, however, may require that a physical examination accompany the interview or necessitate the taking of blood or tissue samples. For these reasons, broad inferences about mortality levels and the general state of health are possible for many developing countries, but detailed empirical descriptions of causes of death and morbidities are simply not available across the board.

4.1. The Epidemiological Transition

Even given the limits on the available data, certain features of morbidity and mortality are readily discerned. As a rule, infant and child mortality risks in the developing world substantially exceed those of developed countries, and the burden of disease is still dominated by communicable causes, although an increasing burden of non-communicable causes is becoming evident. Mathers, *et al.*, (2004) note that of all deaths under age 5 world-wide, 97% take place in the developing countries, where the leading causes of death include perinatal causes (birth asphyxia, birth trauma, and low birth weight), lower respiratory infections, diarrhoeal disease, malaria, measles, and HIV/AIDS. In those developing countries classified by WHO as having high mortality, the leading causes of death for children and adults are roughly as follows: lower respiratory infections (10% of all deaths), HIV/AIDS (9.6), ischaemic heart disease (9.3), perinatal conditions (6.6), diarrhoeal diseases (5.5), cerebrovascular disease (5.3), malaria (4.4), tuberculosis (3.6), chronic obstructive pulmonary disease (2.8), and measles (2.5), as reported by Mathers, *et al.*, (2004). A mix of communicable and chronic, non-communicable causes is evident in these figures.

The epidemiological transition—the process by which non-communicable and chronic diseases come to supplant communicable diseases in cause-of-death distributions and related health indicators—is occurring unevenly across the developing world, and for some time to come most developing countries will grapple with substantial burdens of communicable disease. Nevertheless, there is a perceptible shift underway in which chronic non-communicable diseases are coming to play an increasingly important role. As the WHO (2003) writes,

> The chronic disease problem is far from being limited to the developed regions of the world. . . . Although human immunodeficiency virus/acquired immunodeficiency syndrome (HIV/AIDS), malaria and tuberculosis, along with other infectious diseases, still predominate in sub-Saharan Africa and will do so for the foreseeable future, 79% of all deaths worldwide that are attributable to chronic diseases are already occurring in developing countries. . . . It has been projected that, by 2020, . . . 71% of deaths due to ischaemic heart disease (IHD), 75% of deaths due to stroke, and 70% of deaths due to diabetes will occur in developing countries. . . . Indeed, cardiovascular diseases are even now more numerous in India and China than in all the economically developed countries in the world put together.

4.2. Urban Burdens of Disease

Unfortunately, the WHO's Global Burden of Disease project does not supply separate rural and urban cause-of-death or morbidity estimates, and evidence on the urban component of the epidemiological transition can be pieced together only for selected countries. Considering mortality together with disabilities, Table 1 shows that for Mexico, the 15 leading causes of disability-adjusted life years (DALYs) lost in rural and urban areas are much the same, although they follow a different rank order. Of the top 5 causes in Mexico's urban areas, three (deaths related to motor

Table 1. Disability-Adjusted Years of Life Lost in Mexico by Cause and Residence (1991 Estimates, Expressed per 1000 Population).

Cause	Rural	Rural rank	Urban	Urban rank	Rural/Urban
Diarrhea	12.0	1	2.8	9	4.28
Pneumonia	9.3	2	3.9	7	2.39
Homicide and violence	9.2	3	7.4	2	1.23
Motor vehicle-related deaths	7.9	4	8.3	1	0.95
Cirrhosis	7.5	5	6.3	4	1.19
Anemia and malnutrition	6.8	6	2.4	11	2.86
Road traffic accidents	5.5	7	6.8	3	0.81
Ischemic heart disease	5.1	8	5.3	6	0.96
Diseases of the digestive system	4.7	9	1.7	15	2.74
Diabetes mellitus	4.1	10	5.7	5	0.72
Brain vascular disease	3.0	11	3.0	8	1.02
Alcoholic dependence	3.0	11	1.9	13	1.56
Accidents (falls)	2.8	13	2.6	10	1.09
Chronic lung disease	2.6	14	1.9	13	1.39
Nephritis	2.2	15	2.2	12	1.01

Source: Lozano, *et al.* (1999, 130).

vehicles, homicide and violence, and cirrhosis) are also found among the top five in rural areas. As this table suggests, urban areas do not necessarily present health profiles that are wholly distinct from those of rural areas. In the next section of this chapter, we will take a closer look at some of the important causes of death and disease in urban areas.

As we have argued, though sample surveys of households are not always effective instruments for gathering information on health morbidities and adult mortality, they do open a window on socioeconomic differentials, allowing further insights into these determinants of health. Intra-urban health inequalities—all too often overlooked by development agencies—are clearly apparent in such household survey data. Using some 90 surveys fielded by the Demographic and Health Surveys program in developing countries, the Panel on Urban Population Dynamics (2003) assembled estimates of all-cause infant mortality for the urban poor, other urban households, and all rural households. (See Chapter 17 of the current volume for a discussion of how the authors of this report arrived at an urban poverty classification.) These estimates are summarized in Table 2. As can be seen, the effects of poverty are substantial, indicating that the urban poor face mortality risks that are significantly greater than those facing other urban residents. The estimates shown here place poor urban infants at a point midway in the risk spectrum between the urban non-poor and rural infants. In the 87 surveys for which it was possible to examine the difference in mortality risks between the urban poor and rural children, the risks facing the urban poor were found to be significantly lower in 57 surveys. In 25 of the surveys, however, the urban poor were estimated to face significantly higher mortality risks than rural children. Hence, even the generalization that urban infant mortality is lower than rural needs to be qualified; much depends on whether the urban poor are separated out in urban–rural comparisons.

A similar analysis of children's height for age—an often-used measure summarizing nutrition and disease history—is shown in Table 3 for children in the age range 3–36 months. (The table entries are *Z*-scores, with a value of -100 indicating that a child is one standard deviation shorter, given its age and sex, than the median of an international reference population.) The urban poor are again seen to exhibit worse health than other urban children. When the height of poor urban children was compared with that of rural children, however in almost all surveys (60 of the 67 studied) the poor urban children were found to be significantly taller for their age than were rural children. For this indicator of health, therefore, evidence of urban advantage persists even among the urban poor.

Table 2. Infant Mortality Estimates for Urban Poor, Urban Nonpoor, and Rural, by Region.

DHS surveys in region	Rural	Urban poor	Urban nonpoor
North Africa	0.081	0.060	0.043
Sub-Saharan Africa	0.103	0.089	0.074
Southeast Asia	0.059	0.053	0.027
South, Central, West Asia	0.074	0.069	0.049
Latin America	0.069	0.062	0.039
Total	0.086	0.075	0.056

Source: Panel on Urban Population Dynamics (2003).

Table 3. Height for Age *Z*-scores among Children 3–36 Months of Age, by Residence and Poverty Status.

DHS Surveys in Region	All rural	Urban poor	Urban nonpoor
North Africa	–155.00	–122.35	–86.53
Sub-Saharan Africa	–184.60	–153.64	–125.86
Southeast Asia	–139.01	–106.46	–48.18
South, Central, West Asia	–176.78	–157.95	–120.31
Latin America	–157.09	–130.28	–80.61
Total	–173.51	–145.43	–109.37

Source: Panel on Urban Population Dynamics (2003).

To be sure, these height-for-age estimates refer to all poor urban children, and an analysis of children living in slums and communities of concentrated disadvantage (not carried out by the authors of the 2003 report) might have proven illuminating. (Chapter 17 of this volume presents recent evidence on the health implications of concentrated poverty.) Nor does Table 3 exhaust the possibilities for analyses of poverty in connection with children's age, height, and weight: WHO (2003) emphasizes the need to examine the incidence of over-weight and obesity among urban children in developing countries, with special attention to the implications of poor diet and physical inactivity. (Unfortunately, the age range of children on whom weight and height data are gathered has not generally extended to the late childhood and adolescent ages in the Demographic and Health Surveys program.)

4.3. The Service Environment

The differences between the urban poor and other urban residents evident in these tables arise from many factors, but one important factor is that private providers dominate much of the urban health care system in poor countries. Fee-for-service arrangements are characteristic of urban health care in these countries, whereas rural services are often ostensibly provided free of money cost (or made available for nominal fees) at public healthposts and clinics. (Of course, whatever the regulations may suggest, rural clients may also need to pay significant fees or make side-payments to providers to secure effective access to health care.) In the more monetized urban economy, those among the urban poor who lack sufficient income can find themselves unable to gain access to the modern urban system of hospitals, clinics, and well-trained providers. They may then seek care in other tiers of the urban system, where ill-trained providers make drugs and diagnoses available for lesser fees, and may also pursue traditional practitioners, who can adjust the level and type of payment to the needs of their poor clients. Privatized care is likely to become even more prominent on the urban scene as government health services are decentralized and local governments make arrangements for service provision with a range of private providers.

The money costs of health care clearly affect the urban poor, but as is commonly observed, they are also driven away from the modern health system by the indifference or abuse that they experience at the hands of formal sector health workers. A study of urban Zimbabwe describes the nature of interactions between nurses and women from the community (Bassett, *et al.*, 1997),

> To community women, the expectation of abrupt or rude treatment was the main complaint about the health services. Community complaints were voiced most strongly in the urban areas, where accusations of patient neglect and even abuse suggested a heightened hostility between the clinic and community in the urban setting. Several explanations for nurse behavior were put forward, chief among them was elitism . . . it is in urban areas that class differentiation is most advanced. [The perspective of nurses differed. For them] overwork and low pay promote the adoption of the attitude of an industrial worker—to do what is required and no more. Most nurses work more than one job, not to get rich but to survive.

A related factor (see Panel on Urban Population Dynamics (2003) for discussion) is that much like rural healthposts, urban clinics and hospitals can be afflicted with shortages of drugs and supplies as well as staff absenteeism. Inconvenient hours of operation, the time and money costs of transport, overcrowding of facilities, and long waits for care all present disincentives for the urban poor. In sum, both money costs and the inadequate quality of health care can be expected to discourage the urban poor.

5.0. URBAN HEALTH RISKS AND RISK FACTORS

In keeping with this chapter's focus on social epidemiology, in what follows we highlight health risks for which this perspective might prove especially helpful. As is well known, social epidemiology conceives of several levels or structures of "communicability," including: the air-, water-, and food-borne transmission mechanisms featured in conventional epidemiology; the spread of disease through sexual contacts and sexual networks as well as networks of injectable-drug users; and the beneficial diffusion of health-related information that takes place through a great range of personal social networks, local community and health institutions, and the public health bureaucracy. Less direct social mechanisms have also been identified in the recent literature, with perceived socioeconomic injustices and inequities recognized as factors that might erode individual senses of efficacy and thus discourage health-seeking behavior. Likewise, the concept of collective efficacy—the perceived power of local organizations to effect change—figures prominently in recent social epidemiological thinking. Urban social interaction is something of a common thread in all this, summarizing as it does the many processes by which diverse individuals come into contact, either directly or indirectly through the groups in which they participate, in ways that affect health.

In what follows, we offer a series of remarks on specific features of urban health that warrant closer study, roughly ordering the discussion to proceed from the health issues that are recognized in "conventional" epidemiological perspectives on infectious and communicable disease to those health concerns with a more prominent social component. More detailed discussion can be found in Panel on Urban Population Dynamics (2003), which includes extensive references to other urban health reviews.

5.1. Environmental Threats to Health

As the founders of modern epidemiology well knew, the spatial proximity of city-dwellers, and their dependence on common resources, puts them at risk of several sorts of communicable disease. Although many cities in today's developing world have benefited from the investments in public health infrastructure needed to safeguard the water supply and assure sanitary disposal of waste, these protections have often been only partially extended across and even within cities, leaving substantial numbers of city-dwellers to face risks not unlike those of the nineteenth century. The risks are thought to be especially great in those slum populations where social and economic disadvantages are concentrated.

The inadequacies of water supply and sanitation in developing-country cities are documented in two recent authoritative reviews carried out by UN-Habitat (UN-Habitat, 2003a; 2003b). In its own examination of data from the Demographic and Health Surveys, the Panel on Urban Population Dynamics (2003) showed that household poverty is closely associated with access to piped drinking water and adequate sanitation. Table 4 presents some of this study's findings, comparing poor urban households with other urban households and with households living in rural areas. As can be seen in the table, the urban poor are markedly ill-served by comparison with other urban households, although they generally enjoy better access to services than do rural-dwellers.

5.2. Tuberculosis

The development of the germ theory of disease in the late nineteenth century eventually supplied confirmation of what many public health experts of the time had suspected: the proximity of urban residents places them at risk of contracting air-borne and related diseases. Tuberculosis was then a major cause of death, and even today it is among the leading causes of death among adults in developing countries, killing an estimated 3 million people in 1995 (Boerma, *et al.*, 1999). The interactions between HIV/AIDS and tuberculosis, and the spread of multi-drug-resistant strains

Table 4. Percentages of Poor Urban Households with Access to Services, Compared with Rural Households and the Urban Non-Poor.

DHS Countries in Region		Piped water on premises	Water in neighborhood	Time to water[a]	Flush toilet	Pit toilet
North Africa	Rural	41.6	37.3	33.4	41.3	17.5
	Urban poor	67.3	27.8	23.1	83.7	8.5
	Urban non-poor	90.8	7.8	22.8	96.3	2.6
Sub-Saharan Africa	Rural	7.8	55.7	29.4	1.1	47.6
	Urban poor	26.9	61.6	17.5	13.0	65.9
	Urban non-poor	47.6	45.8	16.9	27.4	67.2
Southeast Asia	Rural	18.6	53.7	13.1	55.5	24.3
	Urban poor	34.0	53.7	9.8	61.8	22.9
	Urban non-poor	55.8	40.1	10.1	89.0	9.4
South, Central, West Asia	Rural	28.1	53.6	26.4	4.3	55.4
	Urban poor	58.0	36.3	20.4	39.8	34.1
	Urban non-poor	80.2	17.7	19.9	64.0	23.2
Latin America	Rural	31.4	36.4	19.9	12.6	44.0
	Urban poor	58.7	35.2	18.8	33.6	47.0
	Urban non-poor	72.7	24.9	18.4	63.7	31.6
TOTAL	Rural	18.5	50.7	26.5	7.5	46.6
	Urban poor	41.5	49.4	18.1	28.3	51.7
	Urban non-poor	61.5	34.0	17.6	48.4	46.5

Source: Panel on Urban Population Dynamics (2003).

of tuberculosis, have generated fears of a global resurgence of this disease. As in the nineteenth century, urban crowding increases the risk of contracting tuberculosis (van Rie, *et al.*, 1999), and high-density low-income urban communities may face elevated levels of risk.

The notion of collective efficacy, which figures so prominently in discussions of social epidemiology, are pertinent here. In a study of tuberculosis in urban Ethiopia, Sagbakken, *et al.*, (2003) have shown how the local social resources of urban communities (organized in "TB clubs") can be marshalled to reduce the stigma associated with the disease and encourage patients to adhere to the demanding short-course regimen of treatment. As with the malaria program in Burkina Faso to be described below, this urban intervention was informed by earlier program efforts that were set in the rural areas of Ethiopia (Demissie, *et al.*, 2003). Similar interventions have been fielded in urban India, as described by Barua and Singh (2003), using community health volunteers to identify local residents with symptoms of tuberculosis and refer them to hospitals for diagnosis; local health workers attached to the hospitals then provide follow-up care and lend support during treatment. A still more elaborate system of care, involving multiple urban community and health service associations in Lima, Peru, is described in Shin, *et al.*, (2004).

5.3. Indoor and Outdoor Air Pollution

Among other air-borne threats to urban health, the risks presented by indoor air pollution are being increasingly recognized. Recent estimates suggest that world-wide, more than 2 billion people rely on solid fuels, traditional stoves, and open fires for their cooking, lighting, and heating needs (Larson and Rosen, 2002). These fuels generate hazardous pollutants—including suspended particulate matter, carbon monoxide, nitrogen dioxide, and other harmful gases—that are believed to substantially raise the risks of acute respiratory infections (ARI) and chronic obstructive pulmonary disorders. Such fuels are often used by the urban poor, who must cook in enclosed or inadequately ventilated spaces. The health burdens associated with indoor air pollution are likely to fall heavily upon women, who spend much of their time cooking and tending fires, and also afflict the children who accompany them.

The Latin American literature is especially rich in scientific analyses of outdoor urban air pollution and its effects on respiratory illness via the intake of airborne particulates and other pollutants emitted by industry and vehicles. Ribeiro and Alves Cardoso (2003) provide a thorough review of such studies for São Paulo; for Mexico City, Santos-Burgoa and Riojas-Rodríguez (2000) have assembled and reviewed a great range of studies. The literature presents a number of studies in which children and the elderly are the subjects of interest.

5.4. Urban Malaria

Although malaria has often been regarded as problem afflicting rural populations, and rural rates of transmission are known to be markedly higher than urban rates, there is clear evidence that malaria vectors have adapted to urban conditions in sub-Saharan Africa (Modiano, *et al.*, 1999) and some evidence suggestive of urban risks has emerged for parts of Asia as well. (Hay, *et al.*, [2004] present a global overview of changes over time in the spatial range of malaria.) As Hay, *et al.*, (2004) argue, urban population growth in Southeast Asia, as well as sub-Saharan Africa, may be contributing substantially to the global burden of malaria morbidity.

Keiser, *et al.*, (2004) note that although the higher-income areas of sub-Saharan African cities generally present few sites where mosquitos can breed, in the lower-income areas breeding sites are provided by the presence of small open bodies of water, nearby swamps and marshes and water standing in ditches, canals, and construction pits; certain urban agriculture practices also supply breeding sites. This paper contains extensive references to the urban malaria literature for sub-Saharan Africa.

These authors calculate that in urban sub-Saharan Africa, some 200 million city dwellers face appreciable risks of malaria, and they estimate that 25–100 million clinical episodes of the disease occur annually in the region's cities and towns. Indirect estimates suggest wide variations in prevalence by site, even within small geographic areas, with higher prevalence in the suburbs and city peripheries (especially when these are adjacent to wetlands) than in city centers. For example, a detailed, time-series study of Dar es Salaam, Tanzania (Caldas de Castro, *et al.*, 2004), which relies on an unusual combination of high-resolution aerial photography and extensive ground validation, depicts the micro-zones of high malaria risk within this country. In 1994, Guiguemde and colleagues studied the impact of malarial fevers on family health expenditures in Bobo-Diouslasso, a secondary city of Burkina Faso, and found that prevention efforts (via mosquito coils, sprays, and purchase of insecticide-treated bednets) and treatment absorb about 5% of family money income over the six-month malarial transmission season.

Pictet, *et al.*, (2004) describe a recent urban intervention program mounted in Ouagadougou, Burkina Faso's capital, which aimed to make use of the social resources of urban communities to provide care in uncomplicated cases of child malaria. Inspired by a rural program that yielded good results, this urban program enlisted local community residents ("health agents"), gave them training in the recognition of malarial symptoms in young children, and supplied the agents with packets of chloroquine and paracetamol in age-appropriate doses. (In Ouagadougou, a high fraction of malaria cases still respond to chloroquine, although the parasite's resistance is evidently growing.) In cases of childhood fevers, it has been common practice for residents of the Ouagadougou slums to buy chloroquine tablets (or drugs that give the appearance of being similar) in local markets and use these to medicate their ill children. Preliminary research showed, however, that the residents had little knowledge of the dosages or lengths of treatment appropriate for their children. Thus, when judged against the medication practices that were already widely prevalent in these communities, the program intervention was expected to improve the standard of malaria care.

When pilot-tested in two communities in Ouagadougou, the malaria intervention showed the expected positive results in the lower-income community, which was located on the fringes of the city and somewhat isolated from sources of modern health care. Of the two study communities, this was the more homogeneous in social and economic terms, and it exhibited evidence of greater "neighborliness" and other forms of social interaction through which information about the intervention might have circulated. In the other pilot community, however, easier access was already available to modern health clinics and reputable pharmacies, and more residents could afford to pay for their own care. In this middle-income site it proved difficult to sustain community interest in the intervention.

In the Ouagadougou project, the local health agents expressed concern about how to establish their legitimacy as informal health providers and thus differentiate themselves from the itinerant drug sellers who roam through many neighborhoods proffering cures for fevers and other ailments. This concern, we suspect, will often surface in attempts to exploit the informal social resources of urban communities. The social trust that can sometimes be taken as a given in small rural villages may need to be established more explicitly—perhaps through public endorsements by local community leaders—in urban settings.

5.5. HIV/AIDS

An enormous literature is now available on the social epidemiology of HIV/AIDS in both developing and developed countries. Researchers soon recognized the social components implicated in the spread of the virus, and emphasized the importance of social and sexual networks in shaping its transmission dynamics (Morris, 1993). Friedman and Aral (2001) give a succinct and valuable introduction to the use of social network concepts and methods in the study of HIV/AIDS, other sexually-transmitted diseases, and their linkages to networks of drug users and similarly high-risk behavioral groups. Where urban social resources are concerned—the matrix of formal organizations and informal associations that are often described as urban social capital—some insights are to be found in a recent World Bank report (World Bank, 2003), which documents how local urban governments can marshal resources needed to fight HIV/AIDS in their communities.

Despite the quantities of research underway on HIV/AIDS, much remains to be learned about its social components. Indeed, although HIV/AIDS is commonly thought to be more prevalent in urban than rural areas, the scientific basis for this belief is surprisingly thin (UNAIDS, 2004). As noted by UNAIDS, in only a few developing countries are community-based studies of prevalence available that can quantify the urban–rural differences. (Country profiles are available at http://www.census.gov/ipc/www/hivaidsn.html, but these profiles are worked up from the reports of selected clinics and various sentinel sites, which do not necessarily yield statistically representative portraits for urban or rural populations.)

Figure 5 presents recent findings from several nationally representative community-based studies in which prevalence is estimated from blood samples taken in connection with household-level demographic surveys. In these three cases—Mali, Kenya, and Zambia—urban prevalence rates are clearly much higher than rural rates. Where HIV/AIDS is concerned, therefore, one sees little evidence of the "urban advantage" expected in other domains of health, and as the epidemic proceeds in southern Africa, and begins to affect large populations in India and China, an erosion of urban health advantages in these countries may also take place. However, circular and urban-to-rural migration is a factor that is contributing to the spread of disease in rural areas (UNAIDS, 2004), and many observers foresee an upcoming era of rising rural incidence and prevalence.

5.6. Reproductive Health

Maternal mortality risks offer a revealing entry-point for the study of the broader field of urban reproductive health. Because it is difficult to predict whether life-threatening problems will emerge in the course of a woman's pregnancy, delivery, and the aftermath, maternal mortality risks depend crucially upon having fast access to emergency care. It might be thought that cities, which offer many more transport options than do rural areas, would exhibit much lower levels of maternal

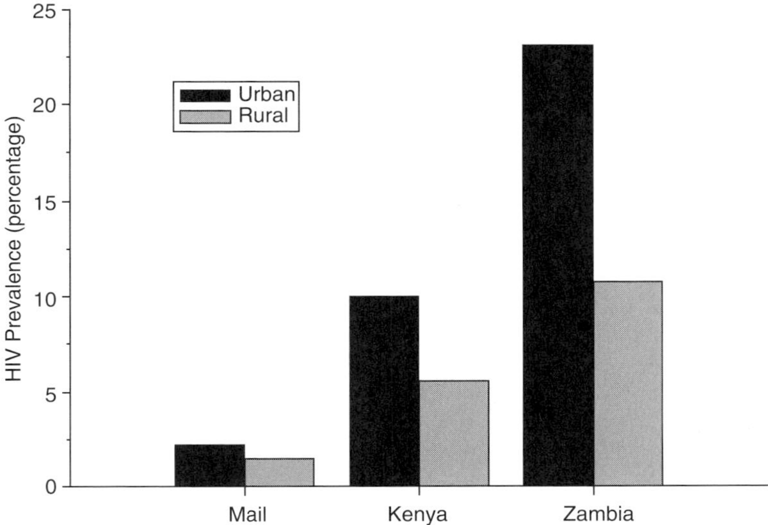

Figure 5. Estimates of Urban and Rural Prevalence of HIV from the Demographic and Health Surveys: Mali, 2001; Kenya, 2003; and Zambia, 2001–2002 (*Sources*: Mali Ministère de la Santé [2002]; Kenya Central Bureau of Statistics [2003]; Zambia Central Statistical Office [2003]).

mortality. The cases in which the expected urban advantage does not emerge are therefore especially revealing about the circumstances of the urban poor.

Fikree, *et al.*, (1997) compared maternal mortality rates in the low-income communities of Karachi with rates in six rural districts elsewhere in Pakistan. Estimates of maternal mortality ratios (MMRs), together with their confidence bands, are shown in Figure 6. Although the MMR estimate for Karachi is the lowest among all sites, the rural estimates are significantly higher than Karachi's only for the remote districts of Loralai and Khuzdar. It appears that Karachi's poor suffer from maternal health disadvantages not unlike those that afflict Pakistan's rural dwellers.

Why did the urban health advantage not prove greater in this case? In the poor communities of Karachi, some 68% of births are delivered at home and 59 % are attended by traditional birth attendants (TBAs). Yet rural women are even more likely to deliver at home and to have family members or TBAs in attendance. Another study of Karachi slums (Fikree, *et al.*, 1994) identifies the core of the problem: When acute pregnancy and delivery complications arise in these communities, there can be critical delays in locating male decision makers and obtaining their consent to hospital care. It has not been customary in these communities for husbands or other men to be present at the time of childbirth. Delays in initiating the search for care are compounded by the tendency for poor Karachi families to pursue local care first, going from place to place in the neighborhood before making an effort to reach the modern health facilities located outside the neighborhood. Fikree, *et al.*, (2004) illustrates these care-seeking patterns in a study of postpartum morbidities in the Karachi slums.

Mayank, *et al.* (2001), who studied poor urban women in a New Delhi slum, find that women and their families possess strikingly little information about the risks of pregnancy and birth, and on their part, local antenatal clinics do little to fill

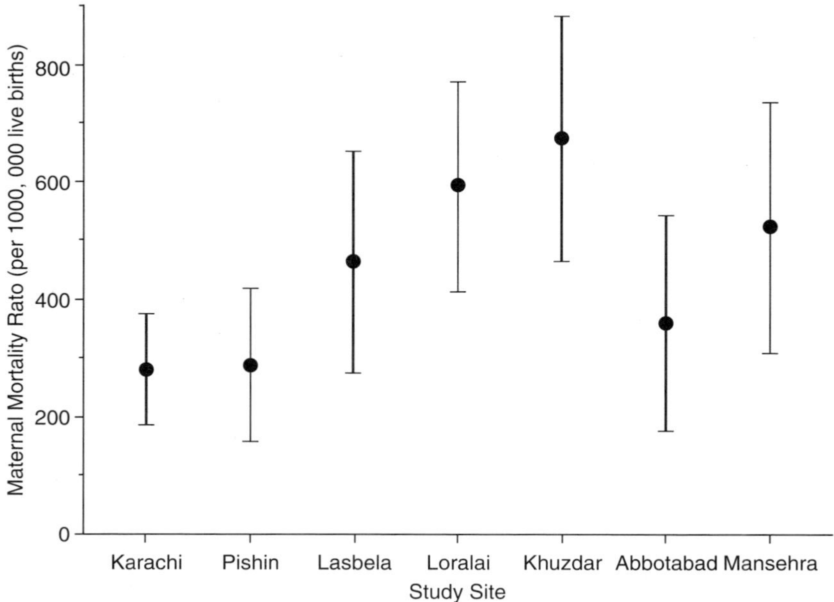

Figure 6. Maternal Mortality Ratios in Karachi and Six Rural Sites (*Source*: Fikree, *et al.* [1997]).

the gap. The maternal mortality rate in this urban sample was estimated at 645 deaths per 100,000, a rate not much different from that prevailing in rural India. A number of pregnant women suffered from potentially serious ailments—over two-thirds were clinically diagnosed as anemic, and 12% were found to be seriously anemic. Yet relatively few understood that high fevers and swelling of the face, hands, or feet might be symptoms of conditions that could endanger their pregnancy. In this community, antenatal care is provided free of charge in the local health clinic, and the vast majority of women made use of this care. However, the quality of the care the women received is grossly inadequate; for example, fewer than 10% of women attending the local clinic were given any advice about the danger signs of pregnancy.

5.7. Obesity and Related Chronic Diseases

Diabetes, obesity, cardiovascular disease, cancers, and coronary heart disease are sometimes termed chronic "lifestyle" diseases, in the sense that they are at least partly attributable to behavior. Undernutrition, food insecurity, dietary excess, and obesity often coexist in urban populations. In many developing countries, substantial proportions of the population are either underweight or overweight, with the increase in the overweight percentage being a recent and worrisome development. Obesity tends to appear first among the affluent and then among low-income groups, including young children and teenagers. Its main causes include the adoption of lipid-rich diets and (more importantly) the reduction in physical activity that often accompanies city life. Malnutrition during fetal development and early childhood are predisposing factors for later obesity.

Popkin (1999) shows that more urbanized developing countries exhibit higher per capita consumption of sweeteners and fats, noting that "a shift from 25% to 75%

urban population in very low income countries is associated with an increase of approximately four percentage points of total energy from fat and an additional 12 percentage points of energy from sweeteners." In several of the developing countries he studies, obesity is markedly higher in urban areas than in rural. Monteiro, *et al.*, (2000) find that in urban Brazil, it is the city residents with more education who are less likely to be overweight. Much the same pattern has been observed in South Africa (South African Department of Health, 1998). As a result of these and other studies, there is an emerging consensus that obesity is a significant problem facing the urban poor (WHO, 2003; Du, *et al.*, 2004), and is increasingly evident among urban children.

5.8. Accidents, Violence, and Injuries

Drawing on a DALYs analysis, Zwi, *et al.*, (1996) draw attention to the effects of injuries on health and well-being:

> [W]orld-wide, intentional injuries (suicide, homicide and war) account for almost the same number of DALYs lost as either sexually transmitted diseases and human immunodeficiency virus (HIV) infection combined, or tuberculosis. Unintentional injuries cause as many DALYs lost as diarrhea, and more than those lost from cardiovascular disease, malignant neoplasm, or vaccine-preventable childhood infections. In developing regions of the world, in 1990, injuries in males aged 15-44 years led to 55 million DALYs lost, over one-third of those lost from all causes in this sex and age group.

Bartlett (2002) provides a discussion of other injuries affecting children and adults, drawing on hospital and community-based studies. He gives particular attention to how poverty and gender affect these risks, and how time pressures on urban parents limit the effort they can devote to closely supervising their children.

Traffic accidents—a category that includes pedestrian injuries—are a major but often overlooked cause of urban death and injury (Mock, *et al.*, 1999; Kayombo, 1995; Byarugaba and Kielkowski, 1994). Urban residents are often thought to face higher risks of accident than rural residents, but higher rural accident rates have sometimes been recorded (see Table 1 and Odero, 1995; Odero, *et al.*, 1997; Mock, *et al.*, 1999). One estimate suggests that traffic accidents account for a significant percentage of all trauma-related hospital admissions (Odero, *et al.*, 1997). Híjar, *et al.*, (2003) conducted a detailed analysis of pedestrian injuries over a three-year period in Mexico City, where pedestrian death rates are estimated at three times those of Los Angeles. Using a mix of spatially-coded quantitative data and qualitative methods, these authors developed portraits of drivers and victims that underscore the importance of several mutually reinforcing risk factors: poverty, a lack of understanding of how drivers are apt to react, inattention by drivers and pedestrians to risky conditions, insufficient public investment in traffic lights, and dangerous mixes of industrial, commercial, and private traffic.

As the quotation above indicates, violence is one of the major causes of injuries in poor countries. Much of the empirical work on violence has been carried out in Latin America and the Caribbean. This is for good reason: Latin America has the world's highest burden of homicides, which occur at a rate of 7.7 per 1000 population, more than twice the world average of 3.5 per 1000. Approximately 30% of all homicide victims in Latin America are adolescents, and young men are the most affected group (as cited in Grant, 1999).

Violent crime is particularly prevalent in Latin America's large cities, and in these cities, it disproportionately affects men living in low-income neighborhoods (Barata, *et al.*, 1998; Grant, 1999). Data collected between 1991 and 1993 in São Paulo suggested that men aged 15–24 in low-income areas were more than 5 times likelier to fall victim to homicide than were men of the same age in higher-income areas (Soares, *et al.*, cited in Grant, 1999).

Gender roles and relations put men and women at risk of different types of violence. Higher rates of homicide are reported for men, but rape and domestic violence rates are higher for women. Heise, *et al.*, (1994) reviewed community-based data for eight urban areas from different regions of the developing world and found that mental and physical abuse of women by their partners was common, with damaging consequences for women's physical and psychological well-being.

5.9. Mental Health

The World Health Organization has been placing increasing emphasis on mental health, underscoring its importance to the burden of disease in developing as well as developed countries (WHO, 1996; 2001). Community-based studies of mental health in developing countries suggest that 12% to 51% of urban adults suffer from some form of depression (see 16 studies reviewed by Blue, 1999). Although these studies employ a range of samples, definitions, and instruments, their conclusions underline the importance of mental ill-health in the urban spectrum of disease. Day-to-day life in poor communities can subject their residents to sustained, chronic stress. Poor urban residents often show great resilience and creativity in meeting such challenges. Nevertheless, they can be beaten down by the demands of poverty and wearied by the constant need to improvise new coping strategies.

Anxiety and depression are typically found to be more prevalent among urban women than men and are believed to be more prevalent in poor than in nonpoor urban neighborhoods (Almeida-Filho, *et al.*, 2004). In a study of Mumbai, Parkar, *et al.*, (2003) give an evocative account of the stresses that affect men and women in a slum community just north of the city. Men in this community are deeply frustrated by the lack of work, and seeing few prospects of improvement, many of them fall into a pattern whereby idleness is mixed with helplessness and hostility. This has increased the burdens on women, especially when their spouses retreat into alcoholism or lash out in episodes of domestic violence, infidelity, and deliberate humiliation.

For both women and men, the stresses of slum life may well undermine the physiological systems that sustain health. Boardman (2004) explains the mechanism, which has to do with "allostatic load," a phrase referring to the debilitating effects stemming from the release of cortisol and other hormones in stressful situations. Those suffering from stress may be able to call upon various forms of emotional support from family and neighbors, as well as material support in the form of goods, services, and information. Such social resources can help in coping with stress and mitigating its damage (Thoits, 1995; Kawachi and Berkman, 2001). Even routine interactions with neighbors may provide a sense of coherence and consistency (Boardman, 2004). In empirical analyses, differences in social support—the degree to which basic social needs are gratified through interaction with others—have been estimated to account for 5% to 10% of the variance in levels of mental ill-health (of all types) in different areas (Harpham, 1994; Committee to Study Female Morbidity and Mortality in Sub-Saharan Africa, 1996; Aidoo and Harpham, 2001; Harpham and Blue, 1995).

In recent research, Harpham, *et al.*, (2004) make use of the WHO's self-reporting questionnaire—a bank of 20 items designed to detect depression and anxiety—to study the mental health of adolescents in Cali, Colombia. In this city, girls were found to be three times more likely than boys to exhibit signs of ill-health; and multivariate analyses showed that being female, having no schooling or incomplete primary (relative to secondary) are associated with greater likelihood of illness, as are reported family violence, being a victim of violence, and perceptions that violence affects the community. Despite expectations, however, measures of trust and other cognitive expressions of social capital did not emerge as significant factors with controls for violence in place.

Evidently, then, the posited connections between social capital and mental health need to be confirmed with attention to violence and social disorder (Boardman, 2004). In low-income urban communities, social capital has been found to weaken as households' ability to cope decreases and community trust breaks down, and to be severely eroded by various forms of violence (Moser and McIlwaine, 1999). Strong social capital has been linked to reduced mortality at the state level in the United States (National Research Council, 2000). However, most of the available research on mental health and social support is cross-sectional, leaving open the possibility that mental illness itself reduces social support and that the positive relationship between social support and mental health may have been somewhat overstated (Kawachi and Berkman, 2001).

6.0. CONCLUSION

Although our sketch of urban health in developing countries cannot substitute for the full treatment that the issues deserve, we hope that at least it may at least suggest the unexploited potential of social epidemiological research to illuminate urban health risks and behavior in these countries. The compartmentalization of health research to which we referred at the outset is both unfortunate and unnecessary. As we will discuss further in Chapter 17, there is no reason not to apply concepts such as neighborhood effects, personal and collective efficacy, and health externalities in studies of the cities of poor countries, and the research methods developed with Western cities in mind may well be put to good use in African, Asian, and Latin American cities. The spectrum of disease and health behavior evident in developing-country urban populations differs in many ways from what is seen in high-income countries, of course, but there are also broad similarities that should invite comparison. Ample material exists to enliven a global conversation on urban health research.

REFERENCES

African Population and Health Research Center. (2002). *Population and Health Dynamics in Nairobi's Informal Settlements: Report of the Nairobi Cross-Sectional Slums Survey (NCSS) 2000.* African Population and Health Research Center, Nairobi.

Aidoo, M., and Harpham, T. (2001). The explanatory models of mental health amongst low-income women and health care practitioners in Lusaka, Zambia. *Health Policy and Planning* 16(2):206–213.

Almeida-Filho, N., Lessa, I., Magalhães, L., Araújo, M. J., Acquino, E., James, S. A., and Kawachi, I. (2004). Social inequality and depressive disorders in Bahia, Brazil: Interactions of gender, ethnicity, and social class. *Soc. Sci. Med.* 59(7):1339–1353.

Barata, R. B., Ribeiro, M. C., Guedes, M. B., and Moraes, J. C. D. (1998). Intra-urban differentials in death rates from homicide in the city of São Paulo, Brazil, 1988–1994. *Soc. Sci. Med.* 47(1):19–23.

Bartlett, S. N. (2002). The problem of children's injuries in low-income countries: A review. *Health Policy and Planning* 17(1):1–13.

Barua, N., and Singh, S. (2003). Representation for the marginalized—Linking the poor and the health care system. Lessons from case studies in urban India, Draft paper. World Bank, New Delhi.

Bassett, M. T., Bijlmakers, L., and Sanders, D. M. (1997). Professionalism, patient satisfaction and quality of health care: Experience during Zimbabwe's structural adjustment programme. *Soc. Sci. Med.* 45(12):1845–1852.

Blue, I. (1999). Intra-Urban Differentials in Mental Health in São Paulo, Brazil, PhD thesis. South Bank University, London.

Boardman, J. D. (2004). Stress and physical health: The role of neighborhoods as mediating and moderating mechanisms. *Soc. Sci. Med.* 58:2473–2483.

Boerma, J. T., Nunn, A. J., and Whitworth, A. G. (1999). Spread of HIV infection in a rural area of Tanzania. *AIDS.* 13:1233–1240.

Byarugaba, J., and Kielkowski, D. (1994). Reflections on trauma and violence-related deaths in Soweto, July 1990–June 1991. *S. Af. Med. J.* 84(9):610–614.

Caldas de Castro, M., Yamagata, Y., Mtasiwa, D., Tanner, M., Utzinger, J., Keiser, J., and Singer, B. H. (2004). Integrated urban malaria control: A case study in Dar es Salaam, Tanzania, Working paper. Office of Population Research, Princeton University, Princeton, NJ.

Committee to Study Female Morbidity and Mortality in Sub-Saharan Africa. (1996). In: Howson, C.P., Harrison, P.F., Hotra, D., and Law, M. (eds.), *In Her Lifetime: Female Morbidity and Mortality in Sub-Saharan Africa.* National Academy Press, Washington, DC.

Demissie, M., Getahun, H., and Lindtjørn, B. (2003). Community tuberculosis care through `TB clubs' in rural North Ethiopia. *Soc. Sci. Med.* 56(10):2009–2018.

Du, S., Mroz, T. A., Zhai, F., and Popkin, B. M. (2004). Rapid income growth adversely affects diet quality in China—particularly for the poor!. *Soc. Sci. Med.* 59(7):1505–1515.

Fikree, F. F., Gray, R. H., Berendes, H. W., and Karim, M. S. (1994). A community-based nested case-control study of maternal mortality. *International Journal of Gynecology & Obstetrics* 47:247–255.

Fikree, F. F., Midhet, F., Sadruddin, S., and Berendes, H. W. (1997). Maternal mortality in different Pakistani sites: Ratios, clinical causes and determinants. *Acta Obstetricia et Gynecologica Scandinavica* 76:637–645.

Fikree, F. R., Ali, T., Durocher, J. M., and Rahbar, M. H. (2004). Health service utilization for perceived postpartum morbidity among poor women living in Karachi. *Soc. Sci. Med.* 59:681–694.

Frenk, J., Londoño, J. L., Knaul, F., and Lozano, R. (1998). Latin American health systems in transition: A vision for the future. In: Bezold, C., Frenk, J., and McCarthy, S. (eds.), *21st Century Health Care in Latin America and the Caribbean: Prospects for Achieving Health for All.* Institute for Alternative Futures (IAF) and Fundacion Mexicana Para la Salud, Alexandria, VA and Mexico, DF, pp. 109–142.

Friedman, S. R., and Aral, S. (2001). Social networks, risk-potential networks, health, and disease. *J. Urban Health* 78(3):411–418.

Grant, E. (1999). *State of the art of urban health in Latin America, European Commission funded concerted action: 'Health and human settlements in Latin America.'* South Bank University, London.

Guiguemde, T. R., Dao, F., Curtis, V., Traore, A., Sondo, B., Testa, J., and Ouedraogo, J. B. (1994). Household expenditure on malaria prevention and treatment for families in the town of Bobo-Dioulasso, Burkina Faso. *Trans. R. Soc. Trop. Med. Hyg.* 88: 285–287.

Harpham, T. (1994). Urbanization and mental health in developing countries: A research role for social scientists, public health professionals and social psychiatrists. *Soc. Sci. Med.* 39(2):233–245.

Harpham, T., and Blue, I. (eds). (1995). *Urbanization and Mental Health in Developing Countries.* Aldershot, Avebury.

Harpham, T., Grant, E., and Rodriguez, C. (2004). Mental health and social capital in Cali, Colombia. *Soc. Sci. Med.* 58:2267–2277.

Hay, S. I., Guerra, C. A., Tatem, A. J., Noor, A. M., and Snow, R. W. (2004). The global distribution and population at risk of malaria: Past, present, and future. *Lancet Infectious Diseases* 4:327–336.

Heise, L. L., Raikes, A., Watts, C. H., and Zwi, A. B. (1994). Violence against women: A neglected public health issue in less developed countries. *Soc. Sci. Med.* 39(9):1165–1179.

Híjar, M., Trostle, J., and Bronfman, M. (2003). Pedestrian injuries in Mexico: A multi-method approach. *Soc. Sci. Med.* 57(11):2149–2159.

Kawachi, I., and Berkman, L. F. (2001). Social ties and mental health. *J. Urban Health* 78(3):458–467.

Kayombo, E. J. (1995). Motor traffic accidents in Dar es Salaam, *Tropical Geography and Medicine* 47(1): 37–39.

Keiser, J., Utzinger, J., Caldas de Castro, M., Smith, T. A., Tanner, M., and Singer, B. H. (2004). Urbanization in sub-Saharan Africa and implications for malaria control, Working paper. Office of Population Research, Princeton University, Princeton, NJ, and the Swiss Tropical Institute, Switzerland.

Kenya Central Bureau of Statistics., (2003). Kenya Demographic and Health Survey 2003: Preliminary report. Central Bureau of Statistics, Nairobi, Kenya.

Larson, B. A., and Rosen, S. (2002). Understanding household demand for indoor air pollution control in developing countries. *Soc. Sci. Med.* 55:571–584.

Lozano, R., Murray, C., and Frenk, J. (1999). El peso de las enfermedades en Mexico. In: Hill, K., Morelos, J.B., and Wong, R. (eds.), *Las Consecuencias de las Transiciones Demografica y Epidemiological en América Latina*, El Colegio de México, Mexico City.

Mali Ministère de la Santé. (2002). *Enquête Démographique et de Santé Mali 2001.* Ministère de la Santé [Mali] and ORC Macro, Calverton, MD.

Mathers, C. D., Bernanrd, C., Moesgaard Iburg, K., Inoue, M., Ma Fat, D., Shibuya, K., Stein, C., Tomijima, N., and Xu, H. (2004). Global Burden of Disease in 2002: Data sources, methods and results, Global Programme on Evidence for Health Policy Discussion Paper no. 54, World Health Organization, Geneva.

Mayank, S., Bahl, R., Rattan, A., and Bhandari, N. (2001). Prevalence and correlates of morbidity in pregnant women in an urban slum of New Delhi. *Asia-Pacific Population Journal* 16(2):29–45.

Mock, C. N., Abantanga, F., Cummings, P., and Koepsell, T. D. (1999). Incidence and outcome of inquiry in Ghana: A community-based survey. *Bull. World Health Org.* 77(12):955–964.

Modiano, D., Sirima, B., Sawadogo, A., Sanou, I., and Paré, J. (1999). Severe malaria in Burkina Faso: Urban and rural environment. *Parassitologia* 41:251–254.

Monteiro, C. A., Benicio, D. A., Conde, W. L., and Popkin, B. M. (2000). Shifting obesity trends in Brazil, *European Journal of Clinical Nutrition* 54(4):342–346.

Morris, M. (1993). Epidemiology and social networks: Modeling structured diffusion. *Sociol. Methods Res.* 22(1):99–126.

Moser, C. O. N., and McIlwaine, C. (1999). Participatory urban appraisal and its application for research on violence. *Environ. Urban* 11(2):203–226.

National Research Council. (2000). *Beyond Six Billion: Forecasting the World's Population, Panel on Population Projections.* Committee on Population, National Academy Press, Washington, DC.

Odero, W. (1995). Road traffic accidents in Kenya: An epidemiological appraisal, *East Af. Med. J.* 72(5):299–305.

Odero, W., Garner, P., and Zwi, A. (1997). Road traffic injuries in developing countries: A comprehensive review of epidemiological studies. *Tropical Medicine and International Health* 2(5):445–460.

Pan American Health Organization (PAHO) (1996). *Adolescent Programme Health Situation Analysis (Technical health information system mortality database).* PAHO, Washington, DC.

Pan American Health Organization (PAHO). (1998). *Health in the Americas.* 1998 PAHO, Washington, DC.

Panel on Urban Population Dynamics. (2003). *Cities Transformed: Demographic Change and Its Implications in the Developing World.* M. R., Stren, R., Cohen, B., and Reed, H., (eds.). National Academies Press, Washington, DC. Montgomery,

Parkar, S. R., Fernandes, J., and Weiss, M. G. (2003). Contextualizing mental health: Gendered experiences in a Mumbai slum. *Anthropology & Medicine* 10(3):291–308.

Pictet, G., Kouanda, S., Sirima, S., and Pond, R. (2004). Struggling with population heterogeneity in African cities: The urban health and equity puzzle, Paper presented to the 2004 annual meetings of the Population Association of America, Boston, MA.

Popkin, B. M. (1999). Urbanization, lifestyle changes and the nutrition transition. *World Development* 27(11):1905–1916.

Ribeiro, H., and Alves Cardoso, M. R. (2003). Air pollution and children's health in São Paulo (1986–1998). *Soc. Sci. Med.* 57(11):2013–2022.

Sagbakken, M., Bjune, G., Frich, J., and Aseffa, A. (2003). From the user's perspective—A qualitative study of factors influencing patients' adherence to medical treatment in an urban community, Ethiopia, Paper presented at the conference *Urban Poverty and Health in Sub-Saharan Africa*, African Population and Health Research Centre, Nairobi. Faculty of Medicine, University of Oslo, Norway.

Santos-Burgoa, C., and Riojas-Rodríguez, H. (2000). Health and pollution in Mexico City Metropolitan Area: A general overview of air pollution exposure and health studies, Presentation to the Panel on Urban Population Dynamics. U.S. National Research Council, Mexico City.

Shin, S., Furin, J., Bayona, J., Mate, K., Kim, J. Y., and Farmer, P. (2004). Community-based treatment of multidrug-resistant tuberculosis in Lima, Peru: 7 years of experience. *Soc. Sci. Med.* 59(7):1529–1539.

South African Department of Health: 1998, *South African Demographic and Health Survey 1998*, South African Department of Health, Pretoria.

Thoits, P. A. (1995). Stress, coping, and social support processes: Where are we? What next?. *J. Health Soc. Beh.* Extra Issue, 53–79.

United Nations Department of Economic and Social Affairs/Population Division. (2003). World urbanization prospects: the 2003 revision. United Nations; http://www.un.org/esa/population/publications/wup2003/2003WUPHoghlights.pdf

UN-Habitat. (2003a). *The Challenge of Slums: Global Report on Human Settlements 2003.* Earthscan, London.

UN-Habitat (2003b). *Water and Sanitation in the World's Cities: Local Action for Global Goals.* Earthscan, London.

UNAIDS. (2004). *2004 Report on the Global AIDS Epidemic*, UNAIDS, New York.

United Nations: 2002, *World Urbanization Prospects: The 2001 Revision. Data Tables and Highlights*, United Nations. Department of Economic and Social Affairs, Population Division, New York.

van Rie, A., Beyers, N., Gie, R. P., Kunneke, M., Zietsman, L. and Donald, P. R. (1999). Childhood tuberculosis in an urban population in South Africa: Burden and risk factor. *Archives of Disability in Children* 80(5):433–437.

WHO. (1996). *Investing in Health Research and Development: Report of the Ad Hoc Committee on Health Research Relating to Future Intervention Options.* World Health Organization (WHO), Geneva.

WHO. (2001). *The World Health Report 2001. Mental Health: New Understanding, New Hope.* World Health Organization, Geneva.

WHO (2003). Diet, nutrition and the prevention of chronic diseases. Report of a joint WHO/FAO expert consultation, WHO Technical Report Series 916. World Health Organization, Geneva.

World Bank. (2001). *World Development Report 2000/2001: Attacking Poverty.* Oxford University Press, Oxford and New York.

World Bank. (2003). *Local Government Responses to HIV/AIDS: A Handbook.* The World Bank, Washington, DC.

Zambia Central Statistical Office. (2003). *Zambia Demographic and Health Survey 2001–2002.* Central Statistical Office [Zambia], Central Board of Health [Zambia], and ORC Macro, Calverton, MD.

Zwi, A. B., Forjuoh, S., Murugusampillay, S., Odero, W., and Watts, C. (1996). Injuries in developing countries: Policy response needed now. *Trans. R. Soc. Trop. Med. Hyg.* 90(6):593–595.

Chapter 11

Perspectives on the Health of Populations in Nepal

Tej Kumar Karki

1.0. URBAN POPULATION AND HEALTH

Nepal is primarily a rural nation but is rapidly urbanizing. Nepal's average annual growth rate of the urban population is 6.65% compared to the national population growth rate of 2.25 % (Population Census 2001; 2002). At present, there are 58 municipalities, and a total urban population of 3.28 million urban residents or 13.9% of the national population. Should this trend continue, half of the population of Nepal will be living in urban areas by the year 2035 (Asian Development Bank, 2000). About 23% of the total urban population or three fourth of a million people in Nepal are urban poor. It is estimated that this figure will reach 15 million by 2035 (Bryld, 2001).

The present status of urban services such as water supplies and access to electricity is far from satisfactory. Less than half (46%) of the population of Nepal has private water supply connection (Table 1). It is estimated that 33% of the population does not have access to toilet facilities, 20% have no electricity, 80% are not served by waste collection services, 79% do not have telephone connection, and 5% of the population still have to walk half an hour to reach an asphalted road.

The infant mortality rate per 1000 live births in urban areas is 50.1 deaths, mortality rates for children under five years old is 16.7 deaths and child mortality under five per 1000 live births is 65 deaths (Table 2). About 5.37% of the urban population has had chronic illnesses (Adhikari, 1999).

The rapid rate of urbanization during the past two decades has created unprecedented pressure on Kathmandu and a number of cities in the plains (Ministry of Health, 2004). The incapacity to manage these pressures have spurred various environmental and health problems in cities and towns of Nepal.

In the next sections we discuss some of the key determinants of poor health in Nepal's urban areas.

Table 1. Status of Access to Basic Services to the Urban Population of Nepal

Types of services	Percent of population
Without private water supply connection	54
Without access to toilet	33
No waste management	80
No electricity	20
Without private telephone	88
Population walking half an hour to reach a metalled road	5
Illiterate population	63

Source: World Bank, 1999.

Table 2. National Health Determinants of Nepal

Determinants	National	Urban	Rural
Infant Mortality rate/1000 live births	64	50.2	79.3
Child Mortality rate under 5 years of age/1000 live births	91	65.9	111.9
Maternal Mortality rate/100,000	415		
Crude Birth rate/1000	34		
Crude Death Rate/1000	10		
Average life expectancy/years	61.9		

Source: National Planning Commission's Document, 2002, Nepal Demographic and Health Survey 2001.

2.0. CITY ROAD NETWORK, TRANSPORTATION, AND HEALTH

2.1. Inefficiencies in City Road Networks

Growth of cities in Nepal has been up to now, mostly unplanned. One of the repercussions of cities that are not designed is the inadequate intra-city road networks and road width. In the past decades, the traditional walkways in the Kathmandu Valley were widened and renovated into vehicular roads (Japan International Cooperation Agency, 1993) which has taken much planning. This is not an easy task. Urban roads in Nepal are limited by various deficiencies of urban planning. The deficiencies include building material dumping areas in the roads, vehicular parking, hawker display space, periodic market places on streets, and space for public interaction which block the improvement of roads and the use of roads.

In addition, mixed movement of vehicles (slow and fast) on the road slows all vehicular movement; the average speed of most of the vehicles in Kathmandu Valley was 35–50 kilometers per hour (Adhikari, 1999). The rapid growth of the number of vehicles in the valley further compounds the problem, increasing at a rate of 16% per year (Nepal Health Research, 2004). Kathmandu Valley had 224,098 registered vehicles and a total road network of only 1339 kilometers in 2003.

2.2. Pollution

One obvious outcome of this phenomenon (growth of vehicles, inadequate road network and slow vehicular movement) is the rapid increase in vehicular emission. The vehicles contributed about 31 thousand tons of pollutants in 1996. Carbon monoxide constituted about 60% of the total vehicular emission (Adhikari, 1998). It was found that the dust particles in the air of Kathmandu valley was high due to increased traffic, extension of dirt road and scattered garbage disposal and building materials (Environmental Management Action Group, 1992). The existence of one third of the air polluting industries of the nation being located in Kathmandu Valley makes an additional contribution to the air pollution of the region (Industrial Census, 1992).

During the dry season (March to May) Particulate Matter of size less then 10 microns (PM10) along busy roads of Kathmandu Metropolitan City* has been measured as being above the national standard of 120 micrograms per cubic meter, and its concentration has tripled in the last 10 years (Tuladhar, 2004).

2.3. Health Consequences

The recent urban health data reconfirmed the rising level of air pollution in urban areas of Kathmandu Valley. Air pollution, which has long been linked to respiratory problems and complications (e.g., Dockery et al. 1993), could be contributing to health problems among the inhabitants of Kathmanu Valley. Chronic Obstructive Pulmonary Disease (COPD) is the number one cause of mortality in Bir Hospital (Figure 1) and the respiratory disease was the number two cause of mortality in Kanti Children Hospital (Department of Health Services, 2003). The number of patients admitted to Patan hospital with Chronic Obstructive Pulmonary Disease (COPD) has doubled in the past five years (Kathmandu's Air Quality, 2003). Similarly the number of COPD patients as a percentage of the total medical patients being admitted to the hospital increased from 19% in 2052 to 27% in 2002 (Tuladhar, 2004).

Likewise, 18% of deaths of urban children below five years of age were due to respiratory infection (Central Department of Population Studies, 1997). The number of urban children reporting respiratory related cases in Kanti Children Hospital, Kathmandu was higher than rural children (LEADERS Nepal, 1998).

Indoor smoke pollution also plays a crucial role in urban Nepal. About 39.1% of the urban population in Nepal use firewood (Nepal Demographic and Health Survey 2001:409) and 35.8% use kerosene as a source of fuel. As a result, nearly 11% of the bronchitis cases were due to indoor smoke pollution in urban areas of Kathmandu (Pandey and Basnet, 1987).

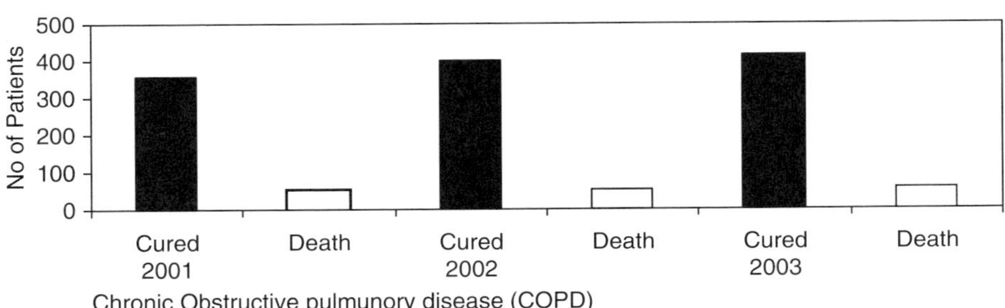

Figure 1. Trend of COPD Disease in Bir Hospital of Kathmandu Metropolitan City (*Source*: *Hospital Record* [2003]).

* KMC is one of the five municipalities of Kathmandu Valley and it is also the capital city

2.4. Estimated Health Cost of Air Pollution

It has been estimated that reducing PM2.5 level in Kathmandu Valley by just half (by 47.4mg/cum) would reduce daily mortality by 7% and hospital admissions by 24% (Kathmandu's Air Quality, 2003). Likewise, the reduction of PM2.5 levels in KMC by half (by 63.4 mg/cum) would reduce mortality by approximately 10% and hospital admissions by 32%.

Similarly, reducing the annual average PM10 level in Kathmandu to the international standard (50mg/mcu) has been estimated to avert over 2000 hospital admissions, over 40,000 emergency room visits, over 135,000 cases of acute bronchitis in children, over 4,000 cases of chronic bronchitis and half a million asthma attacks. A World Bank study in 1990 estimated the total cost of the health impacts of PM10 to be approximately Nrs (Nepalease Rupee) 210 million in Kathmandu (Sah, 1996).

Likewise, preliminary estimates suggest that reducing the annual average PM10 levels in Kathmandu to international standards (50mg/mcu) will save approximately Nrs 30 million in just hospital admission costs (Kathmandu's Air Quality, 2003). However, the hospital admission cost is only 0.02 percent of the total cost of health effects of air pollution according to a World Bank study. Therefore, it is safe to assume that Nrs 150 billions could be saved by reducing Kathmandu's PM10 levels to that of international standards (Tuladhar, 2004).

2.5. Noise Pollution

Noise can cause hearing impairment, interfere with communication, disturb sleep, cause cardiovascular and psycho-physiological effects, reduce performance, and provoke annoyance responses and changes in social behavior (World Health Organization, 2001). The main social consequence of hearing impairment is the inability to understand speech in normal conditions, which is considered a social handicap. Noise levels surveyed at four major city locations of Kathmandu had exceeded the standards of 85 – 90 dB* (A) (Ojha, 1995).

3.0. URBAN RESIDENTIAL PLANNING AND HEALTH

In the absence of zoning and subdivision regulations, city growth and expansion occur through the informal land development process led by the land brokers. The process is neither logical nor orderly. People first purchase land on an urban fringe, build houses and then attempt to bring in basic services and infrastructure. They do this through the uncoordinated individual decisions and, parcel by parcel development of land.

This has resulted in erratic patterns of street layout, often causing drainage problems, making the extension of infrastructure tedious and inhibiting the entry of emergency vehicles. This hodgepodge process also does not ensure the provision of parks and open spaces in the developing areas; children are often observed to be playing in the streets and the elderly are deprived of such space.

On the other hand, the already developed or semi developed urban communities are found to have inadequate basic services. For example, they have clogged drains, unpaved streets, courtyards without street lights. The old traditional houses

* dB is a decibel, a unit to measure the loudness of sound. Loudness doubles everything three decibels. So 93 decibels is actually twice as loud as 90 decibels.

of Kathmandu city are dark, damp and made up of bricks and mud mortar and without proper waste disposal. Public land and open spaces are gradually disappearing due to their encroachment by surrounding residents.

In recent years, a number of private land and housing development projects have emerged but their projects are scattered in inappropriate locations (low lands and flood plains and in pockets of land surrounded by narrow roads) causing a threat to the urban physical environment and the safety of residents.

We know of no studies on the impact of lack of open space on the urban community in Katmandu or Nepal. Congested living in haphazardly developed residential areas without greenery and open space has been associated with mental distress in other contexts (Evans, 2003). Damp, dark and cold areas may human health. Lack of physical activity due to insufficient spaces or parks for recreation may also encourage indoor living, further limiting the capabilities of those with physical disorders.

4.0. URBAN POOR SETTLEMENTS AND HEALTH

Urban poor communities have rapidly grown in the towns and cities in Nepal. At present, there are about 63 squatter settlements in Kathmandu Valley which accommodate 2,600 families or nearly 15,000 people and are growing at the rate of 25% per year (Pradhan, 2003). Most squatters are located along the flood prone polluted river banks (Shakya, 2003). The squatter sheds are susceptible to roof leakage, wall wetting and room flooding in the rainy season. Three to nine people live in two rooms which have no ventilation. None of the households have sanitary toilets and the toilet effluents are directly discharged into the river. Availability of drinking water is about 24 liters per family per day. Even these water samples are found unfit for drinking in most of the cases. The water samples show fecal contamination of 56 to 260 Coliform/100ml water. Firewood is the dominant form of cooking energy in most of the squatter sheds which are mostly unventilated. Cold, cough, fever, diarrhea and headache are the most common diseases in the squatter settlements. In developing countries, environmental hazards in urban areas mainly affect low income people, especially women, children and migrants, that is the people who are least able to avoid the hazards and or least able to deal with the illness or injury they cause (Commonwealth Consultative Group on Environment, 2004).

5.0. THE CITY AND SOCIAL HEALTH

The inadequate urban built environment in developing world cities leads to congestion and pollution, unemployment, and deterioration of social support. Noise, overcrowding, inappropriate urban design, and stresses contribute to the growing psychosocial health problems of many urban dwellers in developing countries, especially of adolescents and young adults (Commonwealth Consultative Group on Environment, 2004).

Suicides in Kathmandu, Lalitpur and Bhaktapur were 237, 49 and 48 respectively in 2002. Likewise, there were 30 homicides, 57 theft cases, and 25 robbery cases in Kathmandu district. The national prevalence rate of HIV/AIDS is estimated to be 0.5% in 2001 (Nepal Country Reports, 2001). Likewise, there were 58,000 people estimated to be living with HIV AIDS in Nepal and about 2400 deaths were HIV related. The urban HIV/AIDS data is not available but it is likely that urban areas account for a large share of HIV/AIDS cases in Nepal.

6.0. URBAN SERVICES AND HEALTH

6.1. Solid waste management

Although private and public waste management systems exist in the Kathmandu valley, waste disposal practices of local residents are not suitable. Throwing household wastes into local streams has affected the quality of water in local streams as well as the aesthetics value of the cities of Kathmandu Valley (Pradhan, 1998). The solid waste pollutes the land and contaminates the ground water and wells. About three million urban residents in 1999 in Nepal generated an estimated amount of 426,500 tones of waste and 29% of it was produced by the Kathmandu Metropolitan City alone according to the Minority of Local Development.

Segregation of hospital infectious waste is not practiced in a systematic way. Considering the population growth rate of 4.8% per annum in Kathmandu, hospital waste in 1990 was estimated to be 679 tons/annum or 1.86 tons/day (National Review Committee, 1992). A total of 6251 hospital beds in Nepal generated approximately 500 tons of hazardous waste per year.

Most of the waste is mixed with other garbage and is either dumped or burned in ordinary kilns (Tuladhar, 1999). There has been little study on the health impact of poor waste management, although its health impact was likely substantial for the waste management workers, scavengers and river users.

6.2. Sanitation and Water Quality

About 33% of the urban population has no access to toilet facilities in Nepal. They use river banks, ponds and urban fringe land for ablution. Cities have inadequate number of toilets in public areas and people use public roads and park corners, which pollutes the city areas and contaminates ground and surface water. Only half of the total urban population is served by piped drinking water supplies (Nepal Demographic and Health Survey, 2001).

Drinking water in Kathmandu Valley is unsafe throughout the year. The samples of water supplied by the Nepal Water Supply Corporation have up to 180 plus coliform organism per 100 ml of water (Himalayan Times, 2004). In Kathmandu Valley only 29.4 % of households boil the government supplied water before its use according to government statistics (His Majesty's Government in Nepal, 2000).

The fecal and pathogen contamination of drinking water causes diarrhea, gastroenteritis, infectious hepatitis, typhoid, paratyphoid, cholera, bacillary dysentery, amoebic dysentery, and giardiasis. Hospital records of Kathmandu city in 2003 revealed that gastroenteritis was the number two cause of morbidity in Kanti Children hospital and number one in Sukraraj Tropical Infectious Disease (STID) Hospital. The second and third causes of morbidity in the STID hospital were enteric fever and hepatitis respectively. Likewise, Hepatitis was the leading cause of mortality in STID Hospital. A hospital record survey of 2002 revealed that diarrhea (1960), typhoid (322), and hepatitis (160) were the three major diagnoses among those admitted to the STID hospital (Figure 2). Similarly, diarrhea (2036) and typhoid (170) were the major diagnoses among those admitted in Kanti Children's hospital in 2002 (Department of Health Services, 2003).

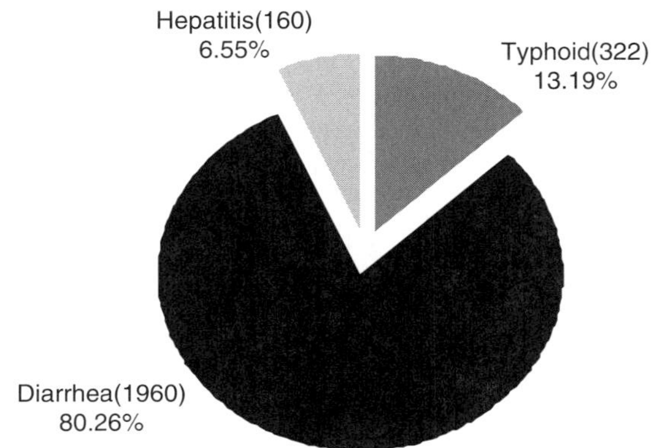

Figure 2. Pattern of Disease Recorded in STID Hospital, Kathmandu City (*Source*: *Hospital Record*, 2003).

6.3. Ground Water Contamination

Ground water contains high concentrations of iron, manganese and ammonia in Kathmandu Valley (Tamrakar, 1995). A more serious issue is the arsenic poisoning in the ground water of Tarai (plain area) towns of Nepal. About 30,000 shallow tube wells have been tested for arsenic and 7% were found to contain arsenic exceeding the national guideline: 50 parts per billion (ppb) (Shrestha, *et al.*, 2004). About 435 arsenicosis patients were identified by a study conducted in four districts of Tarai (plains): Nawalparasi, Parsa, Bara and Rautahat (Pradhan, et al., 2004).

6.4. River Water Pollution

Kathmandu Valley hosts more than 72% of the country's water polluting industries (Devkota and Neupane, 1994). Many of these discharge effluents to the rivers accounting for about 7% of the total effluents (domestic and industrial) in Kathmandu Valley. Rivers and ground waters are also polluted due to haphazard disposal of sewerage, waste water and solid wastes. The study by Devkota and Neupane in 1994 indicates that about 93% of the pollution load is from domestic sewage and the remaining 7% from the industrial effluent.

The health impact of this is on the residents of the nearby settlements; children who play with these water, women who wash their clothes and vegetable produce. The washed vegetables on these rivers would also eventually affect the health of the urban consumers.

7.0. FOOD QUALITY AND HEALTH

About 10.6 % of the food samples inspected in 2003 by the Department of Food Technology and Quality Control in Kathmandu Valley were found to be substandard. There has been an increasing prevalence of zoonotic diseases in Nepalese cities in the past few years. Staphylococcus, tuberculosis and brucellalocis were found in meat products and salmonella in fish and prawns (Ministry of Population and Environment, 1999). Many food items including ice cubes, meat products, fish, prawns and butter collected from hotels and restaurants were found to be contaminated with coliform bacteria above permissible and safe limits (His Majesty's Government/WHO, 1993).

An examination of 184 pasteurized milk samples of different brands by the Department of Food Technology and Quality Control found 66.8 % to be coliform positive. Twenty nine out of 70 samples of mineral and processed drinking water had higher mesopholic count and three of them had coliform bacteria. Street food vendors usually sell low quality food, which is a serious public health concern as the most vulnerable individuals are children and people with low incomes. Farmers wash carrots and other root crops in polluted rivers before they reach vegetable markets. There are serious health implications of the quality of food in urban areas of Nepal. However, an impact study of food quality on health in urban residents has yet to be carried out.

8.0. NATIONAL INSURGENCY AND HEALTH

The impact of terror on the mental health of the Nepalese has not yet been assessed but it is likely that ongoing low-intensity conflict has had substantial impact on the mental health of the general population, particularly women and children. Bombing, shooting, kidnapping and slaughtering are the events that have taken place in rural areas and towns of Nepal in recent years. Thousands of people have fled from rural areas to safer towns or abroad. The insurgency has produced thousands of widows and orphans; haphazard disposal of explosives has killed many children. Evidence from other countries suggests that there is an association between the experience of mass trauma and mental health suggesting that there is a substantial, undocumented, mental health burden in Nepal in general and in cities in particular (Galea, *et al., 2002)*.

9.0. POTENTIAL STRATEGIES FOR IMPROVING THE HEALTH OF PEOPLE IN CITIES OF NEPAL

9.1. Urbanization and Health

The process of rapid urban growth is inevitable in Nepal but it should be harnessed in a planned way to ensure a safe urban environment as well as the health and well being of urban citizens. Therefore, health concerns should be the heart of urban planning and urban environmental management practices. Environmentally friendly urban planning and healthy city programs should be the key to planned development and management of urban growth. The Health Impact Assessment of urban policies, programs, and development projects would be a good starting off point to ensure healthy urban environment.

Growth of poor communities in cities and towns of Nepal is an inherent byproduct of urbanization. These are vulnerable communities prone to urban health risks without an adequate history of municipal infrastructure to adjust to the city market forces. Thus, government should take special efforts to address the employment, basic services, and environmental and health concerns of these urban poor communities. Government should initiate pro-urban health programs for the poor to monitor, evaluate, and improve the health of these people.

9.2. City Transportation and Health

To reduce air pollution and minimize respiratory diseases in cities and towns of Nepal, an appropriate city level transportation policy has to be adopted. The government should ensure a congestion-free city-wide transportation network through a well developed road master plan. It is also important to enforce strict traffic management rules to avoid slow vehicular movement and air pollution. Improvement of roads and foot paths with pavement is equally essential to achieve dust free streets in cities and towns.

It also is timely to regulate the growth of vehicles by banning air polluting vehicles, discouraging small private vehicles such as motor bikes and taxis that have unsafe exhaust and encouraging mass transporting public vehicles. We suggest promotion of electric vehicles wherever applicable and measures to reduce fuel adulteration. We also suggest development of pedestrian lanes, bicycle lanes, parks and green belts to enhance the road environment. The available evidence lends itself to the argument that a combination of urban design, land use patterns, and transportation systems that promotes walking and bicycling will help create, healthier, and more liveable communities (Handy, *et al.*, 2002).

There needs to be effective implementation of emission standards for air quality. As well as, the indoor air pollution and its health hazard should be minimized through reduction in the use of firewood. Enforcement of noise standards in cities and towns is also essential to minimize its negative impact on health. A mechanism of monitoring of heart, respiratory, and other air pollution related disease in towns and cities particularly at the community and ward level is essential.

9.3. Urban Community and Health

Appropriate zoning and subdivision regulations should guide the urban development and planning of cities and towns of Nepal in order to enhance better physical environment and health of urban communities. The residential development should ensure adequate open space for children, elderly and youth for their physical, recreational and social activities and emergency relief purposes. Urban planning should include infrastructure upgrading programs particularly for degraded and older urban communities. The emerging private land developers should implement incentives to create environmentally friendly and healthy planning through the enforcement of planning codes. A community-level health examination and monitoring program should be launched on a regular basis to understand the causes of health degradation in urban communities.

The majority of residents in urban poor communities live in illegally occupied marginal land. They do not improve their living environment due to the potential threat of eviction. Thus, government should have a policy to provide some form of security of tenure on land so that the residents can take initiatives to improve their environment. This will also legalize the concerned agencies to work toward upgrading, rehabilitation and resettlement for urban poor community. The government should pay special attention to providing clean drinking water, sanitary toilet facilities and health services such as health check ups, health education and medicines to the poor communities. The urban poor should have better access to low cost housing and rental provisions.

The urban poor are prone to health risk and the appropriate services available in the market are unaffordable if not inaccessible to them. Thus, the state or government has a unique role in making available social and health services that can provide assistance to Nepal's poorest families.

A city planning framework that promotes space in urban communities that provides a sense of belonging to the residents, where neighbors gather and interact, is critically needed as a means of promoting discourse and social contact within Nepal's cities (Semenza, 2003).

9.4. Urban Services and Health

Waste management system should ensure reductions in contamination of land, ground, surface water, and rivers. The solid waste management system should ensure that it takes care of the health of waste workers and scavengers. Solid waste should be disposed in the sanitary land fill site. Special arrangements for disposal should be made for the hospital and hazardous waste and it should not be treated as any other normal waste.

High priority should be given to improve the sanitation and water quality of urban communities. Adequate public toilet provisions should be made, including the introduction of community level toilets, pay toilets and credit support for making residential toilets. The government should carry out drinking water quality improvement programs such as water treatment facilities. It is also important that the piped drinking water leakage be improved and the chances of contamination reduced. Systematic testing and monitoring of water quality is necessary to take appropriate preventive measures.

Similarly, appropriate testing and treatment of ground water is essential before it is used for drinking purposes. Special treatment programs and awareness program should be launched in the urban areas where people are using arsenic contaminated ground water. Regular study of the trend of water borne disease in urban areas of Nepal is essential to develop appropriate health and urban policies. Urban water borne disease control programs should be launched for appropriate mitigation.

Discharging of untreated domestic waste water, sewerage, and industrial effluents directly into the river should be prohibited. Disposing of wastes into the river should be prevented. Programs of river bank cleaning, protection and greening programs should be launched. River users and river front residents should be educated and motivated for cleaning the river. Likewise, river water quality monitoring system should be established.

Urban residents largely depend upon the market supplied food and its quality directly affects the health of urban residents. Therefore, strict and regular inspection of urban food sources (including the street food vendors) in cities and towns should be made by the food inspecting agencies. The quality of the inspected food should be tested and its quality should be publicized. Those sellers who do not comply with the food quality standards should be penalized. A general awareness of food hygiene among both consumers and sellers has to be made in cities and towns by the Department of Food Technology and Quality Control.

Urban health is also affected by the growing terrorism nationally and - internationally. Peace and counseling centers should be established. Relief programs for victims should be launched. Rehabilitation and resettlement programs for the insurgency affected families should be launched. Moral, spiritual, emotional and confidence building programs also are essential in the towns and cities of Nepal too.

9.5. Role of Institutions

Last and not least, without the appropriate role of institutions it is difficult to achieve the health objectives of cities and towns of Nepal. Urban health is a broad issue and it encompasses large number of sectors and agencies such as Department of Health (DOH), Department of Urban Development and Building Construction (DUDBC), Department of transport and traffic management (DTTM), Department of Road (DOR), Department of Water Supply and Sewerage (DWSS), Department of Food Technology and Quality Control (DOFTQC). Therefore, coordination and cooperation amongst these agencies is essential to develop a national urban health policy. Based on this systematic overall policy, respective agencies should launch their coordinated health and sanitation programs.

At the local level, the capacity of the municipalities and the urbanizing Village Development Committees should be upgraded for better monitoring and facilitating urban health programs. Urban health education campaigns should be launched at all levels: community level, ward level and municipal level. The local clubs, community based organizations and Non Governmental Organizations, schools and colleges should also be motivated to play an instrumental role in enhancing urban health in Nepal.

REFERENCES

Adhikari, A. P. (1998). Urban and Environmental Planning in Nepal, IUCN, Kathmandu, Nepal, (September 15, 2004); http://www.panasia.org.sg/nepalnet/mahilaweb/environment/reports_summary/urban_and_environment_planning_in_nepal.htm

Adhikari, A. (1999). *Air Pollution Situational Analysis and Management Plan, World Health Organization/Department of Water Supply and Sewerage, unpublished report.* Kathmandu, Nepal.

Asian Development Bank (2001). Nepal Urban Sector Strategy, His Majesty's Government of Nepal and the Asian Development, Bank Volume 1, TA 3272 (Report July 2001).

Bal Kumar, K.C., Dev Pant, P., Subedi, G., and Veer Shakya, D. (1997). *Birth, Death and Contraception in Nepal.* Central Department of Population Studies Tribhuvan University, Kathmandu, Nepal.

Bryld, E. (2001). Problems and Potentials with an Urbanizing Nepal, an unpublished Paper.

Commonwealth Consultative group on Environment. Effective partnerships in the areas of human settlements, water sanitation and waste management, (September 15, 2004); http://www.thecommonwealth.org/shared_asp_files/uploadedfiles/%7BE44377F4-04E8-4560-B9D1-D863225DECC7%7D_CCGE(04)1_Effective%20Partnerships.pdf

Department of Health Services. (2003). *Annual Report of His Majesty's Government of Nepal.* Ministry of Health/UNFPA, Kathmandu.

Devkota, S. R., and Neupane, C.P. (1994). *Industrial pollution inventory of the Kathmandu Valley and Nepal Report HMG/MOI/UNIDO/91029.* Industrial and Pollution Control Management Project, Ministry of Industry, Industrial Pollution Control Management Project, Kathmandu, Nepal.

Dockery, D.W., Pope, C.A. 3rd, Xu, X., Spengler, J.D., Ware, J.H., Fay, M.E., Ferris, B.G. Jr, and Speizer, F.E. (1993). An association between air pollution and mortality in six U.S. cities. *N. Engl. J. Med.* 9(24):1753-9.

Environmental Management Action Group. (1992). Environmental Problems of Urbanization and Industrialization: The existing situation and the future direction, report prepared for UNDP.

Evans, W. E. (2003). The Built Environment and Mental Health. *J. Urban Health* 80:536-555.

Galea, S., Ahern, J., Resnick, H., Kilpatrick, D., Bucuvalas, M., Gold, J., and Vlahov, D. (2002). Psychological sequelae of the September 11 terrorist attacks in New York City. *N. Engl. J. Med.* 346(13):982-7.

Handy, S.L., Boarnet, M.G., Ewing, R., and Killingsworth, R.E. (2002). How the built environment affects physical activity: views from urban planning. *Am. J. Prev. Med.* 23(2 Suppl):64–73.

Himalayan Times. (2004). *Coli-form organism found in drinking water in valley, published in the Himalayan Times, Kathmandu, 29 July, 2004,* (September 16, 2004); http://www.thehimalayantimes.com/

fullstory. asp?filename=aCXatKsbrzqda9Sa8ta6HNamal&folder=aCXatK&Name=City&dtSiteDate=20040730&sImageFileName.

His Majesty's Government of Nepal. (2000). Report on the Situation of Women, Children and Households published in collaboration with UNICEF Nepal.

His Majesty's Government/WHO, (1993). Collaborating Program on Protection and Promotion of Health and Environment, Bexmal Jon.

Hunter College, The Impact of Noise on Health, the center for occupational and environmental health, 1999, New York (September 16, 2004); http://www.hunter.cuny.edu/health/coeh/publications/Awarecu. ric_HTML/HEALTHEF01.htm

Industrial Census. (1992). Report prepared by His Majesty's Government of Nepal.

Japan International Cooperation Adgency, Kathmandu Valley Urban Road Development, report prepared for Department of Road in Nepal, 1993, Nepal, (September 16, 2004); http://www.jica.go.jp/english/evaluation/report/expost/14-4-41.html.

Kathmandu's Air Quality. (2003). Clean Energy Nepal and Environment and Public Health Organization, 2003. Health Impact of Kathmandu's Air Pollution, Factsheet 1, pp 1–4.

LEADERS Nepal, (1998). A citizen report on air pollution in Kathmandu Valley: Children's health at risk. Kathmanudu, Nepal.

Ministry of Health of Nepal, 2004, Kathmandu, Nepal, (September 16, 2004); http://www.moh.gov.np/generalinfo/countryprofile.htm

Ministry of Local Development, (2000). Municipal Population estimation, unpublished document.

Ministry of Population and Environment, 1999, Kathmandu, Nepal. (September 16, 2004); http://www.mope.gov.np/index.php

National Planning Commission, 2002, Tenth Five Year National Plan Document published by His Majesty's Government of Nepal, Kathmandu, (September 16, 2004); http://www.npc.gov.np/tenth-plan/approach_paper_in_english.htm

Nepal Country Reports, Kathmandu, Nepal, 2001, (September 15, 2004);http://countryreports.org/content/nepal.htm

Nepal Demographic and Health Survey, 2001. (2002). Family Health Division, Ministry of Health, Kathmandu, Nepal.

Nepal Health Research. (2004). Assessment of Ambient Air Quality in Selected Urban Areas of Nepal, (September 15, 2004); http://www.cleanairnet.org/caiasia/1412/article-58901.html

National Review Committee. (1992). *New Era, National Report on United Nations Conference on Environmental and Development (UNCED).* Kathmandu, Nepal.

Ojha, S. (1995). Regulating Growth: Kathmandu Valley, Public Health, Annex 10, unpublished report.

Pradhan, B. (1998). *Water quality assessment of Bagmati River and its Tributaries, the Kathmandu Valley, Nepal.*, Vienna: Institute of Water and Waste water engineering, BOKU.

Pradhan, P.M.S, and LUMANTI Support Group for Shelter, June 30, 2003. Housing the poor: Providing Access to Land for Poor Families in Kathmandu, (September 16, 2004); http://www.lumanti.com.np/nav.php3?view=newsArt1

Pradhan, B., Shrestha R., Shrestha MP., Maskey A., Dahal, B., Gorkhali M., Dangol, B., Tuladhar P., and Gorkhali, L. (2004). Effects of Arsenic Mitigation Measures on Arsenicosis Patients in Tarai Districts, Nepal published in Environment and Public Health Organization Magazine.

Pandey, M., and Basnet, B. (1987). *Chronic Bronchitis and Cor Pulmonale in Nepal, A Scientific Epidemiological Study Monograph*. Mrigendra Medical Trust, Kathmandu.

Population Census 2001. (2002). *National Report; UNFPA Nepal for National Planning Commission Secretariat.* Central Bureau of Statistics, Kathmandu.

Sah, R.C. (2003). *Advocating and Enforcing Air-Quality Standards in Nepal, Kathmandu Valley Report, URBAIR.* Environmental Law Alliance Worldwide, Eugene, Oregan.

Schuster, M. A., Stein, B.D., Jaycox, L.H., and Collins, R. (2001). A national survey of stress reactions after the September 11, 2001, terrorist attacks. *N. Engl. J. Med.* 345(20); 1507–1512.

Semenza, J. C. (2003). The intersection of urban planning, art and public health: the Sunnyside Piazza. *Am. J. Public Health* 93(9):1439-41.

Shakya, S. (2003). Environmental Implication of poverty in the selected squatter settlements of Kathmandu and Dharan, preliminary report of the MSC School of Environment and Sustainable Development, Pokhara University, unpublished thesis.

Shrestha., R. M., and Raut, A. K. (2002). Air quality management in Kathmandu better air quality to Asian and Pacific cities, RAQ 2002. Hong Kong, PRC.

Shrestha, R., Ngai, T., Dangol, B., Dahal, B., and Paudyal, U. (2004). Arsenic Biosand Filter: A Promising Technology for Removal of Arsenic in Nepal, Environment and Public Health Organization Magazine.

Tamrakar, (1995). Regulating Growth: Kathmandu Valley, Water Resources, Annex, 3, unpublished report.

Tuladhar, B. (1999). Hazardous waste management, Nepal country report, Kathmandu: WHO.

Tuladhar, (2004). Breathing Kathmandu's Air can be dangerous, an article on Environment and Public Health Organization Magazine.

World Health Organization, 2001. Occupational and community noise Fact Sheets No. 258 (September 16, 2004); http://www.who.int/mediacentre/factsheets/fs258/en/.

Chapter 12

Integrative Chapter

The Health of Urban Populations

The Editors

The preceding ten chapters have each considered the health of a particular urban population, ranging from homeless persons to sexual minority groups, and through the use of Nepal as a case study, to persons in urban areas in developing countries. In this brief integrative chapter we do not aim to summarize what the authors of each chapter have already presented. Rather, we offer our synthesis of common elements that cross chapters, important differences, and more importantly, the implications of these chapters for the study of urban health.

In reading this first section on urban populations, it appears to us that the clearest message to emerge across chapters is the fact that rather than being different, these populations are in many ways similar. Across these different populations, there are urban exposures including pollution, foodstores, traffic, and elements of the built environment, all of which may affect the health of most, if not all, of the key populations in urban areas (young, old, poor, homeless, substance users, and immigrants). Some authors chose to use our formulation (discussed in Chapter 1) of the physical environment, social environment, and health and social services to organize these themes, while others focused principally on the elements of the urban environment that were particularly salient for the population group with which they were concerned. More importantly, these chapters show that while the impact of each of these characteristics of the urban environment on each population (however categorized) may be the same, they also may differ in terms of the specific aspects of health and well-being that are affected by a particular feature of the urban environment, the magnitude of the effect, or in terms of a unique relationship between an element of the urban environment and an aspect of health in a particular group. For example, several of the chapters note the relation between urban design/planning and the likelihood of physical injury in different groups. However, it is likely that air pollution plays a particular role in childhood asthma, hence making that aspect of the urban physical environment particularly important when considering the health of cities in urban areas. More dramatically, although availability of affordable housing recurs as an important determinant of the health of urban populations, it clearly is particularly important in the context of the health of homeless persons. We suggest that this observation, that is the commonality of urban exposures that may affect the health of urban populations applies equally well to groups not discussed here. For example, these chapters, informed by the roots of public health as a discipline that concerns itself primarily with the health of vulnerable populations, do not consider the health of more wealthy, middle aged, stably housed persons. We leave it up to future reviews and empiric work to assess the extent to which the characteristics of the urban environment discussed here are also important for other groups that constitute the entirety of the population of cities.

Indeed, another point that emerges from these chapters is that they are describing different urban populations less than they are describing groups that are all part of one dynamic, and inter-related, urban population. That these groups are characterized by differences is self-evident, but perhaps it is the similarities between these groups that are ultimately more important to consider. Fundamentally, the authors of all chapters are discussing populations that are not only affected by their urban environment, but in many ways are brought together by their urban environment. Thus, perhaps paradoxically, the heterogeneity of urban populations itself contributes to a homogenization of the urban environment that in turn affects all groups living in urban areas. For example, we saw in the preceding chapters how marginalized groups (e.g., persons who are lesbian, gay, bisexual, or transgendered) within cities have made outsize contributions to cities' cultural life. In turn, this very diversity of cities makes urban areas particularly attractive to a range of other groups, including older adults who increasingly are settling in cities during their retirement. The presence of older adults then is likely to increase demand for sophisticated health services that may change service provision for all urban residents. The careful reader can draw several similar observations from the preceding ten chapters. It appears then that rather than separate urban populations, we are dealing with a *mosaic* of urban groups, all of which constitute an urban population whole that might well behave in ways that are inscrutable if we are to consider only its parts.

An important corollary to this point concerns the reciprocal nature of the relationship between populations in urban areas and the urban environment itself. Therefore, while features of the urban environment may shape the health of urban populations, it is of course urban populations that shape their environment. While at first glance this observation may seem self-evident, it has important implications for how we consider cities and their role in determining population health. Adults in cities make decisions that form urban characteristics (e.g., contribute to decisions about placement of parks, or influence their social networks about a particular behavior) that in turn have a direct bearing on their own health, and that of others (e.g., their own children) in cities. This observation is perhaps most starkly illustrated in the chapter that presents the health of urban populations in Nepal. The author here provides clear proscriptions for changes in the urban environment, ranging from individual, to municipal, to federal changes that are likely to improve the health of Nepalese urban residents. The evident need for these changes then suggests the importance of ensuring that urban residents are empowered to affect these changes.

Another point that readily emerges, not inconsistent with the principal point being discussed here, is that group "membership" is a limited tool in terms of helping us understand the health of individuals within cities. Indeed almost all chapters discuss the range of factors across levels (e.g., individual characteristics like behaviors and features of their social environment) that likely affect the health of persons in cities, and group identity (e.g., elderly, homeless) is merely one such characteristic that at best modifies the relationship between the fundamental determinants of health, many of which are rooted in the urban context. Further driving home this point is the observation, made by many of the preceding chapters, that membership in the groups discussed here is far from "exclusive", and individuals frequently belong to multiple groups (e.g., minority elderly) and change "group membership" over time (e.g., persons enter and exit periods of economic disadvantage in their time). It is in this context then that consideration of the urban environment and the context within which individuals live may more fruitfully allow us to understand the interventions that might best improve population health.

These chapters then suggest that we might be on the threshold of understanding not only the relevant exposures that affect health in cities across different groups, but also to start refining our theory and empiric work that considers how modifications of the urban environment can be made that have a far-reaching impact on the health of urban populations as a whole. We return to this point in Chapter 29 were we offer our synthesis of Part III of this book.

Part II

Methods

Chapter 13

An Anthropological Perspective on Urban Health

Frances K. Barg and Jane Kauer

1.0. INTRODUCTION

An anthropological focus on urban health is a necessary part of an in-depth understanding of the ways that social and cultural factors affect humans and human behavior in the urban environment (Obrist, *et al.*, 2003a; 2003b). Anthropology is the study of human evolution, variation, and behavior in an environmental context (Campbell and Loy, 2000). The various aspects of anthropology (biological, cultural, linguistic, and archaeological) share a core focus on human thought and behavior and together attempt to create an integrated perspective on human experience. Medical anthropology and human biology in particular have focused on bringing the theoretical and methodological perspectives of anthropology at large into the public discourse on health, medicine, healthcare, wellness, and illness.

Anthropology can have a significant impact on urban health by providing a theoretical perspective on human prehistoric environments and through the employment of methods used commonly by anthropologists, especially in the fields of cultural and medical anthropology. Whereas for most of human history as a species we have adapted to a broad range of ecological situations, only recently have human beings had to cope with the various stressors (and resources) of urban living (Satterthwaite, 2000; Obrist, *et al.*, 2003b).

In this chapter, we will first discuss how human adaptation to prehistoric environments affects our ability to function in the present-day urbanized context. Second, we will show how anthropology provides a unique combination of theory and practice at the nexus of culture and biology that may help us understand the variation we observe in heterogeneous modern urban environments. Third, we will explore ways that race categories are used in urban health research, noting the pitfalls that such received categories create.

Anthropologic field methods incorporate qualitative and quantitative methods for studying health. In doing so, anthropologic methods offer ways to understand the context in which health and illness occur as well as the distribution and frequency of different illnesses in the urban setting. We conclude this chapter with several examples of mixed-methods studies that demonstrate how blending methods can enhance the understanding of health in urban areas.

2.0. HUMAN ADAPTATION

2.1. Changes in Human Settlement Patterns

Ongoing massive migration into the world's cities during the 20th and early 21st centuries has resulted in a major shift in human settlement patterns. There is a significant difference between the manner in which human populations lived during the last 50,000 years, and present-day settlement patterns. Humans did not evolve in the context of urban environments. Over the last several tens of thousands of years, our human ancestors have had to cope with a variety of environmental constraints arising from changes in both the climate and in human cultural evolution.

As of about 12,000 years ago, when humans practiced a variety of food acquisition strategies that often involved some amount of travel on a seasonal basis, humans began using agricultural techniques that increased the reliability of the food supply, enabling some populations to settle in a single location. Over the past 12,000 years, depending on their environmental and cultural context, human populations have slowly shifted, from a generally hunting and gathering lifestyle to one which relied more heavily on management of livestock, often in the context of a nomadic lifestyle. In many populations, this combination of nomadism and pastoralism has slowly yielded to an increased reliance on agricultural products and a more settled lifestyle. Thus, a great deal of environmental and cultural change has occurred in little more than ten thousand years.

At the beginning of the 21st century, humans, as a species, live predominantly in cities (Vlahov and Galea, 2002). Moreover, the majority of the urbanization has occurred in the last 100 years, and by the end of the first decade of the 21st century the majority of the world's population will be living in cities (Obrist, *et al.*, 2003b). In essence, this means that from now on, the majority of human beings will be living in a type of environment for which they are not adapted, in the evolutionary sense. This is important because in thinking about the effects of living in urban environments, anthropologists need to take into account not just direct costs and stressors, but also those that are built into our human biology. People living in urban environments have direct stressors to cope with, as well as the indirect – and perhaps more cryptic – costs of being organisms adapted to a significantly different environment. There is, then, an implicit tension between the urban environment and the set of current human cultural and biological adaptations. It is hard for evolution, in the form of genetics, to 'catch up' with this change from humans as hunter-gatherers to humans as predominantly urban residents. Certainly changes in the cultural context can take place relatively rapidly to help people work with, understand, and adapt to their surroundings. This is not true of human biology, which is not able to change radically with great shifts in the environment. Although it has taken place over thousands of years, the transition in human settlement patterns from low population density to high population density and from rural to urban settings, has affected a shift from a pre-modern diet to a modernized diet that has greatly affected human health. It is the results of this shift itself, and the underlying tension with human biology, that current work in urban health needs to address. Urban health and anthropology can address together how this complex of biology and culture affects human life and health presently.

2.2. How Do Humans Adapt to the Stressors and Resources of Urban Environments?

Human biologists and medical anthropologists generally situate the effects of the environment on humans in two (admittedly highly simplified) categories: stressors and resources. In the context of urban health, we are concerned with how humans adapt to the stressors and unique resources of urban environments (Schell and Ulijaszek, 1999). How do these stressors and resources affect human health, and what are the various factors that are part of this system? It has been pointed out that while cites – especially the megacities of the late 20th and early 21st centuries – are generally seen as sources of social, physical, and economic problems, they are also places where resources are concentrated (Satterthwaite, 2000; Obrist, *et al.*, 2003b). Indeed, this combination of the specific environmental context, the people, the stressors, and the resources comprise the context of work for urban health researchers and practitioners. In particular, recent research into the relationships between health and culture has indicated that in both domains – clinical practice and research – a critical component is attention to the immediately local context (Obrist, 2003; Parkar, *et al.*, 2003; van Eeuwijk, 2003; Obrist, *et al.*, 2003a).

2.3. Discussion of Anthropological Work on Urban Stressors

Stressors specific to the urban environment – either because they are uniquely urban, or because they are uniquely presented or concentrated in the urban setting – are discussed briefly in this section. While many disciplines address the interrelationships among features of the urban environment and health, anthropologists in particular have contributed to our understanding related to population density, infectious disease, social stress, nutrition, and air and noise pollution. We discuss each in turn.

2.3.1. Population Density

By definition, urban areas have more people per unit area than non-urban areas and population density is directly related to a number of other traits of urban settings. Anthropologists have examined various aspects of population density, with a variety of emphases. Some have examined the relationship between the perceived permanence of residence and urbanism, doing ethnographic research on what may be referred to as peri-urban communities such as trailer parks and squatter communities (Huss-Ashmore and Behrman, 1999). Depending on the manner in which cities are constructed, the built environment and individual activity and time budgets may also inhibit people's ability to get adequate physical exercise (Ulijaszek, 1999), thereby compounding the effects of other stressors, such as nutritional quality of the diet and air quality (Epstein and Rogers, 2004).

2.3.2. Infectious Disease

Medical anthropology and human biology have a long history examining disease states and their biocultural context in human beings. In the 21st century, with increasing urbanization, the specifics of this inquiry require some rethinking. Over the course of the last two centuries, settlement patterns that accompanied industrialization concentrated people in cities and overwhelmed resources so that infectious diseases remained a public health problem in cities until the beginning of the Sanitary Awakening in the mid to late 19th century. Since that time, a major epidemiological transition has occurred in which infectious disease has less of an impact on mortality and non-infectious disease has a greater impact on human mortality. This remains true in urban settings, but there are some caveats.

First, in the last few decades there have been some significant dents put in the argument that infectious disease does not have as much of an impact as it used to – the global HIV epidemic is one example. Second, while people may live longer, the impact of noninfectious diseases and other negative effects on human quality of life are concentrated in cities. For example, the chronic degenerative disease states (so-called 'diseases of civilization') include hypertension, cancer, cardiac illness, obesity and Type II diabetes and have far-reaching effects across the society. In addition, urban settings also have more violent crime, which undermine social cohesion in neighborhoods (Wright and Fischer, 2003), and result in greater rates of homicide.

There has recently been an increased focus on the relationship between microbial 'cleanliness,' and the rising incidence of asthma, allergies, and infectious disease. Several studies have indicated that one factor in the variance of rates of overall childhood infection is degree of exposure to agents that stimulate the immune system early in life. While not isolated to cities, the increase in asthma itself has been shown to be much higher in inner cities. Also, livestock, putative sources of immune stimulation early in life, are relatively rare in urban environments (Bach, 2002; Weiss, 2002; Braun-Fahrlander, *et al.*, 2002), and greenhouse warming effects and climate change have differential effects on urban health (Epstein and Rogers, 2004).

Finally, urban centers serve as a nexus for trade and transportation. As such, cities are often the points of entry for new infectious agents. Furthermore, population density and concentrated poverty serve as fertile ground for transmission of these agents within the population (Acevedo-Garcia, 2000).

2.3.3. Social Stress

Although not unique to the urban environment, social stress is concentrated in urban contexts. Social stress may arise from a combination of specific factors, including high population density, lack of traditional social networks, degraded family structure, inadequate housing, and insufficient privacy. Social stress may arise from the necessity to manage numerous 'selves' or social roles (Goffman, 1959). Not only are there more people to deal with in a given time, there are more types of people (professions, social relationships, and economic relationships) with whom to interact. This may be more necessary in the human heterogeneity of urban settings than in rural settings (Goffman, 1959; Pollard, 1999). At the same time, cities are often diverse enough to have the ability to generate new social networks that are more specialized. For example, gays and lesbian groups or immigrant groups may invest a great deal in developing local relationships with strong social ties (Berkman and Clark, 2003; Finkelstein, in this book). Dressler has explored the concept of status incongruity in the context of modernization (1999) as a source of stress. By using a measure he calls "cultural consonance," Dressler has demonstrated effects of a particular type of social stress on hypertension (Dressler and Bindon, 2000).

People in urban settings also have higher rates of mental illness (e.g., Parkar, *et al.*, 2003) and crime compared with other settings, making aspects of these behaviors sources of information for urban health practice (Weiss, 2001; Obrist, *et al.*, 2003b). Anthropologists try to understand which features of the urban environment (e.g. concentration of population, proximity to stressors, anomie, and noise) contribute to these higher rates, examining the effects of the 'built environment' on human behavior and biology (Evans, 2003).

2.3.4. *Nutrition*

As the process of globalization occurs, so too does urbanization. Though the exact relationship may not be clear, it is obvious that these are related events. With globalization comes increasing 'modernization' of diets in large urban settings (Sobal, 1999). Modernization of global diets towards a Western model of eating is more common in cities around the world than it is in more rural, outlying areas. Therefore, although food may be highly available, it is also more processed, creating food stuffs that are likely to have higher ratios of simple sugars, 'bad' fats, and lower fiber content (Drewnowski, 1999).

Globalization has also resulted in a reduction in the availability of time, which may contribute to the use of both processed foods and foods prepared outside of the home becoming a greater part of the diet (Bell and Valentine, 1997). In addition, because processed food is less recognizable as a particular organic product, it may increase reliance on processed foods and reduce the likelihood of preparing foods in the home. Food insecurity can be quite high in cities. Few inner-city dwellers have access to garden space that is sufficient to generate a substantial amount of edible produce. Types of stores and store inventory are also an issue. Healthy food choices are often less available in urban settings (LaVeist and Wallace, 2000; Morland, *et al.*, 2002; Sloane, *et al.*, 2003).

Another way nutrition plays a role in urban health is in its effects on children's physical and mental growth and development (Johnston, 1993). While these effects may be more concentrated in urban settings in developing countries, the issues are also present in the developed world (Johnston and Gordon-Larsen, 1999). The effects of nutritional stressors may be additive with other factors, such as pollutants and toxic materials in the built environment (Schell, 1997).

Finally, food insecurity itself is known to be associated with higher rates of obesity, which itself is associated with higher risk of morbidity and mortality from a variety of sources (Centers for Disease Control and Prevention, 2003). Having said this, it is not clear that in all cases the nutritional quality of the diet either does or has to decline in the context of urbanization. Increasingly in the U.S. there are grassroots movements to bring locally grown produce to urban dwellers through farmers' markets and other forms of community supported agriculture (CSA) (Sobal, 1999).

2.3.5. *Culture as a Stressor/Cultural Products (Pollution, Noise)*

If we define environment broadly as the entire context of human experience – geographical, physical, social, and psychological aspects of life – then we can talk about culture as acting as an intermediary between humans and this environment. Culture may thus be viewed as both a product and a producer of the urban environment (Schell, 1997). Urban environments are at the crossroads of human physical and cultural variation and they encompass a great deal of economic and social difference. Socially defined groups (e.g., ethnic groups, the "poor," "minorities," and "homeless") are created through cultural consensus about what is acceptable, right, and normative. There is economic variation across these groups of people, with some having much more than others, and urban environments are loci where there is great disparity among groups of people living in proximity (Aday, 2001; Nguyen and Peschard, 2003; *Panel on ethnic and racial disparities in medical care convened by Physicians for Human Rights*, 2003).

Additionally, cities are complex settings in which many toxic materials – some hazardous in small amounts, some only hazardous when concentrated – are present. The distribution of toxic pollutants may compound disparities in the distribution of social and economic resources, so that the people who have the least social power often end up living in the most toxic environments. Schell (1997) calls this process "risk focusing" and describes ways that toxins accumulate in geographic areas populated by disenfranchised people. In particular, where the large proportion of the risk associated with toxic materials (e.g., lead, PCBs, DDT, mercury, and dioxins) is associated with socioeconomically disadvantaged people, a positive feedback system for increasing social stratification is created. The result of this is that people who already lack social and economic power lose further opportunities due to their higher burden of risk of contact with hazardous materials (Schell, 1997; Litt and Burke, 2002; Schell and Denham, 2003).

Similar to stressors such as chemical or particulate pollutants, noise has also been demonstrated to exert a significant effect on human life (Schell and Denham, 2003). Urban areas are differentially noisier than non-urban areas, due to the population density of city dwellers, use of industrial machinery, sound reflectance from the built environment and the ever-present vehicles of transportation (Chang and Hermann, 1974; Fidell, 1978; Tobias, *et al.*, 2001; Knauss, 2002; Matheson, *et al.*, 2003).

3.0. HUMAN VARIATION

Humans are enormously varied in their appearance, their social systems, and their cultures. It is important to understand human variation and to appreciate the enormous disparities we see in rates of illness among population groups (*Panel on DHHS Collection of Race and Ethnicity Data*, 2004). In the context of human variation, people are also subject to uneven distribution of resources and stressors in their environments that can lead to health disparities. There are numerous levels at which this inequality of distribution of access and provision of healthcare are manifest. Initially, apart from individuals, we can talk about humans as aggregating in communities. A community may be defined as a group of people who share a common identity or interest, who may be thought of as behaving according to a set of unwritten 'rules.' There are a number of different factors used to define communities, including physical factors (geography and topographical features), sociocultural factors (history, politics, and economics), and macro-cultural factors (geo-politics and -economics).

In addition to considering community-level processes affecting healthcare, it is necessary to contextualize health problems as being part of larger global and regional systems; people and communities do not exist in isolation. Social structures should be considered not only in terms of their geographical and environmental contexts, but also in terms of the broader geopolitical and economic variables exerting pressure on human populations. In particular, ethnographic data have shown that the history underlying present-day social structures and concepts is an important part of any holistic understanding of those structures. Therefore, the temporal context may be important in order to grasp an understanding of social variables and cultural variation that affects individual and group decision-making about health and healthcare choices (Nguyen and Peschard, 2003). What is also clear, however, is that it is important to keep in mind the historical, economic, and political contexts of communities; it is services, programs and initiatives which focus on the local context that are, in practice, often most effective (for example, see Kai and Drinkwater, 2004). Therefore, in urban health research there is the need for a fine-tuned comprehension of the relatedness between local and global systems.

At the local level, there are a large number of factors operating to define socio-cultural influences on health. These include health beliefs, social class, social status, and relations with health care providers and institutions. People have a wide range of health beliefs, not just definitions of "wellness" and "illness," but also of what constitutes treatment and competence in health practitioners (Kleinman, 1980). Thus, individuals and communities have particular explanatory models about health and illness that have a direct impact on urban health provision.

Social class is also a major source of variation in healthcare in urban settings. To the extent that globalization results in greater social stratification and that this is concentrated in cites (Schell, 1997), differences in social class greatly affect the distribution of healthcare resources (Link, *et al.*, 1998; Aday, 2001). In addition to the external effects of social class on individuals and communities, people's perceptions of their 'position' in the social system will affect how they (and whether they) engage with urban health sources and practitioners (Fullilove, 2001). Disadvantaged, disempowered people may be less likely to seek out a relationship with a healthcare practitioner or program if the perception is that they will be entering into yet another relationship where they lack authority or agency.

People use a variety of medical systems, aside from the standard Western medical model. This use of 'alternative' or complementary medical resources is common in urban settings where there are people living together from a great variety of cultural backgrounds. Alternative medical practices are often seen by people as forming part of the normative medical practice, and therefore it is important to be aware that patients may be using not only standard medical diagnosis and treatment options, but complementary ones as well (Adler, 2001). Additionally, some people are less likely to consider that they need any medical care at all, and may 'refer' themselves only to family members or close friends, or even keep their own 'medical' counsel. Where there is a great deal of explicit cultural variation, it may be assumed that there is also a wide variety of perspectives on what constitutes 'medical' or 'health' care (Pachter, *et al.*, 1998; Plotkin and Post, 1999; Gomez-Beloz and Chavez, 2001).

Medical anthropologists acknowledge that Western biomedicine is as "cultural" as other less familiar forms of medicine. Common to all medical systems is a relationship between the patient and their healer. In most cultures, the patient – practitioner relationship is a fairly unique one in its combination of intimacy, authority and expertise (Wylie and Wagenfeld-Heintz, 2004). While this structural relationship differs across cultural lines, and has been changing in the West in the last few decades, it still underlies many if not all healthcare interactions (Martin, 1984; Ramirez, 2003). In urban settings, where members of many cultural groups interact, one significant influence on health is the expression and perception of prejudice in a given community. Prejudice here describes all bias against persons because of some perceived trait, or some group identification (e.g., racism, ageism, and sexism) (Bailey, 2000; Aday, 2001; Nguyen and Peschard, 2003). Prejudice may affect the practice of urban health by operating to create bias against a patient, or against a practitioner/researcher. If a patient perceives that she is treated differently than others because of prejudice on the part of a healthcare provider or investigator there may be a profound effect.

Aday points out that the groups most vulnerable to health risks in present-day American society are those where a number of the high-risk traits intersect, as in low-income single young black mothers (2001). Table 1 contains many variables

Table 1. Possible Categorization of Individual-Level (Micro-cultural) Variables Influencing Health: An Example from the U.S.

Gender, Age, Ethnicity	"Minority" Non-"minority"	
Language	English is first language Speak English, not first language Do not speak English	
Religiosity	Organized religion	Major world religions Less known religion/faith Attend services Do not attend services
	Individualized faith No religion	
Citizenship / Immigration status	Citizen Non-citizen Legal Illegal Temporary Permanent	
Poverty level	Poor Not poor	
Social class	Lower class Middle class Upper class	
Income	Income level Income stability	
	Source/type of income	Employment Public assistance / welfare Disability Social security Pension / retirement income
Education	No high school High school incomplete High school degree College, some College degree Graduate/Professional degree	
Marital status	Married / Civil union Established relationship (no legal contract) Widowed Separated	

Table 1. (Continued)

	Divorced	
	Single	
Occupation	Risk / hazard level	
	Income level	
	Stability	
	Commute or travel	
	No commute or travel	
	Retired	
Residence status	Residence stability	Stable residence
		Unstable residence
	People in household	Living alone
		Living with others
		Homeless
	Control over residence	Own
		Rent
	Squatting	
	Homeless	
	'Crashing' in others' residence	
Health status	'Healthy'	
	'Not healthy'	
	Chronic illness	
	Acute illness	
	Terminal illness	
Health coverage	Health insurance	Private, self-paid
		Private, employer-paid
		Public/Governmental
	No health insurance	
Physical activity	Physical exercise frequently	
	Physical exercise infrequently	
	No physical exercise	

that are used by individuals and groups in identification in the U.S. This is not an exhaustive list by any means, but it is intended to draw attention to the immense variety of individual level variables influencing health and healthcare. This table is not intended to show all variants or options, but to illustrate the complexity of categories commonly used in grouping people.

4.0. CONTRIBUTIONS OF ANTHROPOLOGY TO THE STUDY OF URBAN HEALTH

Anthropology provides three important perspectives that can inform urban health research: 1) the consequences of using "race" as a variable in research; 2) the benefits derived from an emic, or within-a-culture point of view as well as an etic, or external point of view; and 3) the importance of using appropriate research methods (both qualitative and quantitative) to understand the biopsychosocial factors that affect health.

4.1. Race: The Pitfalls of "Natural" Categories

Race is one of the most common ways of categorizing people in biomedical and health research. However, epidemiologists are joining with anthropologists to question the use of the concept of race in research (Fullilove, 1998; Bhopal and

Donaldson, 1998; Cooper, 2000). This is an important consideration in urban health research, both because in large urban areas there is an increasingly complex mix of people from many geographic, national, and linguistic groups, and because the category race/ethnicity is often used to define groups in medical research.

As we understand it in anthropology, there is no such thing as biological race. There are no clear lines of demarcation, such that there is any way in which one could use biological data to sort humans in to distinct groups (Lewontin, 1972; Owens and King, 1999). This is true of skin color, hair type, UV sensitivity, body shape, and size (Miranda, *et al.*, 2003). Anthropologists consider that variation in these traits – those traits used visually to define 'race' – change gradually across geographic regions. Importantly, because the biological variation in these traits is as great within so-called 'race' groups as it is between them, it is an unacceptable marker of similarity or difference. There is certainly measurable genetic variation in human beings; one requires a very large number of genetic markers to be able to distinguish a large group of people by shared geography (history) (Bamshad and Olson, 2003). Although we reject the concept of biological race, as anthropologists working in the context of human health, 'race' is certainly a very important social construct. Humans do use physical (visual) markers of 'race' or 'ethnicity' such as skin color, eye color, hair color and texture, and facial features to categorize people. This is not a statement of racism, but of the recognition that there is obvious physical variation in the human species. That these categories may be and have been used in malicious ways is a fact. However, the supposed opposite of this is also true. That is, race/ethnicity is also used as a concept for categorizing people for what are presumed to be non-malicious, beneficial reasons, such as defining groups for analysis in epidemiological or medical anthropology studies (Bailey, 2000). One of the projects of medical anthropology is to be able to acknowledge human variation at both biological and social levels in research without reifying social constructs as if they were biological ones (Osborne and Feit, 1992; Bailey, 2000; Bamshad and Olson, 2003).

A logical result of this should be that we do not consider race to be an adequate marker of different groups of people for biological purposes in the context of biomedical and health-oriented research. There is a recent and ongoing disagreement among biomedical researchers as to the utility of 'race' as a group-defining characteristic (Osborne and Feit, 1992; Burchard, *et al.*, 2003). A public discussion about the use of 'race' as a category in biomedical research can yield a useful lesson, deriving from anthropology's distinction between the social construct 'race,' and so-called biological race. It is important to understand, or access the emic (within-a-culture) perspective of a given concept or topic. Fullilove (1998) suggests that a public health appreciation for the limits of the concept of race might benefit from two complementary anthropologic research strategies: 1) ethnography and; 2) evolutionary/ecological analyses to understand geographic, cultural, historic and adaptive contributions to human phenotypic variation.

4.2. Anthropology in Urban Health

4.2.1. Anthropology Uses a Combination of Emic and Etic Perspectives

Anthropologists investigate cultural phenomena from the point of view of an external observer (an etic perspective) and from the point of view of individuals who live within the culture (an emic perspective). Since the time of Bronislaw Malinowski in the early 20th century, anthropologists have been aware of the fact that experts who study a culture may or may not have the same view about the culture as do individuals who live in that culture. This may be evident in particular in studies of health and illness. Scientific classification systems (about causes of illnesses, meaning of illness, manifestations of illness, or treatment of illness) may vary greatly from local classification systems. Lambert and McKevitt (2002) argue that, for health related research, taking an emic as well as an etic approach furnishes an empirically based example of the context-specific nature of social processes. By looking at the meanings of illness and the way that illnesses are classified in a local sense, and comparing the results with investigator-defined understandings, anthropologists can help to understand the links between what people say and what they do.

4.2.2. Cultural Epidemiology

Although anthropologic and epidemiologic research are often complementary (Wiebel, 1988), historically, anthropology and epidemiology have had a somewhat contentious relationship (Trostle and Sommerfeld, 1996). On the surface, this is often attributed to a divergence in methods, but there are also fundamental differences in the types of questions each discipline asks. Both disciplines address the frequency and distribution of disease at the community or group level. Anthropologists, especially medical anthropologists, also describe the distribution of meaning related to illness and then relate that to a biological and cultural context. Epidemiology is oriented around the questions of the distribution of disease and its association with place, time, population, and behavior. The traditional methods employed in epidemiology are those of biomedical science, the use of objective measures combined with statistical relationships. Epidemiologists also consider cultural effects on illness, but often consider culture one "variable" among many that affect health and illness (DiGiacomo, 1999; Weiss, 2001). Anthropologists' methods may be qualitative or quantitative and often involve immersion, or long-term engagement in the culture under study.

4.3 The Anthropologist's Toolkit

Anthropologists use a wide variety of methods to study people within their cultural context. Anthropologists are perhaps best known for their use of participant observation in the process of doing ethnography. Participant observation is a research strategy in which the researcher spends an extended period in the research setting observing (in a number of different ways) actual day-to-day behaviors and practices (Schensul, *et al.*, 1999). Prolonged engagement in the setting allows the observer to observe daily life in a naturalistic (as opposed to laboratory) setting. It also enables the observer to "blend in," to a certain extent, thus minimizing the effect of the researcher on the observations. Ethnography is both the research process (doing ethnography) and the research product (one writes an ethnography). While doing ethnography, the researcher might conduct individual, open-ended interviews with key informants, implement community wide surveys, conduct focus groups, explore archival records (such as birth or death records), or conduct individual case studies. Historically, anthropologists conducted ethnographic work in isolated foreign cultures. More recently, however, many anthropologists study people that live side by side with people from other cultures in local or foreign settings (Inhorn and Buss, 1994; Kauffman, 1995; Higgins and Learn, 1999; Thompson and Gifford, 2000; Kane and Mason, 2001;

Monaghan, 2002; Goldman, *et al.*, 2003; Chapman, 2003; Bourgois, 2003; Larson, *et al.*, 2004; Goldman and Risica, 2004; Wind, *et al.*, 2004; Wacquant, 2004).

A main feature of much anthropologic research is its inductive character. That is, hypotheses and conclusions emerge from the data after they have been collected or during data collection. This can be contrasted with hypothetico-deductive (quantitative) research strategies that operate from an *a priori* set of assumptions about the subject matter.

4.3.1. Mixed Methods Research

Urban health research requires a combination of epidemiologic observations, ecological characterization, and a description of the lived experience of individuals living in a given environment. This type of holistic description affords opportunities for measurement and analysis at the individual level, the community level, and the macrosocial level. Thus, urban health research can benefit from a mixed methods approach (Creswell, 1995; Tashakkori and Teddlie, 1998; Creswell, *et al.*, 2003; Borkan, 2004) in which qualitative and quantitative approaches are used to study health problems. Borkan (2004) states that mixing qualitative and quantitative methods in a single study combines the benefits of generalizability with the interpretation of experience.

Data from standardized instruments may be combined with ethnographic findings to understand the nature of health disparities. Although the health inequalities between social groups are important factors affecting the practice of urban health, they are simultaneously difficult to measure, especially across locations (Murray, *et al.*, 1999). This is an important point in considering study design, as it is directly relevant to planning any study that has some comparative component. Using an anthropological approach to urban health might result in collaboration among researchers from a variety of fields, for example: medicine, biostatistics, epidemiology, anthropology, sociology, and psychology (although this is not without its problems, see Schell and Stark, 1989).

4.3.2 Examples of Mixed Methods Research

Anthropologists are joining with colleagues in other disciplines to study urban health problems using mixed methods. For example, Brett, Heimendinger, Boender and colleagues (Brett, *et al.*, 2002) conducted open-ended interviews with key informants to understand the social/structural and cultural factors that affect regular exercise and good nutrition. These data were then used to develop and test, through quantitative means, an intervention to improve diet. Goldman and colleagues conducted individual interviews with key informants to understand cultural factors that affect the likelihood of cancer screening among Dominicans and Puerto Ricans in Rhode Island (Goldman, *et al.*, 2003). This qualitative study was then coupled with quantitative screening results to understand the epidemiology of screening among diverse population groups. Goldman also used life-history interviews to understand the cultural context in which a cancer prevention intervention was developed and tested (Goldman and Risica, 2004).

The Spectrum Study is an example of a study in which a mixed methods approach was used to understand the clinical and public health implications of depression among older adults; 355 older adults (with and without depression) were followed for 12 months. Quantitative data relating to depression status, physical co-morbidities, cognitive status, personality traits, and service utilization were gathered at three time points over a 12 month period (Gallo, 1000; Bogner, 2004; Barg, *et al.*, 2004). From the original group of 355, 160 people are now participating in qualitative interviews in which they discuss and describe their own experiences with depression and their impressions of other people with depression. By taking the data from semi-structured, qualitative interviews and the results of discourse analysis, and combining these with data from existing structured, quantitative interviews, this study will help elucidate the epidemiology and experience of depression in late life, highlighting social and cultural meanings of depression among black and white American older adults. Using mixed methods helps us to understand the meanings that people associate with depression and its treatment, and to understand how those meanings might vary depending upon the time in history in which one was born, the presence or absence of depression in the family, the role that spiritual explanations play in one's understanding of depression, the concept that one has about treatment, or one's perception about the seriousness of a disease such as depression. In order for depression treatment to be adopted, it must make sense to people in the context of their everyday lives (Hohmann, 2002). A mixed methods approach that incorporates the perspective of the person experiencing the problem with the perspective of experts provides the multiple points of view and the multiple channels for intervention that will be needed to make the intervention successful.

5.0. CONCLUSION

Anthropology brings a useful suite of tools and concepts to urban health research. Mixed-methods approaches can embrace both objective and more subjective ways of understanding human adaptation to and variation within the urban context. There have been many productive interactions among anthropologists and various disciplines studying health over the course of the 20th century and into the 21st. At the beginning of the 21st century, we are poised to enhance our ability to understand urban health contexts through effective collaboration among anthropologists and other disciplines studying urban health.

REFERENCES

Acevedo-Garcia, D. (2000). Residential segregation and the epidemiology of infectious diseases. *Soc. Sci. Med.* 51:1143–1161.

Aday, L. A. (2001). *At risk in America.* Jossey-Bass Publishers, San Francisco.

Adler, S. R. (2001). Intergrating personal health belief systems: Patient-practitioner communication. In: Brady, E. (ed.), *Healing logics: culture and medicine in modern health belief systems.* Utah State University Press, Logan, UT, pp. 115-128.

Bach, J. F. (2002). The Effect of Infections on Susceptibility to Autoimmune and Allergic Diseases. *N. Engl. J. Med.* 347:911–920.

Bailey, E. J. (2000). *Medical anthropology and African American health.* Bergin & Garvey, CT.

Bamshad, M. J., and Olson, S. E. (2003). Does race exist? *Sci. Am.* 289(6):78–85.

Barg, F. K., Murray, G. M., Huss-Ashmore, R. A., Bogner, H., Wittink, M., and Gallo, J. J. (2004). Using mixed methods to understand depression in older adults. Journals of Gerontol: Social Sciences. In press.

Bell, D., and Valentine, G. (1997). *Consuming geographies: we are where we eat.* Routledge, London.

Berkman, L. F., and Clark, C. (2003). Neighborhoods and networks: The construction of safe places and bridges. In: Kawachi, I. and Berkman, L.F. (eds.), *Neighborhoods and health.* Oxford University Press, Oxford, pp. 288–302.

Bhopal, R., and Donaldson, L. (1998). White, European, Western, Caucasian, or What? Inappropriate labeling in research on race, ethnicity and health. *Am. J. Public Health* 88:1303–1307.

Bogner, H. R., Wittink, M., Merz, J. F., Straton, J., Cronholm, P., Rabins, P., and Gallo, J. J. (2004). Personal characteristics of older primary care patients who provide a buccal swab for APOE testing and banking of genetic material: The Spectrum study. In press.

Borkan, J. M. (2004). Mixed methods studies: A foundation for primary care research. *Ann. Fam. Med.* 2:4-6.

Bourgois, P. (2003). *In search of respect: Selling crack in el barrio.* Cambridge University Press, Cambridge.

Braun-Fahrlander, C., Riedler, J., Herz, U., Eder, W., Waser, M., Grize, L., Maisch, S., Carr, D., Gerlach, F., Bufe, A., Lauener, R. P., Schierl, R., Renz, H., Nowak, D., and von Mutius, E. (2002). Environmental exposure to Endotoxin and its relation to asthma in school-age children. *N. Engl. J. Med.* 347:869–877.

Brett, J. A., Heimendinger, J., Boender, C., Morin, C., and Marshall, J. A. (2002). Using ethnography to improve intervention design. *Am. J. Health Promot.* 16:331-340.

Burchard, E. G., Ziv, E., Coyle, N., Gomez, S. L., Tang, H., Karter, A. J., Mountain, J. L., Pérez-Stable, E. J., Sheppard, D., and Risch, N. (2003). The importance of race and ethnic background in biomedical research and clinical practice. *N. Engl. J. Med.* 348:1170–1175.

Campbell, B. G., and Loy, J. D. (2000). *Humankind emerging.* Allyn and Bacon, Boston.

Centers for Disease Control and Prevention. (2003). Self-reported concern about food security associated with obesity – Washington, 1995-1999. *MMWR.* 52:840–842.

Chang, H. C., and Hermann, E. R. (1974). Acoustical study of a rapid transit system. *AIHA. J.* 35:640-653.

Chapman, R. R. (2003). Endangering safe motherhood in Mozambique: prenatal care as pregnancy risk. *Soc. Sci. Med.* 57:355–374.

Cooper, R. (2000). A note on the biological concept of race and its application in epidemiologic research. In: LaVeist, T. (ed.), *Race, Ethnicity, and Health.* Jossey Bass, San Francisco, pp. 99–114

Creswell, J. W. (1995). *Research design: Qualitative and quantitative approaches.* Sage Publications, Inc., CA.

Creswell, J. W., Clark, V. L. P., Gutmann, M. L., and Hanson, W. E. (2003). Advanced mixed methods research designs. In: Tashakkori, A, and Teddlie C. (eds.). *Handbook of mixed methods in social and behavioral research.* Sage Publications, Inc., CA, pp. 209–240.

DiGiacomo, S. (1999). Can there be a cultural epidemiology? *Med. Anthropol. Q.* 13:436–483.

Dressler, W. (1999). Modernization, stress, and blood pressure. *Hum. Biol.* 71(4):583–605.

Dressler, W. W., and Bindon, J. R. (2000). The health consequences of cultural consonance: Cultural dimensions of lifestyle, social support, and arterial blood pressure in an African American community. *Am. Anthropol.* 102:244–260.

Drewnowski, A. (1999). Fat and sugar in the global diet: dietary diversity in the nutrition transition. In: Grew, R. (ed.), *Food in global history.* Westview Press, Colorado, pp. 194-206.

Epstein, P. R., and Rogers, C. (2004). Inside the greenhouse: The impacts of CO_2 and climate change on public health in the inner city. Center for health and the global environment, Harvard Medical School, MA.

Evans, G. W. (2003). The built environment and mental health. *J. Urban Health* 80:536–555.

Fidell, S. (1978). Nationwide urban noise survey. *J. Acoust. Soc. Am.* 64:198–215.

Fullilove, M. T. (1998). Comment: Abandoning "race" as a variable in public health research – An idea whose time has come. *Am. J. Public Health* 88:1297–1298.

Fullilove, M. T. (2001). Root shock: the consequences of African American dispossession. *J. Urban Health* 78:72–80.

Gallo, J. J., Bogner, H. R., Straton, J. B., Margo, K., Lesho, P., Rabins, P. V., and Ford, D. E. (2004). Patient characteristics associated with participation in a practice-based study of depression in late life: The Spectrum study. *Int. J. Gen. Psychiatry* In press.

Goffman, E. (1959). *The presentation of self in everyday life.* Doubleday, New York.

Goldman, R., Hunt, M. K., Allen, J. D., Hauser, S., Emmons, K., Maeda, M., and Sorenson, G. (2003). The life history interview method: applications to intervention development. *Health Educ. Behav.* 30:564–581.

Goldman, R. E., and Risica, P. M. (2004). Perceptions of breast and cervical cancer risk and screening among Dominicans and Puerto Ricans in Rhode Island. *Ethn. Dis.* 14:32–42.

Gomez-Beloz, A., and Chavez, N. (2001). The botanica as a culturally appropriate health care option for Latinos. *Journal of Alternative and Complementary Medicine* 7:537–546.

Higgins, P. G., and Learn, C. D. (1999). Health practices of adult Hispanic women. *J. Adv. Nurs.* 29: 1105–1112.

Hohmann, A. A. (2002). Community based intervention research: Coping with the "noise" of real life in study design. *Am. J. Psychiatry* 159:201–207.

Huss-Ashmore, R., and Behrman, C. (1999). Transitional environments: health and the perception of permanence in urban micro-environments. In: Schell, L.M., and Ulijaszek, S.J. (eds.), *Urbanism, Health and Human Biology in Industrialized Countries.* Cambridge University Press, Cambridge, pp. 67–84.

Inhorn, M. C., and Buss, K. A. (1994). Ethnography, epidemiology and infertility in Egypt. *Soc. Sci. Med.* 39:671–666.

Johnston, F. E. (1993). The urban disadvantage in the developing world and the physical and mental growth of children. In: Schell, L.M., Smith, M.T., and Bilsborough, A. (eds.), *Urban ecology and health in the Third World.* Cambridge University Press, Cambridge, pp. 26–37.

Johnston, F. E., and Gordon-Larsen, P. (1999). Poverty, nutrition, and obesity in the USA. In: Schell, L.M., and Ulijaszek, S.J. (eds.), *Urbanism, health, and human biology in industrialised countries.* Cambridge University Press, Cambridge, pp. 192–209.

Kai, J., and Drinkwater, C. (2004). *Primary care in disadvantaged communities.* Radcliffe Medical Press, United Kingdom.

Kane, S., and Mason, T. (2001). AIDS and criminal justice. *Annu. Rev. Anthropol.* 30:457–479.

Kauffman, K. S. (1995). Center as haven: Findings of an urban ethnography. *Nurs. Res.* 44:231–236.

Kleinman, A. (1980). *Patients and healers in the context of culture: An exploration of the borderland between anthropology, medicine, and psychiatry.* University of California Press, California.

Knauss, D. (2002). Noise mapping and annoyance. *Noise Health* 4:7–11.

Lambert, H., and McKevitt, C. (2002). Anthropology in health research: from qualitative methods to multidisciplinarity. *BMJ.* 325:210–213.

Larson, A., Bell, M., and Young, A. F. (2004). Clarifying the relationships between health and residential mobility. *Soc. Sci. Med.* 59:2149–2160.

LaVeist, T. A., and Wallace, J. M. Jr. (2000). Health risk and inequitable distribution of liquor stores in African American neighborhood. *Soc. Sci. Med.* 51:613–617.

Lewontin, R. C. (1972). The apportionment of human diversity. *Evol Bio.* 6:381–389.

Link, B. G., Northridge, M. E., Phelan, J. C., and Ganz, M. L. (1998). Social epidemiology and the fundamental cause concept: on the structuring of effective cancer screens by socioeconomic status. *Milbank Q.* 76:375–402.

Litt, J. S., and Burke, T. A. (2002). Uncovering the historic environmental hazards of urban brownfields. *J. Urban Health* 79:464–481.

Martin, E. (1984). Primary care in two cultures. *J. R. Soc. Med.* 77:379–383.

Matheson, M. P., Stansfeld, S. A., and Haines, M. M. (2003). The effects of chronic aircraft noise exposure on children's cognition and health: 3 field studies. *Noise Health* 5:31–40.

Miranda, J., Nakamura, R., and Bernal, G. (2003). Including ethnic minorities in mental health intervention research: A practical approach to a long standing problem. *Culture, Medicine & Psychiatry* 27:467–486.

Monaghan, L. F. (2002). Opportunity, pleasure, and risk -An ethnography of urban male heterosexualities. J. *Contemp. Ethnogr.* 31:440–477.

Morland, K., Wing, S., Diez Roux, A., and Poole, C. (2002). Neighborhood characteristics associated with the location of food stores and food service places. *Am. J. Prev. Med.* 22:23–29.

Murray, C. J. L., Gakidou, E. E., and Frenk, J. (1999). Health inequalities and social group differences: what should we measure? *Bull. World Health Organ.* 77:537–543.

Nguyen, V.K., and Peschard, K. (2003). Anthropology, inequality, and disease: A review. *Annu. Rev. Anthropol.* 32:447–474.

Obrist, B. (2003). Urban health in daily practice: livelihood, vulnerability and resilience in Dar es Salaam, Tanzania. *Anthropology & Medicine* 10:275–290.

Obrist, B., Tanner, M., and Harpham, T. (2003a). Engaging anthropology in urban health research: issues and prospects. *Anthropology & Medicine* 10:362–371.

Obrist, B., van Eeuwijk, P., and Weiss, M. G. (2003b). Health anthropology and urban health research. *Anthropology & Medicine* 10:267-274.

Osborne, N. G., and Feit, M. D. (1992). The use of race in medical research. *JAMA.* 267:275–279.

Owens, K. and King, M. C. (1999). Genomic views of human history. *Science* 286:451–453.

Pachter, L. M., Sumner, T., Fontan, A., Sneed, M., and Bernstein, B. A. (1998). Home-based therapies for the common cold among European American and ethnic minority families: the interface between alternative/complementary and folk medicine. *Archives of Pediatric and Adolescent Medicine* 152:1083–1088.

Panel on DHHS Collection of Race and Ethnicity Data. (2004). *Eliminating Health Disparities: Measurement and Data Needs.* National Academies Press, Washington, D.C.

Panel on ethnic and racial disparities in medical care convened by Physicians for Human Rights. (2003). The right to equal treatment: An action plan to end racial and ethnic disparities in clinical diagnosis and treatment in the United States. Boston, MA.

Parkar, S. R., Fernandes, J., and Weiss, M. G. (2003). Contextualizing mental health: gendered experiences in a Mumbai slum. *Anthropology & Medicine* 10:291–308.

Plotkin, S. R., and Post, R. (1999). Folk remedy use in the inner city. *South Med. J.* 92:795–798.

Pollard, T. M. (1999). Urbanism and psychosocial stress. In: Schell, L.M. and Ulijaszek, S.J. (eds.), *Urbanism, Health and Human Biology in Industrialised Countries.* Cambridge University Press, Cambridge, pp. 231–2249.

Ramirez, A. G. (2003). Consumer-provider communication research with special populations. *Patient. Educ. Couns.* 50:51–54.

Satterthwaite, D. (2000). Will most people live in cities? *BMJ.* 321:1143–1145.

Schell, L. (1997). Culture as a stressor: A revised model of biocultural interaction. *Am. J. Phys. Anthropol.* 102:67–77.

Schell, L. M., and Denham, M. (2003). Environmental pollution in urban environments and human biology. *Annu. Rev. Anthropol.* 32:111–134.

Schell, L. M., and Stark, A. D. (1989). Biomedical anthropology in a multidisciplinary, multi-institutional research project: the Albany lead study. *Med. Anthropol. Q.* 3:385–394.

Schell, L. M., and Ulijaszek, S. J. (1999). Urbanism, urbanisation, health and human biology: an introduction. In: Schell, L.M. and Ulijaszek, S.J. (eds.), *Urbanism, Health, and Human Biology in Industrialised Countries.* Cambridge University Press, Cambridge, pp. 3–20.

Schensul, S. L., Schensul, J. J., and LeCompte, M. D. (1999). *Essential Ethnographic Methods.* Alta Mira Press, California.

Sloane, D. C., Diamant, A. L., Lewis, L. B., Yancey, A. K., Flynn, G., Nascimento, L. M., McCarthy, W. J., Guinyard, J. J., Cousineau, M. R., and for the REACH Coalition of the African American Building a Legacy of Health Project. (2003). Improving the nutritional resource environment for healthy living through community-based participatory research. *J. Gen. Intern. Med.* 18:568–575.

Sobal, J. (1999). Food system globalization, eating transformations, and nutrition transitions. In: Grew, R (ed.), *Food in global history.* Westview Press, Colorado, pp. 171–193.

Tashakkori, A., and Teddlie, C. (1998). *Mixed Methodology.* Sage Publications, Inc., California.

Thompson, S. J. and Gifford, S. M. (2000). Trying to keep a balance: The meaning of health and diabetes in an urban Aboriginal community. *Soc. Sci. Med.* 51:1457–1472.

Tobias, A., Diaz, J., Saez, M., and Alberdi, J. C. (2001). Use of poisson regression and box-jenkins models to evaluate the short-term effects of environmental noise levels on daily emergency admissions in Madrid. *Eur. J. Epidemiol.* 17:765–71.

Trostle, J. A., and Sommerfeld, J. (1996). Medical anthropology and epidemiology. *Annu. Rev. Anthropol.* 25:253–274.

Ulijaszek, S. J. (1999). Physical activity, lifestyle and health of urban populations. In Schell, L.M. and Uliaszek S.J. (eds.), *Urbansim, Health and Human Biology in Industrialised Countries.* Cambridge University Press, Cambridge, pp. 250–279.

van Eeuwijk, P. (2003). Urban elderly with chronic illness: local understandings and emerging discrepancies in North Sulawesi, Indonesia. *Anthropology & Medicine.* 10:325–341.

Vlahov, D., and Galea, S. (2002). Urbanization, urbanicity, and health. *J. Urban Health* 79:S1-S12.

Wacquant, L. J. D. (2004). *Body & Soul: Notebooks of an Apprentice Boxer.* Oxford University Press, Oxford.

Weiss, M. G. (2001). Cultural epidemiology: an introduction and overview. *Anthropology & Medicine* 8:5–29.

Weiss, S. T. (2002). Eat dirt – The hygiene hypothesis and allergic diseases. *N. Engl. J. Med.* 347:930–931.

Wiebel, W. W. (1988). Combining ethnographic and epidemiologic methods in targeted AIDS interventions: the Chicago model. *NIDA. Res. Monogr.* 80:137–150.

Wind, S., Van Sickle, D., and Wright, A. L. (2004). Health, place and childhood asthma in southwest Alaska. *Soc. Sci. Med.* 58:75–88.

Wright, R. J., and Fischer, E. B. (2003). Putting asthma into context: Community influences on risk, behavior, and interventions. In: Kawachi, I., and Berkman, L.F. (eds.), *Neighborhoods and Health.* Oxford University Press, Oxford, pp. 233–264.

Wylie, J. L., and Wagenfeld-Heintz, E. (2004). Development of relationship-centered care. *Journal of Healthcare Quality* 26:14–21.

Chapter 14

Epidemiology and Urban Health Research

Sandro Galea and David Vlahov

1.0. WHAT IS EPIDEMIOLOGY AND WHAT ROLE CAN IT PLAY IN URBAN HEALTH RESEARCH?

"Epidemiology" is derived from the Medieval Latin term "*epidemia*," meaning an epidemic, and reflects the origins of epidemiology as the discipline concerned with tracking and controlling disease epidemics. Modern epidemiology has expanded its scope and many definitions for epidemiology have been suggested, some at odds with one another (Swinton, 2004). Most epidemiologists might characterize their discipline as the study of the distribution of disease and of the causes (or determinants) of that distribution (Lilienfeld, 1978). Congruent with this definition, the American Heritage Dictionary defines epidemiology as "The branch of medicine that deals with the study of the causes, distribution, and control of disease in populations" (American Heritage Dictionary, 2000). Therefore epidemiology provides the empiric tools that inform both medicine and public health and epidemiologic method are critical to the study of disease distribution, cause, and subsequently control.

Broadly speaking, we can think of two principal roles for epidemiology. First is a descriptive role, often referred to as disease surveillance. Here epidemiology helps to describe the frequency of disease, both overall, but also in different groups, including, for example, gender, race/ethnicity, geographic groups, or over time. Description of disease is a critical function epidemiology plays to inform public health policy and practice. For example, the recent documentation of the growing prevalence of obesity throughout the U.S. has fuelled national interest in the obesity epidemic and the development of national and regional initiatives aimed at reducing obesity and associated morbidity (Katz, 2003; Wang, *et al.*, 2002). In local public health departments, epidemiologic surveillance of infectious diseases serves to identify infectious disease outbreaks, a core function of both local and federal public health agencies.

Second, epidemiology plays a critical role in understanding disease etiology, or identifying causes of diseases. Classically, epidemiology has concerned itself with identifying different factors, often called "exposures" or "risk factors" that are associated with categorical disease outcomes. Both observational and experimental methods have been employed to this end. Historic examples of this include the identification of smoking as a risk factor for lung cancer and cardiovascular disease and the absence of folic acid as a risk factor for neonatal neural tube defects. In the context of public health practice, epidemiology contributes methods that aid in the search for causes of infectious disease epidemics. For example, outbreak investigations include both the description of the increase in incidence of a particular disease and also the search for the cause, or of the mechanisms of transmission of a well-known cause, of the same disease. Both these traditional roles of epidemiology have concerned themselves with individual disease expression and with the individual factors (including behaviors or exposures to toxins or other possibly harmful substances) that contribute to the development of disease.

Recently there has been an expansion in the role of epidemiology both in terms of the outcomes as well as with the exposures of interest. In terms of outcomes, epidemiologists have broadened their scope to consider not only disease but also health and well-being. In addition, there has been increasing interest in considering the health of populations, not simply of individuals, and in understanding that population health is not an aggregate of the health of independent individuals, but rather a product of inter-dependent individuals who influence one another's health and disease status (Koopman and Lynch, 1999). In terms of exposures or risk factors, modern epidemiologic thinking has expanded its scope beyond intrinsic individual factors or behaviors to consider factors exogenous to the individual (e.g., socio-economic status), individual inter-connections (e.g., social networks and social supports), and contextual factors that are not characteristics of any one individual (e.g., social capital) (Kaplan, 1999). In broadening its scope to include these factors modern epidemiology has made its task, the description or characterization of states of health and the determinants of those states, considerably more complex than it was a few decades ago. The development of epidemiologic methods (e.g., regression techniques, hierarchical analysis) that can account for increasing analytic complexity both has made it possible to meet the challenges introduced by this broader scope and raised new questions in its own right (Oakes, 2003).

As discussed in many chapters in this book, the study of urban health encompasses a broad range of questions, exploiting, and challenging the epidemiologic armamentarium. In this chapter we will first discuss the different perspectives that have been employed in the epidemiologic literature that explores questions relevant to urban health, second we will consider various aspects of epidemiologic techniques and how they can be applied to questions in urban health, and third we will discuss key challenges facing epidemiology in the study of urban health. We will conclude with directions for epidemiologic inquiry in urban health. We note that we do not here attempt to explain epidemiologic methods, instead referring the reader to standard epidemiologic textbooks for explanation of epidemiologic techniques (Rothman and Greenland, 1998; Gordis, 2000). Instead, we consider how epidemiologic approaches may illuminate questions in urban health research and potentially guide intervention. This chapter draws on our other published work that presents some of the issues discussed here in more detail (we refer the reader to Galea and Vlahov, 2004; Galea, *et al.*, 2005; Galea and Schulz, 2006).

In order to illuminate some of the points being made in this chapter, we will refer throughout to an example that we hope will be illustrative of the role epidemiologic methods can play in urban health research. Recently, there has been growing interest in the possible role that the built environment may play in shaping health (Jackson, 2003). For example, specific features of the built environment including density of development, mix of land uses, scale of streets, aesthetic qualities of place, and connectivity of street networks, may affect physical activity (Handy, *et al.*, 2002). In turn, low levels of physical activity are a well-established risk factor for cardiovascular disease and all-cause mortality in urban areas (Diez-Roux, 2003; Pate, *et al.*, 1995). Other work has shown that a deteriorating built environment is associated with greater incidence of sexually transmitted diseases (Cohen, *et al.*, 2000). Considering the role of the built environment is clearly a priority of studies that consider the relations between living in urban areas and health. Several chapters in this book discuss the multiple potential roles of the built environment in shaping health. Heavily built environments are the hallmarks of many urban areas, and urban residents are in greater contact with the built environment on a daily basis than are non-urban residents. Therefore, if the built environment is a determinant of human health it is likely to play an important role in shaping the health of urban populations. We will consider different aspects of questions related to the urban built environment and health throughout this chapter.

2.0. DIFFERENT PERSPECTIVES ON THE EPIDEMIOLOGIC STUDY OF URBAN HEALTH

The study of urban health thus far has fallen to work in multiple different disciplines, each employing methods that are particular to a specific field. Epidemiologic methods have been employed in some of this work, occasionally in concert with methods from other disciplines. However, in general, we can consider three types of studies that have applied epidemiologic methods to address questions relevant to urban health. These are: studies comparing rural and urban communities, studies comparing cities within countries or across countries, and studies examining intra-urban (e.g., neighborhood) variations in health. We will discuss each of these types of studies briefly highlighting the methodological issues inherent to each type of study.

Until recently, studies that have compared rates and prevalence of morbidity and mortality in urban and rural areas were probably the most common application of epidemiologic techniques to urban health, although these studies have become less common in recent years. Following the two different roles of epidemiology discussed earlier, these urban vs. rural comparisons largely fall in the category of descriptive, or surveillance, epidemiology. These studies typically contrast several urban areas with rural areas in the same country, or consider morbidity and mortality in urban vs. non-urban areas, the latter frequently being defined as all areas that do not meet "urban" criteria. These studies are typically cross-sectional studies, considering both the characteristics of the urban and rural areas and the prevalence of morbidity and mortality rate at one point in time. These studies are best suited to address questions about *whether or not urban areas are characterized by different burden of disease than are non-urban areas.* Such urban-rural or urban-non-urban comparisons may also draw attention to particular features of urban areas that may be associated with health and that merit investigation. However, these studies are limited in their ability to shed light on what these features may be and on how urban areas may affect the health of the residents within them.

Considering the example introduced earlier about assessing the role of the built environment in shaping health, urban-rural comparisons can shed little light on whether the built environment actually is associated with a particular morbidity. Urban-rural comparisons could be employed to assess if cardiovascular disease is more prevalent in urban verses rural areas (e.g. Keil, *et al.*, 1985). For example, a study could collect data from several urban and non-urban areas and compare cardiovascular disease mortality between the two types of areas. Demonstrating that there is a higher prevalence of cardiovascular disease mortality in urban areas then might alert us to something about the urban context that may predispose urban residents to higher cardiovascular disease than their non-urban counterparts. However, urban-rural comparisons are not able to suggest whether it is the built environment, or other characteristics of urban areas (e.g., air pollution) that are contributing to cardiovascular disease. More sophisticated analyses are needed to attempt to deduce reasons for any observed urban-rural difference in morbidity.

Given these limitations, that different urban-rural comparisons have provided conflicting evidence about the relative burden of disease in urban and non-urban areas is not surprising (Galea and Vlahov, 2004). Changing conditions within cities over time, and differences in living conditions between cities suggest that at best these studies provide a crude snapshot of how the mass of urban living conditions at one point in time may be affecting population health. These studies may be most relevant in areas where urbanization is still proceeding rapidly (e.g., China or India), helping public health officials to predict changing national health profiles as the proportion of the population living in urban areas increases (e.g., Zhao, 1993).

The second type of study that attempts to address how cities affect health involves comparisons of health between cities, either within a country or between countries (e.g., Levine, *et al.*, 1989). Using the city itself as the key unit of analysis, these studies compare different cities in order to reach conclusions about urban characteristics associated with health. Although these studies can play a surveillance role, they also may begin to generate etiologic hypotheses that may explain *why* differences in health and disease exist between urban areas. These studies contribute to the ability to discern features of cities that may promote or harm population health and may suggest practices at the city level that are amenable to intervention that improves population health. These studies are best suited to ask *which characteristics of cities as a whole may be associated with specific health-related outcomes.* Returning to our running example, cross-urban comparisons can test associations between the quality of the built environment and health in cities. Therefore, a study that collects information about the quality of buildings in different cities and then uses statistical testing to determine if there is an association between quality of buildings in a city and the prevalence of sexually transmitted diseases can suggest that the quality of the built environment may influence behavior, or facilitate disease transmission. Urban-urban comparisons also can be used to assess inter-urban differences in health service delivery and to assess the relations between these differences and health outcomes (Rodwin and Gusmano, 2002). Comparisons of health risk factors within three cities in China (Beijing, Shanghai, and Hong Kong) have shown different risk profiles between cities (Fu and Fung, 2004).

However, by considering the city as the unit of analytic interest, these studies implicitly assume that aggregate behaviors or characteristics at the city level are equally important for all residents of those cities. This limits the consideration of how cities may affect the health of urban residents to an analysis of city-wide characteristics that may, or may not, affect all urban residents equally. In addition, demonstrated cross-sectional disparity in risk factors and morbidity between urban areas may equally be due to some causal difference in the urban context as it may be due to other factors, such as selective migration in specific cities. Epidemiologic methods, including stratification, restriction, or regression modeling can be applied to adjust for such potential confounders. However, even after adjustment for confounding, observed urban-urban disparities may not necessarily reflect a relation between the urban context and individual health. Inference documented through ecologic studies cannot be extended to the individual-level and as such, these studies cannot be used to infer relations between the urban context and the health of individuals (this has been referred to as the "ecologic fallacy"; see Lilienfeld, 1983; Diez-Roux, 2000).

A third group of studies has employed epidemiologic techniques and has contributed to our understanding of how city living may affect health. This group of studies has become more common in the past decade and has frequently included studies of how living in particular urban communities may be associated with health. Most commonly, these studies focus on spatial groupings of individuals (typically conceived as "neighborhoods", although several studies assess the contribution of administrative groupings that are not necessarily meaningful to residents as neighborhoods) and typically consider the role of one's community of residence within an urban area on individual health. *These studies then are suited to assessing questions related to which characteristics of areas within cities may be associated with individual health.* These studies are more suited to considering questions of disease etiology than are any of the two other study designs discussed here. Returning to the example of the built environment, several studies have shown that the quality of neighborhood sidewalks is associated with the likelihood of physical activity among urban residents (Sharpe, *et al.*, 2004; De Bourdeaudhuij, *et al.*, 2003). Intra-urban analyses may thus assess how the quality of buildings in one's neighborhood of residence is associated with individual health behavior or disease status. In addition, and importantly, multi-level analytic techniques can allow the consideration of these associations while taking into account both potential group-level and individual-level confounders. Although this work by and large has thus far been carried out using cross-sectional study designs, recent work has employed other epidemiologic study designs including case-control studies and longitudinal studies to test multi-level hypotheses (Galea, *et al.*, 2003a; Windle, *et al.*, 2004; Sundquist, *et al.*, 2004; Marinacci, *et al.* 2004). These study designs, as discussed later, allow us to avoid problems with reverse causality that are inherent to cross-sectional study designs. However, it is important to note that while these studies contribute important insights about urban conditions and their implications for health they may be difficult to generalize to other cities, or to urban areas more broadly.

3.0. EPIDEMIOLOGY AND URBAN HEALTH

Multiple epidemiologic methods lend themselves to the study of urban health and, as discussed above, different methods may be more applicable to different questions in the field. We discuss here three epidemiologic approaches to questions that may pertain to the study of urban health and then present particular considerations that may influence both the choice of epidemiologic method employed and the interpretation of results from the studies employing each of these methods.

3.1. Epidemiologic Approaches

A number of epidemiologic approaches can be used to examine urban health issues. Here we present three broad approaches, namely, ecological, contextual, and hierarchical approaches. The purpose of these analyses is to identify factors associated with place (i.e., cities) that can affect the health of urban residents.

Ecologic analyses consider associations between factors at the group or aggregate level. For example, ecologic analyses can consider the association between population density and all-cause mortality rates across cities. Simple correlations can suggest features of cities that co-vary with measures of population health at the city level while more sophisticated techniques such as regression analyses can consider how particular factors co-vary with others while accounting for the contribution of potentially important variables. Ecologic analyses provide an opportunity to document how characteristics of cities are related to population health in the aggregate and have historically been the primary method used in urban-rural and inter-urban comparisons discussed above (e.g., Schouten, *et al.*, 1996; Douste-Blazy, *et al.*, 1988; Hersh, *et al.*, 1992). The primary current use of ecologic analyses in the study of urban health is to generate hypotheses about features of cities that may affect health; in the context of the examples discussed above, urban-rural and urban-urban comparisons typically make use of ecologic analyses. Returning to our running example, ecologic analyses can assess whether availability of park space is associated with the prevalence of cardiovascular disease mortality in city neighborhoods.

However, ecologic analyses, while potentially useful in identifying features of cities that may shape population health, have limited usefulness in determining *how* these characteristics of cities may be associated with individual health. Causal inferences at the individual level cannot be drawn from ecological associations. For example, ecologic observation that show cities with lower availability of park space have higher cardiovascular disease mortality rates say little about the individual use of park space, or individual exercise patterns, and whether there are causal links between access to park space, health behavior, and cardiovascular disease mortality. This inability to draw cross-level inference limits interpretations that can be drawn from ecologic observations. However, ecologic analyses will probably continue to play a role in urban health primarily in hypothesis generation and in suggesting characteristics of cities that may influence population health. Ecologic analyses are not limited to inter-urban comparisons, but can equally generate hypotheses about features of intra-urban units that may shape population health (e.g., neighborhoods, social networks).

Contextual analyses assess how urban living, as a characteristic of the individual, is associated with health. Contextual analyses, together with ecologic analyses, have been most commonly employed in the studies of urban vs. rural (or non-urban) health discussed above. Thus, contextual analyses attribute to the individual a variable that represents whether or not one lives in an urban vs. rural context and then analytic methods, ranging from contingency tables to regression analyses, are applied to determine if an individual's likelihood of having a particular health status (including the presence or absence of disease or morbidity from a particular disease) is higher or lower in urban individuals compared to non-urban individuals. Contextual analyses consider urban as a variable with a fixed effect on individuals, i.e., that the urban variable has the same effect on all individuals in an analysis. Simple methods can consider the association of the urban variable with health status without controlling for the role of other potentially confounding or modifying variables, while more sophisticated methods (e.g., Mantel-Haenzel adjustment, multiple regression) can assess the role of the urban variable while taking into account other potentially important variables (e.g., gender). Extending the park space analysis discussed above, contextual analyses can attribute to the individual an area-level variable representing urban park space availability and can assess if this variable is associated with individual risk of cardiovascular disease while controlling for potential individual behaviors or characteristics that may confound the relation of interest.

Although relatively common in urban health research, the inferences that can be drawn from contextual analyses about how urban living can affect health are limited. Contextual analyses assume that the import of a given urban characteristics in a given city is the same for all individuals in the analyses. This obscures the fact that some individuals may have more or less *access* to the park pace that is available to everyone. Access to park space may be determined by individual proximity to such space, socio-economic barriers to park space use, or any number of factors that are not accounted for by the attribution of a simple measure of park space availability to all individuals equally in an analysis. Overall urban contextual analyses fail to provide insight into *how* cities may affect health and contextual analyses within cities remain limited to an assessment of a few key variables in isolation. As such, the role of contextual analyses in urban health studies is limited primarily to descriptive summaries of the burden of health in specific urban contexts. While this may be useful in advancing urban health as a topic for investigation or intervention, contextual analyses has limited utility in scientific inquiry that attempt to understand disease etiology.

Relatively new to the study of urban health, multilevel analyses allow the consideration of how characteristics of cities, or of units within cities, contribute to individual health independent of the contribution of other individual and contextual variables. For a full review of the methods behind multilevel analyses we refer the reader to other published work (Diez-Roux, 2001; Langford, *et al.*, 1999). Specific considerations with respect to multilevel urban studies are discussed in the next chapter ("Design and analysis of group (or neighborhood) level urban studies") in this book. In brief, multilevel analyses consider the contribution of variables at multiple levels to the variability in a particular individual-level dependent variable. In its simplest application to urban health, a multilevel analysis uses data from individuals in multiple cities (or from multiple areas within a city) to consider whether city living independently explains inter-individual variability in health status after controlling for other relevant individual characteristics. More useful to the study of urban health however is the consideration of how different *characteristics* of urban living at multiple levels may be associated with health. For example, multilevel analysis can test whether social capital at the city level is associated with individual mental health while controlling for social ties at the neighborhood level and for individual characteristics (Kawachi and Berkman, 2001). In our running example, multilevel analysis can be used to test whether living in neighborhoods characterized by deteriorating buildings is associated with individual behavior or disease outcomes while taking into account individual demographic characteristics.

Multilevel analyses also allow the investigator to consider the possibility that urban living has a different effect on individuals in different urban communities by introducing random slopes that allow for variable strengths of the association between urban characteristics and health. For example, multilevel analyses may show that the salutary effect of green space is different in different areas of a particular city (Takano, *et al*,. 2002; Tanaka, *et al*,. 1996). Therefore, multilevel methods allow for the analysis of how characteristics of urban living may affect health and how these associations may differ in different urban communities, taking into account factors at other levels that may be important determinants of health. If applied in inter-urban datasets, multilevel methods can assess the role of city-level variables as well as of variables at different levels within cities. These methods hold much promise in urban health research.

3.2. Study Design

The three broad categories of epidemiologic methods discussed here can be applied in a variety of different contexts and in conjunction with multiple study designs. There are several considerations, pertaining both to the particular research questions of interest and to each of the analytic methods discussed here, that merit discussion as we consider the role of epidemiologic methods in urban health.

The methods summarized above may be applied to several study designs. Cross-sectional studies are the basis of most of the existing urban vs. non-urban contextual analyses and also represent the most common study design for multilevel analyses. The ubiquity of cross-sectional study designs primarily reflects the fact that cross-sectional studies are easier and less expensive to design and execute than longitudinal studies. Also, analyses relevant to urban health have tended to rely on publicly available community level indicators to characterize urban and intra-urban areas and as such are constrained by the fact that these data are usually collected at infrequent intervals. Multilevel analytic methods while comfortably developed for cross sectional analyses have been somewhat more complicated for prospective data that involves possible changes at each and across all levels. However, longitudinal study designs are becoming more important to advance hypothesis testing in urban health (e.g., Molnar, *et al.*, 2004). While cross-sectional studies can document associations between characteristics of urban living and health, they cannot provide information about the temporal relations between characteristics of urban areas and the onset of disease, an essential step in causal inference. For example, a cross-sectional multilevel study can establish that living in urban neighborhoods characterized by a deteriorating built environment is *associated* with greater sexual risk behavior (Cohen, *et al.*, 2000), but cannot establish that the urban built environment *causes* riskier behavior. It is equally plausible that persons who engage in risky sexual behavior migrate to neighborhoods where deteriorating buildings are the norm (and are potentially cheaper to live in). Longitudinal studies (or well-designed case control studies that mimic longitudinal studies through careful control selection) are needed to advance thinking about how urban characteristics may cause different health behaviors and outcomes and ultimately to suggest which urban characteristics can fruitfully be subject to intervention. It is also worth noting that new research suggests that longitudinal research that takes into consideration life course perspectives, i.e., how exposures in one's early life may affect subsequent health, (Lawlor, *et al.*, 2003) may have a particular contribution to make in considering the role of urban living in shaping population health.

More challenging, but potentially even more useful, experimental studies that manipulate characteristics of the urban environment in a controlled fashion can help isolate and establish how features of the urban environment may affect health. Although examples of experimental studies in urban health are uncommon, a few examples have shown promising results. For example, in Chicago, specific housing projects were landscaped while others were not, through a natural experiment, and investigators were able to show that persons living in the upgraded housing projects had improved functioning, fewer episodes of interpersonal violence, and better concentration than persons in the control group (Kuo, 2003). Such studies can convincingly demonstrate the role that particular aspects of the urban environment play in shaping health and, perhaps more importantly, identify avenues for intervention.

Important considerations in selecting a study design are limitations regarding sample size and the statistical power available for multilevel or intra-urban analyses. The size of the analytic sample both at the individual level and at the group level becomes a relevant concern for multi-level designs. Power calculations for multilevel analyses remain limited, but it is clear that in order to carry out meaningful comparisons of the role of group-level variables, sufficient numbers of groups must be included for a particular study, requiring larger study samples and more complex study designs (Hoover, 2002).

3.3. Analytic Considerations

Epidemiologic analyses frequently rest on translating broad concepts into operational variables that can then be analyzed using some of the methods discussed earlier. Although this is true of all quantitative analyses it may be a particularly important issue in urban health studies. In urban health studies variables need to be specified that represent complicated constructs often with varying meaning in different contexts. "Urban", while referred to throughout this chapter as a potential variable of interest, is challenging to define, and definitions vary between countries and between studies (Galea and Vlahov, 2004). This variation limits inter-study comparisons and generalizations. Clear and reproducible definitions of urban may facilitate such comparisons. More saliently, specification of the "exposures" of interest is a critical issue in all quantitative urban health research. Throughout this chapter we have discussed how constructs at multiple levels (e.g., qualities of the built environment, social ties) may be assessed in urban health studies. Several chapters in this book elaborate further about what these constructs are and how they may influence health. Recognizing that the role of specific constructs may be different across urban contexts makes the careful specification of the key exposures of interest critical. Therefore, while we encourage consideration of multiple levels of potential influence in the urban context, we also note that more work needs to be done on appropriate specification of important urban constructs before convincing quantitative work can assess whether these constructs influence health.

Another consideration in thinking about quantitative analyses in urban health pertains to the complexity of urban living as a variable of interest. We discussed earlier how contextual urban vs. non-urban analyses are frequently not replicable, probably reflecting the complexity of each individual urban setting and the inability of a single "urban" variable to summarize multiple relevant dimensions. However, summarizing all the variables of interest in the urban context can be daunting and fully representing the key relations between urban constructs that shape health beyond the capability of commonly used analytic techniques. It is likely that many characteristics of cities affect health by modifying the effect of other factors that are causally linked to health. For example, transportation routes may not be causally linked to cardiac arrest survival, but the efficacy of emergency medical services systems in reducing cardiac arrest mortality may be different in neighborhoods with easy ambulance access compared to neighborhoods that do not have easy ambulance access. Studies that are adequately powered to detect effect modification across levels need to have larger sample sizes than conventional studies aimed strictly at detecting associations.

In addition to the modifying role that characteristics of cities may play, characteristics of cities at different levels may also mediate or confound relations between other characteristics and health. For example, while municipal-level spending on public hospitals within a city may be associated with health in the aggregate, it is likely that this relation is modified by baseline quality of care in the public hospitals and mediated by access that persons with substantial morbidity have to hospital care. This latter consideration reflects the complex causal chain that most accurately reflects how urban characteristics may influence health. Ultimately, most epidemiologic analyses in urban health and across disciplines rely on assumptions of linearity for hypothesis testing. However, in complex systems, non-linear associations are common. The application of innovative methods that take into account non-linear relations may be particularly important in considering how cities may affect health (e.g., qualitative loop analysis, see Levins and Lopez, 1999).

4.0. KEY CHALLENGES FACING EPIDEMIOLOGIC STUDY OF URBAN HEALTH

Forging urban health into a coherent discipline, and advancing epidemiologic studies of how urban living may affect health, requires an appreciation of the complexities inherent to urban health research (Vlahov and Galea, 2003). As interest in urban health grows, several conceptual frameworks have been presented that suggest that a full understanding of how cities affect health may not necessarily lend itself to the easy application of a single empiric method (Vlahov and Galea, 2002). This complexity, and the features that make the study of urban health challenging, in many ways are not unique to urban health but rather are characteristics shared by the study of complicated human systems in general. In considering such systems, simple paradigms of single exposure and disease, traditionally the "bread and butter" of epidemiology, are inadequate. We consider here these challenges in the context of urban health research and discuss how they may influence the choice and application of research methods.

4.1. Specification of Research Question

Clear specification of a research question is the necessary first step in all etiologic and interventional epidemiologic research and is often one of the hardest. More specifically, the greatest challenge in the epidemiologic study of urban health is in adequate specification of research questions that address how and why urban living may affect health.

There are three primary reasons why this task may be particularly challenging in urban health. First, much of what may be considered urban health research in the literature thus far has arisen from different disciplines, using different theoretical frameworks (or sometimes from an a theoretical perspective), and applying different disciplinary orientations and terminologies. For example, in demography and epidemiology, research into the role of urbanization in shaping health may focus on how population change in cities, resulting from migration and population growth, may influence the distribution of diseases (e.g., Yusuf, *et al.*, 2001; Peters, 1999). In contrast, the study of urbanization in sociology may focus on social activities and social organization in cities and their association with changing behaviors and their consequences. Clearly, in considering how urban living may affect health the study of both changing urban population size and of how individuals acquire different urban lifestyles are important. Useful epidemiologic research should help us understand the role of each in influencing health and behavior; however few researchers have posed questions that enable them to consider both these perspectives.

Second, many questions in urban health research do not meaningfully exist in isolation (Israel, *et al.*, 1998). Understanding how urban living affects health requires consideration of multiple, often competing, influences. Broadly speaking there may be factors in urban areas that are detrimental to health (this has previously been referred to as the "urban health penalty", see ACP, 1997), while other factors may confer "an urban health advantage" (Vlahov, *et al.*, 2005). For example, while social capital associated with group membership may be salutary (Kawachi, 1999), identification with tightly knit homogenous ethnic communities may result in spatial racial segregation that has been associated with poor health (Acevedo-Garcia, *et al.*, 2003). Continuing to consider the example of urbanization, different disciplines might study various aspects of urbanization that coexist and potentially exert varying effects on population health. This interdependence of research questions complicates the empiric task of assessing how cities may affect health and suggests that while epidemiologic contributions to the study of urban health can be invaluable, in isolation these contributions are unlikely to extend our understanding of the field. Specification of relevant research questions in epidemiologic research must at least acknowledge, if not take into account, the interrelated processes that ultimately determine health in cities and take into account the contribution that may be made by other disciplines both to framing the epidemiologic question of interest and to aiding in the interpretation of the empiric observations within their appropriate context.

Third, as is the case with all research, clear specification of a research question rests, at least implicitly, on the acknowledgement of a theoretical framework that suggests how and why the characteristics of interest may affect health. The absence of a single, agreed upon framework in the study of urban health complicates the specification of research questions in the field, as well as the interpretation of research findings. In recent years several investigators have proposed more comprehensive models that may help to unify these different strands of urban research (Northridge, *et al.*, 2003; Galea, *et al.*, 2005).

4.2. Definitions of Urban, Intra-urban Spaces, and Urbanization

Epidemiologic research is predicated to a large extent on the appropriate operationalization of the constructs of interest into simple variables. In the context of urban health research, definitional issues become critical to permit empirically rigorous analyses that are generalizable across studies. The definitions of import differ, depending on the research question being investigated (as discussed above) and whether the research in question is concerned with inter- or intra-urban comparisons. Starting with the most basic definitions, there are multiple, and inconsistent definitions of what constitutes "urban", thus complicating and limiting the generalizability of inter-urban comparisons. No definition of urban places has been universally adopted and multiple, inconsistent definitions of urban are used by different countries, and at times within countries. For example, the U.S. Bureau of the Census defines an urbanized area in the following way: "An urbanized area comprises a place and the adjacent densely settled surrounding territory that together comprise a minimum population of 50,000 people. . . . The 'densely settled surrounding territory' adjacent to the place consists of territory made up of one or more contiguous blocks having a population density of at least 1,000 people per square mile". However, this definition is not consistent in other countries and in fact, among 228 countries on which the United Nations has data, about half use administrative definitions of urban (e.g., living in the capital city), 51 use size and density, 39 use functional characteristics (e.g., economic activity), 22 have no definition of urban, and 8 define all (e.g., Singapore) or none (e.g., Polynesian countries) of their population as urban. Official statistics (i.e., all the statistics above) rely on country-specific designations and do not use a uniform definition of urban. In specific instances, definitions of "urban" in adjacent countries vary tremendously. For example, urban definition in Bolivia includes localities with 2,000 or more inhabitants. In neighboring Peru, populated centers with 100 or more dwellings grouped contiguously and administrative centers of districts are considered urban. Compounding the difficulties in considering "urban" as a consistent definition, definitions of urban have changed over time in different ways in different countries and these differences are frequently embedded in calculations about changing urban proportions. Thus, what we may call urban in different settings may include what might otherwise be construed as city centers, peri-urban fringe cities, and densely populated isolated regions.

Intra-urban research in turn relies on the appropriate specification of intra-urban units that are theoretically meaningful to residents within cities. As discussed earlier, intra-urban spaces are typically conceived of as "neighborhoods". Conceptually, there is likely no "one" neighborhood unit that is important to the exclusion of all other units. For example, while a person may be influenced by her immediate environment (few blocks) in choice of foods purchased, it is equally plausible that safety in the larger neighborhood determines whether the same person exercises on a regular basis. Previous research has confirmed this thinking and shown that different social and environmental measures operate at different levels. For example, studies of social capital and health have been conducted at both the small neighborhood scale in Chicago and at the statewide level across the U.S. (see Sampson, *et al.*, 1997; Kawachi and Kennedy, 1997). Poverty at the state, county, city, and neighborhood levels has been linked to poor health status.

Implicit in these different contextual units of analyses is the lack of a clear consensus on the appropriate definitions of relevant intra-urban units of theoretical and empiric interest. Existing research has utilized various definitions of neighborhoods, including communities as identified by their residents, block groups, census tracts, and clusters of census tracts. Measures of neighborhood probably should be homogeneous enough to make measures such as median household income meaningful, but also be heterogeneous enough to be able to observe the effects of this variation (Pickett and Pearl, 2001). Unfortunately, as these studies have used different measures of the relevant intra-urban unit of analysis, generalizations from these observations become difficult. Further conceptual and empiric development will be necessary to clarify the appropriate use of intra-urban units of analysis and to advance our understanding of the role of specific urban characteristics that may affect population health.

Definitions of "urban" or of the relevant intra-urban units of analysis are important aids to analysis that deal with cities at one point in time. However, it is *change* in cities over time that may be an equally, if not more important determinant of population health. "Urbanization", generally considered to refer to "population growth in cities" is also complex to measure and different methods of measuring urbanization. At its simplest level, there are several ways to measure growth in cities that in different ways may affect health. Overall, these may include the absolute annual increase in urban population size, the urban population growth rate, the level of urbanization, and the rate of urbanization. Urbanization, at its simplest level, may be calculated as the change in the proportion of the national population that is urban. However, this change in proportion is dependent both on the urban population growth, and on the relative growth of the rest of the country. There are different implications for countries and cities where urbanization is driven by rural-urban migration or international migration, compared to other countries where urbanization is largely driven by natural growth of cities. Together with changing urban proportions, changes in the absolute number of urban residents are also meaningful. Thus, while countries of vastly different sizes can share urbanization rates, these urbanization rates can represent vastly different absolute numbers of urban residents. Also, the percent of national growth that's influenced by growth in urban areas ultimately also is reliant in the change of the overall national population. So, net urban growth is again differently meaningful in the context of larger and smaller countries.

Further development in urban health requires careful consideration of how key epidemiologic units of interest–cities themselves, units within cities, and the changes in cities over time, are measured both within and across studies and what the implications are for different methods of assessment.

4.3. Cities Are Complex and Multiple Competing Influences May Be Important Determinants of Health

As discussed in several chapters in this book, cities are complex communities of heterogeneous individuals and multiple factors may be important determinants of population health in cities. For example, in order to understand the role that racial/ethnic heterogeneity plays in shaping the health of urban populations, it is important to understand both the role of segregation in restricting access to resources in urban neighborhoods (Acevedo-Garcia, *et al.*, 2003) and the potential for greater tolerance of racial/ethnic differences in cities compared to non-urban areas. Assessing how urban living may affect health raises challenges and introduces complexity that is often not easily addressed through the application of simple epidemiologic methods.

Recent epidemiologic thinking has introduced the notion that epidemiologic analyses should consider the complexity of factors that can shape individual and population health. Several observations suggest that human populations behave as complex systems. First, there are multiple examples of discontinuous changes in health in relation to monotonic changes in exposures facing human populations (Philippe and Mansi, 1998). For example, the relation between population health and several environmental exposures encompass threshold and sigmoid curves, both hallmarks of nonlinear dynamics (Maynard, *et al.*, 2003). Second, the effects of particular exposures on human populations can linger well beyond removal of the exposure. For example, the population mental health consequences of disasters are well known to persist beyond the disaster itself (Galea, *et al.*, 2003b). Third, multiple diseases, including infectious diseases and neoplastic diseases, frequently share determinants that are affected by common environmental exposures (Koopman and Lynch, 1999; Koopman and Longini, 1994). Although none of these observations in and of themselves *define* complex systems, they provide empiric evidence that human populations exhibit complex system behaviors and as such, that epidemiologic assessment of the role of complex environments such as urban environments might benefit both from considering the contribution of disciplines such as ecology that have long considered the contribution of complex determinants and non-linear system dynamics.

4.4. Cities Are Different from One Another and May Change Over Time

Epidemiologic inquiry in health presupposes that there are identifiable (and modifiable) factors that influence health. Typically, public health studies imply, for example, that we can generalize about how different foods will affect health across individuals, at least within the confines of effect modification across groups (e.g., age groups)) or under different circumstances (e.g., at different levels of caloric intake). However, cities are characterized by multiple factors (e.g., size, population density, heterogeneity etc.) that in many ways make each city unique. The complexity of cities and of city living may mean that urban characteristics that are important in one city may not be important in others, limiting the generalizations that can be drawn about how urban living influences health. Further complicating this task is the fact that cities change over time with implications for the relative contribution of different factors in determining health in cities. For example, municipal taxation of alcohol and cigarettes may be an important determinant of alcohol and cigarette consumption in a particular city at one point in time (Grossman, 1989). However, changing social norms around smoking and alcohol use may either obviate or reinforce the influence of taxation. Returning to our built environment and health example, it may not be the quality of the built environment at one point in time that is associated with infectious disease, as much as it is the pace at which buildings are erected (or abandoned) that disrupt disease vectors and facilitate the transmission of infectious disease in urban areas. For example, it has been shown in several developing world cities, where much of the growth in urban areas is taking place, that rapid (and uncontrolled) building in dense urban areas is associated with increasing breeding grounds for mosquitoes and an increase in mosquito-borne diseases such as malaria and dengue fever (Sutherst, 2004). As such, epidemiologic inquiry into urban characteristics that affect health may do well to note both the prevailing context within which such characteristics operate and that the role of these characteristics may change over time.

5.0. THE FUTURE: WHAT IS THE ROLE OF EPIDEMIOLOGY IN THE STUDY OF URBAN HEALTH?

As we have discussed throughout this chapter, in thinking about health in cities, the perspective of urban epidemiology needs to be based on an appreciation of the complexity of living conditions and how, as an array, they affect health. In epidemiologic studies, the traditional predominant approach to causal inference is to isolate exposures and outcomes, controlling or adjusting for confounding factors or revealing interactions. When thinking about the health of populations in cities, establishing these associations in isolation of other factors that may be equally important is problematic. The range and overlap of exposures in cities is more complex than would be suggested by inference drawn from individual risk factor-disease associations, and the degree to which they are left unconsidered makes results and priority setting incomplete. An urban epidemiology shifts the focus to how associations reported in simpler settings are observed within a more complicated urban setting that embeds multiple physical and social factors that may determine population health. In so doing, urban epidemiology must draw both on different fields of epidemiology, including categorical and exposure-based expertise, and on different disciplines including ecology, sociology, and mathematical modeling. This obviously presents challenges and frustrations.

However, this approach also has tremendous potential. We argue that the study of urban health lends itself to the creative application of methods from multiple disciplines and the nuanced appreciation of the role of multiple factors that may determine population health in cities. With the rapidly growing predominance of cities worldwide we can ill-afford to avoid focusing attention on how the complexities of urban living may affect population health. We suggest that an agenda for urban epidemiologic research, including theoretical frameworks and methodologic development, is urgently needed.

REFERENCES

Acevedo-Garcia, D., Lochner, K.A., Osypuk, T.L., and Subramanian, S.V. (2003). Future directions in residential segregation and health research: a multilevel approach. *Am. J. Public Health* 93(2):215–21.

Andrulis, D.P. (1997). The urban health penalty: new dimensions and directions in inner-city health care. In: *Inner City Health care.* American College of Physicians, Philadephia, PA.

American College of Physicians. (1977). Inner-City Health Care. *Ann. Intern. Med.* 127:485-490.

The American Heritage® Dictionary of the English Language, 2000, Fourth Edition (August 26, 2004), http://www.bartleby.com/61/69/E0176900.html.

Bond, K.C., Valente, T.W., and Kendall, C. (1999). Social network influences on reproductive health behaviors in urban northern Thailand. *Soc. Sci. Med.* 49(12):1599–614.

Bruce, M.L., Smith, W., Miranda, J., Hoagwood, K., and Wells, K.B. (2002). NIMH Affective Disorders Workgroup. Community-based interventions. *Ment. Health. Serv. Res.* 4(4):205–14.

Cohen, D.A., Spear, S., Scribner, R., Kissinger, P., Mason, K., and Wildgen, J. (2000). Broken windows and the risk of gonorrhea. *Am. J. Public Health* 90(2):230–236.

De Bourdeaudhuij, I., Sallis, J.F., and Saelens, B.E. (2003). Environmental correlates of physical activity in a sample of Belgian adults. *Am. J. Health Promot.* 18(1):83–92.

Diez-Roux, A.V. (2003). Residential environments and cardiovascular risk. *J. Urban Health* 80(4): 569–89.

Diez-Roux, A.V. (2001). Investigating neighborhood and area effects on health. *Am. J. Public Health* 91(11):1783–9.

Diez-Roux, A.V. (2000). Multilevel analysis in public health research. *Ann. Rev. Public Health* 21: 171–92.

Douste-Blazy, P., Ruidavets, J.B., Arveiler, D., Bingham, A., Camare, R., Schaffer, P., Aby, M.A., and Richard, J.L. (1988). Comparison of cardiovascular risk factor levels in two French populations: Haute-Garonne (Toulouse) and Bas-Rhin (Strasbourg). *Acta. Med. Scand. Suppl.* 728:137–43.

Fu, F.H., and Fung, L. (2004). The cardiovascular health of residents in selected metropolitan cities in China. *Prev. Med.* 38(4):458–67.

Galea, S., Ahern, J., Vlahov, D., Coffin, P.O., Fuller, C., Leon, A.C., and Tardiff, K. (2003b.) Income distribution and risk of fatal drug overdose in New York City neighborhoods. *Drug Alcohol Depend.* 70(2):139–48.

Galea, S., Freudenberg, N., and Vlahov, D. (2005). Cities and population health. *Soc. Sci. Med.* 60(5): 1017-1033.

Galea, S., and Schulz, A. (2006). Methodologic considerations in the study of urban health: How do we best assess how cities affect health? In: Freudenberg, N., Galea, S., and Vlahov, D. (eds.)., *Cities and the Health of the Public.* Vanderbilt University Press, Forthcoming.

Galea, S., and Vlahov, D. (2004). Urban Health: Evidence, challenges and directions. *Ann. Rev. Pub. Health.* Epub instead of print, (August 18, 2004); http://arjournals.annualreviews.org/doi/abs/10.1146/annurev.publhealth.26.021304.144708.

Galea, S., Vlahov, D., Resnick, H., Ahern, J., Susser, E., Gold, J., Bucuvalas, M., and Kilpatrick, D. (2003a). Trends in probable posttraumatic stress disorder in New York City after the September 11 terrorist attacks. *Am. J. Epi.* 158:514–524.

Gordis, L. (2000). *Epidemiology.* W.B. Saunders, 2000, Philadephia.

Grossman, M. (1989). Health benefits of increases in alcohol and cigarette taxes. *Br. J. Addiction* 84:1193–1204.

Handy, S.L., Boarnet, M.G., Ewing, R., and Killingsworth, R.E. (2002). How the built environment affects physical activity: Views from urban planning. *Am. J. Prev. Med.* 23(2S):64–73.

Hersh, B.S., Markowitz, L.E., Maes, E.F., Funkhouser, A.W., Baughman, A.L., Sirotkin, B.I., and Hadler, S.C. (1992). The geographic distribution of measles in the United States, 1980 through 1989. *JAMA.* 267(14):1936–41.

Hoover, D.R. (2002). Power for T-test comparisons of unbalanced cluster exposure studies. *J. Urban Health* 79(2):278–94.

Israel, B.A., Schulz, A.J., Paker, E.A., and Becker, A.B. (1998). Review of community-based research: assessing partnership approaches to improve public health. *Annu. Rev. Public Health* 19:173-202.

Jackson, R.J. (2003). The impact of the built environment on health: an emerging field. *Am. J. Pubic Health* 93(9):1382–1384.

Kaplan, G.A. (1999). What is the role of the social environment in understanding inequalities in health? *Ann. N. Y. Acad. Sci.* 896:116–9.

Katz, D.L. (2003). Pandemic obesity and the contagion of nutritional nonsense. *Public Health Rev.* 31(1):33–44.

Kawachi, I., and Kennedy, B.P. (1997). The relationship of income inequality to mortality: Does the choice of indicator matter? *Soc. Sci. Med.* 45:1121–1127.

Kawachi, I. (1999). Social capital and community effects on population and individual health. *Ann. N. Y. Acad. Sci.* 896:120–30.

Kawachi, I., and Berkman, L. (2001). Social ties and mental health. *J. Urban Health* 78(3):458–67.

Keil,J.E., Saunders, D.E. Jr., Lackland, D.T., Weinrich, M.C., Hudson, M.B., Gastright, J.A., Baroody NB., O'Bryan, E.C. Jr., and Zmyslinski, R.W. (1985). Acute myocardial infarction: period prevalence, case fatality, and comparison of black and white cases in urban and rural areas of South Carolina. *Am. Heart J.* 109(4):776–84.

Kessler, R.C., McGonagle, K.A., Zhao, S., Neson, C.B., Hughes, M., Eshleman, S., Wittchen, H., and Kendler, K.S. (1994). Lifetime and 12-month prevalence of DSM-III-R psychiatric disorders in the United States. *Arch. Gen. Psych.* 51:8–19.

Koopman, J.S., and Lynch, J.W. (1999). Individual causal models and population system models in epidemiology. *Am. J. Public Health* 89:1170–4.

Koopman, J.S., and Longini, I.M. (1994). The ecological effects of individual exposures and nonlinear disease dynamics in populations. *Am. J. Public Health* 84:836–842.

Kuo, F. (2003, October 16). *Why urban health research matters: A view from inner-city Chicago.* Paper presented at the Second International Conference on Urban Health at the New York Academy of Medicine, New York City, New York.

Langford, I.H., Leyland, A.H., Rasbash, J., and Goldstein, H. (1999). Multilevel modeling of the geographical distributions of diseases. *J. R. Stat. Soc. Ser. C. Appl. Stat.* 48(2):253–68.

Lawlor, D.A., Davey Smith, G., and Ebrahim, S. (2003). Life course influences on insulin resistance: findings from the British Women's Heart and Health Study. *Diabetes Care* 26(1):97–103.

Levine, R.V., Lynch, K., Miyake, K., and Lucia, M. (1989). The Type A city: coronary heart disease and the pace of life. *J. Behav. Med.* 12(6):509–24.

Levins, R., and Lopez, C. (1999) .Toward an ecosocial view of health. *Int. J. Health Serv.* 29(2):261–93.

Lilienfeld, D.E. Definitions of epidemiology. (1978) *Am. J. Epidemiol.* 107(2):87–90.

Lilienfeld, A.M. Practical limitations of epidemiologic methods. (1983). *Environ. Health Perspect.* 52 3–8.

Lynch, J.W., Kaplan, G.A., Pamuk, E.R., Cohen, R.D., Heck, K.E., Balfour, J.L., and Yen, I.H. (1998). Income inequality and mortality in metropolitan areas of the United States. *Am. J. Public Health* 88(7):1074–80.

Lynch, J., Smith, G.D., Harper, S., Hillemeier, M., Ross, N., Kaplan, G.A., and Wolfson, M. (2004). Is income inequality a determinant of population health? Part 1. A systematic review. *Milbank Q.* 82(1):5–99.

Marinacci, C., Spadea, T., Biggeri, A., Demaria, M., Caiazzo, A., and Costa, G. (2004). The role of individual and contextual socioeconomic circumstances on mortality: analysis of time variations in a city of north west Italy. *J. Epidemiol. Community Health* 58(3):199–207.

Maynard, R., Krewski, D., Burnett, R.T., Samet, J., Brook, J.R., Granville, G., and Craig, L. (2003). Health and air quality: directions for policy-relevant research. *J. Toxic. Environ. Health* Part A, 66:1891–904.

Molnar, B.E., Gortmaker, S.L., Bull, F.C., and Buka, S.L. (2004). Unsafe to play? Neighborhood disorder and lack of safety predict reduced physical activity among urban children and adolescents. *Am. J. Health Promot.* 18(5):378–86.

Northridge, M.E., Sclar, E.D., and Biswas, P. (2003). Sorting out the connections between the built environment and health: a conceptual framework for navigating pathways and planning healthy cities. *J. Urban Health* 80(4):556–68.

Oakes, J.M. (2004). The (mis)estimation of neighborhood effects: causal inference for a practicable social epidemiology. *Soc. Sci. Med.* 58(10):1929–52.

Pantoja, E. Exploring the concept of social capital and its relevance for community-based development: The case of coal mining areas in Orissa, India. World Bank; Social Capital Working Paper series. (August 30, 2004); http://www.worldbank.org/poverty/scapital/wkrppr/sciwp18.pdf

Pate, R.R., Pratt, M., Blair, S.N., Haskell, W.L., Macera, C.A., Bouchard, C., Buchner, D., Ettinger, W., Heath, G.W., King, A.C., Kriska, A., Leon, A.S., Marcus, B.H., Morris, J., Paffenbarger, R.S., Patrick, K., Pollock, M.L., Rippe, J.M., Sallis, J., and Wilmore, J.H. (1995). Physical activity and public health: A recommendation from the Centers for Disease Control and Prevention and the American College of Sports Medicine. *JAMA.* 273:402–407.

Paykel, E.S., Abbott, R., Jenkins, R., Brugha, T.S., and Meltzer, H. (2000). Urban-rural mental health differences in Great Britain: findings from the National Morbidity Survey. *Psych. Medic.* 30:269–280.

Peters, J. Urbanism and health in industrialized Asia. (1996). In: Schell, L.M., and Ulijaszek, S.J. (eds.), *Urbanism, health and human biology in industrialized countries.* Cambridge University Press, Cambridge, MA.

Philippe, P., and Mansi, O. (1998). Nonlinearity in the epidemiology of complex health and disease processes. *Theoretical Medicine and Bioethics*, 19:591–60.

Pickett, K., and Pearl, M. (2001). Multi-level analyses of neighborhood socioeconomic context and health outcomes: a critical review. *J. Epidemiol. Community Health* Feb;55(2):111–22.

Rodwin, V.G., and Gusmano, M.K. (2002). The World Cities Project: rationale, organization, and design for comparison of megacity health systems. *J. Urban Health* 79(4):445–63.

Rothman, K.J., and Greenland, S. (eds.). (1998). *Modern Epidemiology.* Lippincott_raven Publishers, Philadelphia, PA, pp. 201–230.

Sampson, R.J., Raudenbush, S.W., and Earls, F. (1997). Neighborhoods and violent crime: a multilevel study of collective efficacy. *Science* 277(5328):918–24.

Sampson, R.J. (2003). The neighborhood context of well-being. *Perspect. Biol. Med.* 46(3 Suppl): S53–64.

Schouten, L.J., Meijer, H., Huveneers, J.A., and Kiemeney, L.A. (1996). Urban-rural differences in cancer incidence in The Netherlands 1989-1991. *Int. J. Epidemiol.* 25(4):729–36.

Sharpe, P.A., Granner, M.L., Hutto, B., and Ainsworth, B.E. (2004). Association of environmental factors to meeting physical activity recommendations in two South Carolina counties. *Am. J. Health Promot.* 18(3):251–7.

Sundquist, K., Malmstrom, M., and Johansson, S.E. (2004). Neighborhood deprivation and incidence of coronary heart disease: a multilevel study of 2.6 million women and men in Sweden. *J. Epidemiol. Community Health* 58(1):71–7.

Sutherst, R.W. (2004). Global change and human vulnerability to vector-borne diseases. *Clin Microbiol Rev.* 17(1):136–73.

Swinton, J. A dictionary of (ecological) epidemiology, (August 30, 2004); http://www.swintons.net/jonathan/Academic/glossary.html#E

Tanaka, A., Takano, T., Nakamura, K., and Takeuchi, S. (1996). Health levels influenced by urban residential conditions in a megacity -Tokyo. *Urban Stud.* 33(6):879–894.

Takano, T., Nakamura, K., and Watanabe, M. (2002). Urban residential environments and senior citizens' longevity in mega-city areas: the importance of walkable greenspaces. *J. Epidemiol. Community Health* 56:913–918.

Vlahov, D., and Galea, S. (2003). Urban health: a new discipline. *The Lancet* 362:1091–1092.

Vlahov, D., and Galea, S. (2002). Urbanization, urbanicity, and health. *J. Urban Health* 79 Suppl 1:S1–S12.

Vlahov, D., Galea, S., Freudenberg, N. (2005). The urban health advantage. *J. Urban Health* 83(2):1-4.

Wang,Y., Monteiro, C., and Popkin, B.M. (2002). Trends of obesity and underweight in older children and adolescents in the United States, Brazil, China, and Russia. *Am. J. Clin. Nutr.* 75(6):971–7.

Windle, M., Grunbaum, J.A., Elliott, M., Tortolero, S.R., Berry, S., Gilliland, J., Kanouse, D.E., Parcel, G.S., Wallander, J., Kelder, S., Collins, J., Kolbe, L., and Schuster, M. (2004). Healthy passages; A multilevel, multi-method longitudinal study of adolescent health. *Am. J. Prev. Med.* 27(2): 164–72.

Yusuf, S., Reddy, S., Ounpuu, S., and Anand, S. (2001). Global burden of cardiovascular diseases: Part I: general considerations, the epidemiologic transition, risk factors, and impact of urbanization. *Circulation* 104(22):2746–53.

Zhao, D. (1993). The epidemiology of coronary heart disease (CHD) in 16 provinces of China. Multiprovince Cooperative Group of Cardiovascular Disease Surveillance (MONICA Project). *Zhonghua Liu Xing Bing Xue Za Zhi.* 14(1):10–3

Chapter 15

Design and Analysis of Group (or Neighborhood) Level Urban Studies

Donald Hoover

1.0. INTRODUCTION

By necessity and convenience, urban health observational and interventional studies are often conducted using samples composed of groups of related persons, often persons living in the same neighborhoods (Cochran, 1977; Cornfield, 1978; Korn and Graubard, 1999). While most related group studies in urban health involve persons living in the same neighborhoods, there are other types of Group Studies, such as of groups of persons related because they receive behavioral intervention from the same teaching class or cycle. While this chapter emphasizes neighborhood studies which are more frequent in urban health, the methods presented here apply to all types of Group Level studies including group behavioral interventions.

As the methods for "group" level studies differ from those of traditional studies of completely unrelated (independent) subjects, this chapter is written to help readers better understand articles written on urban group level studies and to be an introductory, but not complete, tool for design and analysis of urban group level studies. Basic issues of design and analysis of group studies are presented on mostly conceptual levels with references for further details. Some sections assume a background in statistics up to and including linear regression, logistic regression, and/or survival analysis, but this is not necessary to understand much of the chapter.

2.0. TYPES OF GROUP LEVEL STUDIES USED IN URBAN HEALTH

We start with the standard analytic setting where it is of interest to determine whether an exposure X is related to an outcome Y (also see Dixon and Massey 1968,

Dunn and Clark 1974). In general, the outcome *Y* could be either continuous (number of cigarettes per day smoked), binary (smoking cigarettes yes/no), or censored binary (time to cessation of smoking). The exposure *X* could be either continuous and/or binary. Furthermore, *X* could measure an existing condition (such as gender, race, weight) or a new intervention (such as a new treatment Vs placebo) or even be a vector of multiple exposures. A given number (say *N*) of subjects are measured for *X* and *Y*, and statistically compared to determine if *X* is related to *Y*. Either a hypothesis testing or inferential statistical estimation approach may be used.

If feasible, when *N* observations (or persons) are obtained for analysis, they all should be independent of each other as this increases precision of inferences. However, as noted earlier, urban health studies often must be conducted using groups, (or clusters) of related (non-independent) persons in settings where a non-ignorable group effect exists (Cochran, 1977; Cornfield, 1978). Sometimes the direct effects of interest in the research are mediated through the group itself. Other times, for cost, convenience or constraint reasons it is necessary to sample subjects by groups. In a Group Level Study, *k* groups are randomly chosen or formed and a certain number n_k subjects are randomly selected for each group often the study is planned for the same $n_k \equiv n$ to be randomly chosen from or placed in each group.

2.1. Group Mediated Effects Are of Interest

Several settings occur where the effect being studied is mediated through a neighborhood or group and there are a limited number of these groups/neighborhoods to study. For example, smoking cessation classes are often taught to classes (i.e. groups) of ~15 students and it may be of interest to know if positive and/or negative synergies form from interactions among the students in the same class. Or a city may have *k* (e.g., *k*=59) distinct neighborhoods. It may be of interest to know whether the neighborhood a person lives in (or characteristics of that neighborhood) is related to his or her level of depression.

2.2. Cost, Convenience, and/or Constraint Group Sampling

Sometimes people must be sampled by groups and are influenced by common group effects (even if those group effects are not of primary interest to the investigators). Suppose a city has 50 neighborhoods and each neighborhood has its own local medical care (i.e. doctors, clinics, etc.). A study to examine if there are underlying gender differences (male versus female) on opinions about the adequacy of medical care in that city is being conducted among 400 men and 400 women. But clearly the specific medical care available in local neighborhoods might (even differentially) influence gender opinion. Some neighborhoods for example, could be less female oriented (i.e. have fewer female doctors, obstetricians, etc.) than others. If the entire sample was obtained by taking eight men and women each from the 50 neighborhoods, then the 16 persons (eight men and eight women) from each neighborhood would be a structural "Group Level Sample". It might cost substantially less to sample 400 men and women from a randomly chosen 25 neighborhoods (i.e. 32 persons per neighborhood, rather than having to travel to all 50 neighborhoods to achieve 400 men and 400 women.)

Three types of "Group Level" Study Designs are commonly used in Urban Health Research, each of which tends to have different design and analysis properties. These are: *Exhaustive Neighborhood Samples*, *Partial Neighborhood Samples*, and *Group Interventions*.

2.2.1. Neighborhood Samples (Exhaustive and Partial)

This occurs when subjects already live in or are otherwise treated in neighborhoods. A study therefore obtains its subjects from these already previously formed correlated neighborhoods such as a particular borough of the city or a specific hospital where persons seek treatment (in this case the hospital can be thought of as a neighborhood). In an *Exhaustive* sample, all available neighborhoods are sampled from. In a *Partial* sample only a randomly chosen subset of the neighborhoods are sampled from.

While nonrandom subsets of neighborhoods or networked neighborhoods can be chosen as well (sometimes referred to as *Convenience Samples*) this is less desirable statistically since now the overall sample is no longer random and we do not focus on this type of design here. However, while it is beyond the scope of this chapter, in some settings where it is impossible to obtain a complete listing of the population, but where networked referrals from previous participants to new participants can be given, Markov chain approaches can be used to obtain unbiased point estimates and error bounds (also see Heckathorn, 2002).

To obtain a neighborhood sample, the neighborhoods must first be identified. Then a sampling frame(s) of persons from within the neighborhoods (or from the neighborhoods that have been randomly chosen to participate in the study) is obtained and used to randomly sample persons within the neighborhoods.

For example, let City X have 100,000 blacks and 200,000 whites. These persons live in 30 neighborhoods, 10 of which are almost exclusively black and 20 of which are predominantly white. Each of these neighborhoods has its own unique social, health and crime environment that influences its members. For simplicity, let's now assume each neighborhood has the same number of persons (i.e. 10,000 persons each).

In an *Exhaustive Neighborhood Sample* of 300 persons, in order to be sure that each neighborhood is proportionately represented, 10 persons would be randomly chosen from each neighborhood. But if some neighborhoods were larger than others, the numbers sampled from each neighborhood could be made proportional to neighborhood size. The sampling schemes could be even more complicated, as described later, involving stratification and possibly weighted samples. If the 300 subjects had been randomly sampled from the entire city population of 300,000 rather by using neighborhood sampling, then the neighborhoods would probably not be equally represented since by chance alone, 20 persons could have been taken from one neighborhood and five from another. As each neighborhood may have its own effect on the outcome, balancing the sample by neighborhood helps to appropriately average neighborhood effects to obtain better estimates of the overall city average.

A *Partial Neighborhood Sample* could be done if there was only enough money/time to drive to 15 neighborhoods; 15 neighborhoods would be randomly chosen from the 30 within the entire city and 20 persons each would be randomly chosen from these neighborhoods. While a Partial Neighborhood Sample is statistically less desirable than an exhaustive sample, the partial sample is still random and representative. Statistical methods exist to account for non-exhaustive nature of partial samples (also see Cochran, 1977; Korn and Graubard, 1999; SAS 2002; Shah, *et al.*, 1996; STATA 2004; SPSS 2004). If maintaining the same racial representation as for the entire city was important, the neighborhoods could be chosen for the Partial Neighborhood Sample using a *stratified* scheme that ensured five of the 10 exclusively black and 10 of the 20 predominately white neighborhoods would be taken.

2.2.2. *Group Intervention*

An intervention is delivered to an entire neighborhood or perhaps more often to a "Teaching Group" of persons that initially were unrelated prior to the intervention (Cornfield, 1978; Hoover, 2002b). Independently of the intervention, the group itself may exert some effect on the outcome and/or the intervention may be delivered with differing effectiveness to different groups. For example (since it costs too much to treat each person one on one) an alcohol cessation program is delivered to classes of 15 students. The students within the same classes may be correlated with each other if they have positive or negative interactions with each other. Also, if the teacher of a given class is good, then all students in that class will do better.

Ideally when intervention group studies are used, subjects should be randomized into the intervention groups. For example assume two behavioral interventions (A and B) against alcohol use are being compared. Each is given to classes of 15 students with 150 students given Intervention A in 10 teaching groups and 150 given Intervention B in 10 teaching groups. If the 300 students are randomly recruited, it is best to randomly assign them to the 20 intervention groups so that at least these groups will not have any pre-intervention correlation. Often this may not be feasible. For example, if the behavioral intervention is given to networks (i.e. groups of friends and/or relatives) then the classes of 15 must be subjects of interrelated networks who will have pre-existing correlation in addition to shared teaching effects from the intervention class.

3.0. STATISTICAL PROPERTIES AND DESIGNS OF GROUP LEVEL SAMPLES

Observations from the same group are by design potentially correlated as persons (for example) living in the same neighborhoods, or taking the same intervention class, are correlated with each other due to shared common effects (Cochran, 1977; Cornfield, 1978). However, the correlation is not 100%; it is possible for one person in a smoking cessation class to dramatically reduce smoking cigarettes, yet another person in the same class to increase smoking. Thus, for example, if 400 people are taken from 40 neighborhoods, there are not 400 independent observations, but instead are 40 independent clusters (or groups) of correlated observations. Standard statistical analyses assuming that each of these 400 observations is independent are therefore not appropriate, but instead, as described in Section 6, nested or multi-level statistical analyses that allow for a neighborhood effect are needed.

The magnitude of intra-group (or intra-neighborhood) correlation of persons in typical urban studies is not known and is an important area for further research

(Donnar and Klar, 1994). What little information that is available often comes from large neighborhoods and suggests that intra group or "intraclass" correlation (ICC) is usually less than 0.05 (Hansen, *et al.*, 1953; Campbell, *et al.*, 2000; Smeeth and Ng, 2002) meaning that neighborhood (and perhaps other group) effects usually explain less that 5% of the population variance of an outcome. Typically, the larger the size of a neighborhood or group, the smaller the intra-neighborhood correlation is (Hansen, *et al.*, 1953), but much interest in urban health is dealing with smaller "neighborhoods". Nothing to date has been published on intraclass correlation between outcomes of students being treated in the same behavioral intervention teaching group (Hoover, 2002a).

Unfortunately, intraclass correlations of even less than 0.05 can still dramatically increase the standard deviation of test statistics beyond that of independent observations; particularly if n_k, the number of subjects sampled from the same group is large (Donnar, *et al.*, 1981; Donnar and Klar, 1994). For example, let ρ be the intra-group (or intraclass) correlation and the same $n_k. \equiv n$ individuals be sampled from each group for an outcome with population variance σ^2. If the n persons within the group were treated as independent, then the perceived (i.e. naively calculated) variance of the group mean would be σ^2/n. But because these observations are correlated, the true variance of the group mean is $[\rho+(1-\rho)/\text{n}]\ \sigma^2$ (Donnar, *et al.*, 1981). This makes the ratio of the true to perceived variance $\rho + (1-\rho)$. Thus if $\text{n}\equiv 20$ subjects are taken from a neighborhood and the overall variance of the outcome Y is 100 with an intraclass correlation of 0.05, the true variance of the observed mean $\bar{Y}$ from 20 the neighborhood members is $9.75 = [0.05 + 0.95/20]^*100$. This is almost twice as large as the naive variance of $\bar{Y}$; $5 = 100/20$ that is estimated assuming the 20 persons from the same neighborhood are completely independent. Thus if a Group Level study is undertaken with 20 subjects sampled from several neighborhoods, analysis by statistical methods that naively assume subjects from the same neighborhood are independent will underestimate true variance of parameter estimates by a factor of 0.5 and give anticonservative P-values and confidence limits.

Unfortunately, this bias is often ignored in the literature with analyses of group level studies being conducted as if the members of the same group were independent often being published (Simpson, *et al.*, 1995; Hoover, 2002a). Section 6.0. describes the appropriate statistical tests to analyze, continuous, binary and censored outcomes for group level data.

3.1. It Is Often Difficult to Determine Whether or Not There Is a Group Level Effect

Often it has been argued that there is no group effect and that special analyses of Group samples thus not needed . . . i.e., just because persons live in the same neighborhood may not necessarily influence their opinion on medical care in the city. But unfortunately this conjecture is usually difficult to test. If Y_{kl} denotes a continuous outcome from the lth person in the kth group then a simple decomposition of Y_{kl} is $Y_{kl} = u + \Delta_k + \varepsilon_{kl}$ where Δ_k is a random group effect distributed normally with mean 0 and variance σ^2_Δ, ε_{kl} the random within group individual error is normally distributed with mean 0 and variance σ^2_P and the intraclass correlation is $ICC = \sigma^2_\Delta/(\sigma^2_\Delta + \sigma^2_P)$. While it is possible to test the null hypothesis that $\Delta_k \equiv 0$ (or equivalently $\sigma^2_\Delta = 0$) (also see Dunn and Clark, 1974), the power to reject this H_o is very limited for even very substantial levels of *ICC* (Donnar, *et al.*, 1994) especially when there are smaller numbers of groups (i.e. $k < 30$) in the study. However, as was just shown, the impact of even small undetectable group effects on hypothesis testing is to inflate the True Type 1 error far above the nominal level α. Thus for most urban group studies it will be necessary to conservatively assume that a neighborhood effect exists even if uncertainty about this exists and tests fail to find a statistical group effect.

4.0. SOME MORE TERMINOLOGY FOR GROUP LEVEL SAMPLES

We have so far presented a simple picture of neighborhood/group level effects which in fact may be largely adequate for group based interventions but not for large neighborhood based surveys. While the full details of very complicated Neighborhood Level sampling are beyond the scope of this introductory chapter, the reader may encounter these in designing or reading neighborhood studies. These include *Clusters, Strata* and *Weights. Clusters* is another name that is commonly used to denote what this chapter refers to as *Groups*; basically (more or less random) geographical, teaching or other groups (or neighborhoods) within which the observations are self correlated. We now describe *Strata* and *Weighted Sampling.*

Strata denote a larger fixed categorical structure either at the neighborhood or individual level at which large effects are potentially exerted. These could either be *Individual Level Strata* – (such as race) or *Neighborhood Level Strata* such as geographic region (East, South, Central, West). Strata are often included in the sampling design of a study for a variety of reasons and add an additional layer of non-randomness that must be accounted for in study planning and data analysis. While it is sometimes difficult to distinguish a *Strata* from a *Cluster* (or *Group*), Strata generally represent well defined general fixed characteristics (i.e. race, sex, etc.) while Clusters/Groups denote random convenience sampling units (i.e., neighborhood, hospital, teaching class). Ideally all Strata should be represented in a sample while often it is acceptable (and often practical) to only include some of the available Clusters (i.e., Groups) in a sample.

4.1. Stratified Sampling by Individual Level Strata

Sometimes it is either of primary interest to compare two different individual strata and/or to obtain an "appropriate balance" between the number of observations from different strata. For example, consider a study of attitudes towards government where Republicans and Democrats are believed to have different opinions with a plan to sample 400 subjects from 20 neighborhoods. Even though there are twice as many Democrats as Republicans living in the city, it is deemed equally important to know the attitude of each political group so the entire sampling frame population is stratified into two parties and from these strata, 200 Republicans and 200 Democrats chosen proportionately to their respective population sizes in each of the 20 neighborhoods.

4.2 Stratified Sampling at the Neighborhood Level

Sometimes it is important to obtain a predetermined balance of different neighborhood types. For example consider an American study of cities where each geographical region is equally important making it desired to have ¼ of the cities chosen each to be from the East, South, Central and West. If 40 cities total are randomly chosen, then 10 each will be chosen from the following regional city strata; East, South, Central and West.

From a design standpoint it only makes sense to think of stratified sampling when subsets (rather than all) of the individuals or neighborhoods being stratified on are chosen. Also, when a stratified design is used, then (as described in Sections 6.4 and 6.5) a stratified analysis that includes the neighborhood strata in the analytical methods must also be used.

4.3. Weighted Observations

Numbers that can be assigned to individuals to undo imbalances created either in stratified sampling or in the response rate are referred to as *Weights*. For some statistical analyses the weight is used to inversely adjust the observation relative to the increased chance to be in the sample. In the previous example where the race-stratified sample was deliberately evenly split into 200 Republicans and 200 Democrats, suppose that the overall population of the city this came from was 100,000 Republicans and 200,000 Democrats (i.e. and no independents). Then Republicans are over-represented in the sample (50% of the sample but only 33% of the city population) A Republican had twice the chance (200/100,000) of a Democrat (200/200,000) to be chosen.

To make up for this imbalance, a Republican in the sample will be assigned a sampling weight of 0.5 and a Democrat a sampling weight of 1. For example in an analysis to obtain a city mean from the sample of 200 Republicans and 200 Democrats; due to over sampling of Republicans, observations from Republicans would be multiplied by the sampling weight 0.5 while Democrats would be multiplied by 1.0. Most software packages (Shah, *et al.*, 1996; SPSS 2004; SAS 2002; STATA 2004) can be instructed to do this and will obtain appropriate standard deviations of estimates and P-values. However, some caution is needed when doing this since as described later in Section 6.3, the default for some statistical software is to consider weights as repeated observations with the same values rather than as an over-sampling adjustment factor.

Sometimes weights will be needed to adjust for unplanned imbalances due to differential contact or response rates. For example, assume there are 30,000 adults in the neighborhood; 10,000 (33.3%) are unmarried and live alone in a house with a telephone and 20,000 (66.7%) are married with each couple living at households with one telephone number. So there are 20,000 telephone numbers 10,000 (50%) for single adults and 10,000 (50%) for married couples. For economic and access reasons the survey must be conducted by telephone. So 200 telephone numbers are randomly dialed and then when a telephone is answered, an adult in that household is randomly selected. Of the 200 numbers dialed, ~100 (50%) will be answered at a household with only one person and 100 (50%) will be answered at a household with a married couple of whom one person will be randomly chosen.

So the final sample will be 50% single and 50% married which over-represents single persons. This is because (even though the study was not deliberately planned that way) a married person had a 100/20,000 = 0.5% chance to be chosen which was half that for an unmarried person to be chosen 100/10,000 = 1.0%. To counterbalance this sampling bias, respondents are asked how many people live in the household; and from the answer a weight of 2 is assigned to each married person (and a weight of 1 to each single person) in the sample. This effectively turns the

100 observations from married persons into 200 (2×100) relative to the 100 from single persons 1×100 and an expected 66.7% of the weighted sample (~200/300) should married, the same as in the neighborhood.

From a statistical standpoint, weighted sampling (i.e. oversampling of some groups and undersampling of others) is suboptimal as it generally results in larger standard deviations of estimates compared to obtaining a random sample where everyone has the same probability to be included. Therefore, weighted sampling should only be done when there are important small strata (such as American Indians) for which an unweighted random sample would select too few persons to be able to perform a meaningful analysis on the strata, or as was the case with the number of telephones per household, it is impossible to take an un-weighted sample.

In some settings where an equal probability random sample was initially obtained, but persons with certain characteristics were more likely to drop out, persons who remained in the study and had the same characteristics as the dropouts are assigned weights to make up for the dropout. For example, if a sample of 100 men and 100 women were obtained with all 100 women providing data but 20 men being lost before the data was obtained, observations from the 80 remaining men could be weighted by 1.25 (1.25*80 = 100) to "re-obtain the entire 100 men" with the 20 lost men being assumed proportionately similar to the 80 men who remain.

4.4. Complex Survey Designs

In large nationwide studies it is possible to combine several levels of sample selection (or multistage sampling) to get what is known as a *Complex Survey Design*. For example, in a nationwide American study of attitudes towards government; at the *First Level,* 10 cities could be randomly selected from the East, North, Central and West. In fact, since some cities have more people than others, within each region the probability for a city to be chosen could be made proportional to its population. At the *Second Level,* persons could be selected from the cities chosen at the first level stratified by party affiliation according to a scheme that ensured the final sample consisted of an equal number of Republicans and Democrats. Sampling weights could then be generated to inversely adjust the contribution from both parties according to their representation in the sample versus the overall populations of the selected cities. Such designs can get very complicated with several levels of clusters, strata, weights, etc. In particular large public use national databases (also see Olin, *et al.*, 1996) are often built this way. We focus on simpler designs here but introduce some concepts that are relevant to more complicated designs that the reader may encounter.

One limitation to designing urban sample studies is obtaining a *sampling frame* that provides both an enumeration and methods to contact all individuals in the study population. While *sampling frames* to identify neighborhoods and higher levels are usually good (i.e. from census data) there are often problems with identifying and establishing methods to contact individuals. Developing a scheme to randomly and unbiasedly identify individuals often constitutes much of the effort needed to design survey samples. For example, as noted before, telephone number directories are often used as a sampling frame, but persons who have multiple numbers are overrepresented in telephone directories and those without telephones are not represented at all. Particularly with increasing regulations towards privacy such as the

2003 Health Insurance Portability and Accountability Act and no call telephone lists this may become a greater problem in the future.

One important term for complex survey design is *Primary Sampling Unit* which denotes the highest level (i.e. cluster or Group) at which random selection occurs. For example in the previously described sample of Republicans and Democrats from randomly selected cities stratified by regions, the city represents the highest level where random selection occurs and as such is the *Primary Sampling Unit.* Often the complicated statistical procedures (for example Shah, *et al.*, 1996; SAS 2002; SPSS 2004; STATA 2002) used to analyze multilevel samples anchor at the *Primary Sampling Unit* and from this can calculate robust-conservative estimates (Diggle, *et al.*, 1994) of variability and P-values.

5.0. CONTEXTUAL SETTINGS AND ANALYSES OF INTEREST

Predictor or exposure variables of interest for a study can occur either at the *Group (or Neighborhood) Level*, the *Individual Level*, or both. For *Group Level* exposures, all persons in the same group share the same value for that exposure while *Individual Level* exposures can vary among different people in the same Group.

For example let the question of interest be whether the "ratio of the number of policemen to people" in a neighborhood is associated with that neighborhood's members level of fear of violent crime. Then the exposure variable "ratio of number of policemen to people" occurs at the *Group Level*" since this variable takes on the same value for all persons who live in the same neighborhood. Or for a group behavioral intervention let the question of interest be whether "the number of years a teacher has led alcohol use cessation classes" influences the success of the students in the class. The "number of years a teacher has led alcohol use cessation classes" is a Group level variable since this takes on the same value for all persons in the same intervention class.

On the other hand, if the exposure of interest is income of the person then this is an *Individual Level* variable since income differs among those living in the same neighborhood (or taking an alcohol cessation class). Similarly *age* is also an individual level variable; ages of persons in the neighborhood or taking the same behavioral intervention class differ.

But, this leads to the question of whether the Group Level effects are something one wishes to adjust for or in fact are part of the outcome of interest. For example, if latinos have poorer health than other ethnic groups does it matter that this could be explained by the fact that latinos live in neighborhoods (i.e. in Group Levels) where there are fewer doctors. Perhaps once this Group Level Effect; number of doctors in the neighborhood is adjusted for, the disparities between latinos and others would diminish dramatically. Should the overall health status of latinos versus others comparison be adjusted for the number of doctors in the neighborhood? Many persons would argue "no". If latinos have poorer health, this needs to be addressed whether or not it is due to living in neighborhoods with fewer doctors. What is most important then is comparing the health status of latinos (i.e. to white non-latinos) and to see if this disparity exists irrespective of whether it is due to Group Level factors.

But consider a different study of whether latinos are more insecure than non-latino whites due to intrinsic (i.e. perhaps cultural based) reasons. In this setting, would it matter if latino had more insecurities because of the fact they come from neighborhoods where poverty and violence are more common? Many now would argue that here one should adjust for the Group Level factors neighborhood violence and poverty characteristics if the study is whether there is something inherent to latino culture that causes insecurity.

6.0. STATISTICAL ANALYSIS OF GROUP LEVEL STUDIES

We present here the basic elements for statistical analyses of group level studies. The full range of possible analyses involving clusters, strata, weights and contextual settings is quite complicated. We thus give details for more simple designs and discuss their extensions. For more details there are several references such as Cochran (1977) and Korn and Graubard (1999). Continuous outcomes are the main focus in this presentation but equivalent procedures for binary and censored outcomes are also mentioned.

For this Section, consider a Study with K neighborhoods and J strata with a given continuous outcome Y. Let X be a single covariate of or a vector (collection of covariates) that may influence the outcome and u denote the true overall population mean for an outcome if X=0. Let k=1,...,K enumerate the neighborhoods and Δ_k be a random neighborhood effect with Δ_k being normally distributed with mean 0 and variance σ^2_Δ. Let j=1,... ,J enumerate strata and st_j denote a fixed strata effect with $\sum_{j=1}^{J} st_j = 0$. Assume that n_{jk} persons are sampled from cluster (or group) k and strata j. If there are no strata in the study, then n_k persons are sampled from cluster k and if the same number of persons are always sampled from each cluster-strata combination then the common number is denoted n. For $l = 1,\ldots n_{jk}$ let jkl denote the lth person taken from the kth cluster in the jth strata and X_{jkl} denote the value of the covariate for that person. If X is a group level covariate, it can be further denoted X_k^{GL} (where GL denotes "Group Level"). In a linear model, the outcome Y_{jkl} from a person taken from cluster (group) k and strata j can be represented as $Y_{jkl} = u + bX_{jkl} + \Delta_k + st_j + \varepsilon_{jkl}$ where b is the true linear relation between X and Y and ε_{jkl} is the person measurement error and is distributed normally with mean 0 and variance σ^2_ϵ. The strata effect is st_j where strata j, could be based on one or multiple individual and/or group level variables. The goal of the analysis often is to obtain $\hat{b}$ an estimator of b and statistically test if b=0.

6.1. Analysis of Individual Effects in (Clustered) Group Level Designs

Let's begin with an unstratified (i.e. no strata) group study which is testing a new group intervention against alcohol abuse (i.e. a Group Level variable X_k^{GL} =0 for those given Program A, X_k^{GL}=1 for those given Program B). Four classes using Program A are taught to $n_k = n$ =15 students each for 60 students total, and 4 classes using Program B are taught to $n_k = n$ =15 students each for 60 students total. So there are a total of K=8=(4+4) teaching groups. For each person, the outcome Y_{kl} is average number of drinks (i.e. wine glass equivalents) of alcohol per week the subject consumes. Since there are no strata (and assuming that no individual level covariates are included in the model), the previously defined model reduces to $Y_{kl} = u + b^{GL} X_k^{GL} + \Delta_k + \varepsilon_{kl}$ where b^{GL} indicates the parameter is for a Group Level variable; $X_k^{GL} = 0$ for classes given Program A, $X_k^{GL} = 1$ for classes given Program B, u is the mean number of drinks consumed by students from Program A, and b^{GL} is the mean difference between Programs A and B. The ability of the teacher and class bonding could directionally influence the outcome of each of the students in the class through Δ_k.

Since there are no strata (i.e., j=1), a naïve analytical approach to test b=0 would be a two-sample t-test of the overall mean results for the 60 persons treated with Program A, $\bar{Y}_A = \sum_{\text{k given A}} \sum_{l=1}^{15} Y_{kl}/60$ Vs for those treated with Program B, $\bar{Y}_B = \sum_{\text{k given B}} \sum_{l=1}^{15} Y_{kl}/60$ and the standard deviation of an observation estimated by a pooled variance $s_p^2 = [\sum_{\text{k given A}} \sum_{l=1}^{15}(Y_{kl} - \bar{Y}_A)^2 + \sum_{\text{k given B}} \sum_{l=1}^{15}(Y_{kl} - \bar{Y}_B)^2]/[120-2]$. The standard error of the difference $\bar{Y}_A - \bar{Y}_B$ is estimated as $s_p\sqrt{2/60}$ since the variance of both $\bar{Y}_A$ and $\bar{Y}_B$ are modeled to be $s_p^2/60$. However, due to the shared Δ_k within the same teaching groups the true variances of $\bar{Y}_A$ and $\bar{Y}_B$ are each $(\sigma_\Delta^2/4 + \sigma_\in^2/60)$ since within each Treatment Arm, there are only 4 independent Δ_k being averaged. However, $s_p^2/60$ estimates a smaller number $(\sigma_\Delta^2/60 + \sigma_\in^2/60)$ by effectively assuming that the Δ_k component for each person is independent. This results in the naïve two-sample t-test having anticonservative (larger than nominal) Type-1 error.

We will now assume n_k is the same size n across all clusters and begin with the simplest approach to compare Program A and Program B. Under this setting, if we look at the mean for all persons in the same teaching Cluster k, $\bar{Y}_k = \sum_{l=1}^{15} Y_{kl}/15$ then the expected value of $\bar{Y}_k$ is u if the teaching group was given Program A and $u + b^{GL}$ if the teaching group was given Program B. Irrespective of treatment, the variance of $\bar{Y}_k$ is $\sigma_\Delta^2 + \sigma_\in^2/15$ and since Δ_k is assumed independent across treatment groups, the $\bar{Y}_k$ are all independent of each other. Therefore, since the treatments are Group Level we can take the averages of the Group means $\bar{Y}_k$ within each treatment group and compare $\bar{Y}_{GL\_A} = \sum_{\text{k given A}} \bar{Y}_k/4$ to $\bar{Y}_{GL\_B} = \sum_{\text{k given B}} \bar{Y}_k/4$ by a two sample t-test $[\bar{Y}_{GL\_B} - \bar{Y}_{GL\_A}] / [\sqrt{2}s_{p,GL}]$ (where the Group Level $s_{p,GL}$ is defined below). Since the $n_k \equiv n$ for all clusters here, it can easily be shown that $[\bar{Y}_{GL\_B} - \bar{Y}_{GL\_A}] = [\bar{Y}_B - \bar{Y}_A]$ (but that is not true if the n_k differ). The pooled variance of the neighborhood mean differences is $s_{p,GL}^2 = [\sum_{\text{k given A}}(\bar{Y}_k - \bar{Y}_{GL\_A})^2 + \sum_{\text{k given B}}(\bar{Y}_k - \bar{Y}_{GL\_B})^2]/[8-2]$ which estimates $(\sigma_\Delta^2 + \sigma_\in^2/15)/4 = (\sigma_\Delta^2/4 + \sigma_\in^2/60)$ which is the true variance of each of the means; $\bar{Y}_{GL\_A}$ and $\bar{Y}_{GL\_B}$. Since there were only 8 intervention groups, the degrees of freedom for $s_{p,GL}^2$ was only 6, even though there were 120 subjects. A more general formulation of this test for differing numbers of groups per intervention arm is given in Section 7.

The small degrees of freedom seen here (i.e., 6) reflect the fact that there were only eight group means and the treatment being studied was delivered at the group level. Degrees of freedom for statistical analyses of group level variables are always less than the total number of groups.

While the two sample t-test provides a good illustration of the fallacy of the naïve approach, it is difficult to use this approach for statistical testing in more general settings when stratified sampling is used, where n_k's (or n_{jk}'s) have varying sizes and/or there are multiple group level or individual level variables of interest. To handle such settings, a class of models known as general linear models have been developed, the simplest of which is known as analysis of variance (Dunn and Clark, 1974) and the more complicated which are known as nested-Mixed and Robust Covariance models (Diggle, *et al.*, 1994).

While the full analytical details of these approaches are beyond this chapter, to illustrate their application we return to the more general model presented earlier $Y_{jkl} = u + bX_{jkl} + \Delta_k + st_j + \varepsilon_{jkl}$ and partition the variables in X_{jkl} into Group Level variables X_{jk}^{GL} and Individual Level (IL) variables X_{jkl}^{IL} to reformulate this model as $Y_{jkl} = u + st_j + (b^{GL} X_{jk}^{GL} + \Delta_k) + (b^{IL} X_{jkl}^{IL} + \varepsilon_{jkl})$ to estimate and test hypotheses on neighborhood level effects X_{jk}^{GL} and on the Variance components Δ_k and ε_{jkl}. In this partitioning, Δ_k reflects the residual Group level effects after adjusting for the covariates in

X^{GL} while ε_{jkl} reflects residual individual effects after adjusting for Δ_k and the covariates in X^{GL} and X^{IL}. Since the group level variables are nested within group (i.e. take the same value for all observations in the same group) a better designation of the model is:

$$Y_{ijk} = u + (b^{GL} X_{jk}^{GL}) + \Delta_k + b^{IL} X_{jkl}^{IL} + s_j + \varepsilon_{jkl} \tag{1}$$

where dropping the subscript l in $(b^{GL} X_{jk}^{GL})$ denotes that some of those effects are exerted through nested group level variables X_{jkl}^{GL}. We also separate the strata effects (st_j) out in this model, since they were part of the sampling design although they can also be predictor variables of interest (including subdivision into Group Level and/or Individual level Strata).

The analytical details of obtaining estimates from models in (1) is beyond the scope of this chapter and are covered elsewhere (also see Diggle, *et al.*, 1994; Korn and Graudard, 1999), but some practical and heuristic details are important for the reader to know. The dual sources of random variance from Δ_k and ε_{jkl} complicates the model fitting as it is analytically and computationally difficult to model both sources of error. In addition, for some studies, potentially unknown correlation structures within a group k may exist (for example subgroups of people may attend the same churches in a given neighborhood and thus have additional subgroup correlation from this source, while other people in that neighborhood do not attend these churches and thus don't share this additional correlation) which are even harder to model.

A *Mixed Model* (including *Hierarchical Models*) approach will directly try to model the heterogeneity of Δ_k and ε_{jkl}. This is often the best approach to use to estimate and test hypotheses on the b (i.e. b^{GL}) for Group Level Effects with small (i.e. <60 groups) and on σ_Δ^2. However, a mixed model may not be optimal if the within group correlation can not be specified correctly due to known or even unknown neighborhood sub-clustering such as among people attending the same churches as described earlier. The simplest mixed model is a nested ANOVA which, for example, could be used instead of a two sample t-test to compare Program A to Program B in the alcohol cessation study described earlier particularly if n_k differed among the teaching classes (for an example see Dunn and Clark, 1974).

A *robust covariance* (also known as *General Estimation Equation or GEE*) approach does not try to directly model the intra-group correlation, but rather uses robust methods to estimate the variance of test statistics and parameters which give conservative results (making it less likely to reject the null hypothesis) when unmodeled covariance structure within the groups exist (Diggle, *et al.*, 1999). While full details are beyond this chapter, the analyst can identify the lowest level of independent clusters. (In our previous examples this would be neighborhood or behavioral intervention teaching class). He/she can then attempt to specify the best correlation structure for repeated observations within these clustered (i.e. the correlation structure of repeated persons, or even person-visits, within a Group). However, a robust covariance that gives conservative results (i.e., less likely to reject null hypothesis when H_o true and gives wider than actual confidence limits) is utilized so if the covariance structure is misperceived, the nominal Type-1 error is not exceeded (although the Type-2 error may be penalized).

If the groups (or individuals within a group) are selected using a stratified scheme then the model declaration is more complicated. The robust covariance approach is best used when complicated or unknown intra-group correlation structures exist and in particular when comparing variances of group level effects is not of interest. But robust covariance models cannot estimate and test for random group level effects i.e. ($\sigma_{\Delta}^2 > 0$) as well as Mixed Models can. But another advantage of the robust covariance model is that it has been more widely applied to binary outcomes (using the logit link) and to censored survival outcomes than have Mixed Models.

6.2. Analysis of Group Mediated Effects in Group Level Designs

Special attention is needed in statistical analysis of Group Level exposures as these should be fit nested within the Group. For example, if there are K groups in the study, then there are at most K different values for a group level variable. But, more importantly, all persons from the same group who share the same value for a Group Level variable also share the same common group effect (Δ_k) mediated in the random error. This means that the maximum degrees of freedom for testing a group level effect is K which can limit power when the number of distinct groups is small. Hence if group level effects are important, one should emphasize sampling from greater numbers of groups within other limitations and study constraints.

6.3. Analysis of Weighted Samples

When it is necessary to use weights to adjust for differential sampling and obtain overall population estimates, the relative weighting must be specified in the statistical analysis. For example, if W_i is the weight of the ith observation to adjust for its sampling probability, then the overall sample mean is $\bar{Y} = \sum W_i Y_i / \sum W_i$ and the variance of this overall mean can be estimated by $\hat{\sigma}^2 = \sum W_i (Y_i - \bar{Y})^2 / \sum W_i$. Similar adjustments for weights are made for other procedures such as multivariate linear/logistic regression and survival analysis when clustering and strata are involved. Most software packages such as SAS 2002; Shah, *et al.*, 1996; SPSS 2004; STATA 2004) permit this to be done in analyses of continuous, binary and censored data.

Typically, when weights were involved in either the planned or unplanned process of sample selection and retention, weights should be used in both univariate and multivariate analyses of the sample. From a programming standpoint, some caution is needed when using sampling weights as many software packages by default take the weights to denote the number of independent observations rather than as weighting for oversampling; *even when the weights have fractions or decimal values*! For example for a given observation let, $W_i = 2$, Sex = Male, Race = White, Hamilton Score = 3 and Systolic Blood Pressure = 148. When presented with $W_i = 2$, the default of some software is to assume that there are *two independent* white men with a Hamilton score of three and a systolic blood pressure of 148. This assumption of two independent observations deflates the calculated variance of statistical estimators below what it should be. To prevent this from happening, the programmer needs to find and use the software commands that specify the weights reflect over/under sampling rather than independent observations.

6.4. Analyses of Stratified Designs

When strata are used in the design of the sample, then they should also be specified and used in the analysis to improve efficiency and validity. For example, suppose a study of income was done in a city of 20,000 blacks and 20,000 whites.

A proportionate stratified sample of 40 blacks and 40 whites is chosen. Within the strata, for the blacks, mean annual income was $\bar{X}_B$ =\$40,000 while whites mean income was $\bar{X}_W$ =\$60,000. For simplicity let within strata standard deviations of income for both races be s_{st} =\$15,000.

Using a naïve analysis that ignored the strata, overall mean annual income for the city would be \$50,000 = (\$40,000 + \$60,000)/2 with, ignoring some minor adjustments for degrees of freedom, an inflated naive standard deviation of $s_n = \sqrt{(15,000)^2 + 0.5\,(60,000-50,000)^2 + 0.5\,(40,000-50,000)^2} = 18,028$. The naïve standard deviation is based on the difference of each observation from the overall mean rather than from the *mean of its own strata* and thus incorporates differences of the strata mean from the overall mean (i.e. where the $0.5(60,000-50,000)^2 + 0.5(40,000-50,000)^2$ terms are added to the within strata standard deviation. Overall, a point estimate and naïve 95% confidence interval for overall mean income of the city would then be \$50,000 ± 1.96* $18,028/\sqrt{40}$ or (44,413 to 55,587)

However, since a stratified design was used with the knowledge that 0.5 of the residents were black and 0.5 of the residents were white, it follows that $\mu = 0.5\mu_B + 0.5\mu_W$ where μ is he overall city mean and μ_B and μ_W are means for the black and white residents, respectively. Now $\bar{X}_B = 40,000$ estimates μ_B and based on the within strata standard deviation of $s_{st} = 15,000$ has a standard error of $15,000/\sqrt{20}$ while $\bar{X}_W = 40,000$ estimates μ_W and has a standard error of $15,000/\sqrt{20}$. Since $\bar{X}_B$ and $\bar{X}_W$ are independent, $0.5\bar{X}_B + 0.5\bar{X}_W$ is an unbiased estimate of $\mu = 0.5\mu_B + 0.5\mu_W$ and has a standard error of $\sqrt{(0.5)^2(15,000/\sqrt{20})^2 + (0.5)^2(15,000/\sqrt{20})^2} = 15,000/\sqrt{40}$. The point estimate for mean overall income is the same as with the naïve approach $0.5\bar{X}_B + 0.5\bar{X}_W = \$50,000$. But the 95% confidence interval is reduced to \$50,000 ± 1.96* $15,000/\sqrt{40}$ or (45,485 to 54,649).

This reduction in the standard error of the overall mean from $18,028/\sqrt{40}$ in the naïve method to $15,000/\sqrt{40}$ in the stratified design reflects an efficiency of 15,000/18,028 = 0.83 that was gained by using stratified sampling versus random sampling. It holds true not only for the overall mean but also exists for estimates from other statistical analyses. But this will be gained only if the programmer specifies the stratified design correctly when performing the statistical analysis.

6.5. Analyses of Subpopulations in Stratified Designs

Sometimes when stratified samples are obtained from a population, analyses are done where the interest is only on a subpopulation of the original population. For example, if all adults in a city are sampled, but the analysis only focuses on females then women constitute the *subpopulation* of interest. When restricting analysis to a subpopulation from a stratified design, an easy mistake is to eliminate observations from the other subpopulations from the analysis. However, as the next example will show, for many settings it is more appropriate to include all observations in the analysis and use what is known as a *subpopulation statement* to define the subpopulation of interest.

To illustrate why, going back to the previous stratified sample of 40 blacks and 40 whites, suppose we are interested in average income of all women in the city (i.e., the subpopulation of interest is *Females*). Suppose $n_{BF} = 15$ of the 40 blacks were female with a mean income of $\bar{X}_{BF}$ = \$35,000 and $n_{WF} = 25$ of the 40 whites were female with a mean income of $\bar{X}_{WF}$ =\$55,000. To make this example easier to present, assume an extreme setting of where the standard deviation of women's income within each strata is $s_{st} = 0$; that is each black woman had an annual income of 35,000 while each white woman had an annual income of $55,000.

If only the 40 women are subsetted for the analysis (i.e. the 25 black men and 15 white men are excluded and ignored) the estimated mean female income in the stratified design is $\overline{X}_{BF} {}^{*} n_{BF}/(n_{BF}+n_{WF}) + \overline{X}_{WF} {}^{*} n_{WF}/(n_{BF}+n_{WF}) = 35{,}000^{*}15/(15+25) + 55{,}000^{*}25/(15+25)$ = $47,500. The estimated standard deviation for this mean based on the within strata variance of income and the weighted means is $s_{st} {}^{*} \sqrt{\{[n_{BF}/(n_{BF}+n_{WF})]^2[1/n_{BF}] + [n_{WF}/(n_{BF}+n_{WF})]^2[1/n_{WF}]\}} = 0/\sqrt{(n_{BF}+n_{WF})} = 0$. In other words because the income did not vary among women within each racial strata (i.e. $s_{st} = 0$) using a standard stratified approach that ignores the number of men sampled within each racial strata the overall estimate must also have zero variance.

While this reasoning may seem logical at first, it is erroneous since it ignores the fact that within each race strata, *the number of women selected is random,* which contributes to the variance of the estimate (Graubard and Korn, 1996). For example only 15 of the 40 blacks selected were women while 25 of the 40 whites selected were women. This numerical superiority of white women caused the overall mean income of $47,500 to be closer to the mean of white ($55,000) women than to that of black women ($35,000). But if in reality 50% of each racial group were women, then the true overall mean income among women in the city would be $45,000 = 0.5*$35,000 + 0.5*$55,000. Furthermore, if 50% of each racial group were women it would also be possible by chance to obtain 15 women in a sample of 40 blacks and 25 women in a random sample of 40 whites. This randomness of number of women taken within each strata in addition to the within strata standard deviation of income among women must be factored into estimation of the standard deviation of overall mean income of women in a stratified design.

The correct statistical approach to estimation of variance for overall mean income of women is to include all 40 men and women from both strata in the analysis with a *Subpopulation statement* indicating that while only outcomes of women are of interest, the relative numbers of women and men sampled from each strata are also important for estimating strata mediated effects on the variance. Income from men (and all other variables obtained form men) will not be included into the analysis. However, the analysis will note that n_{BF} and n_{WF} are random variables and for our example, $n_{BF}=15$ out of a total number of 40 from the black strata (i.e. or an estimated $p_{bf} = 0.375$ (15/40) of adult blacks were women), while $n_{WF}=25$ out of a total number of 40 from the white strata (or an estimated $p_{bf} = 0.625$ (25/40) of adult whites were women). While the full details are beyond this chapter, the variances of the observed n_{BF} and n_{WF}, and their impact on the overall mean estimated income for women will then be derived and combined with the observed within strata variance, S_{st}, of the outcome among women to estimate the variance for the overall mean income of women based on the stratified design.

We presented a simple example for estimating an overall mean for a subpopulation. However, similar problems will arise when performing more sophisticated analyses within a stratified design restricted to a subset of the original population. When restricting analysis to a subset of a population from a stratified design whose characteristics were not part of the stratification criteria, all observations should be included in the analysis data set with a subpopulation statement indicating the persons the analysis is being restricted to.

6.6. Putting Everything Together for Complex Surveys

As indicated earlier, urban surveys can be conducted using multilevel strata and cluster sampling along with weights. It is statistically possible to simultaneously adjust for all of the effects from each of these components provided the correct sampling design is specified in the analysis. Either robust covariance methods or mixed models can be used. However, when the outcomes are are binary or survival (censored time to event) robust covariance models are better (Diggle, *et al*,. 1994; Shah, *et al.*, 1996). When necessary, as described in sections 6.1 – 6.5, clusters, strata, sample weights, primary sampling units, and/or subpopulations must be specified in the analysis statements.

7.0. PLANNING URBAN GROUP LEVEL STUDIES (SAMPLE SIZE AND POWER)

We assume that the reader has some background on general power and sample size estimation and focus here on issues that are unique to Group Level Urban Studies. Most power estimation approaches have been developed for the simpler settings of group clinical trials where the studies can be controlled and made more balanced (Raab, 2001). While power estimation methods will become more advanced with time, to date only some approaches exist to estimate power/sample size for complex Group Level studies involving strata (Snjiders 1993). Some approaches also exist for Group Level binary (Donnar, 1981; Corle and Lake, 2003) and Group Level censored time to event (Poisson) (Hayes and Bennett, 1999). To date no approaches have been developed to estimate sample size/power for weighted sample designs.

We concentrate on estimation of power for a given sample size although the approach presented here can be modified to estimate minimal sample size or minimal detectable difference. Most current approaches (Donnar, *et al.*, 1981; Hsieh, 1988; Donnar and Donald, 1987; Hoover, 2002a; Hoover, 2002b) focus on comparing the effect of a binary exposure at the Group Level (B denotes an exposed group and A denotes an unexposed group) on a continuous outcome Y with K_B groups exposed and K_A groups not exposed. For example, let Y = {perceived importance of having clean air} among residents of K_B=20 neighborhoods exposed to air pollution compared to K_A = 30 neighborhoods not exposed to air pollution. While it is difficult to ensure this occurs in practice, it is also assumed that within each exposure Group, the number of individuals sampled is constant; i.e., $n_k \equiv n$ persons are sampled from each neighborhood For, example let, n = 10 persons be sampled for each of the 30 neighborhoods in the air pollution study. Approaches exist which allow the number of subjects sampled to differ between exposed and unexposed groups, say n_{k_b} = 12 persons sampled from each neighborhood exposed to air pollution and n_{k_a} = 8 persons sampled from each neighborhood not exposed to air pollution (for an example see Hoover, 2002a).

Expanding on Section 6.1, the null hypothesis of no exposure group difference would be tested with a two sample t-test $[\bar{Y}_{GL\_B} - \bar{Y}_{GL\_A}]/\sqrt{2}s_p, GL]$. Where

$$\bar{Y}_{GL\_A} = \sum_{\text{k Not Exposed}} \bar{Y}_k / K_A,\ \bar{Y}_{GL\_B} = \sum_{\text{k Exposed}} \bar{Y}_k / K_B \text{ and } s^2_{p,\ GL} =$$

$$[\sum_{\text{k Not Exposed}} (\bar{Y}_{GL\_A} - \bar{Y}_k)^2 + \sum_{\text{k Exposed}} (\bar{Y}_{GL\_B} - \bar{Y}_k)^2]/[K_A + K_B - 2].$$

When estimating the Type-2 error β for this test ((1− β) = power), besides K_A, K_B, n and the type-1 Error (α) of the test used, one must also input σ the (ie. estimated) standard deviation of an observation, ρ the (estimated) intraclass correlation of observations and d the expected difference between the real means of the exposed and unexposed groups, $[\mu_{GL\_B} - \mu_{GL\_A}]$ you wish to detect. The power of the study is then (Hoover, 2002a);

$$1-\beta = 1-t^{-1}_{K_A + K_B - 2,\, d/\sigma\sqrt{(1/K_A + 1/K_B)(1/n + \rho(1-1/n))}}[t_{K_A + K_B - 2}(1-\alpha/2)]. \qquad (2)$$

Where $t_{K_A+K_B-2}(1-\alpha/2)$ is the value marking the $[1-\alpha/2]$ cumulative density of a central t distribution with $K_A + K_B-2$ df, and $t^{-1}_{K_A + K_B - 2,\, d/\sigma\sqrt{(1/K_A + 1/K_B)(1/n + \rho(1-1/n))}}[v]$ is the probability for a variable having a non-central t distribution with $K_A + K_B-2$ df and non-centrality parameter $d/\sigma\sqrt{(1/k_A + 1/k_B)(1/n + \rho(1-1/n))}$ to be smaller than the value v. While (2) is somewhat non-intuitive, the non-centrality parameter becomes larger (which means power increases) when d increases, n increases K_A or K_B increases and σ decreases. Software to calculate power is available (Hoover, 2002b; Corle and Lake, 2003), and other packages perform similar analyses with the restriction $K_A = K_B$ (Hintze, 2001). Going to the example of this section with $K_A = 20$ $K_B = 30$ and $n = 10$, if the standard deviation of Y is 15, the intraclass correlation is $\rho = 0.04$, the null hypothesis is tested with a two sided $\alpha=0.05$ and it is desired to detect a mean difference of $d = 2$ between residents of neighborhoods with air pollution and residents of neighborhoods without air pollution, the power of the study will be 99.7%. But for the same study, if it turns out $d = 1$, then there will only be a 66% to statistically detect a difference between the exposure arms.

As noted previously, it is assumed that for all individuals within the same sampling group the intraclass correlation of the outcome Y is some value ρ with $0 < \rho < 1$. The larger ρ is the larger the group effect. While it is very difficult to estimate ρ, as described in Section 3, ρ is usually less than 0.05 (Hansen, *et al.*, 1953; Campbell, *et al*, 2000; Smeeth and Ng, 2002). Some approaches have been developed if the intraclass correlation differs between different groups (Hoover, 2002a). If either n differs between clusters or ρ differs between different individuals in the same cluster the averages $\bar{n}$ and $\bar{\rho}$ may be input into the power estimation formulas used such as (2).

ACKNOWLEDGEMENT: Dr. Hoover would like to acknowledge partial support from NSF grant EIA 02-05116 for this work.

REFERENCES

Campbell, M., Grimshaw, J., and Steen, N. (2000). Sample size calculations for cluster randomised trials. *Health Serv. Res. Policy* 5(1):12–6.

Cochran, W.G. (1977). *Sampling Techniques, Third Edition.* John Wiley & Sons, New York, NY.

Cohen, J. (1988). *Statistical Power Analysis for the Behavioral Sciences, Second Edition.* Academic Press, New York, NY.

Corle, D., and Lake, W. Jr. (2003). *Interactive Power Program Inernational Management Systems and NIH/NCI Biometry, Version July 17, 2003,* Bethesda, MD Version.

Cornfield, J. (1978). Randomization by group: a formal analysis. *Am. J. Epidemiol.* 108(3):100–102.

Diggle, P., Liang, K-Y., and Zeger, S.L. (1994). *The Analysis of Longitudinal Data.* Oxford Press, London.

Dixon, W.J., and Massey, F.M. (1969). *Introduction to Statistical Analysis.* McGraw Hill, New York, NY.

Donner, A., Birkett, N., and Buck, C. (1981). Randomization by cluster, sample size requirements and analysis. *Am. J. Epidemiol.* 114(6):906–914.

Donner, A., and Donald, N. (1987). Analysis of data arising from a stratified design with the cluster as the unit of randomization. *Stat. Med.* 6:43–52.

Donner, A., and Klar, N. (1994). Cluster randomization trials in epidemiology: theory and Application. *J. Stat. Plan. Inf.* 42:37–56.

Dunn, O.J., and Clark, V.A. (1974). *Applied Statistics: Analysis of Variance and Regression.* Wiley and Sons, New York, NY.

Gail, M.H., Byar, D.P., Pechacek, T.F., and Corle, D.K. (1992). Aspects of statistical design for the Neighborhood Intervention Trial for smoking cessation (COMMIT). *Control Clin. Trials* 13(1):6–21.

Graubard, B.I., and Korn, E.L. (1996). Survey Inference for Subpopulations *Am. J. Epidemiol.* 144(1):102–6.

Hansen, M.H., Hurwitz, W.N., and Madow, W.G. (1953). *Sample Survey Methods and Theory. Vol 1. Methods and Application.* Wiley, New York, NY.

Hayes, R.J., and Bennett, S. (1999). Simple sample size calculation for cluster-randomized trials *Int. J. Epidemiol.* 28(2):319–26.

Heckathorn, D.D. (2002) Response driven sampling II: deriving valid population estimates from chain referral samples of hidden populations. *Social Problems* 49(1):11–34.

Hintze, D.J.L. (2000). *Power and Sample Size.* NCSS Trial and PASS Chicago, IL.

Hoover, D.R. (2002a). Clinical trials of behavioral interventions with heterogeneous teaching subgroup effects. *Stat. Med.* 21:1351–64.

Hoover, D.R. (2002b). Power for T-Test comparisons of unbalanced cluster exposure studies *J. Urban Health* 79(2):278–94.

Hsieh, F.Y. (1988). Sample size formulae for intervention studies with the cluster as unit of randomization. *Stat. Med.* 7(11):1195–201.

Koepsell, T.D., Martin, D.C., and Diehr, P.H. (1991). Data analysis and sample size issues in evaluations of neighborhood-based health promotion and disease prevention programs: a mixed-model analysis of variance approach. *J. Clin. Epidemiol.* 44(7):701–13.

Korn, E.L., and Graubard, B.I. (1999). *Analysis of Health Surveys.* John Wiley & Son, New York, NY.

Olin, G.L., Liu, H., and Merriman, B. (1996). *Health & Health Care of the Medicare Population data from the 1995 Medicare Benificiary Survey.* Westat, Rockville, MD.

Raab, G.M., and Butcher, I. (2001). Balance in cluster randomized studies. *Stat. Med.* 20:351–56.

SAS Institute Inc. (2002). *SAS Version 9.0.* SAS Institute, Cary, NC.

Shah, B.V., Barnwell, B.G., and Bieler, G.S. (1996). *SUDAAN User's Manual: Release 7.0.* Research Triangle Institute, Research Triangle Park, NC.

Simpson, J.M., Klar, N., and Donner, A. (1995). Accounting for cluster randomization: a review of primary prevention trials, 1990 through 1993. *Am. J. Public Health* 85(10):1378–83.

Smeeth, L., and Ng ES-W. (2002). Intraclass correlation coefficients for cluster randomized trials in primary care: data from the MRC Trial of the Assessment and Management of Older People in the Neighborhood Controlled *Clinical Trials* 23(4):409–21.

Snijders, T.A.B., and Bosker, R.J. (1993). Standard errors and sample sizes for two level research. *J. Educat. Stat.* 18:237–59.

STATA Inc. (2004). *STATA Base Reference Manuel.* STATA Press, College Station, TX.

SPSS Inc. (2004). *SPSS Version 12.0.* Chicago, IL.

Chapter 16

Health Services Research and the City

Michael K. Gusmano and Victor G. Rodwin

1.0. INTRODUCTION

Health services research is, by nature, multidisciplinary, for it draws on the methods, concepts, and theories of social sciences, which are relevant to the study of how the organization and financing of health services can improve the delivery of health care services (Gray, *et al.*, 2003). While medicine and public health, too, are multidisciplinary enterprises drawing on such disciplines as molecular biology, physiology, anatomy, genetics, epidemiology and more, health services research departs from these disciplines in focusing not on the nature of disease and health but rather on the financing and organization of health systems.

So it is with urban health services research albeit that this field is more narrowly focused on health services in cities. The city focus has resulted in a large body of research on vulnerable groups, barriers to service access, public health clinics and community health centers. Likewise, it has led to important investigations of safety-net institutions, e.g. public hospitals and health centers, which serve a disproportionate share of uninsured and low-income patients. In addition, urban health services research has focused on a host of specific services associated with subpopulations suffering from TB, HIV/AIDS, drug addiction and other social pathologies that are typically associated with the "inner city."

If one views the field of urban health services research through a kind of intellectual telescope, what is most striking are the many issues that have escaped careful scrutiny. The city, after all, is more than a center of disease, poor health and pervasive poverty (Rodwin, 2001; Glouberman, 2003). Since the oracle of Delphi and the miracles of Lourdes, the city has also functioned as an economic base for medical cures. Most large cities serve as headquarters for academic medical centers (Ginzberg and Yohalem, 1974), places where health professionals congregate, and more generally, strategic locations for health promotion (Freudenberg, 2000) as well as the diffusion of healthy lifestyles among the well-to-do. There is a significant literature on academic medical centers, hospitals, health centers and multiple organizational forms of medical practice but most studies do not explore the relationships between these institutions and the city. What is more, there are few comparative analyses of health systems and services among cities (Rodwin, 2005).

These gaps in the field are unfortunate for several reasons. First, they leave open a host of important and unanswered questions. For example, does the density of tertiary health services – academic medical centers, sub-specialists, and state-of-the-art medial technologies – improve access and quality of urban health care? Does it confer any discernable benefits on the health status of the urban populations who reside in their proximity? Do the teaching programs, hospital clinics and affiliated health centers provide significant benefits to those most in need of basic health services, including primary care? What side effects, other than employment (Vladeck, 1999) diffuse down to the most disadvantaged "inner city" populations who live in the shadow of the academic medical center? And what is the optimal location of public facilities for the provision of health services to the most disadvantaged?

Second, given significant differences among cities and their health systems, there are clearly ample opportunities for comparative learning. For example, cities as different as New York, Los Angeles, Chicago, and Houston could clearly learn from one another's experience in organizing their public health infrastructure and providing health services to their residents? Often it is easier to implement policy changes at the local level, particularly when decision-making is decentralized, fragmented and responsive to local preferences, traditions and distinctive conditions. Typically, local authorities are able to move faster than their national governments in learning from city-to-city exchanges (O'Meara, 1999). Thus, it would be fruitful for the field of urban health services research to initiate systematic comparisons of urban health systems – both among cities as well as among neighborhoods within them.

In this chapter, we review some of the more salient studies at the intersection of urban and health services research. In addition, we propose a research agenda to address the gaps noted above. Finally, to illustrate some small steps along an international dimension of the proposed research agenda, we provide some examples of our own on-going urban health services research on world cities.

2.0. URBAN STUDIES AND HEALTH SERVICES RESEARCH

As Scott Greer (1983) observed over two decades ago, "What is striking to those who have been immersed in urban studies and then have become interested in the social response to health and ill health is the extreme segregation of the two areas of inquiry." From the heyday of 19th century European public health movements which focused on the importance of sanitation (clean water supply, sewers and garbage disposal) and improvements in housing conditions, to twentieth century interventions aimed at improving access to health services, the main body of research on public health, as well as on medical care, was largely focused on cities. Moreover, the triumph of public health is largely responsible for making cities more habitable. Yet, the field of urban studies has largely ignored public health (Coburn, 2004), and the field of health services research has followed the growth of the welfare state in veering away from local territorial concerns and focusing largely on statistical aggregates ranging from regions, states and nations.

Urban planners typically study cities from perspectives that span across architecture, urban design, transportation, economic development, the environment, sociology, anthropology, management, and ecology. Even in great syntheses on the state of cities, e.g. Lewis Mumford's *Culture of Cities* (1938), Jane Jacobs's *Death and Life of Great American Cities* (1961) or more recently Peter Hall's *Cities in Civilization* (1998), there is virtually no discussion of the health systems that service their populations. Likewise, in the official annual reviews by the Department of Housing and Urban Development on the State of Cities (HUD, 1999a), there are no chapters on the state of local public health infrastructure or even safety-net services for the uninsured, most of which are left to city and county governments.

In the literature on public health, there are, of course, some classic case histories on the evolution of public health and hospitals in specific cities. For example, on New York City, Duffy's (1974) history of public health or Rosner's (1982) history of New York's hospitals. In the broader field of health services research, however, whenever the city appears as a unit of analysis, there seem to be only two ways to explain it. The investigators are either: 1) focused on "inner city" (often meant to refer to "poor" and "poor minority") populations that happen to be concentrated in specific inner city neighborhoods ("concentrated deprivation"); or 2) have selected, unwittingly, a spatial unit that happens to be a neighborhood, a city, or part of a greater metropolitan region. In both cases, however, their choice was driven more by data availability or other criteria than derived from theoretical or practical considerations about how characteristics of cities are related to different aspects of health care systems.

We propose to review two bodies of urban health services research, which fit either in categories (1) or (2) above, or provide noteworthy exceptions to them: a) health services for "inner city" populations; and b) performance of health systems. All of these areas of research are clear exceptions to our general proposition that health services research has focused largely on national or state levels of analysis. They deserve a good deal of attention because of their significance for the field. But none of them dispel our critique that the dominant approach to health services research has largely ignored the question of how cities and their health systems affect urban health.

3.0. HEALTH SERVICES FOR "INNER CITY" POPULATIONS

The dominant literature on health services in cities focuses on the use of health care among vulnerable populations and the organizations that care for them. Only rarely does this literature discuss the unique challenges associated with addressing the health care needs of vulnerable populations in urban environments. By focusing exclusively on the underserved populations of the "inner city," it fails to provide a complete picture of urban health care systems. Nonetheless, this literature has contributed to our understanding of the health services system for the uninsured and disadvantaged (the so-called "safety net"), the barriers to access faced by vulnerable populations, and the value of innovations in health policy and health care delivery for these populations. Noteworthy examples include single city case -studies of particular populations, programs or safety-net institutions, studies that examine a particular type of program or safety-net institution in several cities and, more rarely, studies that compare health services for vulnerable populations in urban, suburban and/or rural areas. Review of this literature can be organized into lessons about safety net providers and health insurance programs for the poor and underserved.

3.1. Safety-Net Providers

An important cluster of studies on "inner city" populations examines the performance and well-being of health care safety-net institutions in cities. The U.S. relies on a patchwork "system" of safety-net providers for the uninsured, Medicaid recipients, and other medically vulnerable populations. The nature of the patchwork varies considerably from community to community (Grogan and Gusmano, 1999; Lewin and Altman, 2000), but often includes institutions and programs funded, in part, by city and other local governments (National Governor's Association, 2000; Norton and Lipson, 1998a). City and County public hospitals, community health centers, local health departments, and a variety of local programs for the uninsured are usually the "providers of last resort" for individuals in the community who do not qualify for Medicare, Medicaid, or other forms of public health insurance (Salit, *et al.*, 2002). Beyond these formal safety-net institutions, physicians and other health care providers located in low-income neighborhoods represent an important part of the ambulatory care system for poor people.

Concerns about the viability of the health care safety-net have prompted studies that evaluate the health and performance of safety-net institutions in cities (Ambruster and Lichtman, 1999; Felt-Lisk, *et al.*, 2002; Thaver, *et al.*, 1998; Thorpe, 1988). These institutions and programs play a critical role in providing access to care for the uninsured and other medically underserved individuals, but they are threatened by recent changes in the health care system. The growth in the number of uninsured, reductions in payments from public and private payers and greater competition in the health care system have combined to make it more difficult for health care safety-net providers to serve the uninsured (Cunningham, 1998; Iglehart, 1995; Lewis and Altman, 2000). An Institute of Medicine (IOM) report notes that America's health care safety-net is "intact, but endangered" (Lewin and Altman, 2000). Faced with these challenges, cities across the U.S. are working to restructure their health care safety-net systems. This often involves changing the role of government and forming a variety of public-private partnerships (Andrulis, 1997; Felland and Lesser, 2000; Gabow, 1997; Norton and Lipson, 1998b).

Many of the innovations adopted in recent years involve the application of fashionable management technologies and public health ideas to health programs for the poor. In summary, such elements of managed care (Andrulis and Gusmano, 2000) involve the use of primary care gatekeepers, health promotion and disease prevention programs, and careful scrutiny of medical care use. For example, more than 100 health care safety-net institutions created their own Medicaid managed care plans during the 1990s (Freund, 1984; Gray and Rowe, 2000; Gusmano, *et al.*, 2002). Nearly all of these plans are based in cities. They are important because their survival and performance can have dramatic effects on their sponsoring organizations and the populations they serve. Although these plans remain fragile, they are playing an increasingly important role in the Medicaid program of many cities (Sparer and Brown, 2000).

The Agency for Healthcare Research and Quality (AHRQ) has coordinated a number of studies of the urban health care safety-net, which provide a comparative analysis of these institutions, as well as several indices that measure their needs and capacities. As Billings and Weinick (2003), the authors of these reports, have emphasized, "all safety-nets are local," which is why the AHRQ compares safety net institutions in 90 metropolitan areas, including 171 cities. The extraordinary variation in the size, scope and health of the health care safety-net in different parts of the U.S. supports the thesis that "place matters" among and within metropolitan regions (Dreier, *et al.*, 2001). Kawachi and Berkman (2000) have provided a theoretical and empirical basis for research on the impact of neighborhood characteristics, e.g. income, social cohesion and crime on population health status. Billings and Weinick, (2003) show that neighborhood characteristics, not directly related to the health care system, are important because they influence the health care safety-net and are, in turn, influenced by it.

To support such analyses, Billings and Weinick, (2003) include a variety of contextual variables in their data book, including population size, age distribution, racial/ethnic distribution, income, education, living arrangements, home ownership, and crime. This recognition of the relationship between city and neighborhood characteristics and the health care safety-net represents an important and promising direction for a more comprehensive analysis of urban health care systems. Likewise, a recent comparative study of the urban safety net in Baltimore, Detroit, Boston, Oakland, Atlanta and Chicago represents a promising direction for comparative health services research on cities (O'Toole, *et al.*, 2004).

3.2. Health Insurance Programs for the Poor and Underserved

A second topic in the literature on health services for inner city populations is the implementation of Medicaid (health insurance for the very poor), the State Community Health Insurance Program (SCHIP) – a recent program that covers children whose parents' income exceeds Medicaid eligibility levels – and other federal, state and local programs designed to expand access for the poor and underserved. Although most of the literature on Medicaid and SCHIP is focused on national or state levels of government, there are several exceptions. For example, studies that evaluate innovations in Medicaid and SCHIP enrollment (Fairbrother, *et al.*, 2004; Halfon, *et al*, 1997; Haslanger, 2003), access to care for Medicaid and SCHIP enrollees (Fossett, *et al.*, 1992), and the implementation of Medicaid managed care (Delia, *et al.*, 2001; Gabow, 1997; Page, 1999; Perloff, 1996) often examine city-level data.

Cities and other local governments have also adopted their own small programs to extend health care coverage to the uninsured and other vulnerable populations (Hatton, 2001; Norton and Lipson, 1998b). These programs take a variety of forms ranging from physician volunteer efforts supported by a small pool of public funds, to state licensed programs for the uninsured. Like Medicaid and SCHIP, local programs for the uninsured usually involve some role for managed care (Andrulis and Gusmano, 2000). Some programs contract with HMOs or other managed care organizations. Other cities have created quasi-managed care plans for the uninsured. The Boston Medical Center's (BMC) *Boston HealthNet (Pilot) Program*, for example, served as the pilot plan for BMC's Medicaid managed care plan. This program and similar plans in cities across the country, are not state licensed HMOs, but rely on managed care techniques to control costs and encourage primary care (Andrulis and Gusmano, 2000). Such programs are quite fragile due to the uncertainty of the local fiscal environment, and the growing pressures to spend limited resources on different priorities. Their existence highlights the extent to which cities are responsible for the "residual" populations that fall between the cracks of national and state policy (Rodwin and Gusmano, 2005). The limited scope and instability of these programs, however, illustrates the limits that cities face when they try to address these problems – limits in their capacity to raise revenue and reliance on local business to maintain their tax receipts (Elkin, 1987; Peterson, 1981; 1995; Peterson and Rom, 1990; Stone, 1989).

3.3. Programs for Special Populations

Since special populations – for example, ethnic minorities, poor immigrants, and injection drug using (IDU) populations are concentrated in cities, the urban health services research literature includes many studies of programs for these groups (Solomon, *et al.*, 1991; Juday, *et al.*, 2003). Such programs include those for people with tuberculosis and HIV/AIDS (Ryan White) as well as needle exchange and other programs for IDU populations. Infectious diseases like hepatitis, tuberculosis, and HIV/AIDS spread rapidly in densely populated areas and cities are viewed as "breeding grounds," as well, for social pathologies, e.g., drug use (*New York Academy of Medicine*, 2001). Some of this literature explores the prevalence of these conditions and identifies the risk factors for infection, but most studies examine the availability, use and performance of health care and social programs for specific subpopulations. Even broad-based interventions such as the RW Johnson's Urban Health Initiative, tend to focus on specific population groups, e.g. children (Schroeder, 1998).

3.4. Barriers to Services and Insurance

Studies that investigate the use of health services by subpopulation groups identify multiple barriers to access. Not surprisingly, these include barriers that affect other poor and underserved groups including, income, education, insurance and the availability of health care providers. In addition, alcohol use, the presence of minor children, concerns about privacy, trust and stigma also inhibit the use of health care among these special populations (Hutchinson, *et al.*, 2004; Shedlin and Shulman, 2004; Sterk, *et al.*, 2002). Finally, policies designed to provide care can, themselves, represent a barrier if they "impose unrealistic expectations" on the populations they are designed to serve (Van Olphen and Freudenberg, 2004).

3.5. Race, Ethnicity, Culture and Access to Medical Services

Studies that focus on health care for inner city populations often document and explain the relationship between race, ethnicity and access to quality health care. Big cities often serve as the sites for this research because their populations are so diverse. These studies highlight significant barriers to access faced by racial and ethnic minorities (Andrulis, 2000; Garbers, *et al.*, 2004; Kotchen, *et al.*, 1998; Ray, *et al.*, 1998; Seid, *et al.*, 2003).

What accounts for these persistent barriers to access? Language (Seid, *et al.*, 2003), culture (Garbers, *et al.*, 2004; Kosloski, *et al.*, 2002), insurance coverage (Andrulis, 2000), and proximity to medical services (Prinz and Soffel, 2004; Schulz, *et al.*, 2002), all contribute. And one important response to these access barriers faced by racial and ethnic minority residents of cities is the growing push to develop greater "cultural and linguistic competence" among health care providers (Diversity Rx, 2001). AHRQ, the Department of Health and Human Services and the National Institutes of Health, among others, have each called for research and training to improve cultural competence.

4.0. PERFORMANCE OF HEALTH SYSTEMS—PRACTICE VARIATIONS AND AVOIDABLE HOSPITALIZATIONS

John Wennberg's pioneering research on small-area variations in health care delivery, and the subsequent research that it spawned, compares the performance of health care systems across small geographic areas including, but not limited to, cities (Wennberg and Gittlesohn, 1973; Wennberg, Freeman and Culp, 1987). These studies document extensive variations in rates of hospital admission for certain conditions and rates of surgical procedures between areas that have similar demographic characteristics and similar rates of mortality (Perrin, *et al.*, 1990). The findings raise important questions about standards of clinical decision-making and the adequacy of reimbursement mechanisms.

This approach to health services research can also be used to evaluate disparities in care and to investigate problems of access to care for poor, underserved populations in cities. For example, studies of ambulatory sensitive conditions (ASC) often examine the variation in rates of ASC within and across cities. This research suggests that individuals without health insurance are more likely to be admitted to hospitals with ASC because they are less likely to receive appropriate and timely primary care than those with insurance (Billings, *et al.*, 1996; Weissman, *et. al*, 1992; Hadley, *et al.*, 1991). These are diagnoses for which access to timely and appropriate primary care should decrease or avoid the need for hospital admission. High rates of admission for ASC, among residents of an area, may indicate that residents face inappropriate barriers to primary care.

In contrast to many comparisons of the urban health care safety-net or the implementation of Medicaid and other health care programs for the poor, much of the literature on small area variations in health care documents the performance of a local health care system for the entire population, not just the components of the system that address the needs of the poor. The most noteworthy examples of this approach, applied to whole cities, are the comparative analyses of Boston and New Haven (Fisher, *et al.*, 1994; Wennberg, *et al.*, 1987) which suggest that significant differences in population-based patterns of hospital discharges, in these cities, do not appear to reflect differences in population health, as measured by mortality. Such findings are critical to the development of further research on the relationship between city characteristics and their health systems.

5.0. BEYOND "INNER CITY" POPULATIONS AND MEASURING HEALTH SYSTEMS PERFORMANCE

Most of the health services research noted above is related to the city, either because it is focused on poor populations and the organizations and programs that serve them, or because the data were available at the city level. It is not, however, related to the city through criteria that are derived from theoretical or practical considerations about how the organization and financing of health services are tied to intrinsic characteristics of cities.

There are, however, some notable exceptions to this pattern. Andrulis and Goodman (1999) published an impressive compendium on the 100 largest cities in the U.S. with some indicators on the extent of the social safety net. This dataset is noteworthy for it distinguishes suburbs from central cities and documents important dimensions of the urban health penalty (Andrulis, 1997). To date, Andrulis and colleagues have focused primarily on measures of health, including infant mortality and life expectancy, but they also present data on the use of prenatal care in these cities. The next stage of the analysis will extend this work to include information on the use of hospital services. There remain, nevertheless, insufficient data on urban (inner city as well as suburban) and health system characteristics across most cities.

6.0. A RESEARCH AGENDA ON HEALTH SERVICES AND THE CITY

The costs of segregating inquiry among the fields of urban planning and health services research have been increasing along with urbanization. For as we live in a more urbanized world, there is increasing awareness that the city is indeed a strategic unit of analysis for understanding the health sector. Yet most health services research – both in the United States and among international organizations such as the United Nations, the World Health Organization (WHO) or the Organization for Economic Cooperation and Development (OECD) – continues to assume that states or the nation, as a whole, are the most relevant units of analysis for assessing the performance of health systems and health policy. There are many limitations to this view.

First, there are enormous variations in health and health system performance within nations, between urban and rural areas, between large and small cities, and between depressed and prosperous ones. Many studies on urban health have documented evidence of an urban health penalty for subpopulation groups living in cities (Andrulis and Shaw-Taylor, 1996; Geronimus, 1996). Other studies have focused on disparities in health status among different groups (NYCDHMH, 2004). In addition, the RWJ Foundation's Tracking Project has highlighted disparities in resource levels and health system performance among midsize cities across the U.S. (Ginsberg, 1996).

Second, it is exceedingly difficult to disentangle the relative importance of health systems from other determinants of health, including the sociocultural characteristics and the neighborhood context of the population whose health is measured (Ellen, *et al.*, 2001). It is even more difficult to do so at a level of aggregation such as the nation state where important dimensions of health policy are made.

Third, despite the rise of the welfare state, even in the most centralized nations, many dimensions of health and social policy elude national and state levels. Some of the most challenging problems – care for vulnerable older persons, people with severe mental illness, the most economically disadvantaged and the uninsured-fall into a kind of residual category of problems that are passed down to local governments among which city governments bear a disproportionate share (Rodwin and Gusmano, 2005).

For all of these reasons, a good case can be made for integrating inquiry across the fields of urban studies and health services research. Among those concerned with cities, this will require a new focus on the health sector and measures of population health. Among those wedded to health services research, it will require special attention to health systems and population health in cities, which will, in turn, require disaggregated data on health services and health at the city and neighborhood levels. To extend previous inquiries along these lines beyond the dominant literature on "inner cities" and health, it would be helpful to develop a framework that explicitly addresses the broad scope of relationships between cities and health systems.

6.1. A Framework for Comparing Cities, Health Services and Health

Development of such a framework raises a number of important questions: What specific requirements do cities place on their public health infrastructure and the organization and financing of their health services? Conversely, what are the effects of hospitals, academic medical centers, medical research and training activities, and more generally patterns of access to primary care services on the local economy of the city, as well as its population's health? How do national and subnational level patterns of health care financing and organization affect city-level interventions in the health sector? Finally, how do spatial patterns of what Kronick and Enthoven (1999) called "excess and deprivation" in the supply of health services, across city neighborhoods, affect a city's health system and its population's health?

Such questions raise at least two conceptual issues. First, a task in any comparative inquiry is the issue of defining relevant units of analysis. Second, related to the first, is the need to structure comparative analyses around similarities, as well as differences, among these units, so as to encourage the generation of hypotheses about the impact of differences in health services financing and organization across cities that share in common a number of explicit attributes.

With respect to the first issue, although there is a rich literature on the classification of cities (Clark, 1996; Friedmann, 1986) most existing comparisons of health and health care in cities have not paid sufficient attention to this problem. Vlahov and Galea (2002) recognize its importance by highlighting what they call "urbanization" as one of two dimensions in their proposed "urban health framework." By this term, they refer to the broader forces affecting the nature of cities over time. If one were to measure such a concept at one point in time and rely on some crude indicators for characterizing different cities, some obvious ones to consider would be: population size, density, and income per capita. Such indicators allow one to distinguish between major categories of cities: e.g. megacities of the third world, defined by the United Nations as urban agglomerations with a population exceeding 10 million people; global (or world) cities or "city-regions" (Scott, 2001), and mid-size or smaller cities, once again classified by density and income per capita. The mid-size or smaller cities might usefully be classified in relation to their current patterns of economic growth. For example, in the U.S. it is common to distinguish northeastern rust-belt, de-industrializing cities from the rapid growing sun-belt cities of the southwest. Alternatively, the U.S. Department of Housing and Urban Development (HUD, 1999b) distinguished a set of "double trouble" cities due to their high unemployment, significant population loss, and/or high poverty rates; and the RW Johnson Foundation's urban health initiative has selected five "distressed cities" for specific interventions and evaluations of their effectiveness (Weitzman, *et al.*, 2002; Brecher, *et al.*, 2004).

Even with such crude distinctions, however, acceptance of such city "categories," (or others) still leaves unanswered the problem of how to define relevant spatial boundaries for purposes of making comparisons. For example, most United Nations' demographic and housing studies, among cities, refer to the most expansive definitions available. New York is defined even more broadly than the U.S. Census definition of the consolidated metropolitan area (21.2 million) or the tri-state region (19.5 million) with 21 counties in New York, New Jersey and Connecticut, let alone the 8 million that make up the legal entity New York City.

Some of the most important studies of health and quality of life in cities have followed the United Nations in this respect. For example, an important comparison of social and health indicators across the world's largest metropolitan areas draws on these United Nations definitions (Population Action International, 1990). Likewise, the World Bank has collected some basic health and quality of life indicators on large cities around the world (World Bank, 2002). In contrast, an important data collection exercise, initiated by the European Community – Project Megapoles (Bardsley, 1999) – draws on the legal definition of city boundaries for the major capitals of Europe. In this case, the selection criteria for inclusion are not related to population size but rather to their political functions as national capitals. The one exception to this criterion was the inclusion of Lyon for France, instead of Paris because French authorities representing the capital decided not to participate.

With respect to the second issue, structuring comparative analyses around similarities, as well as differences, among city units, even after selecting cities among the same category (in terms of population size and density) and agreeing on relevant criteria to define appropriate units of analysis, it is critical to think about relevant criteria for defining similarities and differences among these units. Once again, Vlahov and Galea's (2002) focus on three dimensions of cities – social environment, physical environment and health and social services – is a useful starting point. But to enable a focus on similarities and differences across cities, these dimensions need to be disaggregated. For example, one would want to have some indicators on the economic base of cities, their physical environment, housing characteristics, transportation, socio-economic, demographic characteristics, and more. To develop an understanding of health and social services, it is important to develop some indicators of health system characteristics. For example, the levels of health care resources, the relative importance of hospitals and academic medical centers in the city, the mix of public and private hospitals and the strength of the social safety net.

In summary, an initial framework for comparing cities, health services and health would begin by distinguishing city categories and spatial units of analysis (Table 1).

Next, it would classify them according to a variety of key urban/neighborhood and health system characteristics, as depicted in Table 2, and explore the impact of cities – their neighborhood and health system characteristics – on two outcomes: the use of health services and health status.

Such a framework would provide a useful foundation on which to develop indicators to compare cities with respect to their health systems, use of health services and population health.

Table 1. A Framework for Comparative Analysis

City Categories
Megacity
World city
Mid-size city
Smaller city
Distressed vs. Prosperous city
Spatial Units of Analysis
Metropolitan region
Urban core
Central business district
Suburbs
Neighborhoods

Table 2. The Relationship between Cities and Health System Characteristics

Urban/Neighborhood characteristics		Health system characteristics
Economic base Housing Transportation Socio-economic and demographic Physical environment	⟷	Health care resources Organizational factors Health insurance coverage Social safety-net

6.2. Development of a Database

One of the nagging difficulties in advancing health services research along the lines of the framework outlined above is the lack of available and comparable data on urban and health system characteristics of cities. In the U.S., the Chicago Department of Health has led the way in collecting basic population health data, on an annual basis, for large cities across the nation (Benbow, 1998) but there are no comparable data for their urban and health system characteristics. The Urban Institute collected data on the 100 largest cities in the U.S., but this dataset contained few indicators on population health and health services (Brookings Institute, 2004). As we noted earlier, the compendium of the 100 largest cities in the United States published by Andrulis and Goodman (1999) includes some indicators on the extent of the social safety net. However, it does not contain sufficient data on urban and health system characteristics (e.g., the current version includes data on the use of prenatal services, the next version will include some additional information about hospitalizations). Another noteworthy contribution to database development on health systems characteristics of mid-size urban communities around the country is the RWJ Foundation's (Ginsberg, 1996) because it provides extensive indicators on health system characteristics. In this case, however, there are insufficient indicators on urban characteristics and population health.

To advance health services research on cities, there is no way to escape the "nitty gritty" work of developing a comparative database along the lines of the framework we have outlined. While it would be imprudent to draw causal inferences from such comparisons, observed differences in health status and the use of health care services among a set of cities from a common category, with comparable units of analysis and a set of similar urban characteristics, but different health systems characteristics, can suggest promising directions for new research. Beyond the research component, such a database can support the study of best practices, as well as interesting failures, when policymakers and program mangers look around for innovations to improve health system organization in their own cities. In comparison to the typical study tour, the combination of such a database with selected cases of urban health care innovations would assist knowledgeable practitioners to interpret what they see.

7.0. THE WORLD CITIES PROJECT (WCP): AN INTERNATIONAL EXAMPLE OF HEALTH SERVICES RESEARCH ON CITIES

The World Cities Project (Rodwin and Gusmano, 2002; World Cities Project, 2004) compares health systems, health and quality of life in the four largest cities of the wealthy nations belonging to the OECD: New York, London, Paris and Tokyo. These cities are surely among the best studied cities in the world. Our principal common units of analysis are their historic urban cores (Figure 1) but often studies extend to their surrounding first rings and greater metropolitan regions. What we have termed their "urban" characteristics have been the subject of serious scholarship, e.g. on their global functions (Sassen, 2001), competitive advantages, politics and planning (Savitch, 1988) transportation infrastructure (Focas, 1988) historical development and architecture (Burrows and Wallace, 1999). Although these cities serve as headquarters of "command and control" for transnational corporations and international financial institutions (Sassen, 1999; Harris, 1997), there are still formidable problems in collecting comparable data about them (Short, *et al.*, 1996).

Despite wide-spread interest in these cities and city-specific data on many dimensions of health and health services, comparative analyses of their health systems are notably absent from the comparative urban literature. Moreover, scholars of urban health and services, in an international context, have not systematically compared world cities (Harpham and Tanner, 1995; Atkinson, *et al.*, 1996). For these reasons, we present the WCP as a way to bridge the gap among these segregated areas of inquiry. In addition, WCP illustrates how health services research can frame a comparative analysis of cities around spatial units deliberately selected to highlight points of similarity as a starting point for generating hypotheses to explain observed differences.

7.1. The Urban Core as a Unit of Analysis

In contrast to studies of health system performance at the national level, comparison of world cities provides spatial boundaries within which to assemble local data on the characteristics of populations, the density of medical resources, the extent of health insurance coverage, and other neighborhood and health system characteristics. For this reason we defined an urban core for New York City, London, the Paris Region, and Tokyo (Figure 1). Our definition of the urban core was guided by five criteria: 1) historic patterns of urban development; 2) population size; 3) population density; 4) mix of high and low income populations; and 5) functions as central hubs for employment and health care resources.

First, with respect to urban development, Manhattan, Inner London, and Paris represent the historic centers from which these metropolitan regions grew (Fig. 1). In Tokyo, the same can be said of its 11 inner wards within the surrounding Yamanote subway line. Second, in terms of population size, Manhattan, Inner London, and Paris range from 1.5 to 2.7 million.

Third, in terms of density, Manhattan and Paris are similar: 66,000 versus 53,000 inhabitants per square mile. Both Manhattan and Paris have almost twice the population density of Inner London. Likewise, however one might define an urban core in Tokyo, the density is much closer to London than to Manhattan or Paris.

Fourth, the urban cores of these cities combine a mix of high and low-income populations. In Manhattan, average household incomes range from $92,876 on the Upper East Side to $23,730 in Central Harlem; in Paris, they range from French Francs (FF) 388,883 in the 8th to FF 131,765 in the 20th *arrondissement*; and in Inner Tokyo they range from 3,791 yen in Chiyoda to 1,782 in Arakawa*. In Great Britain household income data is not available but variations in measures of social deprivation vary widely. For example, among the boroughs of Inner London, the percentage of persons who are "income deprived" ranges from 16.8 % in Kensington to

*Manhattan: Housing and Vacancy Survey, 1996; Paris: Ministry of Finance, 1996

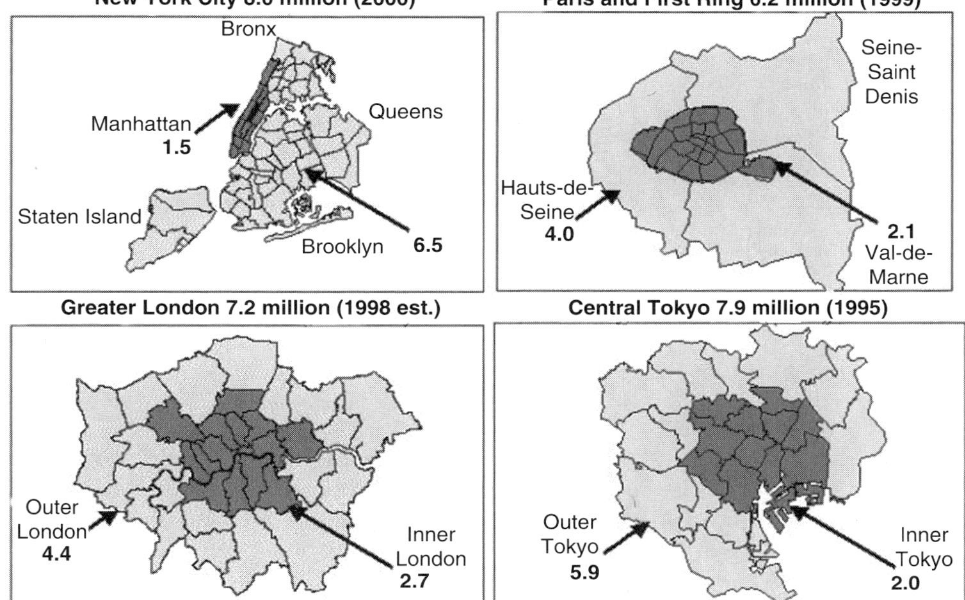

Figure 1. Urban Core and First Ring Populations (Millions).

51.3 % in Tower Hamlets. Tower Hamlet's rank among all 354 local authorities in England is 16, while Kensington's is 177.

Finally, a number of criteria related to their functions as central hubs – what geographers call "central place theory" – suggest three striking parallels among Manhattan, Inner London, Paris, and Inner Tokyo (Berry, 1961; King, 1984).

7.2. Concentrated Employment Centers

These urban cores function as employment centers that attract large numbers of commuters. Approximately one third of the first ring's employed labor force commute to Manhattan, Inner London, Paris, and Inner Tokyo every day.

7.3. Health Care Resources

The urban core as a unit of analysis provides a frame within which to focus cross-national comparisons on a more coherent and discernable set of health system characteristics. For example, with respect to the concentration of medical resources, Manhattan, Paris, and Inner Tokyo are characterized by a high density of physicians (Table 3). Inner London is the outlier. But all four urban cores have a much higher density of physicians than their first rings. The core/first ring ratio of physician density is higher for Inner Tokyo (3.8) and London (3.6) than for Manhattan (2.1) or Paris (2.3).

They also have high levels of acute care hospital beds (public and private combined) with the exception of London (Table 3). Manhattan, Inner London, and Inner Tokyo have 2.5 times as many beds as their first rings; Paris has only 1.5 times as many. These ratios indicate the concentration of acute hospital beds including those among large university teaching hospitals in all of the central cores.

Table 3 Health Care Resources: Manhattan, Inner London, Paris, and Tokyo (1995-2000)

	Manhattan	Inner London	Paris	Inner Tokyo
Number of teaching hospitals	19	13	25	9
Number of medical schools	5	4	7	7
Acute hospital beds per 1000 population	8.9 (1997)	4.1 (1990)	9.6 (1995)	12.8 (2000)[1]
Physicians per 10,000 Population	71.2 (1995)	36.9 (2000)	84.6 (1997)	70.0 (2000)

[1]This figure is an estimate derived by reducing the number of general hospital beds by 30% so as not to include beds in which length of stay is over 30 days.
Sources: Manhattan: New York State Department of Health (NYSDOH), 1998; London: UK Department of Health and Health of Londoners Project; Paris: physicians-Ministère de l'Emploi et de la Solidarité, Direction de la Recherche, des Etudes, de l'Evaluation et des Statistiques (DREES) repertoire ADELI, January 1st 2002; hospitals DRESS, SAE, 2001; Tokyo: "Report on Survey of Physicians, Dentists and Pharmacists 1998", Tokyo Metropolitan Government, Bureau of Public Health, 2000.

In summary, Paris – the city of 2.1 million inhabitants all living within its nineteenth-century walls and the peripheral freeway that surrounds its twenty *arrondissements* – was the prototypical "urban core" against which we selected a comparable urban core for New York, London and Tokyo. The Paris population and area (105 square kilometers) is miniscule in comparison to Greater London's 7.2 million people and 1,590 square kilometers; New York City's 8 million people and 826 square kilometers; and Central Tokyo's 7.9 million people and 616 square kilometers. Paris is comparable to the urban core of these cities (Figure 1). For New York City, this is Manhattan; for London it is the fourteen boroughs known as "Inner London;" For Tokyo, since there is no conventional definition of an urban core, we relied on the five criteria noted earlier and arrived at an urban core comprised of 11 inner wards *(kus)* that have a population of 2 million (1995).

Beyond the selection of four urban cores of New York, London, Paris and Tokyo, WCP illustrates how a comparative inquiry structured around comparable units of analysis can serve to highlight some striking similarities and differences for further investigation.

7.4. Similarities and Differences

All four urban cores have economies based on services and information, which are closely tied to national and international transactions. They are also centers of culture, media, government, and international organizations. And their resident populations include some of the wealthiest and poorest members of their respective nations.

The poverty rate, defined as the percentage of households with income below one-half of the median, is almost twice as high in Manhattan (28.5%) as in Paris (12.8%)†. Although it is impossible to obtain household income data for the United Kingdom, comparison of occupational/class categories defined by the census may

† Poverty level for Manhattan is the percentage of households with income below half of Manhattan median income. For New York City, it is the percentage of households with income below half of NYC median income. The poverty level for Paris is measured as the percentage of households with income below half of Paris median income. For the Parisian agglomeration, it is the percentage of households with income below half of the Parisian median agglomeration income. The area of Paris agglomeration is slightly larger than Paris and its first ring. Data for both cities refer to pretax income; for Manhattan, pretax income includes social security payments and welfare payments but does not include other transfer payments, e.g., food stamps.

Table 4. Measures of Poverty: New York, London, Paris, and Tokyo (1991-1996)

	Urban core	Agglomeration[1]
New York (1994)	28.5%	25.6%
London (1991)	17.0%	14.9%
Paris (1994)	12.8%	10.2%
Tokyo (1996)	2.08%	1.56%

Sources: NYC: Current Population Survey 1994; London: Office of National Statistics (ONS), 1991; Paris: INSEE study on income of Parisian households, carried out by Christine Chambaz; Tokyo: Tokyo Statistical Association (1998); *Tokyo Statistical Yearbook*, 1996.

be used as a proxy for income. Although this is not comparable to the Manhattan and Paris figures, it allows us to observe a similar pattern in all three cities—poverty rates for the population of the urban core are slightly higher than in their first rings (Table 4). In the Paris agglomeration, the poverty rate is 10.2%; in New York it is 25.6%. In Greater London, the share of lower "classes" is 14.9% as opposed to 17% in Inner London. For Tokyo, since we have no data on poverty rates, we examine a proxy indicator of deprivation: the percentage of households receiving public assistance (Figure 2). In 1996 it was slightly higher in the urban core (2.08%) than the periphery (1.56%).

With the exception of Tokyo, a similar pattern holds for the percentage of foreign-born populations. Roughly one-quarter of the population in Inner London and Manhattan, and about 20% of the population in Paris, was born abroad. In Paris and Inner London, this foreign-born population is higher than in the first ring, but in Manhattan the percentage of foreign-born population is lower than in the surrounding boroughs.

Despite their common characteristics, there are some significant differences that make the comparison of these four world cities a promising, if challenging,

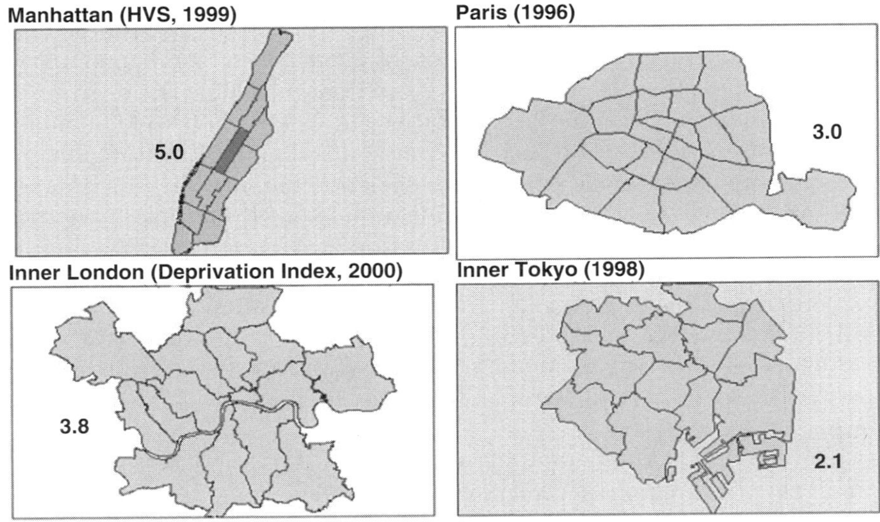

Figure 2. Average Household Taxable Income: Ratio Highest/Lowest Neighborhood.

area for health services research. One of the characteristics of world cities is the polarization between the rich and the poor. Manhattan is characterized by the highest level of inequality in the distribution of income among the four cities. For example, intracity variation in average household income varies from a ratio of 2.1 in Inner Tokyo, 3.0 in Paris, to 5.0 in Manhattan. Opinions differ, however, on the extent to which some of these variations among cities are important (Hamnett, 1994). Paris has been called a "soft" world city in contrast to New York because it provides more family services, income support and health services to the poor (Body-Gendrot, 1996). Tokyo is closer to Paris, based on the above data, and although there is no available household income data on London, studies of London's socio-economic disparities suggest that it resembles New York more closely than Paris or Tokyo.

In addition to income inequality, consider some of the differences among the health systems of these cities. In comparison to Great Britain which assures health care coverage under its National Health Service, and France and Japan, which assure universal coverage under their national health insurance programs, only the U.S. still maintains significant financial barriers to health care access. This is true even in New York City, with its extensive safety net; 28% of the New York City population is uninsured and this remains a significant impediment to health care access. Thus, a reasonable starting hypothesis for distinguishing New York from our other world cities is that the absence of universal coverage exacerbates the problem of access.

7.5. Applying the Framework for Comparing Cities, Health Services, and Health to Four World Cities

WCP has applied elements of the framework presented earlier to study four dimensions of health and access to health care in four world cities: infant mortality, coronary artery disease (CAD), avoidable hospital conditions (AHC), and patterns of aging, quality of life and use of long-term care services.

Our studies of infant mortality across the four cities and their neighborhoods have revealed two findings. First, in comparison to other world cities, Manhattan has more neighborhoods characterized by concentrated poverty and the highest infant mortality rates, and these neighborhoods contribute to Manhattan's citywide high median infant mortality rate (Neuberg and Rodwin, 2002). The degree of consistent spatial inequality over the course of a decade (1988-1997), in Manhattan, far exceeds that of the other cities. Second, after controlling for births, Manhattan is the only city with a statistically significant association between the infant mortality rate and an income (or deprivation) indicator (Rodwin and Neuberg, 2005). Although we do not have sufficient neighborhood data on material conditions, income inequalities, and levels of available health services for mothers to explain the relative importance of these critical variables, we submit the following hypothesis for further study: Manhattan's pattern of spatial inequalities and concentrated poverty combined with its health system characteristics leading to inadequate service provision in the most deprived neighborhoods are the most important factors in accounting for its outlier status.

Our study on the prevalence and treatment of CAD examined mortality, morbidity and treatment patterns for acute myocardial infarction, and other forms of CAD in New York, London, and Paris (Gusmano, *et al.*, 2004). We explored the relationship between the health system and neighborhood characteristics and the prevalence of CAD in New York, London, and Paris. We also examined the relationship between gender and treatment across these cities and their nations (Weisz, *et al.*, 2004). Similarly, our study of avoidable hospital conditions (AHC) compares rates of AHCs by race, and by neighborhood, in these cities (Gusmano, *et al.*, 2003). By comparing the treatment of CAD and rates of AHC for individuals just before and after the age of universal Medicare coverage with treatment for individuals in London and Paris where access to medical care is not conditioned on age, both of these studies allow us to examine the importance of health insurance coverage, income, gender and neighborhood of residence for access to primary and specialty care in these cities.

Finally, in our book on *Growing Older in Four World Cities* (Rodwin and Gusmano, 2005), we found convergent patterns in the share of older persons receiving home help in contrast to divergent patterns in the level of institutional long-term care. Also, we found that there are significantly fewer institutional long-term care beds in the urban cores of these cities than in their surrounding first rings (Figure 1). Land prices make it extraordinarily expensive to build institutional care beds in these urban cores which raises an important policy issue for the future of long-term care in world cities. Can we afford to support the costs of aging in place for the most vulnerable residents?

This question raises a host of issues about the quality of life across diverse neighborhoods in New York, London, Paris, and Tokyo and has led us to investigate the availability and use of health, social and long-term care services within and across these cities. We are particularly interested in the availability of services for isolated older persons. To what extent and how do isolated older persons receive supportive services in their neighborhoods? Third, what explains the gap between eligibility for entitlements and actual use of services by older persons? Is it due to lack of knowledge about available benefits, barriers to access within specific neighborhoods, problems of negotiating bureaucracies, cultural attitudes, including stigma associated with their vulnerable status, fear of losing their assets in order to qualify for benefits; or still other factors? (Gusmano and Rodwin, 2003).

8.0. CONCLUSION

There is a rich and extensive literature on health services in cities. A host of studies explore health services for the urban poor, racial and ethnic minorities and a variety of other "special" populations. A growing number of studies compare health systems across cities, but few provide a comprehensive analysis of urban health care systems. While cities have a disproportionate number of vulnerable populations and organizations that serve them, they also serve as centers of medical excellence with a concentration of academic medical centers, other hospitals, physicians and other health care professionals. We have argued that the field of health services research should adopt a broader perspective on cities and attempt to provide a more balanced assessment of urban health systems. Moreover, we have proposed an initial framework that addresses the relationships between cities and their health systems.

The World Cities Project illustrates this approach to the comparative analysis of urban health systems for an important category of cities. We hope it will stimulate others to extend the approach to these cities and apply it to many more.

ACKNOWLEDGEMENTS: Our own research summarized in this article was supported, in part, by a Health Policy Investigator Award on "Health and Megacities" to Victor Rodwin from the RWJ Foundation; a grant to Gusmano and Rodwin from the Florence Gould Foundation, and general support from the International Longevity Center-USA. We thank Jin Liu for research assistance on this chapter.

REFERENCES

Ambruster, P., and J., Lichtman. (1999). Are school based mental health services effective? Evidence from 36 inner city schools. *Community Ment. Health J.* 35(6):493–504.

Andrulis, D.P. (2000). Community, Service, and Policy Strategies to Improve Health Care Access in the Changing Urban Environment. *Am. J. Public Health* 90(6):858–862.

Andrulis, D.P. (1997). The Public Sector in Health Care: Evolution or Dissolution? Three Scenarios for a Changing Public-Sector Health Care System. *Health Aff.* (July/August):131–140.

Andrulis, D.P., and Goodman, N.J. (1999). *The social and health landscape of urban and suburban America.* Health Forum, Chicago.

Andrulis, D., and Shaw-Taylor, Y. (1996). The Social and Health Characteristics of California Cities. *Health Aff.* (15)1:131–142.

Andrulis, D.P., and Gusmano, M.K. (2000). *Community Initiatives for the Uninsured: How Far Can Innovative Partnerships Take Us?* New York: The New York Academy of Medicine, Division of Health and Science Policy (August), Working paper.

Atkinson, S., Songsore, J., and Werna, E. (1996). *Urban Health Research in Developing Countries: Implications for Policy.* CAB International, Wallingsford, UK.

Bardsley, M. (1999). Health in Europe's Capitals. Project Megapoles: Health indicators. Directorate of Public Health, East London and the City Health Authority, London.

Benbow, N., Wang, Y., and S. Whitman.1998. Big Cities Health Inventory, 1997: The Health of Urban USA. Department of Health, Chicago. *J. Community Health* 23(6):471–89.

Berry, B. (1961). *Central Place Studies; A bibliography of theory and applications.* Regional Science Research Institute, Philadelphia, PA.

Billings, J., and Weinick, R,M., 2003, Agency for Healthcare Research and Quality, Rockville, MD, (October 10, 2004); http://www.ahrq.gov/data/safetynet/databooks/safetynet.htm.

Billings, J., Anderson, G.M., and Newman, L.S. (1996). Recent findings on preventable hospitalizations. *Health Aff.* 15(3):239–249.

Billings, J., Zeitel, L., Lukomnik, J., Carey, T.S., Blank, A.E., and Newman, L. (1993). Impact of socioeconomic status on hospital use in New York City. *Health Aff.* (Spring):162–173.

Body-Gendrot, S. (1996). Paris: a 'soft' global city? *New Community* 22:595–605.

Brecher, C., Searcy, C., Silver, D., and Weitzman, B., 2004, Broookings Institute, 2004, Washington D.C. (September 17, 2004); www.brookings.edu/es/urban/livingcities.htm

Burrows, E., and Wallace, M. (1999). *Gotham: A History of New York City to 1898.* Oxford, New York.

Casanova, C., and Starfield, B. (1995). Hospitalizations of children and access to primary care: A cross-national comparison. *Int. J. Health Serv.* 25(2):283–294.

Chambaz, C., and Office of National Statistics. (ONS). (1991) Paris: National Institute for Statistics and Economics Study on income of Parisian households. Working paper.

Clark, D. (1996). *Urban World/Global City.* Blackwell Publishers, London

Coburn, J. E. (2004). Confronting the Challenges in Reconnecting Urban Planning and Public Health. *Am. J. Public Health.* (94)4:541–6.

Cunningham, P.J. (1998). Pressures on the Safety-Net: Differences in Access to Care for Uninsured Persons by the Level of Managed Care Penetration and Uninsurance. *Health Services Research* 34 (1):255–70

DeLia, D., Cantor, J.C., and Sandman, D. (2001). Medicaid managed care in New York City: Recent performance and coming challenges. *Am. J. Public Health* 91(3):458–460.

Department of Environment, Transportation and Regions. (2000). Indices of Deprivation 2000. Regeneration Research Summary , 31. The Department of Environment, Transporation and Regions, United Kingdom.

Department of Environment and Government Office for London, United Kingdom. 1996. *Four World Cities.* London, UK: Llewelvn-Davies, June.

Department of Human Services, 2004, Victoria, Australia (October 11, 2004); http://www.health.vic.gov.au/ drugservices/pubs/drugstats.htm

Diversity Rx, 2001, New York, (September 16, 2004); www.diversityrx.org

Dreier, P., Mollenkopf, J., and Swanstrom, T. (2001). *Place Matters: Metropolitics for the Twenty-first Century.* Univ. Press of Kansas, Lawrence, KS.

Duffy, J. (1974). *A History of Public Health in New York City.* Russell Sage, New York, NY.

Elkin, Stephen L. (1987). *City and Regime in the American Republic.* The University of Chicago Press, Chicago.

Ellen I, Mijanovich, T, and Dillman, K. 2001. Neighborhood Effects on Health: Exploring the Links and Assessing the Evidence. *Journal of Urban Affairs* 23:391–408.

Fairbrother, G., Dutton, M.J., Bachrach, D., Newell, K.A., Cooper, R., and Boozang, P. (2004). Cost of enrolling children in Medicaid and SCHIP. *Health Aff.* 23(1):237.

Fairbrother, G., Friedman, S., DuMont, K.A., and Lobach, K.S. (1996). Markers for primary care: Missed opportunities to immunize and screen for lead and tuberculosis by private physicians serving large numbers of inner-city Medicaid-eligible children. *Pediatrics* 97(6):785.

Felland, L.E., and Lesser, C.S. (2000). Local Innovations Provide Managed Care for the Uninsured. Issue Brief Findings from the Center for Health Systems Change Report No. 25, (January 2000), pp 1–6.

Felt-Lisk, S., McHugh, M., and Howell, E. (2002). Monitoring local safety-net providers: o they have adequate capacity? *Health Aff.* 21(5):277.

Fisher, E.S., Wennberg, J.E., Stukel, T.A., and Sharp, S.M. (1994). Hospital readmission rates for cohorts of Medicare beneficiaries in Boston and New Haven. *N. Engl. J. Med.* 331(15):989-995

Focas, C. (1988) *The Four World Cities Transport Study.* London Research Center, The Stationery Office, London, England.

Fossett, J.W., Perloff, J.D., Kletke, P.R., and Peterson, J.A.. (1992). Medicaid and access to child health care in Chicago. *J. Health Polit. Policy Law* 17(2):273–297.

Friedmann, J. (1986). The World City Hypothesis. *Dev. Change* 17:69–84.

Freudenberg, N. (2000). Health Promotion in the City: A Review of Current Practice and Future Prospects in the United States." *Annu. Rev. Public Health* (21):473–503.

Freund, D.A. (1984). Medicaid Reform: Four Studies of Case Management. AEI, Washington D.C.

Gabow, P.A. (1997). Denver Health: Initiatives for survival. *Health Aff.* 16(4):24–26.

Garbers, S., Jessop, D.J., Foti, H., Uribelarrea, M., and Chiasson, M.A. (2004). Barriers to breast cancer screening for low-income Mexican and Dominican women in New York City. *J. Urban Health* 80(1):81–91.

Geronimus, A., Bound, J., Waidmann, T., Hillemeier, M., and Burns, P. (1996). Excess Mortality Among Blacks and Whites in the United States. *N. Engl. J. Med.* 335(21):1552–1558.

Ginsberg, P. (1996). The RWJF Community Snapshots Study: Introduction and Overview. *Health Aff.* 15:7–15.

Ginzberg, E., and Yohalem, A. (1974). *The University Medical Center and the Metropolis.* Macy Foundation, New York.

Glouberman, S., 2003, A Toolbox for Improving Health in Cities, Toronto, On, (October 11, 2004); http://www.healthandeverything.org/pubs/index.shtml

Gray, B.H., Gusmano, M.K., and Collins, S. (2003). AHCPR and the politics of health services research. *Health Aff.* Web Exclusive, (June 25, 2003); http://content.healthaffairs.org/cgi/reprint/hlthaff.w3.283v1.pdf

Gray, B.H., and Rowe, C. 2000. "Safety-net health plans: a status report." *Health Aff.* 19(1):185–193.

Greer, S. (1983). Health Care in American Cities: Dedicated Workers in an Undedicated System. In: Greer, A.L., and Greer, S., (eds.), *Cities and Sickness: Health Care in Urban America.* Sage, Beverly Hills, CA.

Grogan, C.M., and Gusmano, M.K. (1999). How Are Safety-Net Providers Faring Under Medicaid Managed Care? *Health Aff.* March/April: 233–237.

Gusmano, M.K., Gray, B.H., Rowe, C., Sparer, M., and Brown, L. (2002). The Evolving Role and Care Management Approaches of Safety-Net Medicaid Managed Care Plans. *J. Urban Health* 79(4):600–616.

Gusmano, M.K., and Rodwin, V.G. (2003). Urban Ecology of Old Age: Social Interaction Among New York Neighborhoods. Presented at the *131st Annual Meeting of the American Public Health Association Conference,* San Francisco, November 17, 2003.

Gusmano, M.K., Rodwin, V.G., and Weisz, D. (2004). L'Affaire du Coeur in the United States and France: The Prevalence and Treatment of Ischemic Heart Disease in Two Nations and their World Cities. Robert Wood Johnson Foundation Scholars in Health Policy Working Paper.

Hadley, Jack, Earl P. Steinberg, and Judith Feder. (1991). Comparison of Uninsured and Privately Insured Hospital Patients. *JAMA.* 265(3):374–379.

Halfon, N., Wood, D.L., Valdez, B., Pereyra, M., and N. Duan. (1997). Medicaid enrollment and health services access by Latino children in inner-city Los Angeles. *JAMA*. 277(8):636–641.

Hall, P. (1998). *Cities in Civilization.* Pantheon, New York, NY.

Hamnett, C. (1994). Social Polarization in Global Cites: Theory and Evidence. *International Journal for Research in Urban and Regional Studies* 31:401—423.

Hatton, D.C. (2001). Homeless Women's Access to Health Services: A Study of Social Networks and Managed Care in the US. *Women & Health* 33(3/4):149.

Harpman, T., and Tanner, M. (1995). *Urban Health in Developing Countries.* Earthscan Publications, London, UK.

Harris, N. (1997). Cities in a global economy: Structural change and policy reactions. *Urban Stud.* 34(10):1693–1705.

Haslanger, K. (2003). Radical simplification: Disaster relief Medicaid in New York City. *Health Aff.* 22(1):252.

Housing and Vacancy Survey, 1996, New York City Department of Housing Preservation and Development, (October, 11, 2004); http://www.tenant.net/Oversight/HVS/

HUD. 1999a. The State of Cities. Washington D.C., (October 11, 2004); http://www.huduser.org/publications/polleg/ tsoc.html

HUD. 1999b. Now is the Time: Places Left Behind in the New Economy. Washington D.C., (October 11, 2004); http://www.huduser.org/periodicals/rrr/rrr6_99art1.html

Hutchinson, A.B., Corbie-Smith, G., Thomas, S.B., Mohanan, S., and del Rio, C. (2004). Understanding the patient's perspective on rapid and routine HIV testing in an inner-city urgent care center. *AIDS Education and Prevention* 16(2):101–114.

Igelhart, J.K. (1995). Health policy report – Academic medical centers enter the market: The case of Philadelphia. *N. Engl. J. Med.* 333(15):1019.

INSEE, National Institute for Statistics and Economics Studies 2004, (October 11, 2004); http://lessites.service-public.fr/cgi-bin/annusite/annusite.fcgi/ nat6?lang=uk&orga=83

Jacobs, J. (1961). *Death and Life of Great American Cities.* Vintage, New York, NY.

Juday, T.R., Wu, A., Celentano, D.D., Frick, K.D., Wang, M.C., and Vlahov, D. (2003). The role of Medicaid HMO enrollment in the longitudinal utilization of medical care services in a cohort of injecting drug users in Baltimore, Maryland. *Subst. Abus.* 24(1):27-41.

Kawachi, I., and Berkman, L. 2000. Social Cohesion, Social Capital and Health. In: Berkman, L., and Kawachi, I., (eds.). *Social Epidemiology.* Oxford: Oxford University Press, pp. 174–190.

Kings Fund, 1998, London, (October 11, 2004); http://http://www.kingsfund.org.uk/PublicHealth/potential_role.html

King, L.J. (1984). *Central Place Theory.* SAGE Publications, Beverly Hills, CA.

Kosloski, K., Schaefer, J.P., Allwardt, D., Montgomery, R.J., and Karner, T.X. (2002). The role of cultural factors on clients' attitudes toward caregiving, perceptions of service delivery, and service utilization. *Home Health Care Serv. Q.* 21(3-4):65–88.

Kotchen, J.M., Shakoor-Addullah, B., Walker, W.E., Chelius, T.H, Hoffmann, R.G., and Kotchen, T.A. (1998). Hypertension control and access to medical care in the inner city. *Am. J. Public Health* 88(11):1696–1699.

Kronick, R., and Enthoven, A. (1989). A Consumer Choice Health Plan for the 1990s: Universal Health Insurance in a System Designed to Promote Quality and Economy. *N. Engl. J. Med.* 320:29–101.

Lewis, M. E., and Altman, S. (2000). *America's Health Care Safety-Net: Intact but Endangered.* Institute of Medicine. National Academy Press, Washington D.C.

Ministère de l'Emploi et de la Solidarité, Direction de la Recherche, des Etudes, de l'Evaluation et des Statistiques (DREES) repertoire ADELI, 2001, France, (January 1, 2002); 2001(Do not see any missing information, but what is SAE?).http://www.travail.gouv.fr/index.asp.

Ministry of Finance, 1996, France, (October 11, 2004); http://www.finances.gouv.fr/minefi/minefi_ang/

Mumford, L. (1938). *Culture of Cities.* Harcourt, Brace & Co, New York, NY.

National Governor's Association, 2000, (October 11, 2004); http://www.nga.org/cda/files/001025HEALTHPRIMER.pdf

National Public Health and Hospital Institute. (1996.) Survey of Managed Care Programs for the Indigent, Report January 1996. Washington, DC.

Neuberg, L., and Rodwin, V. (2002). Infant Mortality in Four World Cities: New York, London, Paris and Tokyo. *Indicators-The J. of Social* Winter(2)1.

New York Academy of Medicine. (2001). Annual Report No. 8. New York Academy of Medicine, New York, NY.

New York City Department of Health and Mental Hygiene (NYCDHMH), 2004, New York, (October 11,2004); (www.nycdoh.gov).

New York State Department of Health, 1998, New York, (October 11, 2004); http:://www.census.gov/mp/www/rom/msrom5a.html

Norton, S.A., and Lipson, D.J. (1998a). *Public Policy, Market Forces, and the Viability of Safety Net Providers.* The Urban Institute, Washington D.C.

Norton, S.A., and Lipson, D.J. (1998b). Portraits of the Safety-Net: The Market, Policy Environment, and Safety-Net Response. Assessing the New Federalism Project Occasional Paper, Report No. 19.

O'Meara, M. (1999). *Reinventing Cities for People and the Planet.* Worldwatch Institute, Washington D.C.

O'Toole, T.P., Arbelaez, J., Haggerty, C., and Baltimore Community Health Consortium. (2004). The urban safety net: can it keep people health and out of the hospital. *J. Urban Health* 81(2):179-90.

Page, L. (1999). Medicaid HMOs limp away from two Ohio cities. *Am. Med. News* 42(14):13–14.

Perloff, J.D. (1996). Medicaid managed care and urban poor people: Implications for social work. *Health Soc. Work* 21(3):189–1995.

Perrin, J.M., Homer, C.J., Berwick, D.M., Woolf, A.D., Freeman, J.L., and Wennberg, J.E. (1990).Variations in rates of hospitalization of children in three urban communities. *N. Engl. J. Med.* 322(3):206–207.

Peterson., P. (1995.) *The Price of Federalism.* Brookings Institution, Washington D.C.

Peterson, P. (1981). *City Limits.* University of Chicago Press, Chicago, IL.

Peterson, P., and Mark, R. (1990). *Welfare Magnets: A New Case for a National Standard.* Brookings Institution, Washington D.C.

Population Action International. (1990). *Life in the World's 100 Largest Metropolitan Areas.* Population Action International, Washington D.C.

Prinz, T.S., and Soffel, D. (2004). The primary care delivery system in New York's low-income communities: private physicians and institutional providers in nine neighborhoods. *J. Urban Health* 80(4):635–649.

Ray, N., Thamer, M., Fadillioglu, B., and Gergen, P. (1998). Race, income, urbanicity and asthma hospitalization in California. *Chest* 113:1277–1284.

Rodwin, V. (2005). Comparative analysis of health care systems in wealthy nations. In: Kovner and Knickman. *Health Care Delivery in the U.S.* Springer, New York. In press.

Rodwin, V. (2001). Urban Health: Is the City Infected? In: Mariner, M., (ed.), *Medicine and Humanity.* King's Fund, London.

Rodwin, V., and Gusmano, K. (eds.). (2005). *Growing Older in World Cities: New York, London, Paris and Tokyo.* Vanderbilt University Press, Nashville, TN. In press.

Rodwin, V., and Gusmano, M. (2002). The World Cities Project: Rationale, Organization, and Design for Comparison of Megacity Health Systems. *J. Urban Health* (79):4.

Rodwin, V., and Neuberg, L. (2005). Infant Mortality and Income in Four World Cities: New York, London, Paris and Tokyo. *Am. J. Public Health.* In press.

Rosner, D. 1982. *A Once Charitable Enterprise.* Cambridge University Press, New York.

Salit, S., Fass, S., and Nowak, M. (2002). Out of the frying pan: New York City hospitals in an age of deregulations. *Health Aff.* 21(1):127–138.

Sassen, S. (2001). *The Global City: New York, London, Tokyo, Second Edition.* University of Princeton Press, Princeton, NJ.

Sassen, S. (1999). Global Financial Centers. *Foreign Aff.* 78:75–87.

Savitch, H. 1988. *Post-Industrial Citie: Politics and Planning in New York, Paris and London.* University of Princeton Press, Princeton, NJ.

Schulz, A.J., Williams, D.R., Israel, B.A., and Lempert, L.B. (2002). Racial and spatial relations as fundamental determinants of health in Detroit. *Milbank Q.* 80(4):677–707.

Schroeder, S. (1998). Urban Health Care: What Works and Why. *J. Urban Health* (75)2:349–355.

Scott, A. (2001). *Global City-Regions: Trends, Theory and Policy.* Oxford University Press, New York, NY.

Seid, M., Stevens, G.D., and Varni, J.W. (2003). Parents' perceptions of pediatric primary care quality: Effects of race/ethnicity, language and access. *Health Services Research* 38(4):1009.

Shedlin, M.G., and Shulman, L. (2004). Qualitative needs assessment of HIV services among Dominican, Mexican and Central American immigrant populations living in the New York City area. *AIDS Care* 16(4):434–445.

Short J, Kim, M., and Wells, H. (1996). The Dirty Little Secret of World Cities Research: Data Problems in Comparative Analysis. *Int. J. Urban Reg. Res.* 20:697–717.

Soloman, L., Frank, R., Vlahov, D., and Sterborski, J. (1991). Utilzation of health services in a cohort of intravenous drug users with known HIV-1 serostatus. *Am. J. Public Health* 81:1285–1290.

Sparer, M.S., and Brown, L.D. (2000). Uneasy alliances: managed care plans formed by safety-net providers. *Health Aff.* 19(4):23–35.

Sterk, C.E., Theall, K.P., and Elifson, K.W. (2002). Health care utilization among drug-using and non-drug-using women. *J. Urban Health* 79(4):586–599.

Stone, C. (1989). *Regime Politics.* University of Kansas Press, Lawrence, KS.

Thaver, I.H., Harpham, T., McPake, B., and Garner, P. (1998). Private practitioners in the slums of Karachi: What quality of care do they offer? *Soc. Sci. Med.* 46(11):1441–1449.

Thorpe, K.E. (1988). Why are urban hospital costs so high? The relative importance of patient source of admission, teaching, competition, and case mix. *Health Services Research* 22(6):821–836.

Tokyo Metropolitan Government. (2000). Report on Survey of Physicians, Dentists and Pharmacists 199. Tokyo Metropolitan Government, Bureau of Public Health, Tokyo, Japan.

Van Olphen, J., and Freudenberg, N. (2004). Harlem service providers' perceptions of the impact of municipal policies on their clients with substance use problems. *J. Urban Health* 81(2):222–231.

Vladeck, B. (1999).The Political Economy of Medicare, "*Health Aff.* (18)1:22-36.

Vlahov, D., and Gallea, S. (2002). Urbanization, Urbanicity and Health. *J. Urban Health* 79 (Supple 1)4:S1-S11.

Wennberg, J.E., and Gittlesohn, A. (1973). Small area variations in health care delivery. *Science* 182: 1102-1108.

Wennberg, J.E., Freeman, J.L. and Culp, W.J. (1987). Are hospital services rationed in New Haven or over-utilised in Boston? *Lancet* 1(8543):1185–1189.

Weissman, J.S., Gatsonis, C., and Epstein, A.M. (1992). Rates of avoidable hospitalization by insurance status in Massachusetts and Maryland. *JAMA.* 268(17):2388–2394.

Weitzman, B., Silver, D., and Dillman, K. (2002). Integrating a Comparison Group Design into a Theory of Change Evaluation: The Case of the Urban Health Initiative. *American Journal of Evaluation* 23(4):371–385.

Weisz, D., and Gusmano, M.K (2005). The health of older New Yorkers. In: Rodwin, V. and Gusmano, K. (eds.), *Growing Older in World Cities: New York, London, Paris and Tokyo.* Vanderbilt University Press, Nashville, TN, In press.

Weisz, D., Gusmano, M., and Rodwin, V. (2004). Gender and the Treatment of Heart Disease among Older Persons in the U.S., England and France: A Comparative, Population-Based View of a Clinical Phenomenon. *Gender Medicine.* In press.

World Bank, 2002, Washington D.C., (September 18, 2004); http://www.worldbank.org/html/fpd/urban

World Cities Project, 2004, New York, (October 10, 2004); http://www.ilcusa.org/prj/research.htm

Chapter 17

Urban Health in Developing Countries

Insights from Demographic Theory and Practice

Mark R. Montgomery and Alex C. Ezeh

1.0. INTRODUCTION

This chapter is concerned with the health of the urban poor in developing countries. In focusing on urban dwellers, we do not mean to overlook the rural poor, but only to acknowledge the seemingly inexorable process of urbanization, whereby steadily greater fractions of national populations are coming to be found in cities. As developing countries continue to urbanize, their national-level dialogues about poverty and health will increasingly have to reckon with urban as well as with rural poverty. In what follows, we identify the gaps in knowledge of urban health that can be addressed in the next generation of research, and examine the conceptual tools and empirical methods that might be brought to bear on the cities of poor countries. To guide the discussion, we draw extensively from the Panel on Urban Population Dynamics (2003) volume, a recent review of urban poverty, demography, and health.

The chapter's principal theme is that a great deal can be learned about health by adopting the perspectives of social epidemiology. It may be helpful to consider why social factors need special consideration. An array of modern health resources—clinics, hospitals, and specialized practitioners—can be found in all but the smallest developing-country cities. Their presence has led both researchers and aid agencies to presume that urban residents must enjoy significant advantages in health by comparison with rural dwellers, from whose villages such resources are generally absent. Indeed, in developing countries such as Bangladesh, primary health care budgets have been largely given over to rural areas on the theory that urban residents already benefit from far easier access to services.

Yet when closely inspected, the health circumstances of the urban poor are often discovered to resemble those of rural villagers, with similarities evident in levels of health risk, in the limits and biases of health knowledge, and in the modes of health-seeking behavior. On the whole, cities are doubtless better supplied than rural areas with modern curative health services, but in many cities the poor are not at all well-supplied with the basic infrastructure needed to protect their drinking water and assure acceptable environmental sanitation. Without such protections, the urban poor can face substantial communicable health risks stemming from spatial proximity and dependence on common resources—as was apparent in the nineteenth century to John Snow (1855) and other founding figures of modern epidemiology. Now as then, the political calculations that exclude the urban poor lie within the broad purview of epidemiology, as do the social factors that give some poor communities the confidence to mobilize and effectively press demands for services.

Social constraints can also undermine the confidence that individuals need to pursue aggressively their own health care needs. For reasons that are not yet well understood, the urban poor often fail to avail themselves of the modern health resources that are distributed about them in the wider urban environment. As Barua and Singh (2003) write for the urban poor of India, even those who have long lived in the city

> are not able to fully decipher the clues that organized, sophisticated institutions present. . . . The poor find the use of health institutions daunting and most poor patients feel out of place when hospitalized. The sense of alienation is compounded by their lack of familiarity with the sophisticated environs of health institutions, which presume a level of *urban literacy* (familiarity with common urban technologies and institutions) and prior experience. . . . In the absence of a more "literate" person to guide them through the intimidating procedure in the government hospitals, they feel particularly vulnerable.

Uneasy about the modern health system and often uncertain of its benefits, the urban poor may meet their health needs by turning to the more familiar providers found in their neighborhoods, including traditional healers, purveyors of drugs in the markets, and local pharmacists or chemists with some form of professed expertise. Like rural villagers, the urban poor often experiment with both modern and traditional remedies, whether in combination or in sequence, as they strive to understand the meaning and origin of an illness and seek the appropriate cure. But unlike rural villagers, the urban poor may have access to many sources of advice and support. The social diversity of urban life can sometimes provide the poor with guidance from the educated members of their social networks, who have greater understanding of the modern health system, and urban diversity may also present them with a range of social reference groups, some of which will illustrate how that system can be approached.

In short, to understand the many constraints facing the urban poor and gain insight into their thinking about health, it is necessary to know something of the multiple social worlds that the poor inhabit. This is far from being a novel or controversial proposition. It is a view that has given impetus to much of the past decade's multilevel health research, in which poor individuals and families are studied in relation to the social structures in which they are embedded—social networks and local associations, neighborhoods, and the wider social and political communities within which neighborhoods are nested.

A remarkable feature of this vigorous literature is the extent to which it has been dominated, thus far, by studies set in the cities of Europe and North America. No comparable surge of research on the cities of poor countries is yet in evidence. How can such an imbalance have come about in research efforts relative to global health needs? The concepts of multilevel health analysis are not obviously parochial in nature; the methods being applied in Chicago and Los Angeles would appear to merit equal consideration in Shanghai and Lagos. Likewise, the health problems arising from poverty and social exclusion would seem to exhibit many common features. To be sure, it can be more difficult to assemble some of the data needed for empirical investigations in developing countries. But we suspect that the crux of the problem lies elsewhere. In urban health as in other scientific fields, compartmentalization is a fact of life, and to date only a few scholars have breached the wall separating research on developing countries from that concerned with developed countries. There are, however, indications of growing recognition and scholarly interest.

1.1. Organization of the Chapter

In the sections of the chapter that follow, we examine the concepts and tools of multilevel health research with an eye to discovering how they may apply to the urban poor of the developing world. "Households, Social Networks, and Neighborhoods" (Section 2.0) is concerned with the theory, that is, with the "micro-mechanisms" of social interaction that influence individual health, taking effect through social networks, the organizational structures of neighborhoods, and the organizational and network ties that cross the urban space. We also address here an important criticism of the current generation of multilevel health research, that it has not given sufficient attention to factors that could induce spurious associations between individual health and neighborhood characteristics (Oakes, 2004a). Much can still be learned about urban health from thoughtful programs of cross-sectional research, but if this criticism is to be addressed, longitudinal (prospective) approaches will also be needed. In concluding this section, we outline the methodological aspects of the argument.

The remainder of the chapter develops these ideas more fully, by considering the difficulties that will confront measurement and fieldwork in these settings. "Assessing Urban Poverty and Living Standards" (Section 3.0) addresses the measurement of urban poverty, with particular emphasis on methods for inferring household living standards from data lacking information on income and consumption. We also briefly survey what is known of neighborhood heterogeneity and the spatial concentration of poverty in developing-country cities. "Urban Social Networks and Social Capital" (Section 4.0) examines the techniques that have been used to map social networks and social capital in developing countries. "What Can Be Learned from Longitudinal Studies" (Section 5.0) investigates the prospects for longitudinal health research, drawing upon the experiences of the African Population and Health Research Center (2002) in the slums of Nairobi. Section 6.0. is the "Conclusion."

2.0. HOUSEHOLDS, SOCIAL NETWORKS, AND NEIGHBORHOODS

In the health literature of the past two decades one sees a mounting interest in the social side of social epidemiology. Motivated by the writings of Wilson, Coleman and like-minded colleagues (Wilson, 1987; Coleman, 1988; Massey, 1990; White, 2001; Sampson, *et al.*, 2002), researchers interested in urban poverty and health have given increasing attention to the health effects of individual social networks, local social capital, social reference groups, and various forms of social comparison. In much of the literature, these concepts are organized under the broad heading of "neighborhood effects," although it is acknowledged that the mechanisms of interest are not necessarily as localized as this phrase would suggest (Wellman and Leighton, 1979). Indeed, one fundamental concern in this literature is how to specify and measure the concept of neighborhood, given that urban dwellers participate in multiple, spatially-distinct groups and communities. Only the core ideas of the literature will be described here.

As this literature matures, it is being confronted with a methodological challenge: how to eliminate selectivity biases in estimating the health effects of neighborhoods and related social mechanisms (Oakes, 2004a). The difficulty is that participation in social networks has a voluntary aspect; so does participation in local community groups; and through decisions about migration and residential mobility, individual households also make choices among alternative neighborhoods. How, then, are estimates of network, group, and neighborhood effects on health to be interpreted? To what extent might such estimates be contaminated by selection bias? In closing the section, we present the methodological arguments that favor longitudinal designs and discuss how to assess the magnitude of bias.

2.1. Theory

In its recent volume on the urban demography of poor countries, the Panel on Urban Population Dynamics (2003) provides an extensive review of neighborhood effects theory and its implications for health and demographic behavior. To briefly summarize this panel's lengthy and complex argument—much of which is dependent on empirical examples from the U.S. experience—one expects neighborhoods to matter for several reasons. Where communicable diseases are concerned, it has long been recognized that the spatial proximity of diverse urban populations can generate negative *health externalities*. As we have seen for Nairobi (discussed in chapter 10), the externalities associated with environmental contamination and communicable disease could cause the health risks of slum life to rival or exceed those of rural areas, despite the generally easier access that urban residents have to emergency transport and modern health services (Harpham and Tanner, 1995; Timæus and Lush, 1995; African Population and Health Research Center, 2002).

Less often recognized, but potentially of equal importance, are the *social externalities* that figure into urban life. Individuals and households are connected to others in their neighborhoods through social network ties, and along these social circuits information may flow about how to recognize and respond to health threats, and where effective services can be found. Of course, social network ties often reach beyond the local neighborhood (Wellman and Leighton, 1979). It has been argued, however, that the social networks of women and the poor are spatially constrained by comparison with those of men and the more affluent. The relative costs of travel may well be greater for the poor, and women with children and domestic responsibilities may find their daily routines largely confined to local neighborhoods (McCulloch, 2003; Panel on Urban Population Dynamics, 2003).

Although we are aware of no recent research on social networks and the diffusion of health information in developing-country cities, the work of Behrman, *et al.*, (2001) and Casterline, *et al.*, (2001) document network effects on contraceptive use in rural and periurban African contexts.* In analyses of mental health (Kawachi and Berkman, 2001; Boardman, 2004) social networks are viewed less as sources of information than as sources of support; in studies of sexually transmitted and contagious disease (Morris, 1993; Friedman and Aral, 2001), networks provide the social mechanisms by which contagion takes place.

On the whole, however, social networks have not received as much attention in the literature as has been given to *social capital* (Kawachi, *et al.*, 1999; Lin, 1999; Putnam, 2000; Sampson and Morenoff, 2000; Swaroop and Morenoff, 2004). Treatments of social capital have generally taken one of two forms.† Some authors stress its structural features, as evident in the range of formal and informal associations in a community and the extent to which residents participate in them. Others emphasize the "cognitive" aspects, that is, the feelings of mutual trust and collective efficacy that are fostered by robust and vibrant local associations (Harpham, *et al.*, 2002).

As with information exchange taking place within social networks, it is likely that information and advice bearing on health circulates within local organizations, such as parent–teacher groups, neighborhood sanitation committees, and local ward associations. To date, however, surprisingly few efforts have been made to measure the health content of exchange in local associations, or to trace the pathways by which generalized feelings of trust or efficacy lead to specific health perceptions and behavior. In a recent exception, Gilson (2003) has invoked the concept of trust to explain attitudes toward health care providers and institutions, which may be of special importance in developing countries where the poor do not necessarily identify with the modern health system and can be apprehensive about the attitudes of its professionals and elites. A related literature in demography explores the connections between *local health services* and health outcomes, with a particular focus on how services may either provide a substitute for, or alternatively complement, the beneficial effects of mother's education. Education is an individual trait that (in this theory) expands the reach of social networks and improves individual capacities to decipher the information provided by modern bureaucratic health institutions. Hence, the presence of health institutions in a community might be thought to add to the advantages already possessed by the educated. However, if health institutions are sensitive to the needs of their illiterate clients, they can provide information in such a way as to disproportionately benefit these clients, thus compensating, at least to a degree, for their lack of "urban literacy". Sastry (1996) gives an insightful review of this literature with attention to such mechanisms.

*One of the most influential randomized interventions in the history of family planning, the Taichung experiment of 1963, found strong evidence of information diffusion along social network lines in this small Taiwanese city (Freedman and Takeshita, 1969). See Casterline (2001) for an excellent summary of related findings on diffusion and social interaction in several areas of demographic research.

†Despite the efforts of theorists to bear down on the distinction, the dividing line between social networks and social capital remains elusive. Some authors have viewed social capital as a feature of neighborhoods rather than individuals, going so far as to construct social capital measures by aggregating individual data. The idea, it seems, is that social capital can function much like a locally non-excludable (i.e., public) good that is accessible, at least in principle, to all local residents. We know of no empirical assessments of this assumption. In any case, as Swaroop and Morenoff (2004) note, individual social networks—such as friendship networks—can assume much of the character of associations if the need arises, such as when perceived threats to the neighborhood cause neighbors to band together in block groups and neighborhood watches. Important dynamic feedbacks also link social networks and capital. For example, local associations facilitate the formation of social network ties among their members, whereas residential mobility, which breaks or stretches such ties, may reduce incentives for participation in community groups (Swaroop and Morenoff, 2004).

Theories of *social comparison and local reference groups* are often invoked in relation to the psycho–social aspects of health. The idea is that individuals may evaluate their own circumstances by comparing them with what can be observed of the circumstances of others (van den Eeden and Hüttner, 1982). Comparisons that are consistently unfavorable may provoke feelings of resentment and injustice, producing stresses and anxieties that undermine mental health. There is reason to think that such mechanisms can affect health more broadly. In the view of Wilkinson (1996),

> It is the social feelings which matter, not exposure to a supposedly toxic material environment. The material environment is merely the indelible mark and constant reminder of one's failure, of the atrophy of any sense of having a place in a community, and of one's social exclusion and devaluation as a human being.

Repeated exposure by the poor to such social inequities could erode their feelings of social confidence, weakening the sense of personal efficacy that is needed to assert claims on health resources and engage in constructive health-seeking behavior.

The role of relative socioeconomic standing, as measured by individual income in relation to the income distribution of the surrounding community or wider social group, is still largely untested in health research, especially for spatial units as small as neighborhoods (Wen, *et al.*, 2003). In North American and European studies, some evidence has emerged indicating that inequality at the county, metropolitan area, and state level is linked to poor health at the individual level. But the literature presents no consensus on these effects—to appreciate its unsettled state, compare Blakely, *et al.*, (2002), Veenstra (2002), Blomgren, *et al.*, (2004), Gerdtham and Johannesson (2004), and Boyle, *et al.*, (2004).

Empirical studies of relative deprivation in developing-country cities are not yet common. For Rio de Janeiro, Brazil, research by Szwarcwald, *et al.*, (2002) examines a type of multilevel model in which infant mortality at the census-tract level is posited to depend on the proportion poor and the dispersion of poverty rates in the larger geographic areas within which tracts are nested. These authors find that the higher the mean poverty rate in the large areas, and the higher the variance, the higher is infant mortality at the tract level. These findings are suggestive of a link between local socioeconomic inequality and health, if not quite as persuasive as estimates from multilevel models with both individual and area characteristics. Other social mechanisms are examined in research on urban and rural India (Kravdal, 2003) which uncovers evidence that community levels of women's education (and autonomy) have a significant influence on child mortality rates with household variables held constant. Kaufman, *et al.*, (2002) find evidence of similar community effects in a study of adolescent reproductive health in urban South Africa.

2.2. What Is an Urban Neighborhood?

The geographical units for which aggregated data are available—in the U.S. these are block groups, census tracts, and the like—have boundaries that need not correspond closely, or indeed at all, with the sociological boundaries of neighborhoods as determined by patterns of social interaction, contagion, and comparison. Writing on health and reference group effects, Wen, *et al.* (2003) acknowledge, "It is not clear what spatial level is appropriate to examine this relationship." For Sweden,

Åberg Yngwe, *et al.*, (2003) define reference groups on the basis of social class, age, and region, rather than in terms of local geography.

Coulton, *et al.*, (1997) and Sastry, *et al.*, (2002) show how difficult it is to mark the boundaries of urban neighborhoods. Coulton, *et al.*, (1997) asked residents of Cleveland to depict their local neighborhoods on maps and found that the perceived boundaries often departed substantially from the boundaries of census-based units. Furthermore, there was a good deal of variation among residents in the spatial extent of their perceived neighborhoods. Despite this variation, when averages of socioeconomic measures (e.g., poverty rates, crime rates) were calculated for the perceived neighborhoods and then compared to figures for the census tracts, the composition of the tracts proved to be similar to that of the units sketched out by local residents. However, Altschuler, *et al.*, (2004) found that residents of Oakland conceived of their neighborhoods as "safe zones" within which daily activities could be carried out without fear of crime or violence. In this way of defining neighborhood, the perimeters are determined by social forces operating across wider geographic areas, and neighborhoods would be expected to show risk profiles quite different from those of the wider areas.

A few studies of health have explored the implications of areal measures defined at varying spatial scales. Examining mortality and cancer incidence in two U.S. states, Krieger, *et al.*, (2002) document the information loss entailed in the use of larger units—measures calculated for these larger units (zip code areas) did not consistently detect the areal effects found to be statistically significant when smaller units (census tracts or block groups) were employed. An example is a study of areal effects on smoking conducted by Diez Roux, *et al.*, in 2003, which found no important differences between estimates based on census tracts and those based on block groups. No larger areal units were examined in this example. But, of course, smaller need not be better—the appropriate spatial scale for any given analysis must depend on the geographic extent of epidemiological and social interaction.

2.3. Neighborhood Heterogeneity

Much of the literature we have reviewed emphasizes the spatial concentration of poverty, but the effects of spatially concentrated affluence are also drawing attention. Wen, *et al.*, (2003) summarize Wilson's work as showing the benefits of economic heterogeneity for urban communities:

> In his [Wilson's] model, the prevalence of middle/upper-income people positively correlates with the material and social resources necessary to sustain basic institutions in urban neighborhoods like the family, churches, schools, voluntary organizations, and informal service programs. . . These institutions are pillars of local social organization that help to nurture neighborhood solidarity and mobilize informal social control.

In their own study, Wen, *et al.* (2003) find that neighborhood affluence exerts a significant positive influence on health net of other covariates, including neighborhood-level poverty, income inequality, aggregated educational attainment, and lagged levels of neighborhood health. However, Pebley and Sastry, (2003) could find no separable, significant effect of neighborhood affluence in their Los Angeles study of children's test scores, given controls for the median level of neighborhood family income, which is a significant positive influence on these scores.

In work on developing country cities, there has been some limited recognition of neighborhood heterogeneity, but as we have mentioned, little by way of quantitative investigation into its extent and nature (UN-Habitat, 2003). In principle, socioeconomic heterogeneity can bring a diversity of urban resources within the reach of the poor. Mixed-income communities may be able to supply more volunteers for community-based organizing activities, and they may also possess a stronger base of local associations. The middle- and upper-income residents of such communities could conceivably serve as "bridges" to politicians, government agencies, and sources of outside funding and expertise. For these reasons, neighborhood social and economic heterogeneity could well amplify the beneficial effects of health program interventions. In theory, at least, programs set in heterogeneous neighborhoods could yield more benefits for the poor than those located in uniformly poor neighborhoods. But there are also risks in situating health interventions in mixed-income communities. Program benefits can be siphoned off by upper-income residents, and it could prove difficult to sustain community motivation for activities for the poor when better-off residents have the private means to purchase health care. These are obviously difficult and situation-specific issues.

The intertwined roles of health programs, social capital, and community mobilization are addressed in a small but growing and highly instructive literature for developing-country cities, much of which has appeared in the journal *Environment and Urbanization*, a steady supplier of evocative case-study material on communities and the urban poor (see in particular its October 2001 issue). As would be expected, there are cases in which well-designed alliances between community organizations of the poor and professional NGOs have proven highly successful (e.g., Appadurai, 2001 for Mumbai) and other instances in which seemingly well-designed efforts could not be sustained (e.g., de Wit, 2002 for Bangalore). The literature on India is especially rich in material of this sort (see, for instance, Burra, *et al.*, 2003 on community sanitation in Mumbai, Kanpur, and Bangalore), but experiences from Africa, Latin America, and other Asian settings also show that poor urban communities are fully capable of mobilizing their social resources and engaging with government and NGOs to improve sanitation, housing, and health. The concept of collective efficacy is, if anything, more vividly illustrated in these cities than in the cities of the West.

2.4. How Strong Is the Empirical Evidence?

Many studies in the emerging multilevel literature on health—though not all, to be sure—have uncovered evidence that community contexts make a difference to health (Timæus and Lush, 1995; Ginther, *et al.*, 2000; Szwarcwald, *et al.*, 2002; Åberg Yngwe, *et al.*, 2003; Drukker, *et al.*, 2003; Wen, *et al.*, 2003; Boyle, *et al.*, 2004; Curtis, *et al.*, 2004). But as evidence of significant community effects has mounted, so has the intensity of criticism. Some critics (notably Oakes, 2004a; 2004b) express doubt as to whether any multilevel study of community factors and health has identified true causal linkages. The essence of the argument is that the vast majority of such studies are cross-sectional "snapshots" of individuals and communities, and such studies cannot control for the many unobserved factors that could generate spurious associations between individual health and observed community characteristics. Similar criticisms have been leveled at studies of group membership, social networks, and other forms of social capital (Manski, 2000; Durlauf, 2000a; 2000b). The problem in teasing out the causal effects of group membership is that unobserved individual-level factors may be expressed in two ways: in propensities for social engagement and in propensities to experience good (or poor) health. The associations that arise from such common unobservable factors are easily mistaken for causal links.

2.4.1. *Addressing Selectivity Bias*

In what follows, we outline how selectivity biases can stem from the choices made by respondents—whether in terms of migration, residential mobility, or group participation—and discuss the statistical tools available to assess the importance of this bias and protect inference against it. Cross-sectional designs provide only a few such tools, whereas longitudinal data much expand the possibilities.

The essence of the problem can be seen in a highly simplified depiction of locational choice. Let the subscript i index individuals and let c=1, . . .,C index communities. Suppose that individuals decide to move to (or remain in) a given community by comparing the well-being ("utility," in the language of economists) they would experience in residing there with what can be attained elsewhere. The utility possibilities are represented in a set of C equations,

$$\begin{gathered} U_{i,\ 1}^{*} = Z_1\,\alpha + u_1 + v_{i,1} \\ = \\ U_{i,\ c}^{*} = Z_C\,\alpha + u_C + v_{i,C} \end{gathered} \tag{1}$$

where $U_{i,\ c}^{*}$ denotes the level of utility that can be attained in community c, which depends in turn on a community characteristic Z_c, a community-specific unobservable u_c, and an idiosyncratic disturbance $v_{i,c}$. If community 1 happens to offer the highest utility in this set, then $Z_1\,\alpha + u_1 + v_{i,1} \geq Z_c\,\alpha + u_c + v_{i,c}$ for all c, or, to put it differently,

$$u_1 + v_{i,1} \geq (Z_c - Z_1)\,\alpha + u_c + v_{i,c} \quad \forall\ c \neq 1.$$

Consider individuals residing in community 1, for whom this relationship holds. The expected value of the composite disturbance $u_1 + v_{i,1}$ conditional on residence in community 1 is a function of Z_1, the observed community variable. With $\alpha>0$, the community variable Z_1 and the composite disturbance $u_1 + v_{i,1}$ will be negatively correlated.

Let the health equation of interest be specified as

$$H_{i,c} = X_{i,c}\,\beta + Z_c\delta + u_c\,\gamma + \omega_i + \varepsilon_{i,c}, \tag{2}$$

such that in addition to the observed individual determinants $X_{i,c}$, health is also affected by the community variable Z_c and the same unobservable u_c that figures into locational choice. We also reserve a role in the health equation for ω_i, a time-invariant individual disturbance, and $\varepsilon_{i,c}$, an idiosyncratic disturbance.

By the argument above, migration-related selectivity causes Z_c and u_c to be correlated, and the parameters of the health equation cannot be estimated consistently without taking this into account. If only cross-sectional data are available, the researcher has three main ways of obtaining consistent estimates of the health equation. One of these is to introduce community-specific dummy variables to control for $u_c\gamma$, the community unobservable that is posited to influence both locational choice and health. Unfortunately, if ω_i is correlated with the $v_{i,c}$ disturbances of the location choice equations (1), the introduction of community dummy variables will not eliminate all sources of selectivity bias.

Instrumental-variables methods can also be deployed, if any variables can be found that meet the demanding requirements for instrument validity. A third strategy is to make use of the structure of equations (1) and (2) to estimate the conditional expectation of the composite disturbance term $u_c\gamma + \omega_i + \varepsilon_{i,c}$ given residence of person *i* in the *c*-th community. This strategy relies upon locational selectivity correction terms—see Schmertmann (1994) and references therein for an application to polytomous logit equation systems.

If longitudinal data are available, a wider array of techniques becomes available. Inserting a time subscript *t* in the health equation, so that

$$H_{i,c,t} = X_{i,c,t}\beta + Z_{c,t}\,\delta + \omega_i + u_c\,\gamma + \varepsilon_{i,c,t}, \tag{3}$$

and taking first differences within individual records, we obtain

$$H_{i,c,t} - H_{i,c,t-1} = (X_{i,c,t} - X_{i,c,t-1})\,\beta + (Z_{c,t} - Z_{c,t-1})\,\delta + \varepsilon_{i,c,t} - \varepsilon_{i,c,t-1}, \tag{4}$$

an expression from which the fixed individual factor ω_i and community factor $u_c\gamma$ are eliminated. Boyle, *et al.*, (2004) apply this first-differences technique to good effect in their longitudinal analysis of health in an English sample. Unfortunately, the differencing method sweeps away all time-invariant individual and community determinants of health, and some of these will be of prime substantive interest. (Interactions between time-varying and time-invariant variables remain.) Even so, the differences approach can provide useful diagnostic information. With consistent health equation estimators from equation (4) in hand (though only for a subset of the β and δ parameters), Hausman, (1978) tests can be applied to determine whether the correlation between $Z_{c,t}$ and the health equation composite disturbance $u_c\gamma + \omega_i + \varepsilon_{i,c,t}$ brings about any significant inconsistencies. In this way, one can gauge whether the selectivity bias criticism is indeed of substantive importance.

To be sure, if the unobserved factors governing locational choice and health (u_c and ω_i in our illustrative model) vary over time, or if there is reason to suspect the $\varepsilon_{i,c,t}$ component of the health equation disturbance of being correlated with $v_{i,c}$, the utility disturbance in the location equations, further adjustments are in order. Instrumental variables methods may still be required. (See Baltagi, (1995) for a review of dynamic panel data instrumental variables models, and Maluccio *et al.*, (2000) for an application to the role of social capital in determining household consumption expenditures in South Africa.) Our point is that while access to longitudinal data does not eliminate the need to think carefully about selectivity bias, it greatly expands the set of tools that can be brought to bear on the problem.

3.0. ASSESSING URBAN POVERTY AND LIVING STANDARDS

The discussion thus far has been concerned with the organizing concepts of multilevel health research, the working assumption being that these concepts have broad applicability to urban populations in poor countries. Because the multilevel literature has been tilted so heavily toward developed-country urban research, much remains to be learned about applicability. In this and the next two sections of the chapter, we consider the empirical tools that have been developed for three key areas of multilevel health research: measures of poverty and living standards; measures of social networks and social capital; and techniques for gathering longitudinal data on these domains. Although much of our discussion of poverty measurement is focused on its household-level manifestations, we also describe empirical efforts to map poverty at the level of neighborhoods.

3.1. Overview

Much as in the U.S. and Europe, the official measures of poverty employed in developing countries are often framed in terms of income- or consumption-based poverty lines—in developing countries, however, these lines have been defined mainly with reference to food (Satterthwaite, 2004). The general approach is to specify a "basket" of basic food needs and calculate the money income required to purchase this basket at prevailing prices. With the food poverty line thus established, an allowance for all non-food items is then added (typically in an ad hoc fashion, without reference to a basket of non-food needs as such) to determine the overall poverty line. As Satterthwaite argues, there is good reason to question whether such procedures give sufficient consideration to the non-food needs of city dwellers. It is not unusual for the urban non-food allowance to be only 30–40 % of poverty-level food expenditures in developing countries, whereas the implied allowance is typically much greater in the poverty definitions adopted in the West.

A deeper concern is that real income and consumption expenditure offer only one perspective on the multiple dimensions of poverty. In developing countries a household whose money income exceeds the poverty line may not be able to secure access to a steady supply of electricity, or assure itself of safe drinking water, decent environmental sanitation, and protection from crime and violence (Mitlin, 2003). Table 1 outlines some of the elements of the more expansive view of poverty that is coming to be characteristic of research in the developing world. The central roles of income and consumption are duly recognized here, but additional dimensions of poverty are also highlighted. As we will discuss, several of the elements listed in the table—household assets, access to adequate infrastructure, even political voice—could well be measured in the course of household surveys focused on health. By contrast, dedicated surveys are needed to gather reliable data on income and consumption, with interview times running to several hours at the minimum. As a result, much of what is known from survey data on the relationship of living standards to health is based on proxy measures for income and consumption.

In what follows we briefly discuss the use of monetized poverty measures using income or consumption data, and then describe the conceptual and statistical issues that arise when proxy measures are employed in their place. We proceed to outline efforts currently underway to quantify several of the elements of Table 1 in the form of questions suitable for household surveys, and ask whether these measurement tools can be expected to register changes in household living standards over time. This section closes with an examination of the multiple levels of poverty, drawing attention to what little is known of the associations between household and neighborhood living standards.

Table 1. The Multiple Dimensions of Urban Poverty

Income and consumption
Poverty is conventionally defined in terms of incomes that are inadequate to permit the purchase of necessities, including food and safe water in sufficient quantity. Because incomes can be transitory and are difficult to measure, levels of consumption are often used as indicators of the longer-term component of income.

Assets
The nature of household assets also bears on the longer-term aspects of poverty and the degree to which households are shielded from risk. A household's assets may be inadequate, unstable, difficult to convert to monetized form, or subject to economic, weather-related, or political risks; access to credit may be restricted or loans available only at high rates of interest. For many of the urban poor, significant proportions of income go to repay debts (see, e.g., Amis and Kumar, 2000).

Time costs
Conventional poverty lines do not directly incorporate the time needed for low-income households to travel to work or undertake other essential tasks. Such households often try to reduce their money expenditures on travel by walking or enduring long commutes (Moser, 1996). Time costs also affect the net value of some goods and services.

Shelter
Shelter may be of poor quality, overcrowded, or insecure.

Public infrastructure
Inadequate provision of public infrastructure (piped water, sanitation, drainage, roads, and the like) can increase health burdens, as well as the time and money costs of employment.

Other basic services
There can be inadequate provision of such basic services as health care, emergency services, law enforcement, schools, day care, vocational training, and communication.

Safety nets
There may be no social safety net to secure consumption, access to shelter, and health care when incomes fall.

Protection of rights
The rights of poor groups may be inadequately protected, there being a lack of effective laws and regulations regarding civil and political rights, occupational health and safety, pollution control, environmental health, violence and crime, discrimination, and exploitation.

Political voice
The poor's lack of voice, and their powerlessness within political and bureaucratic systems, may leave them with little likelihood of receiving entitlements and little prospect that organizing and making demands on the public sector will produce a fair response. The lack of voice also refers to an absence of means to ensure accountability from public, private, and nongovernmental agencies.

Source: Panel on Urban Population Dynamics (2003).

3.2. Monetized Measures of Poverty

Researchers investigating the determinants of urban health in the U.S. or Europe often take for granted the availability of income data for households and aggregated data on median incomes, rates of poverty, and the like for census tracts and other geographic entities. In developing countries, however, data such as these are seldom available in general, and are almost never available from censuses. In part this is because wage and salary work is far from being the dominant form of employment in such economies, and it is a difficult and error-prone exercise to estimate income net of costs for those who are self-employed, engaged in family business, or working in several occupations. Detailed multiple-round surveys, such as those of the World Bank's Living Standards Measurement Surveys (LSMS) program, are required to assemble defensible estimates of household net incomes and consumption expenditures. (Basic documentation on this program of research can be found in Grosh and Glewwe from 1996. For an updated description and access to many of the surveys, see http:// www.worldbank.org/lsms/.)

Even where such data are available, considerable caution is needed in interpreting them. Measurement error is one source of concern. Another is the extent of locational differentials in prices, which in developing countries stem from pervasive market imperfections and the higher relative costs of transport and communication. Since prices cannot be assumed to be uniform across the urban space, household survey data on nominal income and consumption must be supplemented with detailed location-specific price data. In the LSMS program, these data are gathered through spot surveys of local retail markets, conducted so as to ensure that the prices refer to goods of similar quality across markets and with enough items included to constitute a sensible "basket of goods" for urban dwellers. But retail markets inevitably give something less than the full picture. City residents face charges for rent, transport, and many other non-food items that are not purchased in organized retail markets. It is difficult enough to devise a means of collecting prices for these heterogeneous items, let alone to account for their differences by neighborhood within cities. (Imputing the rental equivalent of owner-occupied housing is just one of the many difficulties). Prices can also vary considerably across cities, according to city size and related factors.

Further effort is needed to establish with tolerable accuracy the prices that poor households must pay, especially when the poor are spatially concentrated in slums. The urban poor often lack the ability to buy in bulk, and they can face prices for staples that can be well above those prevailing in areas frequented by the urban middle class (Satterthwaite, 2004). Poor households living in poorly-serviced neighborhoods may be forced to buy essential items that are provided by the public sector in better-serviced neighborhoods. (For instance, water may need to be purchased from vendors or tanker trucks.) Relatively few developing countries have addressed these issues in defining urban poverty, and researchers should therefore exercise caution in making use of the official poverty lines.

3.4. Measures Based on Proxy Variables

As we have noted, much of what is known of health conditions and poverty in developing countries comes from surveys that do not collect income and consumption data as such. The DHS program is perhaps the most prominent example of a survey design that gives detailed attention to health but must pass lightly over the measurement of living standards in order to do so. The Multiple Indicator Cluster Surveys (MICS), which is Unicef's survey program, has adopted a similar approach. (For more information on the MICS program and access to its survey datasets, see http://www.childinfo.org/MIC2/MICSDataset.htm). In surveys such as these, measures of poverty and living standards must be fashioned from what is, typically, a very small set of proxy variables. The living standards indicators common to most surveys in the DHS program include ownership of a car, television, refrigerator, radio, bicycle, and motorcycle; most surveys also record the number of rooms the household uses for sleeping and whether finished materials are used for flooring. These are the standard indicators available in the "core" questionnaires, but some surveys supplement them with additional consumer durable items and, on occasion, with queries about land or producer durables. Also, many DHS surveys have included a question on the time required for households without piped water to reach a source of drinking water and return—this is a measure of the time costs and can also be interpreted as a proxy for water quantity.

A lively literature has emerged in the past few years on the merits of various statistical techniques that make use of such proxies (Montgomery, *et al.*, 2000; Sahn and Stifel, 2000; Filmer and Pritchett, 1999; 2001; Montgomery and Hewett, 2004). Interest has centered on two main approaches: principal components analysis, a very simple but atheoretical method for reducing multiple proxies to one or more indices, and several varieties of factor analysis, which is a better-structured but computationally demanding approach to much the same end. To touch on the essential features of this debate, we briefly describe the so-called MIMIC method ("multiple indicator, multiple cause"), which is a variant of confirmatory-factor analysis (Montgomery and Hewett, 2004).

The MIMIC approach assumes (as does the principal components approach) that a household's standard of living is a theoretical construct that cannot be directly observed, but whose relative level may be inferred from a set of proxy indicators and determinants. Letting f denote the (unobserved) living standards factor, the link to the determinants X is specified as $f = X' \gamma + u$. The probable level of f is signaled through the values taken by $\{Z_k\}$, a set of K indicator variables, such as the ownership of a car, refrigerator, and the like. As in these examples, the indicators are typically yes–no variables, and it is conventional to represent them in terms of latent propensities Z_k^*, with $Z_k = 1$ when $Z_k^* \geq 0$ and $Z_k = 0$ otherwise. We write each such propensity as $Z_k^* = \alpha_k + \beta_k F + v_k$, and, upon substituting for f, obtain K latent indicator equations,

$$Z_1^* = \alpha_1 + X' \gamma + u + v_1$$

$$Z_2^* = \alpha_2 + \beta_2 \cdot X' \gamma + \beta_2 u + v_2$$

$$Z_K^* = \alpha_K + \beta_K \cdot X' \gamma + \beta_K u + v_K. \tag{5}$$

In this set of equations, the β_k parameters show how the unobserved factor f takes expression through each indicator. (Take note that No β_1 coefficient appears in the first of the indicator equations: it is normalized to unity). The estimation of systems such as these, which involve multiple binary indicator variables, is a nontrivial computational exercise, but estimation routines are available in commercial software. With estimates of equations (5) in hand, a predicted $\hat{f}$ factor score can be calculated for each household to serve as a summary measure of its standard of living. As with other approaches based on proxy variables, the MIMIC specification yields a relative measure of living standards.

To implement the approach, the researcher must decide how the X variables, that is, the determinants of living standards, are to be distinguished from the $\{Z_k\}$ variables that serve as indicators of living standards. With proper consumption data lacking, it would seem reasonable to define the set of living standards indicators in terms of consumer durables and housing quality; taken together, these items are at least loosely analogous to measures of consumption. Producer durables should be excluded from the $\{Z_k\}$ set, because while they may help determine final consumption, producer durables are not themselves measures of that consumption. They are better viewed as inputs, or enabling factors, in household production functions.

Some publicly provided services can be viewed as inputs into consumption—notably, the provision of electricity—and these can also be grouped with the X living standards determinants. Adult education can be likened to a producer durable, and on these grounds the set of determinants should include the education (and age) of the household head and other household adults.

Montgomery and Hewett (2004) have estimated MIMIC models of this kind and found that the household living standards score $\hat{f}$ is strongly related to several measures of health. Similar specifications using the principal components approach have also yielded strong predictors of health, access to public services, and children's schooling (Filmer and Pritchett, 1999; 2001; Hewett and Montgomery, 2001; Panel on Urban Population Dynamics, 2003). But much remains to be learned about the meaning of these generally strong empirical associations. According to the findings of Montgomery and colleagues (2000) and Sahn and Stifel (2001), the correlations between the proxies-based living standards scores and consumption expenditures are, though positive, not as high as might be wished. Possibly measurement error in consumption data biases downward its influence on health; for this and other reasons, perhaps, the proxy methods somehow succeed where consumption fails in identifying the core elements of the living standards concept. It is also possible, however, that upward biases are embedded in the proxy variables approach.

3.5. New Strands of Research on Measurement

Table 2 which is adapted from work currently being undertaken by Shea Rutstein of ORC/Macro, and which also draws from the questionnaire fielded by Harpham, *et al.*, (2004) in Cali, Columbia, a survey on social exclusion in Fortaleza, Brazil (Verner and Alda, 2004), and the World Bank social capital questionnaire presented in Grootaert, *et al.*, (2004), illustrates survey questions that could further this line of research. The questions are divided into four sets: qualitative assessments of consumption; additional consumption indicators and determinants; measures that include elements of both consumption and health; and questions that go beyond consumption to probe into additional dimensions of well-being.

Qualitative, subjective assessments of consumption are being explored in a newly-developed and promising line of research, in which the household head (or another member) is simply asked for an assessment of the adequacy of consumption overall and adequacy of food, housing, and clothing consumption. When such subjective measures are compared with monetized measures based on consumption or income data in data sets that have both—ingenious statistical methods are required to establish a basis for comparison—the two approaches are found to agree reasonably well in identifying the households that are poor. It seems, however, that to be properly interpreted the subjective measures need to be adjusted for factors such as urban or rural residence, education of household adults, household size, and the like. Evidently this is because "adequacy" is a subjective concept much influenced by current standards of living and current income. With such adjustments, the subjective method closely resembles the MIMIC factor-analytic approach that was described above, although with fewer indicators. Only a few subjective–objective comparisons of this sort have been made to date (Pradhan and Ravallion, 2000; Lokshin, *et al.*, 2004; Carletto and Zezza, 2004) but if these early studies are any guide, the subjective approach may well provide a useful alternative to detailed consumption and income modules.

Table 2. Supplemental Survey Questions on Living Standards

	Subjective Assessments of Consumption
Adequacy of consumption	Concerning your family's food consumption over the past one month, which of the following is true: It was less than adequate for your family's needs, just adequate, more than adequate? (Similarly for housing, clothing, health care, children's schooling, and overall standard of living.) In each case, "adequate" means no more and no less than what the respondent considers to be the minimum consumption needs of the family. (Pradhan and Ravallion, 2000; Ravallion and Lokshin, 2002; Lokshin *et al.* 2004; Carletto and Zezza, 2004).
	Additional Indicators and Determinants of Consumption
Electricity	Is electricity normally available all day? In the last two weeks, was it unavailable for an entire day or longer?
Quality of housing	How many rooms does this household occupy, not counting bathrooms, closets, and passageways? How many rooms are used for sleeping? Is there a separate kitchen or a room used mainly for cooking?
Consumer durables	Ownership of a functioning radio, television, mobile telephone, other telephone, refrigerator, clock, watch, fan, bicycle, motorcycle or motor scooter, car or truck; the number of tables, chairs, sofas, and beds.
Producer durables	Ownership and amount of agricultural land (by type, e.g., irrigated, wet or dry crop land); amount of non-agricultural land; availability of a room or property that can be rented.
	Ownership of a cart, sewing machine, grain grinder, electric generator, boat with motor, and livestock.
Financial assets	Does any member of the household have a bank account? A pension? Health insurance? Life insurance?
	Indicators of Both Living Standards and Health
Drinking water	Is water normally available all day from this source? In the last two weeks, was water unavailable for an entire day or longer?
Water storage	Do you store the water for drinking? (Examine container) Do you do anything to the water to make it safer to drink? What do you do?
Toilet facilities	Where is this facility located? Does your household share this facility with other households? How many?

Hygiene	Where do members of this household wash their hands? (Examine and record presence of water, soap, hand cleanser, basin, clean towel or cloth.)
Disposal of food wastes	What is the principal way you dispose of garbage? How frequently is the garbage collected?
Air quality	Does your household cook mostly indoors or outdoors? What type of fuel does your household mainly use for cooking? (Record the number of windows and whether they are covered by screens or glass.)
	DIMENSIONS OF LIVING STANDARDS OTHER THAN CONSUMPTION
Eviction risk	How likely is it that you could be evicted from this dwelling? Would you say that it is very likely, somewhat likely, or not at all likely?
Crime	In general, how safe from crime and violence do you feel when you are alone at home? How safe do you feel when walking down your street alone after dark? In the past year, has any member of this household been the victim of a violent crime, such as assault or mugging? How many times? In the past year, has your house been burglarized or vandalized? How many times?
Political voice	To what extent do local government and local leaders take into account concerns voiced by you and people like you when they make decisions that affect you?
	Do local residents frequently talk to authorities or local organizations about local problems? Do people in this area actively participate in elections for the neighborhood and borough committees?
	Does the health center provide a service whenever the community needs it? Do the police provide a service whenever the community needs it? Does the borough committee provide a service whenever the community needs it?
Expectations	Do you think that over the next 12 months, you and your family will live better than today, about the same, or worse?

Substantial efforts are also underway to understand the merits and limitations of abbreviated versions of consumption expenditure schedules. In a rural study Morris, *et al.*, (1999) show that the measures of consumption derived from such short forms are reasonably highly correlated with the totals from fully-elaborated consumption modules. The abbreviated measures are not substitutes for full consumption expenditures, because by construction they understate totals (Pradhan, 2000). But like the proxy variables methods described above, the short-form consumption schedules are of potential value in defining relative measures of living standards and in testing hypotheses about the effects of living standards on health.

A number of the items in Table 2 add to the number of indicators already gathered in demographic surveys—e.g., the elaborated lists of consumer and producer durables, the inclusion of service adequacy indicators for electricity, water supply, and sanitation. These questions are likely to show variation across urban neighborhoods and households, and should reveal inadequacies in service delivery that would not otherwise be apparent. In some countries, employees of government and formal-sector firms will have health insurance and some form of pension; even in a Côte d'Ivoire slum, some 10% of households were found to have health insurance (Bossart, 2003). Much more could be done to assess the productive value of urban housing and the economic benefits derived from security of tenure (Field, 2003). Useful survey questions and methodological tools might also be drawn from the literatures on microfinance and program targeting; see Falkingham and Namazie (2002) for an introduction. These literatures offer a range of techniques for assessing household living standards, including both simple and elaborate forms of means-testing, community appraisals of relative living standards, and systems for classifying household living standards on the basis of age, gender of head, land ownership, and household demographic composition (Coady, *et al.*, 2004; Zeller, 2004).

The third set of questions in the table is as closely tied to health as to the household's standard of living. If an index of living standards includes such items, it should not be employed as a determinant of any closely-related health behavior or risk. Circular reasoning is a concern here, as is statistical endogeneity. The remaining set of items measure aspects of poverty and living standards that have not yet featured in much survey research—e.g., questions on the perceived likelihood of eviction, and insecurities related to violence and crime.

Notably missing from Table 2 are questions touching on perceptions of inequality and social exclusion. A large literature on such topics exists in the field of social psychology (see Walker and Smith, 2002), but the empirical approaches pursued in this literature do not appear to have been systematically exploited in studies of health. Much of this literature is concerned with the conditions under which relative deprivation is interpreted in strictly personal terms or is understood in terms of groups. As Tyler and Lind (2002) explain,

> If people feel that they are not doing well relative to other people, they [may] react in individualistic ways. If they think change is possible, they might go to school or work harder. If they think change is not possible, they might drink or use drugs. In either case, they respond to feelings of deprivation by taking individual actions. . . In contrast, if people feel that their group is deprived relative to other groups, they are more likely to become involved in actions that focus on changing the situation of their group. It is of particular interest if they engage in collective behavior. . .

The concept of relative deprivation thus touches on personal as well as collective efficacy. According to Wright and Tropp (2002), the way in which individuals interpret deprivation and form a response to it depends on their sense of whether individual upward mobility is possible. Smith and Ortiz (2002) argue that deprivation interpreted in personal terms may bring on physiological stress, reduce self-esteem, and induce depression.

An important distinction in this literature, which comes to the fore when individuals engage with institutions, is between relative deprivation in outcomes as against deprivation in procedures (Tyler and Lind, 2002). It is especially interesting to consider the procedural injustices experienced by the urban poor—long waits for care, the dismissive or abusive attitudes exhibited by staff—when they seek care from the modern health system. Differences in health treatments and procedures experienced in the modern system may be viewed by the poor as unjust and illegitimate, whereas the poor might well tolerate substantial inequalities in health outcomes if they believed that they have been treated fairly and impartially.

Much of the theory of relative deprivation has been developed in the context of racism in the U.S. As far as we are aware, the core concepts have not been explored in any depth in empirical studies of health in developing countries. A South African study of the attitudes of blacks, Afrikaans whites, and English whites (Duckitt and Mphuthing, 2002) gives one example of the empirical approaches that might be pursued. Respondents were asked to place each of these groups on a rung of a socioeconomic ladder, and also to indicate where the group should be placed if it were to receive its fair and rightful share of the wealth of the country. The differences in ranking were taken to be a measure of group deprivation.

3.6. Monitoring Change Over Time

Little is yet known of the dynamics of poverty in the cities of developing countries. The study of change requires longitudinal data, and, as we discuss later in the chapter, such data are far from being common in the developing world. But longitudinal studies are now beginning to appear in greater numbers. Although the literature on poverty dynamics has been dominated by studies of rural areas thus far (for an introduction, see Baulch and Hoddinott, 2000), urban poverty dynamics are also coming into focus.

In some recent research, full-scale income and consumption expenditure modules have been fielded for urban populations.* The results indicate that household transitions into and out of poverty are common in urban as well as rural areas. In the Herra and Roubaud (2003) comparison of urban Peru and Madagascar in the late 1990s, for example, some 40% of initially poor urban Peruvians were found to have escaped poverty one year later, whereas 13–20% of those initially nonpoor had fallen into poverty. The corresponding transition rates for urban Madagascar were 10 % for exiting poverty and 33–40% for entry. In KwaZulu–Natal (South Africa), a panel study conducted over a 5-year interval found that roughly two-thirds of households in the bottom two quintiles of the 1993 income distribution had graduated to

*See Maluccio et al. (2000) and Bigsten et al. (2003) for recently published work. A number of studies on this theme were presented at a 2003 University of Manchester (UK) conference on chronic poverty (Amis, 2003; Henry-Lee, 2003; Herra and Roubaud, 2003; Kedir and McKay, 2003; Lalita, 2003; Mitlin, 2003; Parnell and Mosdell, 2003; Pryer et al., 2003; Stevens, 2003; Woolard and Klasen, 2003).

higher quintiles by 1998 (Woolard and Klasen, 2003). If figures such as these are broadly characteristic of urban dwellers in other settings, they would suggest a good deal of volatility in urban standards of living.

As Herra and Roubaud (2003) note, the literature has been less successful in isolating the determinants of transitions than in identifying the factors producing chronic poverty. (Among other things, errors in measuring consumption and income can mislead by masking real transitions to and from poverty or giving the appearance of such transitions when none occurred. The authors Woolard and Klasen in a paper from 2003 lead a discussion in this.) Education seems to exert something of a protective effect in urban settings, making transitions to poverty less likely and reducing the length of spells in poverty. The demographic composition of households, which can be remarkably fluid, also affects poverty dynamics through routes such as the addition or loss of an adult income-earner and changes in household dependency rates (Woolard and Klasen, 2003). Just how these changes in living standards influence health is not yet known. Some reciprocal influence is to be expected—adult ill health or death can precipitate a household economic crisis, and of course poor households will tend to face higher health risks. (For example, in Pryer, *et al.*, (2003), an examination of both causal pathways in the slums of Dhaka, Bangladesh is examined.)

In circumstances where full income and expenditure data cannot be gathered, the measurement of change in living standards can be expected to present difficulties. It is unlikely that brief inventories of consumer durables and housing quality will exhibit sufficient variability over time to track changes in household standards of living. More extensive lists of consumer items, as itemized in Table 2 are perhaps more likely to register change. Attention needs to be given to supplementing these proxies with indicators that are apt to vary over time with the household's standard of living. For example, the household head might be asked whether, over the past weeks, any member has had to forego a full day of meals for lack of income, or whether the household has had to borrow food. Likewise, the household could be queried on whether it has been forced to sell assets or has taken on additional debt to cover living expenses (examples of such coping strategies are given in CARE/Tanzania, 1998). Simple, subjective measures of change also merit consideration, such as whether in the view of the head or another member, the household is better off than it was a year ago. There is ample scope here for creative application of both qualitative and quantitative techniques (Lalita, 2003; Pryer, *et al.*, 2003; Stevens, 2003). But caution is also in order—Kedir and McKay (2003) find that subjective measures of change in household well-being are only weakly correlated with changes in income and consumption.

Another over-time dimension needing study is the cumulative exposure by households (or their individual members) to the risks that are presented by poor neighborhoods. It is unusual for demographic surveys to collect information on residential mobility; the DHS program, for instance, limits attention in its migration histories to moves into and out of cities and does not inquire about moves taking place within cities. But the implications of short-term spells of residence in poor neighborhoods could be quite different from the implications of prolonged exposure to neighborhood disadvantage. Even if households are to be followed prospectively in a health study, there may be a need to devise retrospective questions that probe into residential mobility and ascertain, up to the limits of respondent recall, something of the character of the neighborhoods inhabited earlier.

3.7. Measuring Neighborhood Poverty and Affluence

The discussion has been mainly concerned with the measurement of living standards at the household level. But with reference to the point just made, how might similar techniques be employed to define relatively poor and relatively advantaged neighborhoods and communities? As with the household-level analyses, it must be taken as given that income and consumption data from censuses will generally be lacking.* One might have thought that, in view of the frequency with which the term "slum" appears in the urban poverty literature, a substantial body of research would provide guidance on precisely this issue.

In fact, as UN-Habitat (2003) makes clear, there is a surprising dearth of quantitative research bearing on slum definitions and assessing the internal composition of slums. It is not known, for example, what proportion of the developing-country urban poor live in slums or what proportion of slum dwellers can be counted as poor in terms of income and other socioeconomic criteria. These gaps in understanding are acknowledged by the UN-Habitat (2003): "[S]lum dwellers are not a homogeneous population, and some people of reasonable income live within or on the edges of slum communities. . . . In many cities, there are more poor people outside the slums than within them."

The extent of heterogeneity within slums is of prime importance to health program targeting. If slums are heterogeneous, then geographically-targeted programs may not distribute program resources effectively. (Although this research does not have any specific focus on slums, the work-in-progress by Fenn, *et al.*, (2004) shows lower than expected levels of spatial clustering in child nutrition, calling into question the benefits of geographic targeting.) In the next stage of urban multilevel health research, it will be vitally important to gain insight into the socioeconomic diversity marking slums and other neighborhoods of the urban poor.

Figures 1 and 2, taken from Montgomery and Hewett (2004), convey a sense of this heterogeneity. In this research, household living standards were estimated using the MIMIC approach described above, and both households and their neighborhoods were placed in quartiles based on their factor scores, with poverty defined in terms of the lowest quartile and affluence in terms of the uppermost quartile. Figure 1 characterizes the neighbors of poor households. If poor households were indeed generally surrounded by other poor households—as in the images of slums and shantytowns that are invoked in so many discussions of urban poverty—then we would expect to find that their neighbors are predominantly poor. As the figure shows, however, this is far from being the case. In Latin America, the average poor household lives in a neighborhood in which about 44 % of its neighbors are poor. To be sure, this is well above the percentage of poor in the urban population as a whole (25% by the relative defini-

*Recent research on poverty mapping has explored the possibilities of combining census data with data from household surveys that have detailed information on income and consumption. The essential idea is to estimate models of income or consumption with the survey data, using as explanatory factors the variables that are also collected in the country's census. The coefficients from the estimated models are then applied to the census data to generate estimates of consumption (or related measures of poverty) on an areal basis. See Henninger and Snel (2002) for an accessible treatment and Lanjouw et al. (2002) for an application to Nairobi and other developing-country urban areas. The method appears highly promising; unfortunately, the number of cases in which it can be used have been limited by the reluctance of national statistical agencies in developing countries to release census microsamples.

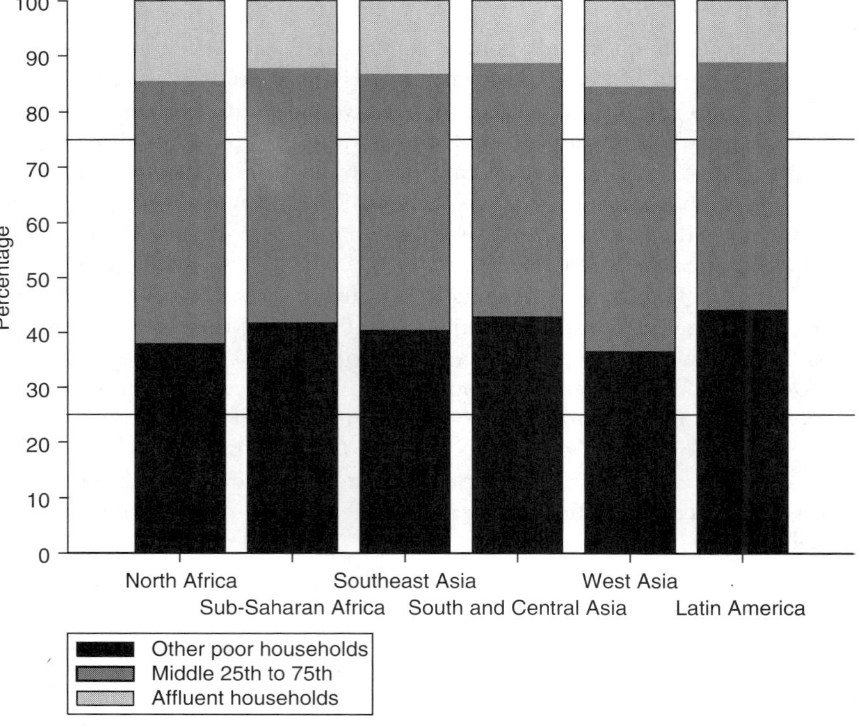

Figure 1. Who Are the Neighbors of the Urban Poor?

tion of poverty adopted here), but it leaves substantial room for neighbors who are in the 25th–75th percentiles of the living standards distribution (in Latin America, this "middle" group accounts for about 45% of a poor household's neighbors) and even for neighbors who are affluent, those who are in the top-most quartile of the urban distribution. A poor Latin American household has, on average, about one neighboring household in ten that is affluent.

Figure 2 depicts the neighbors of these affluent households. Again, as expected, slightly more of the neighbors are themselves affluent than in the urban population at large, and affluent households have somewhat fewer poor neighbors (who make up about 20 % of the neighbors of affluent families). But a household's affluence is not strongly predictive of its neighborhood composition—these are minor departures from the 25th and 75th percentile benchmarks. The spatial concentration of affluence is less clearly evident than would be anticipated given the images of extreme social–spatial polarization that appear so often in the literature.

Figure 3, which summarizes predictions from multivariate models, illustrates the impact of household and neighborhood living standards on one measure of health, whether a woman's labor is attended by a doctor, nurse, or trained midwife. [The figure summarizes estimates from a number of surveys; see Montgomery and Hewett (2004) for the details.] As this figure indicates, with other things held con-

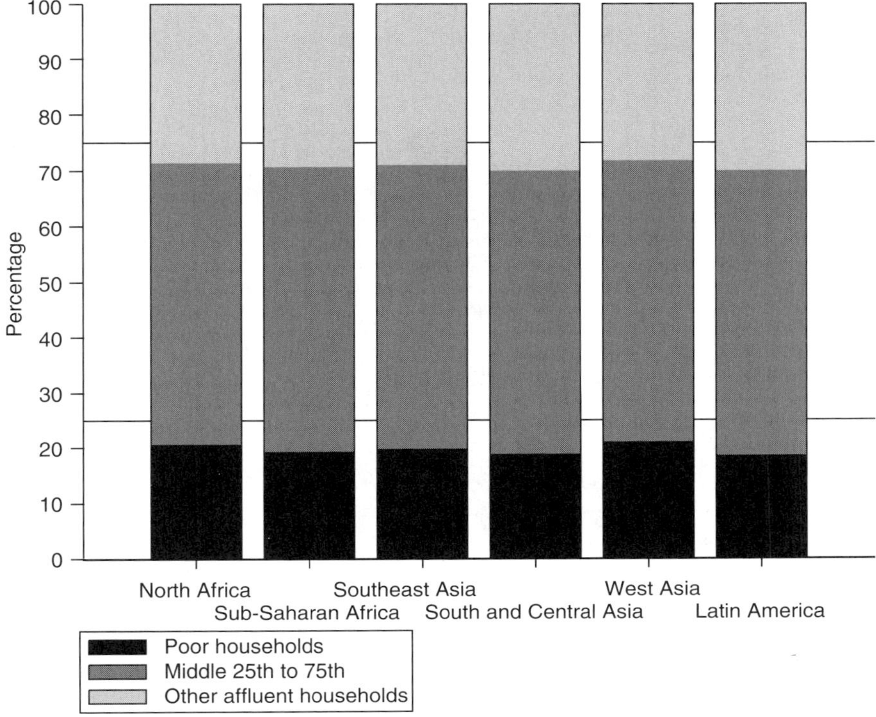

Figure 2. Who Are the Neighbors of the Urban Affluent?

stant, poor women living in nonpoor neighborhoods are much more likely to have their births attended than are poor women in poor neighborhoods. It would appear that social and health resources are available in nonpoor neighborhoods that bring benefits to poor households.

As we have mentioned, little is known about the extent of neighborhood heterogeneity. A detailed study of Cali, Colombia in the mid-1990s (World Bank, 2002) found considerable income heterogeneity within *manzanas*, which are small blocks of housing that are classified into socioeconomic strata for the purpose of targeting subsidy programs and delivering public services. The assumption had been that such strata are internally homogeneous. However, even in the lowest socioeconomic stratum of *manzana* in Cali, one household in five was found to have a per capita income level placing it in the top forty percent of the distribution for the city as a whole. In the highest stratum of *manzana*, about one household in ten had a per capita income in the bottom forty percent of the city income distribution. Unfortunately, detailed studies of neighborhood heterogeneity such as these are not yet widely available for developing countries.

Perhaps it is not, on reflection, greatly surprising that urban neighborhoods in developing countries are heterogeneous. Some of the tools used to enforce social exclusion in high-income countries—i.e., exclusionary zoning—are either unavailable or ineffective in developing-country cities, and affluent families in these cities

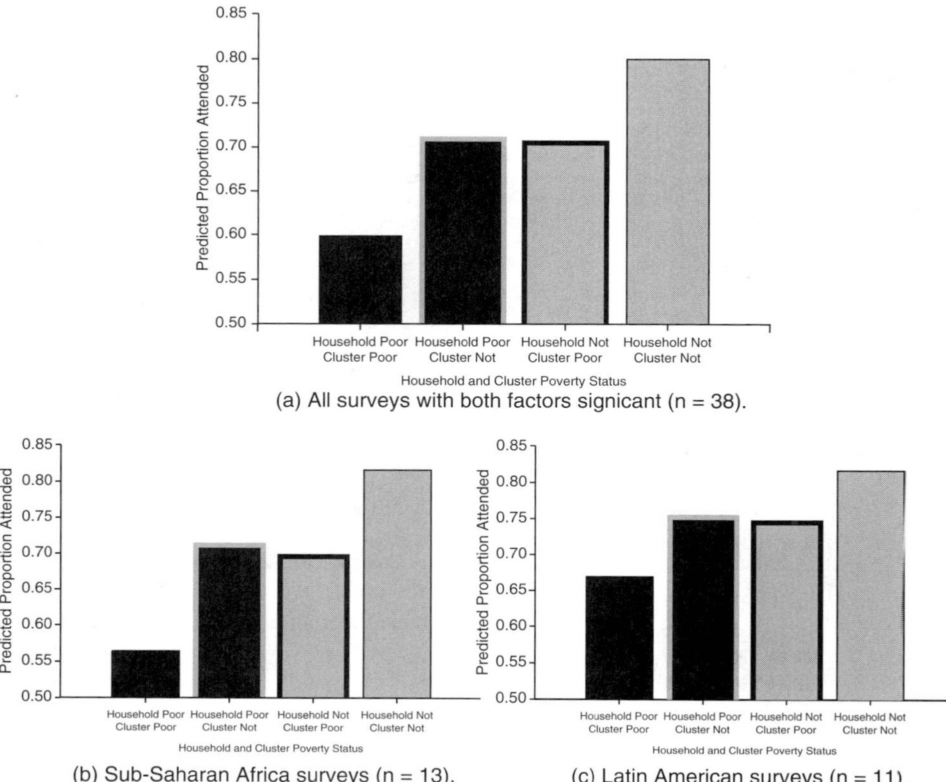

Figure 3. Predicted Proportion of Births Attended by a Doctor, Nurse or Trained Midwife, by Household and Cluster Poverty (*Source*: Montgomery and Hewett [2004]).

benefit from the spatial proximity of the poor, who provide them with a ready source of domestic labor and other services. Moreover, as the Latin American literature shows, social exclusion can be enforced aggressively through non-spatial means (Caldeira, 1999; 2000). Even for the U.S., it has long been known that spatial segregation by income has been less severe on the whole than has segregation by race (e.g., White, 1987; Hardman and Ioannides, 2004).

4.0. URBAN SOCIAL NETWORKS AND SOCIAL CAPITAL

This section is devoted to the tools needed to study social networks and social capital in developing-country cities. Large literatures—mainly though not exclusively concerned with developed countries—have considered social networks and capital, and we will not attempt to give a comprehensive account here. Fuller treatments are available in Panel of Urban Population Dynamics (2003), which explores the implications of social networks and capital for developing-country health and demographic behavior, and in Grootaert, *et al.*, (2004), which offers thoughts on the implications for economic development. Both sources contain extensive references to the social networks literature, which is too large to be adequately summarized here. To bring focus to the discussion, we concentrate mainly on the tools that will be needed in fieldwork and the context-specific difficulties that can be anticipated in the application of such tools.

A recurring theme in what follows is the need to establish plausible mechanisms through which social interaction can affect health. The difficulties in precisely identifying mechanisms is, of course, a longstanding concern in social epidemiology. In studies of sexual networking and HIV-AIDS (Morris, 1993; Friedman and Aral, 2001), the viral transmission mechanism is understood well enough to justify extensive sociological analysis of networks. Pathways for contagious disease—contamination of water or food, airborne transmission—are also sufficiently well established to allow research to concentrate on the kinds of social interaction that raise the risks of contagion. In other dimensions of urban social epidemiology, however, the mechanisms are not yet so well understood. There is a continuing need to explore just how the general factors of interest in social network and social capital research—weak and strong network ties, bridging connections, notions of trust, collective efficacy, and the like—could come to exert an influence on health.

4.1. Measuring Social Networks

The basic elements of a social networks survey module can be thought of as a series of "who, where, when, what" questions, with "what" referring to the health content of interactions in networks. The survey module often opens with a "name-generator" question that elicits the names of the respondent's network partners. This question can be general or it can make specific reference to health. A common strategy is to record as many names as are volunteered, and then to proceed with more detailed queries on a subset of these partners. Because urban dwellers interact in multiple settings within and outside their residential neighborhoods, it is important that each network partner's location be determined in relation to the community in which the respondent lives. This, in turn, means that respondent's own views of community boundaries must be recorded before the social network question sequence begins. The "when" question is also significant. In longitudinal studies, the time since the previous interview establishes a frame that may help respondents to recollect when it was that significant interactions with their network partners took place; otherwise a time frame must be adopted to focus attention.

The respondent-centered approach to delineating networks quickly runs up against the limits of interview time and respondent patience. If, for instance, the respondent has mentioned five network partners and four questions are to be asked about each partner, the interviewer confronts a bank of twenty questions to work through. In the Casterline, *et al.*, (2001) study of social networks in Ghana, it was found that only one set of network questions could be tolerated in any given interview. If the survey is embedded in a larger demographic surveillance system with basic demographic records for all residents (see Section 5), some interview time can be saved by skipping questions for the network partners already covered by the system. For partners living elsewhere, however, there is little alternative but to proceed with all of the questions.

The Casterline, *et al.*, (2001) analysis illustrates how network data can throw light on the health content of social interactions. This study was concerned with modern contraceptive use and how the experiences and views of social network partners affected the motivations of the respondent.* Such information was recorded over seven survey rounds at intervals of about six months. An analysis using statistical methods for longitudinal data uncovered strong evidence that contraceptive use by a respondent's network partners exerted substantial influence on the likelihood that the respondent herself would use contraception. The techniques employed in this study could well be adapted for research on other forms of preventive health behavior.

What roles might urban social networks play in health more generally? Networks could provide their members with information about the location and quality of health services, of both the formal and informal varieties. A member who is ill could turn to her network for advice on interpreting the origin of the illness—e.g., whether the illness is due to "natural" causes of a kind likely to respond to modern-sector care or to other causes requiring traditional interventions—and evaluations of its severity. By sharing their own experiences and those of which they have heard, network partners could estimate the probable effectiveness of various forms of treatment. As Barua and Singh (2003) observe with reference to the urban poor in India, such social groups constitute what has been termed a "lay referral network". As often conjectured in the mental health literature, networks can also make some material assistance available to their members or at least lend to the ill person a measure of comfort and moral support. Furthermore, network partners

*In the opening round of this longitudinal undertaking, a name-generator question referred to conversational networks. Women were given a general frame of reference:

> We all talk to others about important matters in our lives. I would like to ask about the people other than your husband/partner whose opinions are important to you. They are people with whom you discuss your personal affairs or private concerns, such as children's illness, schooling, pregnancy, work, and church. They can live nearby or far away, and you might talk to them frequently or infrequently. Other than your husband/partner, can you please give me the names of people whose opinions matter to you?

In later rounds of the survey, the name-generator question focused specifically on conversations about modern contraception:

> I would like to ask you about the people other than your husband/partner with whom you discuss modern contraception. These are people with whom you have discussed the costs and benefits of modern contraceptive methods, where they can be obtained, their side effects, and how the methods are used. These people can live nearby or far away, and you might talk to them frequently or infrequently. Other than your husband/partner, can you please give me the names of people with whom you have discussed modern contraception in the last 12 months [since the last survey]?

In each case, the interviewer recorded all the names that the respondent volunteered. In the context of general social networks (the names supplied in the first name-generator), the respondent was then asked whether she had discussed childbearing matters with the network partner, whether she felt the network partner approved of modern contraception, and whether she believed the network partner had ever used modern contraception (with a probe into the basis for this belief). In reference to modern contraception networks (second name-generator), the respondent was asked whether she felt the network partner approved of modern contraception, whether she believed the network partner had ever used modern contraception (again with a probe into the basis for the belief), which method she believed the network partner had used, and whether the respondent and network partner had ever encouraged or discouraged each other from using modern contraception.

and others whom they know provide a web of personal connections that may include staff in health clinics and hospitals located throughout the city. Such personal connections take on special importance when healthcare workers have a reputation for exhibiting dismissive, rude, and abusive behavior toward patients they do not know. This discussion has emphasized the connections between individuals and the health system, but social network analysis can also add value to studies of referrals and other linkages among health providers. In research on the slums of Delhi, Jha, *et al.*, (2002) find considerable evidence of interaction between slum households and their local headmen (*pradhans*), other community leaders and elders, and even municipal councilors. The local leaders themselves interact with political and bureaucratic figures across the city. Political connections such as these may offer opportunities for poor households to gain access to health-related public services. A good deal of insight could be secured into the role of "bridging" networks by tracing the connections from households to their local leaders and from these leaders to powerful actors in the wider municipal arena.

Although these propositions about social networks sound plausible enough, their implications for health do not seem to have been investigated empirically. Some conjectures in the literature doubtless overstate the health significance of urban social networks. For example, Janzen (1978) depicted social networks as actively rallying around when a member falls ill. But in an analysis of response to illness in an Abidjan (Côte d'Ivoire) slum, Bossart (2003) found that network members outside the household were not, in fact, much involved in the provision of financial assistance—the obligation to assist in this way fell mainly upon family members in the ill person's household. To be sure, the Abidjan analysis was concerned only with material assistance in times of illness, and left open the possibility of a social networks role in providing information about services and shaping individual interpretations of illness.

Because the empirical literature on the health roles of urban social networks is so thin, new network studies must be preceded by substantial qualitative work. The techniques of urban anthropology (Obrist, *et al.*, 2003a; 2003b; Obrist, 2003) could be usefully brought to bear. Focus group discussions, semi-structured interviews, participant observation, the compilation of community histories, and related methods could reveal the features of social networks that warrant further quantitative study.

4.2. Measuring Social Capital

Much the same preparation would be required for analyses of the structure of local social capital. Before querying individuals about their participation in community groups, a research team will need to take an inventory of the organizations operating in the community, and determine which among these serve as likely forums for exchanges of health information or for collective action (Agyeman and Casterline, 2003; Grootaert, *et al.*, 2004). As Casterline, *et al.*, (2001) discovered in the Ghana study mentioned above, special efforts are required to identify the full range of informal associations in the community. The small villages and peri-urban neighborhoods examined in this study were found to be rife with associations, including many with cultural or religious orientations, occupational and economic groups, various political associations, groups with educational objectives (e.g., parent–teacher associations), general philanthropic and community welfare organizations, and a few groups concerned specifically with health or family life education.

With the organizational terrain thus mapped out, lists of groups in any given community can be incorporated in that community's survey questionnaires. As with the member-by-member inquiries for social networks, the research team will need to decide whether to pursue questions about group participation on an organization-by-organization basis, or to single out only the "most important" organizations. If the latter course is taken, the team will need to consider how importance should be established, given the tendency for organizations to be segregated by sex. An older male household head might have a very different view of organizational importance than a young married woman.

In their work on Chicago, Swaroop and Morenoff (2004) distinguish "expressive" from "instrumental" motivations for community participation and classify community groups accordingly. The expressive motivations have to do with a sense of neighborly identity and obligations, and these motives would be evident in participation in groups that promote social interaction and neighborliness. Examples would include neighborhood religious organizations and those based on ethnicity or (in the case of migrants) regional or national identity. Instrumental motivations, by contrast, arise from desires to protect investments in one's home or local business and to meet threats facing the neighborhood as a whole; these would be evident in involvement in neighborhood watch groups, local sanitation committees, local political organizations, and other types of problem-solving associations.

As Swaroop and Morenoff (2004) observe, it is not easy to understand why it is that one poor community can sustain a rich associational life brimming with energy and collective commitment while another entirely fails to cohere and socially disintegrates. Factors discouraging group participation include the general lack of resources and extra-community ties that may be characteristic of most poor communities; but poor communities also face more threats to health and this should intensify the motivation for participation and collective action. In any case, the fact that participation in some community associations is voluntary, and thus dependent on motivations that go at least partly unmeasured, raises concerns about identifying the causal influence of participation itself on health (Durlauf, 2000a; 2000b).

Substantial knowledge of urban community life may be needed to see how group membership could be related to health. For example, consider a woman who is a member of a rotating savings and credit group (an *esusu* group, as it is known in much of sub-Saharan Africa). This group's main function might seem to be narrowly economic in nature—it helps members to accumulate small amounts of capital and makes modest loans available to members in distress, thus providing a buffer against shocks and risks. How, then, might membership in this group influence individual health? By reducing the anxieties and stress stemming from the anticipation of health shocks and income volatility? By providing material assistance when illness actually strikes? Or might the mechanism be unrelated to the group's main function, having to do instead with the informal exchange of health information and ideas that could take place spontaneously in almost any group setting?

4.3. The Overlap of Social Networks and Capital

In a full portrait of social organization that depicts both individual social networks and community groups, it will be possible to identify mutually reinforcing connections among networks and groups. These connections are illustrated in Figure 4. Respondent 1 (denoted "R1") has a personal network tie to Respondents 2 and 4, and she also participates with Respondent 2 in an informal community group.

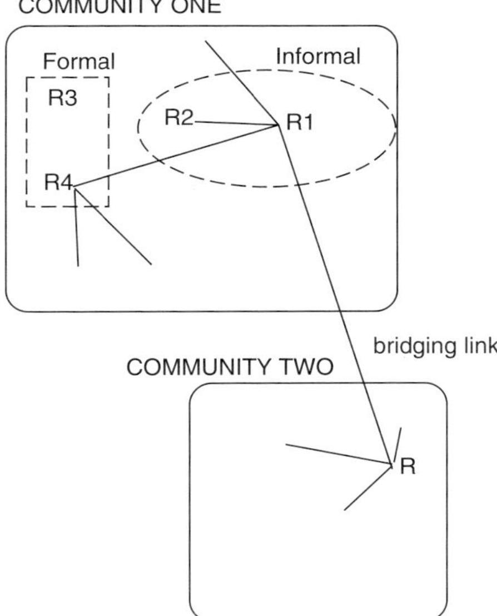

Figure 4. Community Organizations and Personal Networks

Respondent 1 has no direct personal link to Respondent 3, but because Respondents 3 and 4 are both members of a formal community organization, it is possible for information exchanged in this organization to make its way back to Respondent 1 through her R4 network tie. The figure also depicts an outside, or bridging, link between Respondent 1 and a person in another community. One can imagine overlaying the organizational structure of an urban neighborhood on a fully-specified set of social network data such as that shown in the figure, to understand how information may circulate within and across neighborhoods. As far as we are aware, however, no such comprehensive treatment of urban networks and organizations has yet appeared in the developing-country literature.

For at least three reasons, the bridging link shown in Figure 4 is likely to be of considerable significance in urban contexts. First, even poor slum dwellers may have political connections and the sophistication needed to exploit them, which could attract the attention of government and bring health resources to the community (for India, see Parker, *et al.*, 2003; Jha, *et al.*, 2002). However, as we have argued above, mixed-income neighborhoods are likely to have more bridging links of this type (Altschuler, *et al.*, 2004). Second, as Swaroop and Morenoff (2004) note, individual social networks and some community associations can span and thereby link geographically-distinct neighborhoods, providing pathways for information transfer across communities. Moreover, as they suggest, motivation for joining a local association in Community 1 may stem from observation of nearby neighborhoods such as Community 2, which may provide examples of what may befall one's own neighborhood if action is not taken. Third, health interventions in urban communities can deliberately aim to establish bridging links, as embodied in local community health workers whose role is to act as referral agents. Barua and Singh (2003) discuss such "link" workers in the slums of Ahmedabad (India). Here volunteer community workers conduct regular home visits and direct those with the symptoms of tuberculosis to the appropriate health facility in the city; another community agent follows up to encourage compliance with the treatment regimen. A similar strategy is being pursued in efforts to treat malaria in Burkina Faso (Pictet, *et al.*, 2004). In the programs reviewed by Barua and Singh, a community-based organization serves as an umbrella group for these workers and helps to cement their linkages to the formal health system.

4.4. The Cognitive Component of Social Capital

Much of the effort in devising measures of social capital has been devoted to what Harpham, *et al.*, (2002) term the "cognitive component," that is, its manifestations in perceptions of community support and collective efficacy, expectations of reciprocity, and interpersonal trust. The cognitive component is conceptually and empirically separable from membership in organizations—perhaps for the reasons outlined in Swaroop and Morenoff (2004), membership need not be associated with trust in any monotonic fashion. Penetrating discussions of these concepts and suggestions on measurement methods can be found in Harpham, *et al.*, (2002), Harpham, *et al.*, (2004), and Grootaert, *et al.*, (2004), the last of which offers a comprehensive and well-organized list of survey questions on the cognitive component, some of which have been field-tested in developing countries. Some examples include:

Networks: If you suddenly needed a small amount of money, equal to about one week's wages, how many people beyond your immediate household could you turn to who would be *willing* to provide this money? If you suddenly had to go away for a day or two, could you count on your neighbors to take care of your children?

Trust: Agree or disagree: In this neighborhood, one has to be alert or someone is likely to take advantage of you.

Collective efficacy: If there was a water supply problem in this community, how likely is it that people will cooperate to try to solve the problem?

Conflict: In your opinion, is this neighborhood generally peaceful or marked by violence? As noted earlier in this chapter, variants and extensions of such questions were fielded in the Cali, Columbia study of mental health (Harpham, *et al.*, 2004). Presumably the cognitive component influences individual morale and the sense of personal efficacy, and in this way could influence motivations for many forms of health-seeking behavior.

5.0. WHAT CAN BE LEARNED FROM LONGITUDINAL STUDIES?

In research on urban health, longitudinal (prospective) designs offer many advantages over cross-sectional and retrospective designs. We have already discussed some of the methodological benefits in addressing selectivity bias, and in what follows will discuss additional considerations that favor a longitudinal approach. But a longitudinal program of data collection requires heavy resource commitments and faces limitations of its own. Below we describe the benefits and costs in more detail, drawing upon the experiences of the African Population and Health Research Center (2002) in Nairobi, which since the year 2000 has maintained a demographic surveillance system in several of this city's largest slums. In describing this case, we hope to draw out examples and lessons that are of wider applicability.

5.1. The Benefits of Longitudinal Designs

The advantages of longitudinal approaches to health research are well understood, and we need only briefly restate them here. First, longitudinal designs allow the temporal ordering of behavior, exposure to risks, and health outcomes to be established. For instance, the benefits of vaccination for child survival can be traced from the point when a particular child receives the vaccine. During the course of follow-up, a host of time-varying factors may come to impinge on the child's health (stemming from changes in the social, demographic, environmental, or health system environment) and if the dates of each change are recorded, such factors can be incorporated in the analysis of risks and estimates of hazard rates.

Knowing the time-order of events is of particular importance when the nature of an intervention (or illness) makes retrospective recall either impossible or of doubtful value. Where infectious childhood diseases are concerned, the accumulation of risks that comes about through disease synergies (as in cycles whereby infection and nutritional debilitation lead to heightened risks of re-infection) all but demand a prospective approach, because such complex histories are difficult even to describe by other means. In research on reproductive tract infections (RTIs), women are often found to be unaware that they are infected, either because the infection itself is asymptomatic or because its symptoms are not understood by women to indicate disease. Individual recollection can be of little value here. Likewise, mental health is not reliably determined by retrospective methods. Here, too, knowing the sequence of events is critical: without such data, the associations between good mental health and social support networks at a point in time could be attributed not to the protective influence of networks but rather to the withdrawal of those in poor health from social interaction and engagement.

Second, longitudinal designs, can reduce some of the costs of data collection. For health determinants that vary across people but not over time (or which change only occasionally) data-gathering can take place over the course of multiple interviews, whereas in a cross-sectional study all such determinants would need to be addressed in one interview. The ability to stage a sequence of data collection activities can give researchers the luxury of dedicating survey rounds to special topics. A survey round could be largely given over to a detailed examination of household incomes and expenditures, which would have crowded out other high-priority items in a single cross-sectional survey. Also, while data are being collected over time, opportunities will arise to respond to unexpected findings, whether through focused qualitative research or further quantitative probes. On-going data collection programs provide a vehicle to which such investigatory studies can be attached.

Third, a longitudinal approach provides ways of keeping measurement errors and potentially confounding factors in check. Longitudinal questionnaires can be designed so as to concentrate the attention of the field worker and interviewee on the time since the last interview, with the first order of business being to reconfirm the essential items reported in that interview. When combined with appropriately programmed data-entry software, this approach allows cross-checking procedures to be instituted that substantially reduce error. As an example, in Ghana, Casterline, *et al.*, (2001) employed similar procedures in their longitudinal social networks research to determine whether network members mentioned in a given interview had already been mentioned in a previous interview, if so, repetitive questions on the member's age, sex, and education were skipped. See Beckett, *et al.*, (2001) on the use of such methods to aid long-term recall and Pierret (2001) on the loss of information entailed in lengthening the gap between survey rounds. A very important advantage of longitudinal designs—to many researchers this is the decisive advantage, as we discuss below—is that these designs enable statistical controls to be put in place for otherwise unobservable individual, household, and community factors, whose effects might be hopelessly confounded with the effects of interest in a cross-sectional study.

Demographic surveillance systems (DSS) are an important special case of longitudinal designs. (The INDEPTH network links a number of demographic surveillance sites in developing countries, several of which are urban or mixed urban-rural sites. More information on this research network can be found at www.indepth-network.org.) The distinguishing feature of the DSS approach is the collection of data on all individuals (or households) residing in the study sites. Typically these are large undertakings, involving visits to each household every three to six months. The scale of the operation implies that only the most important demographic and health variables can be updated at each round of surveillance. To supplement these data, DSS programs often adopt a hybrid approach whereby more detailed information is obtained through periodic panel surveys administered to a subset of residents.

Surveillance systems offer several advantages. For analyses of the dynamics of disease transmission, the full population coverage achieved by a DSS is obviously very important. Some of the diffusion and "social contagion" mechanisms that were described earlier may also benefit from full coverage. (Not all contagion mechanisms are localized in urban settings.) In addition, because the core household and individual characteristics are gathered in each surveillance round, reliable and up-to-date sampling frames are automatically generated for precisely-targeted studies of population subgroups, such as the elderly or school-age children.

5.2. The Costs of Longitudinal Approaches

None of the advantages from longitudinal research comes without cost, especially if long durations of observation are needed to monitor the health outcomes of interest. Consider studies of seasonal variations in health, the effects of climate or ecological change, mortality and morbidity due to diseases with long latency periods, and the impact of behavioral interventions whose effects are slow to develop. In rich countries such as the U.S., the extra costs have not precluded longitudinal studies of health. Is there any reason to think that the costs might be prohibitive in developing countries? In these settings, what is really entailed in the construction and maintenance of a longitudinal research program?

To begin, there are distinctive demands placed on the research team in the conduct of fieldwork. After multiple rounds of interviewing, respondent fatigue can be expected to set in and some respondents will begin to rebel at the repeated intrusions on their time. The opportunity costs of interview time can be especially high for poor urban dwellers, many of whom must juggle multiple jobs and endure exhausting commutes to work. As the editors of this volume have noted, many health studies have offered modest monetary incentives to compensate respondents for their time. In our experience, urban residents are often aware that they can demand to be compensated for an interview, and the research project may have no alternative but to institute an incentive system to secure cooperation. The many time pressures of urban life can make scheduling interviews exceedingly difficult. Field staff must be ready to call upon all of their reserves of flexibility, tact, and patience to address mounting complaints and to move effectively to defuse hostilities.

If the subjects of the research are to be monitored for any appreciable length of time, rigorous systems for tracking them must be embedded in fieldwork procedures and in the project's management and computer systems. Because telephones and the mail are of little use in developing-country contexts, monitoring is a highly labor-intensive exercise. Intense staff effort and meticulous attention to detail are essential to keep survey attrition in check and to diagnose the root causes of loss to follow-up. DSS programs, in particular, cannot be mounted without the use of sophisticated relational databases, and these require strong statistical and analytical skills on the part of senior staff. The nature of supervision also has some distinctive features. In prospective studies fieldworkers can come to know their respondents all too well and, unless carefully supervised, some will be tempted to substitute their own answers to survey questions for those of the respondent. Acquiescence bias—the tendency for respondents to anticipate what they believe the interviewer would like to hear—is also a mounting risk (Hill and Willis, 2001). Both tendencies can be counteracted, at least to a degree, by judicious reshuffling of interviewer assignments. Specific information about the respondent—such as how to locate the respondent's dwelling, reasons for reluctance to participate in previous waves of the study, and the persuasive techniques used to overcome initial refusals—can be kept in special log files that are transferred to new interviewers. For these reasons, the recruitment and retention of capable fieldworkers, supervisors, and computer staff will almost inevitably require higher levels of compensation than would be needed in one-off, cross-sectional studies.

Even with rapport building, incentives and painstaking supervision, some loss due to attrition must be anticipated. Measures will need to be taken to assess whether the loss threatens the representativeness of the sample. Urban populations are often said to be highly mobile and elusive, a perception that has doubtless dampened enthusiasm for urban longitudinal research. But such perceptions are not always solidly-grounded in field experience (as noted in section 5.6 in this chapter). Some urban longitudinal studies have succeeded in retaining very high percentages of their initial respondents. The Indonesian Family Life Survey (Thomas and Frankenberg, 2001) achieved remarkable rates of retention (over 94% four years after the initial survey) in urban and rural areas alike, in part because this study had the funding and staff resources to trace the initial respondents who moved. A three-year panel study of urban Ethiopia (Bigsten, *et al.*, 2003) lost only 7 percent of its respondents to attrition. A South African study relocated some 90% of its urban residents five years after the initial survey—this despite the fact that the study had not initially been envisioned as a panel (Woolard and Klasen, 2003). In other settings with higher attrition, however, the biases induced by attrition could undermine the statistical foundations of the research. As discussed by Thomas and Frankenberg (2001), longitudinal follow-up rates have been little better than dismal in some West African and Latin American surveys, although it is unclear how much of the problem in these cases stemmed from population mobility and how much from inadequate preparation and fieldwork.

In developing countries, it is difficult to mount any longitudinal research effort that does not in some fundamental way rely on continuing involvement with the communities in which the research subjects reside. At a minimum—for longitudinal and cross-sectional studies alike—local political leaders and other influential persons will need to give permission for the study to proceed in their communities. In longitudinal designs, however, community involvement is also required to establish mechanisms for following individuals over time and to ensure the success of day-to-day fieldwork. Some consultation with local leaders and advice from community members (perhaps in the form of community advisory boards) may be needed to devise workable identification and tracking systems with adequate protections for confidentiality. As fieldwork gets underway, neighbors and others in the community will often be asked for their help in rescheduling interviews of residents who are temporarily absent. If these requests are not carefully framed, they can easily raise suspicions about the true intentions of the project team—especially if that team is also inquiring into the composition of individual social networks. The community may need to be reminded repeatedly of the purposes of the study and the benefits that are expected to come from it, and may also need multiple reassurances about confidentiality.

Given this, longitudinal designs must give careful consideration to the maintenance of community good will. If local residents are hired as survey fieldworkers—a practice that has both benefits and costs—the project will receive some credit for being a steady source of employment. (Among other things, the use of interviewers from the same community can make it difficult to assure confidentiality, so that careful training of staff on confidentiality is important). But further material contributions to the community may well be required to sustain good will, and health research projects will inevitably come under pressure to assist the community in the construction of its health center or its water and sanitation facilities, or to effect improvements in the provision of health information, drugs, and emergency care. Project staff may themselves feel an ethical obligation to respond to the community's needs. A balance will need to be sought between the maintenance of community good will, on the one hand, and the risk of compromising the research design through well-intended assistance, on the other. Still, some form of project investment in the community is likely to be needed in a longitudinal study, and for all but the most lavishly-funded research, this will set strict limits on the number of communities in which the project can reasonably expect to operate.

A central theme in this chapter's discussion is the need to develop multilevel analyses in which careful attention is given to the community features that have a bearing on health, such as the range and diversity of local social networks and the nature of community organizations. If only a few communities can serve as research sites, there may be too little cross-community variation to identify the effects of these features by statistical methods. Of course, other sources of variation could compensate—such as variation within communities in individual social networks or group participation, and over-time variation in certain community-level features. Moreover, the concentration of effort in a few research sites can much enhance a project's ability to provide rich qualitative descriptions of community organization and evocative illustrations of the connections between social organization and individual health. But for a multilevel analysis with a modest budget, it is at least worth asking whether a cross-sectional design involving many communities, with the features of each community being rather thinly characterized, might offer greater initial returns.

5.3. Longitudinal Research in Slums

Many factors will need to be weighed in selecting the communities to serve as study sites. There are considerations of feasibility. In some communities an unfriendly political climate or social disorganization may preclude the possibility of identifying study participants and following them over time; in other communities, the study population may be too mobile or simply too small in total to meet the research goals. (But because residential mobility is often of independent interest in multilevel theories of health, a substantial degree of mobility may have to be tolerated despite the difficulties it entails for fieldwork.) In what follows we consider more closely the rationale for focusing on the health of slum populations, where these and other factors need consideration.

We have already discussed the social and economic heterogeneity that would appear to characterize the neighborhoods of poor urban dwellers in developing countries, and have emphasized how little is known of the overlap between urban poverty and slum residence. Where it is feasible to do so, comparisons of the health of poor households residing in neighborhoods of concentrated poverty to poor households in mixed-income neighborhoods could prove highly illuminating. But fully representative research designs are not necessarily the most efficient designs for understanding the health of the poor. Despite the ambiguity and imprecision that surrounds the term "slum," and the potential payoffs from studying the poor in other types of communities, a focus on slum populations may be well justified.

Among other things, reliable health and demographic data are often lacking for these populations. Furthermore, existing census and survey data (such as provided by the DHS or by health facility data on service availability and utilization) may highlight health disparities that need closer inspection. In the case of Nairobi, for example, DHS survey data from the mid-1990s indicated that some health outcomes were decidedly worse in the slums than in rural Kenyan villages; this was a major motivating factor in the decision to situate the APHRC surveillance sites in the slums. The heterogeneities of slum populations can be exploited, at least to a degree, in choosing among slum research sites. For example, in a qualitative study of slum communities in Uttar Pradesh, India, Parker, *et al.*, (2003) chose sites to obtain variation in several dimensions: city size; the ease of access to employment and public services; the community's legal status (the key distinction being authorized versus illegal squatter settlements); and whether the community was newly settled or long established. Within some slums, smaller enclaves can be found in which residents identify with one another on the basis of ethnicity, religion, or rural village of origin (Jha, *et al.*, 2002). In what follows we summarize some of the lessons learned from recent studies of slum populations.

5.4. Identifying Slum Communities

The maps provided by government agencies do not always depict the geographic extent of slum communities with any accuracy; indeed, in some cases these maps would appear to suffer from systematic omissions. As Parker, *et al.*, (2003, p23) describe their experience in identifying slums in Uttar Pradesh,

> The most significant and serious urban disadvantages were encountered in settlements whose existence is not recognized by government. Many of these settlements are vast and have been in existence for twenty years or more. Officially, however, they do not exist and the land they occupy is identified as "vacant." Since there is officially no one there, local government is under no obligation to provide public services. Water, sewerage, electricity, schools and health facilities are therefore absent from unrecognized settlements except when they have been established by NGOs or community initiatives.

Similar problems are found in many settings. In Indore, the largest city in the Indian state of Madhya Pradesh, a careful census conducted by the research team found there to be 539 distinct slum communities, of which over 100 had gone officially unrecognized (USAID-EHP Urban Health Program, 2004b; 2004c). A similar study of Agra (USAID-EHP Urban Health Program, 2004a) uncovered about as many unregistered as registered slum communities.

If serious biases are to be avoided, such discrepancies from the official accounts must be anticipated and the boundaries of the communities of interest delineated through preparatory fieldwork. A number of useful steps are suggested in USAID-EHP Urban Health Program (2004d), the main one being to comb through all available data sources (census data and maps of enumeration areas, sample surveys, urban planning reports, other geographically-coded data) for clues on the location of communities of the urban poor. Slum residents themselves can provide useful information and help the project team to identify other slum communities not recognized in the official documents. Working together with the project team, local residents can walk the boundaries of their communities and take part in participatory mapping exercises; they can identify health problems that the researchers might have overlooked, clarify the role of local private providers, and point out health facilities situated outside community boundaries to which residents have access. Further insights can be obtained from interviews of officials charged with service delivery, such as municipal water and sewerage authorities. This phase of qualitative research is time-consuming and adds substantial up-front cost to a longitudinal research project, but without it the quantitative phases of the research are likely to founder.

5.5. Understanding Slum Dwelling Units and Households

In order to clearly demarcate household units for its surveillance system, the Nairobi pilot DSS defined households to be groups of individuals who share the same dwelling unit within a given structure. Most slum households in Nairobi occupy a one-room dwelling unit which serves as kitchen, bedroom, and sitting room, but in general, all rooms occupied by the same household within a structure were taken to constitute the residential unit for that household.

As the Nairobi team went into the field with these conventional definitions in hand, it encountered a bewildering variety of exceptions and difficult cases. It proved not uncommon for members of a single slum household to share eating arrangements while living in two distinct but adjoining (or nearby) structures. To handle such cases, in which conventionally artificial definitions of "household" would do violence to the social realities, a field was created in the project's database to allow two households in different dwelling units to be linked for the purposes of analysis.

The difficulties did not end there. To achieve an adequate accounting of who lives where in the Nairobi slums, it proved necessary to assign unique locational identifiers to rooms, which became the lowest-reaching branches in the project's elaborate classification system. Even these small units presented problems—in the clutter and confusion the fieldworkers could not always discern where one room ended and another began. The Nairobi pilot DSS was forced to further elaborate its system and assign unique identifiers to the external doors of each room. (In some cases, thankfully rare, slum residents had built their rooms without any doors, preferring to enter them from the roof or though a window, evidently to avoid being continually disturbed by their neighbors).

Rent difficulties and general flux in household membership caused the number of rooms occupied by a given household to vary considerably from one round of surveillance to the next. Housing structures themselves proved to be far from durable. In Nairobi as elsewhere, slum neighborhoods are continually roiled by waves of construction and demolition. Residents of squatter settlements face frequent destruction of their housing as a result of arson, indiscriminate damage inflicted by government security personnel in pursuit of criminals, and periodic evictions of informal settlers from public or private land designated for other uses. This chaos presents a significant challenge to prospective studies: there is no guarantee that a structure present in one survey round will still be found standing at the time of the next round. As can well be imagined, a highly sophisticated relational database is needed simply to manage demographic data with this degree of complexity.

5.6. Residential Mobility

High residential mobility rates stem from many factors common to slum living conditions, including difficulties in meeting rent payments, job loss, evictions, flooding, and the like. With such high rates of mobility, a sizeable number of residents live for only short durations in the community. Whether such short-term residents ought to be included in a longitudinal research database is not obvious. In the case of the Nairobi DSS, a three-month period of stay was taken to be the minimum spell of residence qualifying for registration in the database, but the researchers understood that substantial numbers of short-term residents would nevertheless be missed.

There is undoubtedly a great deal of variation in mobility rates according to setting and the population age group being studied. For migrant heads of household, a study of Delhi slums (Jha, *et al.*, 2002) found that the median length of residence in the slum community was 13 years, and was 18 years for length of residence in Delhi. Research on adolescents aged 10–14 years in the slums of Allahabad, India, found that from 73 to 90% of girls reported having resided in these slums since birth (Mensch, *et al.*, 2004). The Allahabad figures—which do not include moves taking place within the slums—would seem to suggest relatively low levels of mobility. Yet of the adolescents who were interviewed in a 2001 baseline survey, only about 60% could be located and re-interviewed in a follow-up survey conducted two years later. In the chaotic conditions of the Allahabad slums, even a seasoned survey team found it difficult to track initial respondents moving within the slum communities.

Access to slum respondents can present yet further problems. In the Nairobi slums, where average household sizes are low, fieldworkers arriving for an interview often find no adult present to be interviewed (according to data from the Nairobi pilot DSS, one-third of households contain only one adult, the average number of persons per household being 2.9 for all households and 3.8 for households with at least two persons). The fieldworkers must then rely on the help of neighbors to arrange to revisit the household late at night, very early in the morning, or on weekends. If the interviewer teams had not been drawn from the same slum communities, the costs of all this could well have been prohibitive. In the Nairobi case, the logistical savings achieved by enlisting community members as interviewers outweighed the risks to respondent privacy and confidentiality.

Some of the difficulties inherent in urban longitudinal research are much magnified in studies of slum populations. For example, in the course of its work in the Nairobi slums, the APHRC team faced overwhelming demands from the communities to improve their social and health facilities. Many research groups and NGOs may be operating projects and providing services in the slums, and the residents can feel somewhat under siege from multiple requests for interviews, which contribute to respondent fatigue. Moreover, with multiple interventions underway it can be difficult for a given research project to isolate the connections of greatest interest to it (the "attribution problem"). In addition, some of the social risks facing slum residents can afflict the research team. Slum crime rates are often high and, like the residents, research staff run the risk of being victimized. (This has happened more than once to APHRC fieldworkers in Nairobi; also see Verner and Alda (2004) on the problems posed by gang violence to fieldwork in the slums of Fortalenza, Brazil. In settings such as these, gang leaders are among the local "influentials" whose permission the research team may need to obtain to carry out its work.)

6.0. CONCLUSION

This chapter has reviewed the core concepts of urban multilevel health research and the empirical tools that have been used, mainly in North America and Europe, to shed light on the concepts. When these tools are finally brought to bear on the cities of poor countries, we expect they will unearth many similarities in behavior in rich and poor countries, but also many differences, each having the potential to enrich understanding of urban life and health. Several dimensions of comparison warrant consideration: the situations of large and small cities; the conditions of the urban poor relative to the nonpoor and rural residents; and among the urban poor, the circumstances of those who are spatially concentrated in slums and those who live in more heterogeneous communities.

If progress is to be made in understanding the demographic implications of spatial segregation, urban social networks, social capital, and the like, longitudinal research designs will eventually be needed. We would urge that much more attention be paid to the health implications of neighborhood social and economic composition, as reflected in the percentages of local residents who are educated, for example (Coleman, 1988; Kaufman, *et al.*, 2002; Kravdal, 2003). Theories of urban social and environmental interaction and externalities (Panel on Urban Population Dynamics, 2003) indicate a need for the collection of social network and spatial data that lie well outside the scope of current survey program, and that will require new sorts of surveys to be fielded in the cities of developing countries. There is much could be learned, we believe, through application to these cities of the conceptual and measurement tools now being applied to poor urban communities in the West.

REFERENCES

Åberg Yngwe, M., Fritzell, J., Lundberg, O., Diderichsen, F., and Burström, B. (2003). Exploring relative deprivation: Is social comparison a mechanism in the relation between income and health? *Soc. Sci. Med.* 57(8):1463–1473.

African Population and Health Research Center. (2002). *Population and Health Dynamics in Nairobi's Informal Settlements: Report of the Nairobi Cross-Sectional Slums Survey (NCSS) 2000.* African Population and Health Research Center: Nairobi.

Agyeman, D. K., and Casterline, J. B. (2003). Social organization and reproductive behavior in southern Ghana. In: Agyei-Mensah, S., and Casterline J.B. (eds). *Reproduction and Social Context in Sub-Saharan Africa*, Greenwood Press, Greenwich, CT.

Altschuler, A., Omkin, C. P., and Adler, N. E. (2004). Local services and amenities, neighborhood social capital, and health, *Soc. Sci. Med.* 59(6):1219–1229.

Amis, P. (2003). Chronic poverty in India: Lessons from recent research, School of Public Policy, University of Birmingham, UK. Paper presented at the conference *Staying Poor: Chronic Poverty and Development Policy*, University of Manchester, UK, 7-9 April 2003 (September 23, 2004); http://idpm.man.ac.uk/cprc/Conference/conferencepapers /PhilAmis.pdf

Amis, P., and Kumar, S. (2000). Urban economic growth, infrastructure and poverty in India: Lessons from Visakhapatnam. *Environ. Urban.* 12(1):185–197.

Appadurai, A. (2001). Deep democracy: Urban governmentality and the horizon of politics. *Environ. Urban.* 13(2):23–43.

Baltagi, B. H. (1995). *Econometric Analysis of Panel Data.* John Wiley and Sons, Chichester, England.

Barua, N., and Singh, S., 2003, Representation for the marginalized—Linking the poor and the health care system. Lessons from case studies in urban India, Draft paper, World Bank, New Delhi. Power point presentation, (September 23, 2004); http://www.worldbank.org/urban/symposium 2003/docs/presentations/barua.pdf

Baulch, B., and Hoddinott, J. (2000). Economic mobility and poverty dynamics in developing countries. *J. Devel. Stud.* 36(6):1–4.

Beckett, M., DaVanzo, J., Sastry, N., Panis, C., and Peterson, C. (2001). The quality of retrospective data: An examination of long-term recall in a developing country. *J. Hum. Resour.* 36(3):593–625.

Behrman, J., Kohler, H. P., and Watkins, S. (2001). Social networks, family planning, and worrying about AIDS, Paper presented at the March, 2001*Annual Meetings of the Population Association of America*, Washington, DC.

Bigsten, A., Kebede, B., Shimeles, A., and Taddesse, M. (2003). Growth and poverty reduction in Ethiopia: Evidence from household panel surveys. *World Development* 31(1):87–106.

Blakely, T. A., Lochner, K., and Kawachi, I. (2002). Metropolitan area income inequality and self-rated health—A multi-level study. *Soc. Sci. Med.* 54:65–67.

Blomgren, J., Martikainen, P., Mäkelä, P., and Valkonen, T. (2004). The effects of regional characteristics on alcohol-related mortality–A register-based multilevel analysis of 1.1 million men, *Soc. Sci. Med.* 58:2523–2535.

Boardman, J. D. (2004). Stress and physical health: The role of neighborhoods as mediating and moderating mechanisms. *Soc. Sci. Med.* 58:2473–2483.

Bossart, R. (2003). 'In the city, everybody only cares for himself': Social relations and illness in Abidjan, Côte d'Ivoire. *Anthropology & Medicine* 10(3):343–359.

Boyle, P., Norman, P., and Rees, P. (2004). Changing places. Do changes in the relative deprivation of areas influence limiting long-term illness and mortality among non-migrant people living in non-deprived households? *Soc. Sci. Med.* 58:2459–2471.

Burra, S., Patel, S., and Kerr, T. (2003). Community-designed, built and managed toilet blocks in Indian cities. *Environ. Urban.* 15(2):11–22.

Caldeira, T. P. R. (1999). Fortified enclaves: The new urban segregation, In: Holston J. (ed.). *Cities and Citizenship*, Duke University Press, Durham and London, pp. 114–138.

Caldeira, T. P. R. (2000). *City of Walls: Crime, Segregation, and Citizenship in São Paulo*, University of California Press, Berkeley, CA.

CARE/Tanzania, 1998, Dar-es-Salaam, Tanzania, (September23, 2004); http://www.ifpri.org/themes/mp14/profiles/daressalaam.pdf.

Carletto, G., and Zezza, A., Agricultural and Development Economics Division, Economic and Social Department, the Food and Agriculture Organization, 2004, Italy (September 23, 2004); http://www.fao.org/es/esa/pdf/wp/ESAWP04_12.pdf

Casterline, J. B. (ed.). (2001). *Diffusion Processes and Fertility Transition: Selected Perspectives*, National Academies Press, Washington, DC.

Casterline, J. B., Montgomery, M. R., Agyeman, D. K., Aglobitse, P., and Kiros, G.-E. (2001). Social networks and contraceptive dynamics in southern Ghana. Paper presented at the March 2001 *Annual Meetings of the Population Association of America*, Washington, DC.

Coady, D., Grosh, M., and Hoddinott, J. (2004). Targeting outcomes redux, *World Bank Research Observer* 19(1):61–65.

Coleman, J. S. (1988). Social capital in the creation of human capital, *Am. J. Soc.* 94(supplement): S95–120.

Coulton, C., Korbin, J., Chan, T., and Su, M. (1997). *Mapping residents' perceptions of neighborhood boundaries: A methodological note, Working Paper.* Center on Urban Poverty and Social Change at Case Western Reserve University, Cleveland, OH.

Curtis, S., Southall, H., Congdon, P., and Dodgeon, B. (2004). Area effects on health variation over the life-course: Analysis of the longitudinal study sample in England using new data on area of residence in childhood. *Soc. Sci. Med.* 58:57–54.

de Wit, J. W. (2002). Urban poverty alleviation in Bangalore, *Econ. Polit. Wkly.* 21:3935–3942.

Diez Roux, A. V., Stein Merkin, S., Hannan, P., Jacobs, D. R., and Kiefe, C. I. (2003). Area characteristics, individual-level socioeconomic indicators, and smoking in young adults. *Am. J. Epi.* 157(4):315–326.

Drukker, M., Kaplan, C., Feron, F., and van Os, J. (2003). Children's health-related quality of life, neighbourhood socio-economic deprivation and social capital. A contextual analysis, *Soc. Sci. Med.* 57(5):825–841.

Duckitt, J., and Mphuthing, T. (2002). Relative deprivation and intergroup attitudes: South Africa before and after the transition. In: Walker, I., and Smith, J.H. (eds). *Relative Deprivation: Specification, Development, and Integration*, Cambridge University Press, Cambridge, UK.

Durlauf, S. N. (2000a). A framework for the study of individual behavior and social interactions. Department of Economics, University of Wisconsin at Madison.

Durlauf, S. N. (2000b). *The memberships theory of poverty: The role of group affiliations in determining socioeconomic outcomes.* Department of Economics, University of Wisconsin at Madison.

Falkingham, J., and Namazie, C. (2002). *Measuring health and poverty: A review of approaches to identifying the poor.* DFID Health Systems Resource Center, London.

Fenn, B., Morris, S. S., and Frost, C. (2004). *Do childhood growth indicators in developing countries cluster? Implications for intervention strategies.* Department of Epidemiology and Population Health at the London School of Hygiene and Tropical Medicine, London.

Field, E. (2003). Property rights and household time allocation in urban squatter communities: Evidence from Peru, Economics Department, Harvard University. Paper presented at *2003 Urban Research Symposium.* World Bank, Washington DC.15-17 December 2003.

Filmer, D., and Pritchett, L. (1999). The effect of household wealth on educational attainment: Evidence from 35 countries. *Pop. Devel. Rev.* 25(1):85–120.

Filmer, D., and Pritchett, L. (2001). Estimating wealth effects without expenditure data—or tears: An application to educational enrollments in states of India. *Demography* 38(1):115–132.

Freedman, R., and Takeshita, J. Y. (1969). *Family Planning in Taiwan: An Experiment in Social Change.* Princeton University Press, Princeton, NJ.

Friedman, S. R., and Aral, S. (2001). Social networks, risk-potential networks, health, and disease. *J. Urban Health* 78(3):411–418.

Gerdtham, U.-G., and Johannesson, M. (2004). Absolute income, relative income, income inequality, and mortality. *J. Hum.Res.* 39(1):228–247.

Gilson, L. (2003). Trust and the development of health care as a social institution, *Soc. Sci. Med.* 56(7):1453–1468.

Ginther, D., Haveman, R., and Wolfe, B. (2000). Neighborhood attributes as determinants of children's outcomes: How robust are the relationships? *J. Hum. Res.* 35(4):603–633.

Grootaert, C., Narayan, D., Nyhan Jones, V., and Woolcock, M. (2004). Measuring social capital: An integrated questionnaire, World Bank Working Paper No. 18. World Bank, Washington, DC.

Grosh, M., and Glewwe, P. (1996). A guide to Living Standards Surveys and their data sets, LSMS Working Paper no. 120, Washington, DC: World Bank.

Hardman, A., and Ioannides, Y. M. (2004). Income mixing and housing in U.S. cities: Evidence from neighborhood clusters of the American Housing Survey, Working paper. Department of Economics, Tufts University.

Harpham, T., and Tanner, M. (eds). (1995). *Urban Health in Developing Countries: Progress and Prospects,* St. Martin's Press, New York.

Harpham, T., Grant, E., and Rodriguez, C. (2004). Mental health and social capital in Cali, Colombia, *Soc. Sci. Med.* 58:2267–2277.

Harpham, T., Grant, E., and Thomas, E. (2002). Measuring social capital within health surveys: Key issues, *Health Policy Plan.* 17(1):106–111.

Hausman, J. (1978). Specification tests in econometrics. *Econometrica* 46:1251–1271.

Henninger, N., and Snel, M. (2002). *Where Are the Poor? Experiences with the Development and Use of Poverty Maps.* World Resources Institute, Washington DC, and UNEP/GRID-Arendal, Arendal, Norway.

Henry-Lee, A. (2003) Chronic poverty in the urban ghettos in Jamaica, Sir Arthur Lewis Institute of Social and Economic Studies, University of the West Indies. Paper presented at the conference *Staying Poor: Chronic Poverty and Development Policy*, University of Manchester, UK, 6-9 April 2003.

Herra, J., and Roubaud, F. (2003). Urban poverty dynamics in Peru and Madagascar 1997–1999: A panel data analysis, IRD-INEI, Peru. Paper presented at the conference *Staying Poor: Chronic Poverty and Development Policy,* University of Manchester, UK, 7-9 April 2003.

Hewett, P. C., and Montgomery, M. R. (2001). Poverty and public services in developing-country cities, Policy Research Division Working Paper No. 154. Population Council, New York.

Hill, D. H., and Willis, R. J. (2001). Reducing panel attrition: A search for effective policy instruments, *J. Hum. Res.* 36(3):416–438.

Janzen, J. M. (1978). *The Quest for Therapy in Lower Zaire.* University of California Press, Berkeley, CA.

Jha, S., Rao, V., and Woolcock, M. (2002). Governance in the gullies: Political networks, leadership, and the delivery of basic services to Delhi's urban poor, Work in progress, World Bank, Washington DC.

Kaufman, C. E., Clark, S., Manzini, N., and May, J. (2002). How community structures of time and opportunity shape adolescent sexual behavior in South Africa, Policy Research Division Working Paper No. 159. Population Council, New York, NY.

Kawachi, I., and Berkman, L. F. (2001). Social ties and mental health. *J. Urban Health* 78(3):458–467.

Kawachi, I., Kennedy, B. P., and Glass, R. (1999). Social capital and self-rated health: A contextual analysis. *Am. J. Public Health* 89(8):1187–1193.

Kedir, A. M., and McKay, A. (2003). Chronic poverty in urban Ethiopia: Panel data evidence, Department of Economics, University of Leicester. Paper presented at the conference *Staying Poor: Chronic Poverty and Development Policy.* University of Manchester, UK, 7-9 April 2004 (September 23, 2004); http://idpm.man.ac.uk/cprc/Conference/conferencepapers/kedir&mckay.pdf

Kravdal, Ø. (2003). Community mortality in India: Individual and community effects of women's education and autonomy, East-West Center Working Papers, Population Series, No. 112. East-West Center, Honolulu, HI.

Krieger, N., Chen, J. T., Waterman, P. D., Soobader, M.-J., Subramanian, S. V., and Carson, R. (2002). Geocoding and monitoring of US socioeconomic inequalities in mortality and cancer incidence: Does the choice of area-based measure and geographic level matter? *Am. J. Epidemiology* 156(5):471–2002.

Lalita, K. (2003). Urban chronic poverty in Vijayawada: Insights from household profiles over time, Department of Economics, University of Leicester. Paper presented at the conference *Staying Poor: Chronic Poverty and Development Policy.* University of Manchester, UK, 7-9 April 2004 (September 23, 2004); http://idpm.man.ac.uk/cprc/Conference/conferencepapers/lalitakay.pdf.

Lanjouw, P., Mistiaen, J., and Ozler, B. (2002). Poverty mapping: Methods and experience in urban areas, Presentation to Urban Poverty TG, World Bank, Washington DC.

Lin, N. (1999) Building a network theory of social capital. *Connections* 22(1):28–31.

Lokshin, M., Umapathi, N., and Paternostro, S. (2004). Robustness of subjective welfare analysis in a poor developing country: Madagascar 2001, World Bank Policy Research Working Paper. World Bank, Washington DC.

Maluccio, J., Haddad, L., and May, J. (2000). Social capital and household welfare in South Africa, 1993–98, *J. Dev. Stud.* 36(6):54–61.

Manski, C. F. (2000). Economic analysis of social interactions. *J. Econ. Persp.* 14(3):115–136.

Massey, D. S. (1990). American apartheid: Segregation and the making of the underclass. *Am. J. Soc.* 96(2):329–357.

McCulloch, A. (2003). An examination of social capital and social disorganization in neighborhoods in the British household panel study. *Soc. Sci. Med.* 56(7):1425–1438.

Mensch, B. S., Grant, M., Sebastian, M., Hewett, P., and Huntington, D. (2004). The effect of a livelihoods intervention in an urban slum in India: Does vocational counseling and training alter the attitudes and behavior of adolescent girls? Paper presented at the *2004 Annual Meetings of the Population Association of America,* Boston, MA, 1-3 April 2004.

Mitlin, D. (2003). The economic and social processes influencing the level and nature of chronic poverty in urban areas, Paper presented at the conference *Staying Poor: Chronic Poverty and Development Policy.* University of Manchester, UK, 7-9 April 2003 (September 23, 2004); http://idpm.man.ac.uk/cprc/Conference/conferencepapers/Mitlin%20Diana%2011.03.03.pdf.

Montgomery, M. R., and Hewett, P. C. (2004). Urban poverty and health in developing countries: Household and neighborhood effects, Policy Research Division Working Paper No. 184. Population Council, New York, NY.

Montgomery, M. R., Gragnolati, M., Burke, K. A., and Paredes, E. (2000). Measuring living standards with proxy variables. *Demography* 37(2):155–174.

Morris, M. (1993). Epidemiology and social networks: Modeling structured diffusion. *Sociolog. Methods Res.* 22(1):99–126.

Morris, S., Carletto, C., Hoddinott, J., and Christiaensen, L. J. M. (1999). Validity of rapid estimates of household wealth and income for health surveys in rural Africa, Food Consumption and Nutrition Division Discussion Paper No. 72. International Food Policy Research Institute (IFPRI), Washington, DC.

Moser, C. O. N. (1996). Confronting crisis: A summary of household responses to poverty and vulnerability in four poor urban communities. *Environmentally Sustainable Development Studies and Monographs Series 7.* The World Bank, Washington, DC.

Oakes, J. M. (2004a). The (mis)estimation of neighborhood effects: Causal inference for a practicable social epidemiology, *Soc. Sci. Med.* 58:1929–1952.

Oakes, J. M. (2004b). Rejoinder. Causal inference and the relevance of social epidemiology. *Soc. Sci. Med.* 58:1969–1971.

Obrist, B. (2003). Urban health in daily practice: Livelihood, vulnerability and resilience in Dares Salaam, Tanzania. *Anthropology & Medicine.* 10(3):275–290.

Obrist, B. Tanner, M., and Harpham, T. (2003a). Engaging anthropology in urban health research: Issues and prospects. *Anthropology & Medicine* 10(3):361–371.

Obrist, B., van Eeuwijk, P., and Weiss, M. G. (2003b). Health anthropology and urban health research. *Anthropology & Medicine.* 10(3):267–274.

Panel on Urban Population Dynamics (2003). In: Montgomery, M. R., Stren, R., Cohen, B., and Reed, H., (eds.). *Cities Transformed: Demographic Change and Its Implications in the Developing World,* National Academies Press, Washington, DC.

Parker, B., Kozel, V., and Kukreja, M. (2003). In search of a chance: Urban opportunities, poverty and vulnerability in Uttar Pradesh, India, Paper presented at *World Bank Urban Research Symposium.* 9-11 December 2002.

Parnell, S., and Mosdell, T. (2003). Recognizing, explaining and measuring chronic urban poverty in South Africa, University of Cape Town, South Africa. Paper presented at the conference *Staying Poor: Chronic Poverty and Development Policy.* University of Manchester, UK, 7-9 April 2004 (September 23, 2004); http://idpm.man.ac.uk/cprc/Conference/conferencepapers/parnellsuechronicpovertysouthafrica%2016.03.pdf.

Pebley, A. R., and Sastry, N. (2003). Concentrated poverty vs. concentrated affluence: Effects on neighborhood social environments and children's outcomes, Paper presented at the *2003 Annual Meetings of the Population Association of America,* Minneapolis, MN, 1–3 May 2003.

Pictet, G., Kouanda, S., Sirima, S., and Pond, R. (2004). Struggling with population heterogeneity in African cities: The urban health and equity puzzle. Paper presented to the *2004 annual meetings of the Population Association of America,* Boston MA, 1-3 April 2004.

Pierret, C. R. (2001). Event history data and survey recall: An analysis of the National Longitudinal Survey of Youth 1979 recall experiment. *J. Hum. Res.* 36(3):439–466.

Pradhan, M. (2000). How many questions should be included in a consumption questionnaire? Evidence from a repeated experiment in Indonesia, Cornell Food and Nutrition Program Working Paper No. 112. Cornell University, Ithaca, NY.

Pradhan, M., and Ravallion, M. (2000). Measuring poverty using qualitative perceptions of consumption adequacy. *Rev. Econ. Stat.* 82(3):462–471.

Pryer, J., Rogers, S., and Rahman, A. (2003). Work, disabling illness, and coping strategies in Dhaka slums, Bangladesh, Royal Free and University Medical School, University College London. Paper presented at the conference *Staying Poor: Chronic Poverty and Development Policy.* University of Manchester, UK, 7-9 April 2003 (September 23, 2004); http://idpm.man.ac.uk/cprc/Conference/conferencepapers /Pryer%20Jane%20Workdisab28.02.03.pdf

Putnam, R. (2000). *Bowling Alone: The Collapse and Revival of American Community.* Simon and Schuster: New York, NY.

Ravallion, M., and Lokshin, M. (2002). Self-rated economic welfare in Russia, *Eur. Econ. Rev.* 46:1453–1473.

Sahn, D. E., and Stifel, D. (2001). Exploring alternative measures of welfare in the absence of expenditure data. Department of Economics, Cornell University, New York, NY.

Sahn, D. E., and Stifel, D. C. (2000). Poverty comparisons over time and across countries in Africa. *World Development* 28(12):2123–2155.

Sampson, R. J., and Morenoff, J. D. (2000). Public health and safety in context: Lessons from community-level theory on social capital. In: Smedley B. D., and Syme. S. L. (eds.). *Promoting Health: Intervention Strategies from Social and Behavioral Research.* National Academy Press, Washington, DC, pp. 366–390.

Sampson, R. J., Morenoff, J. D., and Gannon-Rowley, T. (2002). Assessing 'neighborhood effects': Social processes and new directions in research. *An. Rev. Soc.* 28:443–478.

Sastry, N. (1996). Community characteristics, individual and household attributes, and child survival in Brazil. *Demography* 33(2):211–229.

Sastry, N., Pebley, A., and Zonta, M. (2002). Neighborhood definitions and the spatial dimension of daily life in Los Angeles, Paper presented at the *2002 Annual Meetings of the Population Association of America, Atlanta, GA,* 9–11 May.

Satterthwaite, D. (2004). The under-estimation of urban poverty in low- and middle-income nations, Working Paper No. 14. Poverty Reduction in Urban Areas Series, International Institute for Environment and Development (IIED), London.

Schmertmann, C. (1994). Selectivity bias correction methods in polychotomous sample selection models. *J. Econ.* 60:101–132.

Smith, H. J., and Ortiz, D. J. (2002). Is it just me? The different consequences of personal and group relative deprivation. In: Walker, I., and Smith H.J. (eds). *Relative Deprivation: Specification, Development, and Integration.* Cambridge University Press, Cambridge, UK.

Snow, J. (1855). *On the Mode of Communication of Cholera.* John Churchill, London.

Stevens, L. (2003). Chronic poverty in urban informal settlements in South Africa: Combining quantitative and qualitative data to monitor the impact of interventions, Intermediate Technology Development Group, Warwickshire, UK. Paper presented at the conference *Staying Poor: Chronic Poverty and Development Policy.* University of Manchester, UK, 7-9 April 2003. (September 23, 2004); http://idpm.man.ac.uk/cprc/Conference/conferencepapers /Stevens%20Lucy%2005.03.03.PDF

Swaroop, S., and Morenoff, J. D. (2004). Building community: The neighborhood context of local social organization. Population Studies Center Research Report No. 04-549. University of Michigan.

Szwarcwald, C. L., de Andrade, C. L. T., and Bastos, F. I. (2002). Income inequality, residential poverty clustering and infant mortality: A study in Rio de Janeiro, Brazil, *Soc. Sci. Med.* 55(12): 2083–2092.

Thomas, D., and Frankenberg, E. (2001). Lost but not forgotten: Attrition and follow-up in the Indonesian Family Life Survey. *J. Hum. Res.* 36(3):556–592.

Timæus, I. M., and Lush, L. (1995). Intra-urban differentials in child health. *Health Trans. Rev.* 5(2):163–190.

Tyler, T. R. and Lind, E. A. (2002). Understanding the nature of fraternalistic deprivation. Does group-based deprivation involve fair outcomes or fair treatment? In: Walker, I., and Smith H.J. (eds). *Relative Deprivation: Specification, Development, and Integration.* Cambridge University Press, Cambridge, UK.

UN-Habitat, 2003. (2003). *The Challenge of Slums: Global Report on Human Settlements 2003.* Earthscan, London.

USAID-EHP Urban Health Program. (2004a). Agra urban health program: A situation analysis, Presentation to ANE Urban Health Workshop, Agra, India. USAID/India Environmental Health Project, New Delhi.

USAID-EHP Urban Health Program. (2004b). Conducting child health survey in urban slums: Methodology, challenges and lessons learnt, Presentation to ANE Urban Health Workshop, Agra, India. USAID/India Environmental Health Project, New Delhi.

USAID-EHP Urban Health Program. (2004c). Health scenario among urban poor in Madhya Pradesh, Draft paper prepared for ANE Urban Health Workshop, Agra, India. USAID/India Environmental Health Project, New Delhi.

USAID-EHP Urban Health Program. (2004d). Improving the health of the urban poor: Learning from USAID experience, Draft paper prepared for ANE Bureau.

van den Eeden, P., and Hüttner, H. J. M. (1982). Multi-level research. *Current Sociology* 30(3), 1–182.

Veenstra, G. (2002). Social capital and health (plus wealth, income inequality and regional health governance). *Soc. Sci. Med.* 54, 849–868.

Verner, D. and Alda, E. (2004). Youth at risk, social exclusion, and intergenerational poverty dynamics: A new survey instrument with application to Brazil, World Bank Policy Research Working Paper 3296. World Bank, Washington D.C.

Walker, I. and Smith, H. J. (eds.). 2002, *Relative Deprivation: Specification, Development, and Integration,* Cambridge University Press, Cambridge, UK.

Wellman, B. and Leighton, B. (1979). Networks, neighborhoods, and communities: Approaches to the study of the community question. *Uran. Aff. Q.* 14(3):363–390.

Wen, M., Browning, C. R., and Cagney, K. A. (2003). Poverty, affluence, and income inequality: Neighborhood economic structure and its implications for health, *Soc. Sci. Med.* 57(5):843–860.

White, M. J. (1987). *American Neighborhoods and Residential Differentiation.* Russell Sage, New York.

White, M. J. (2001). Residential concentration/segregation, demographic effects of. In: Smelser , N. J., and Baltes, P.B. (eds.). *International Encyclopedia of the Social and Behavioral Sciences,* Vol. 19. Elsevier Science, Oxford, pp. 13250–13254.

Wilkinson, R. G. (1996). *Unhealthy Societies: The Afflictions of Inequality.* Routledge, London.

Wilson, W. J. (1987). *The Truly Disadvantaged: The Inner City, the Underclass and Public Policy.* University of Chicago Press, Chicago, IL.

Woolard, I., and Klasen, S. (2003). Income mobility and household dynamics in South Africa, Human Sciences Research Council, South Africa. Paper presented at the conference *Staying Poor: Chronic Poverty and Development Policy.* University of Manchester, UK, 7-9 April 2002. (September 23, 2004); http://idpm.man.ac.uk/cprc/Conference/conferencepapers /woolard&klasen08.01.pdf

World Bank. (2002). *Cali, Colombia: Toward a City Development Strategy.* World Bank, Washington, DC.

Wright, S. C., and Tropp, L. R. (2002). Collective action in response to disadvantage. Intergroup perceptions, social identification, and social change. In: Walker, I. and Smith H.J. (eds.). *Relative Deprivation: Specification, Development, and Integration,* Cambridge University Press, Cambridge, UK.

Zeller, M. (2004). Review of poverty assessment tools. IRIS Center, University of Maryland, College Park, MD.

Chapter 18

Urban Sociology and Research Methods on Neighborhoods and Health

Joseph A. Soares

1.0. INTRODUCTION

Urban sociologists are very engaged with questions about health. We are more mindful now than ever before that we all live in social landscapes of particular places that have their own power to shelter or harm us. Cities are, as the title of a recent article on urban health puts it, "mosaics of risk and protection" (Fitzpatrick and LaGory, 2003).

Our inquiries on the problem gathered momentum in the 1980s, and then took off in the 1990s. Research questions, methods, and findings flowed together from a wide variety of sources: from work on the impact of social capital on the welfare of communities (Putnam, 1993) and children (Elliot, *et al.*, 1996), from the perception and experience of new "species of trouble" (Erikson, 1994) traumatizing entire communities, from organizational sociologists' attempts to explain the urban patterns of corporate pollution (Grant and Jones, 2003), from the rise of the environmental justice movement (EJM), (Foreman, 1998), a fight to eradicate the racial and social-class penalties of toxic waste in urban areas (Camcho, 1998), from the efforts of urban historical sociologists to understand the "power of place" (Sennett, 1993; Hayden, 1997), from the attempts of business-studies scholars to explain why, in the post-industrial age of internet globalization, geography still matters (Florida, 2002), and even from the study of neighborhoods as sites of consumption by sociologists who pioneered the use of zip code cluster profiles for direct marketing (Weiss, 1988). Those authors and more gave rise to exciting intellectual developments the most promising of which involve the convergence of three factors: substantive questions about health, the exploration of health questions through urban ethnographic and statistical research methods, including multi-level models and geographic information systems, and the effort to use theoretically nuanced models of mechanisms to establish the causal links between the social environment and our health.

If there is a core analytic framework common to those working in this new direction, it is the importance of "neighborhood effects"* (Sampson, *et al.*, 2002). The intellectual move was from a medical-sociological model that prioritized individual-level characteristics, to an urban-sociological model that emphasized community-level effects. To questions about how one's health was influenced by "what one is," were added questions about the effects of "where one lives." Medical sociologists conventionally thought about the "what one is" question in terms of demographic stratification. The idea was to measure the effects of individual attributes, such as income, education, occupation, ethnicity, gender, and age on the individual's health. Then, building on the medical model, urban sociologists began to explore the "where" question with reference to neighborhood or community-level characteristics that have a weight and impact all their own on the individual's as well as the public's health.

Medical sociologists gave us many robust findings on the "what" question. The hypothesis that one's bank account affects one's health, for example, has been abundantly verified. There are few correlations in the field stronger than the link between income and mortality. The association holds up historically and comparatively; the power of money keeps one alive regardless of time period or society (Wilkinson, 1992). The income-mortality correlation is not the only sociological generalization with broad, if not universal, validity – social status works the same way. Separate from income or wealth, people in prestigious positions have better health than those below them (Marmot, 2004). Although prestige rankings lack the obvious physicality and direct resource mobilizing power of money, their effects are just as real and just as quantifiable. Prestige rankings of occupations are a reliable source of demographic information available to health researchers (for an updated rank order see: Nakao and Treas, 1994).

On the "where" question, urban sociologists are now able to demonstrate that neighborhood-level characteristics are important in shaping health patterns. For example, features of one's community, such as its relative number of civic associations, can determine how much pollution there is in the local environment (Grant, *et al.*, 2004; Wakefield, *et al.*, 2001). Even whether or not one lives in a tightly knit community, with dense social ties, matters to the mortality rate of one's locale. Witness Roseto, Pennsylvania, where an Italian-American community for nearly fifty years enjoyed better health than neighboring areas; until it too suffered the effects of declining social ties (Egolf, *et al.*, 1992).

To provide an overview of the sociology of urban health, this chapter will briefly look at the history of the field and the role racial issues played in giving rise to our current focus on neighborhood effects. Then we will discuss the difficulties of doing empirical research on the social and physical environments that affect the health of individuals. It is not easy to distinguish the effects of areas from the attributes of the people who live there. Does a disadvantaged family carry the same burden regardless of location, or does it face additional hurdles if it resides in a disadvantaged community? And how does one measure community disadvantage? The role of particular statistical techniques, mixed or multi-level models, in resolving the neighborhood-effects conundrum will be reviewed. And the importance of researchers knowing how to draw the relevant boundaries of communities, and how to specify the causal pathways between neighborhood characteristics and individuals' health, will be explored in some detail. We will see how the field's most fruitful

*Although some social epidemiologists refer to the move as "ecological" (MacIntyre and Elaaway, 2000), sociologists more commonly use the "neighborhood" trope.

concept, the notion of "social capital" as the resources provided by networks and mutual trust, is used to explain the ties that buffer individuals from harm. In conclusion, we can see that the foundations for the sociology of urban health are well established, but we have some distance to go before our stock of analytical tools and empirical findings rivals those of allied sciences.

2.0. PRECURSORS

The notion that urban life is a source of risk both physical and social has a long history to it (Boyer, 1978). Early examples include W.E.B. Du Bois' 1896 study, *Philadelphia Negro,* which discussed the bad sanitary conditions and death rate in the Seventh Ward (1978). One year later, Emile Durkheim (1951) published the discovery that suicide rates vary in relation to the density and intensity of group ties, as well as between urban and rural areas. And in 1903, Georg Simmel (1997) wrote an essay on the blasé mentality of metropolitan life which over stimulates the nerves and causes an "incapacity . . . to react to new sensations with the appropriate energy".

The premier department of American sociology at the University of Chicago (Park and Burgess, 1967) in its early years focused almost entirely on urban ecology and its social pathologies (Michelson, 1976), which sometimes included references to health issues (Catalano, 1989). The ecological model drew attention to the spatial positioning of different social and ethnic groups in the interconnected social system of the city. New immigrant groups would move from the center to the periphery of the city, as they went in time from poverty to affluence, from group conflict to accommodation to assimilation with the mainstream.

The concentrations of particular groups in certain urban zones lent itself to some of the worst social engineering in the nation's history. Many city leaders drew the simplistic conclusion from urban sociology that "if reformers could only wipe out slums physically, then they would wipe out the social and health problems of the people living there" (Michelson, 1976). From approximately 1949 to 1966, politicians and city planners embraced a form of physical determinism, seeing urban problems as the result of inferior buildings and substandard neighborhoods. Poor black families, for example, would do much better, their children would have fewer colds and their school records would improve, drug use, crime, and mortality rates would go down, if only they could be resettled from private and overcrowded urban dwellings into the vertical grids of sanitary pubic housing (Michelson, 1976). The implementation of "urban renewal" policies destroyed hundreds of poor neighborhoods. Some of those areas were ethnic and working class, such as Boston's Italian West End (Gans, 1962) and Irish neighborhoods in New York's Bronx, but most of them were black. Of the approximately three million Americans forcibly displaced when their homes were declared slums and legally seized by the government, 63% were racial minorities. We know that the forced evacuation did not heal urban America. It did, however, ironically contribute to black urban rebellions in the late 1960s, and cause new health problems, including what was diagnosed as a "grief syndrome" for one's lost home (Michelson, 1976).*

*For a visual record of the history of three urban renewal projects, see my web site, "The Social Life of Cities." http://www.wfu.edu/academics/sociology/sociallifeofcities/urban/urban.html. And for a recent work on the connections between a people and an area, see: Mindy Thompson Fullilove, *The House of Joshua: meditations on family and place,* 1999.

Urban-renewal social engineering in America with its emphasis on social and physical hygiene was unsurpassed for destructiveness. Of analogous historical cases, neither Haussmann's Paris nor or Mussolini's Italy (Kostof, 1994) tore down a relative or absolute number of housing units comparable to New York City. Many scholars attribute the excesses of our public policy on urban areas to the unresolved dilemma of race in the U.S.; the legacy of slavery, Jim Crow apartheid, and racial violence is blamed for our public policy blunders. The blinders were worn by sociologists as well as politicians. Despite one of the Chicago School's founders, Robert Park's, personal commitment to racial equality, the "color line" was the greatest analytic weakness of urban ecology. Park's ecological succession and assimilation model did not fit the experience of black Americans.

The Chicago School was given an intellectual opportunity to address the issue of race, to make what William Julius Wilson calls a "fundamental revision" (Wilson, 1993) of its model, through the efforts of two black sociologists, St. Clair Drake and Horace Cayton (1993). Their comprehensive ethnography of Chicago's black community (1993), published in 1945, exposed the limits of the ecological view on racial matters. Among many injustices, they documented health disparities, measured as infant mortality, death rates, TB, and syphilis rates, between white Chicago and five black neighborhoods, each one defined by geography and social class (Drake and Cayton, 1993).

3.0. NEW DEPARTURES

Drake and Cayton's (1993) research did not immediately reorient urban sociology, but in time it did lead to new departures. Their legacy was picked up and carried forward by others including, most prominently, Elijah Anderson (1978; 1990) and William Julius Wilson (1987; 1996). Anderson spent years doing field work, observing life in bars, shops, and street corners in the most troubled areas of the black community. His vivid ethnographies of black urban life are compelling sociological descriptions of the "codes of the street," the cultural logic of black male self-presentation to negotiate urban zones of potential violence. The clothes, the jewelry, the tattoos, body language and verbal idiomatic sparring are all ways of signifying to others that one is an inside player, capable of taking care of business, by physically defending oneself or inflicting violence on another. Paradoxically, the code enables black men to avoid random physical violence through its ubiquitous symbolic projection. While Anderson's work gets inside the mindset of being on the block, Wilson's work provides the most rigorous empirical account available of the forces that structure life on the block. His research methods and findings have inspired many to join the effort. As the National Research Council and Institute of Medicine's text, *From Neurons to Neighborhoods* puts it, Wilson, "galvanized empirical research on community and neighborhood effects with his description and analysis of conditions in high-poverty, inner-city Chicago" (Shonkoff and Phillips, 2000). Ethnographers and urban sociologists have been looking at the intersection of race, urban life, and health ever since.

3.1. The Disappearance of Jobs is an Urban Health Issue

Wilson's (1996) basic argument drew attention to the way black urban neighborhoods were vulnerable to negative social and health effects due to the disappearance of work. Deindustrialization since 1970, has taken well-paying manufacturing jobs out of the city, away from black males in particular, leaving behind unemployment or low-paying service-sector jobs. And in terms of individual or public health, MacDonald's is no replacement for General Motors.

Wilson's "Chicago Urban Poverty and Family Life Survey," an age cohort study of Chicago's poor neighborhoods where "at least 20 percent of the residents had family incomes below the federal poverty line" (1996), documents the phenomena. By 1980, 55% of Chicago's black families lived in poor urban neighborhoods while only "3% of the non-Hispanic whites" did so (1996). In those urban areas, of the cohort of black men born between 1950 and 1955, employed in 1970 before deindustrialization, 72% of them held down manufacturing jobs; for the cohort born between 1961 and 1969, of those working in 1987, only 21% of them were in industry (1996). Wilson concluded that, "No other male ethnic group in the inner city experienced such an overall precipitous drop in manufacturing employment . . . . Joblessness and declining wages . . . had devastating effects on the social organization of many inner-city neighborhoods" (1996). After 1970, the employment options for urban blacks were fewer and less well-paying, than before. New jobs grew in suburbia, not downtown, creating "a growing mismatch between the suburban location of employment and minorities' residence in the inner city" (1996). The spatial distance between urban blacks and jobs, their declining standards of living, broken families, and "the demise or exodus of the smaller stores, the banks, and other businesses that relied on the wages paid by the large employers" (1996) all contributed to the growth of urban neighborhood disorder.

3.2. The Disappearance of the Urban Black Middle and Working Classes

If that was not enough, an ironic rupture in the social fabric of urban black communities was provided by the exodus of black middle-class and working-class families from the city. Nationally, "from 1970 to 1995 some seven million blacks moved into the suburbs" (Freedman, 2004). Wilson's *The Truly Disadvantaged* (1987) drew attention to the disintegration of urban black communities caused by suburban pull. Middle-class and working-class black families with jobs were taking their skills and experience elsewhere. No longer would they be available as what Wilson calls, "social buffers" (1987), providing network resources or role models for others in difficult times.

The irony was that black families had been confined to the cities by racial apartheid laws and practices that persisted well into the 1960s. During the time period when America's suburbs and their access highways were built, roughly the late 1940s through the 1950s, perpetuating and extending residential racial segregation was the official and legal intent of the Federal Housing Authority (FHA) and the banking industry. The FHA underwrote fully half of all home mortgages issued between 1934 and 1966, and during that time not one FHA loan went to a prospective home buyer, black or white, whose move would integrate a neighborhood (Jackson, 1985; Massey and Denton, 1993). Housing did not exchange in an Adam Smith type of free market, but in quite the opposite. We had a racist political economy where individual preferences and pocketbooks were trumped by racial and social status categories. Sadly, no one has been able to make the case that white homebuyers were ignorant or unwilling accomplices of the apartheid system. The vast majority of whites registered no objections, lawsuits, boycotts, or picket lines, against the racial benefits of government subsidies and higher property values.

Indeed, home ownership is one of the central mechanisms of racial wealth accumulation that has kept whites substantially ahead of blacks (Oliver and Shapiro, 1995; Conley, 1999; Haynes, 2001). And although residential racial segregation has declined since 1980, it remains alive in the land (Iceland, *et al.*, 2002). At the turn of the 21st century, whites still express a preference to flee from neighborhoods where more than 15 percent of the residents are black – even if those black families all positively glow with middle-class respectability (Emerson, *et al.*, 2001).

4.0. NEIGHBORHOOD EFFECTS

Wilson's work helps redirect attention from individual-level investigations to community-level inquiries. The 1990s saw a groundswell in the number of "neighborhood-effects" articles published by academic journals. One review of the phenomenon identified 1995 as the "take-off point" when "about 100 papers per year" on neighborhood effects were being published (Sampson, *et al.*, 2002). One indicator, as well as medium, of the surge was the launch of a new journal in 1995 by social epidemiologists specifically to publish area-effects-on-health studies, *Health & Place*. The journal seeks to advance "sound work which contributes to an understanding of how, why and whether place and context really matter when it comes to health and health care" (Moon, 1995). Reflecting on this new literature, one scientist in the field succinctly described the new paradigm as follows. Morenoff wrote, "The term 'neighborhood effects' generally refers to the study of how local social context influences the health and well being of individuals in a way that is not reducible to the properties of individuals themselves. One of the hallmarks of this research is its attention to the potentially confounding influences of individual-level attributes in making neighborhood-level inferences, either through the use of multilevel research designs and statistical methods or through randomized experimental designs" (Morenoff, 2003).

As Morenoff's comment suggests, community-effects scientists were engaged from the start in a dispute over how to distinguish between compositional and contextual factors. How does one separate out the effects of an area from the characteristics of the people who choose to live there? When, for example, birth weights are too low is that due to the neighborhood, to the family, or to something else? What analytic and explanatory advantage is gained by the search for neighborhood effects?

4.1. Critical Objections

Christopher Jencks, one of the nation's most respected sociologists, co-authored early on, in 1989, a highly critical response to William Julius Wilson's neighborhood-effects thesis. Mayer and Jencks published (1989) an evaluation and rejection of the empirical claims made by researchers working with the new perspective. They selected articles for review that measured neighborhood effects on children's cognitive or behavioral performance. In those studies the researchers all committed what Mayer and Jencks saw as a grave error; they modeled "neighborhood effects" as the average socio-economic (SES) profile of the parents in the area. Disadvantaged areas are filled with poor people, so researchers reasoned that neighborhoods could be described by the average SES of the families living there. When the only variable used to measure "neighborhood-effects" is the mean score of parents' SES in the area, that choice makes it difficult to "distinguish the effects of neighborhoods from the effects of neighbors" (Mayer and Jencks, 1989). It is likely, Mayer and Jencks point out, that the statistical significance of the community variable will be spurious. In a regression model the mean parents' SES score, standing alone as a neighborhood-level variable, will not tell us about community characteristics as much as it will capture unmeasured SES differences between families. They wrote, "the apparent effect of mean SES [the community-effects variable] is likely to be inflated because the neighborhood mean will be a partial proxy for unmeasured differences in individual SES" (Mayer and Jencks, 1989).

If neighborhoods have special structuring powers on some macro- or mezzo-level, as distinct from the micro-level of individual attributes, or put another way, if neighborhoods have contextual effects distinct from compositional effects, then it is nearly impossible for social scientists to prove that, according to Mayer and Jencks. "Because social scientists cannot control where people live, they cannot conduct actual experiments to estimate the effects of neighborhoods" (Mayer and Jencks, 1989). Families "self-select" to move into, remain in, or to leave particular neighborhoods. It is indisputable that the results from a self-selected survey-sample group cannot be applied to a general demographic category. If we are ever going to control for selection bias, Mayer and Jencks argue, social scientists would have to be able to randomly assign families to live in different communities. And without an ability to control for selection bias, one would never be able to build a case about causation. One would not be able to tell whether being in an area causes problems, or whether problem people are just overrepresented in that area.

Even if we could conduct a randomized experiment, with good community-level variables that would capture something distinct from individual characteristics, we would still need something else that is missing from these studies. We would need to specify the mechanism of transmission. Just how do features of neighborhoods affect individual behavior? The studies Mayer and Jencks examined did not theorize or model any links, they merely assumed causation from statistical correlation (1989). What are the mechanisms that translate environmental factors into individual attributes? How are individuals constrained or enabled by the local area?

4.2. Externally Affected Communities or Internal Community Effects?

Mayer and Jencks raise doubts of such a fundamental character about selection bias, variable definition, and unspecified causal mechanisms that one wonders why anyone thought community-effects studies were worth pursuing. It may help us to evaluate the research approach if we reconsider the reasons why Wilson's work put this strategy on the agenda.

Wilson's argument addresses a special kind of community effect, the impact of deindustrialization and suburban flight on pre-existing urban black neighborhoods. Wilson's account of the creation of a black, urban under-class is a story about external forces that transform social relations. The structure of opportunities and the web of social ties were objectively broken, and particular places suffered for it. Analytically and empirically, those processes were macro- or mezzo-level effects distinct from the attributes of the individuals who composed the community. So, does Wilson's work offer us a unique illustration of neighborhood effects mattering when an ongoing community is disrupted by structural forces? Or did he hit on an extreme example of what is in fact a general relationship between place and social behavior? Do neighborhood effects count only in relation to dramatic macro re-structuring that impact old communities? Or are there community effects worth investigating across a range of community types and outcomes?

Mayer and Jencks' criticisms were not really addressed to the "structural impact" type of community effects outlined above. They were making a case against the thesis that particular areas have independent effects on the life chances of people who live there. But their objections did not get at the problem of the effects of structural change, for ill or good, on communities. When, for example, industrial toxic waste dumps proliferate, so do the health risks of people in the area for reasons that have nothing to do with changes in their individual attributes. Nor did Mayer and Jencks' argument address the issue of the relative advantages that may be attached to particular locations. There is such a thing as positive community-level effects. For example, it is a feature of economic life even in the age of globalization that firms of a particular type tend to cluster in particular areas. Firm clustering may provide positive community-effects, such as when employment opportunities and tax revenues go up. The question Richard Florida (2002) attempts to answer, "Why firms cluster?" is another way of thinking about the attractions of location, the positive power of place. The growth of high tech industries in Silicone Valley, California and the Research Triangle in North Carolina provide positive community benefits, at least for the highly educated people Florida describes as the "creative class." But positive effects were not a concern of Mayer and Jencks. Rather, the real issue for them was whether poor people paid a penalty for living concentrated in particular areas that they would escape if they were dispersed and scattered around middle class communities.

4.3. Randomized Experiments

There is evidence on the preceding question that responds to Mayer and Jencks' challenge to correct selection bias by randomly assigning families to particular neighborhoods. Five cities are engaged in applying a scientifically valid, randomized experiment on poor people, their choice of residence, and their behavioral and health outcomes. Sponsored by the U.S. Department of Housing and Urban Development, and begun during the Clinton years, these programs help science to progress, even if at the expense of some poor people in the short term. The Moving to Opportunity (MTO) program takes poor people eligible for welfare housing assistance in Baltimore, Boston, Chicago, Los Angeles, and New York and randomly assigns them to one of three groups: a control group that is denied any change of their circumstances; a group that receives assistance but without any requirement to move; and an experimental group that receives assistance only if they move into a working- or middle-class area with a low level of poverty. As one review of the experiment concludes, "Preliminary evidence is generally positive . . . Generally, families that moved to low-poverty areas experienced improved outcomes vis-à-vis overall health (physical and mental), safety, boys' problem behavior, and well-being" (Sampson, *et al.*, 2002). Thanks to the Clinton welfare reforms, we have had the power of the federal and local government to construct a randomized experiment, with the result suggesting that neighborhoods do matter, and that economic desegregation works.

4.4. Multilevel Models

The government provided an opportunity for social science to verify the existence of neighborhood effects, but how can we study those effects without the powers of the state behind us? Fortunately, the statistical sophistication of behavioral scientists has improved since the time of Mayer and Jencks' critique. It is now widely recognized that multilevel models can sort out the differences between compositional and contextual effects.

The statistical logic of multilevel modeling was discussed in the literature as early as 1984 (Mason, *et al.*, 1984). Subsequently, statisticians have given the technique three different labels: multilevel models (Goldstein, 1995), random coefficient models (Longford, 1993), and hierarchical linear models (Bryk and Raudenbush, 1992; Duncan, *et al.*, 1998). A more theoretical explanation of multilevel modules is also presented in the previous chapter.

Regardless of name, multilevel models enable social scientists to control for bias that comes from having samples of particular populations, such as from people who all live in one area or who all belong to the same organization. The problem is a form of self-selection bias because the responses of those people in the focused sample will be more similar and less random than from a national survey. The homogeneity of the sample, if not controlled for, will distort one's statistical findings and mislead one into "find[ing] differences and relationships where none exist" (Duncan, *et al.*, 1998). And, separate from seeing things as statistically significant when they are not, without multilevel models, one cannot, as already noted, "distinguish the effects of neighborhoods from the effects of neighbors" (Mayer and Jencks, 1989).

In an excellent review article on the application of the technique to urban health research, Duncan and colleagues explain that, "Multilevel modeling does not, however, simply provide a means of assessing the relative contribution of compositional and contextual effects. Importantly, the technique [also] provides a way of showing how, and for which types of people, contextual effects matter" (Duncan, *et al.*, 1998). The characteristics of one's community may have greater effects on the health of those with low incomes than for the affluent. The poor, the elderly, and the undereducated may be more constrained by where they live than their opposites. By placing the attributes of individuals in the context of where they live, we can see a more accurate estimate of the weight each individual-level variable has, such as income or education, than we get by looking at individuals abstracted from their real position in social and physical space (Bourdieu, 1985). And while many multilevel studies look at only two levels, the individual-level and the community-level, there are examples of three-level analyses: individual-level effects, neighborhood-level effects, and neighborhood-cluster effects all in one series of multilevel statistical analyses (Morenoff, 2003; Singer, 1998).

Initially, multilevel modeling flourished in the sociology of education (Duncan, *et al.*, 1998). Researchers wanted to know, for example, how students performed on academic tests in relation to not only their SES, race, and gender but in connection to the type of school attended. Educational sociologists found that some types of schools had better records than others on particular outcomes for certain categories of student. Catholic high schools, for example, had lower dropout rates, especially for black and latino youths, than public schools or non-Catholic private schools. Without multilevel models, the debate on Catholic school effects sparked and fuelled by James Coleman (1988) would have been mired in muddy evidence and ideology (for an example of the literature, see Morgan and Sorensen, 1999). We would not have been capable of resolving whether the low dropout rate was due to the type of families who select Catholic schools, or to some contextual feature of the institution itself. Outside the field of education, other researchers started using multilevel models including criminologists, organizational ecologists, medical sociologists, urban sociologists, and by the 1990s social epidemiologists. As Patricia O'Campo put it in a review on multilevel models and studies of neighborhood effects on health, "In less than 10 years, the field of epidemiology has been transformed. During this time, multilevel modeling has gone from a little-known and perhaps even unwelcome method of analysis to a household name" (2003). Today, multilevel modeling software is widely available; some statistical packages, such as SAS [Proc Mixed], include it and there are web sites that introduce it to researchers and offer technical assistance (see: Singer, 1998; http://gseweb.harvard.edu/~faculty/singer/).

5.0. CAVEATS ON MECHANISMS AND MEASURES

Multilevel models have established, contrary to Mayer and Jencks' expectation, that "neighbourhood effects are fairly consistent across studies" (Pickett and Pearl, 2001). Just because there are such things as "neighborhood effects," however, does not mean that their investigation is unproblematic. There remain a number of underdeveloped aspects of the neighborhood effects strategy that must be addressed.

There is a wide consensus that research on neighborhood health effects is insufficiently theory driven (Diez-Roux, 2000; Duncan, *et al.*, 1998; MacIntryre and Ellaway, 2000; O'Campo, 2003; Pickett and Pearl, 2001; Robert, 1998; Sampson, *et al.*, 2002). Not enough attention is being paid by researchers to specifying two theoretical constructs: What should be the appropriate units of measurement for community-level variables? And what are the causal mechanisms that transfer community effects into individual health outcomes? If one does not have good intellectual reasons for one's measurements of "neighborhood" and for the causal paths and dynamics linking neighborhood to individual health behaviors, one will have no way of evaluating the worth of one's findings. All research produces results, but meaningful results require the theoretical specification of a model, the parameters of the variables, and particular hypotheses on the associations or causal relations one hopes to find. The cliché is true that if you do not know where you want to go, all roads lead you there.

Ideally, good neighborhood-effects research begins with a map that is provided by one's theory, and a clear sense of the desired destination that is provided by one's research question. By "theory" one need not turn to global visions of the way everything micro and macro works in the social world, such as Jurgen Habermas or Michel Foucault offer (Skinner, 1985). While some do produce important work by applying grand theories, such as Aihwa Ong's (2003) brilliant use of Foucault's analytics of bio-power on the process of turning Cambodian refugees in California into U.S. citizens, something more modest is intended here by the term "theory." One needs a theoretical model of the mechanisms linking individuals to environments, mechanisms that make empirical sense of the causal paths between the two levels. The neighborhood effects literature is quite congenial to the attempt to move the social sciences forward by sidestepping grand theoretical debates through the identification of middle range paths and mechanisms (Hedstrom and Swedberg, 1998) that explain particular social outcomes.

5.1. Mechanisms: Example of Neighborhood Birth Weight

It may help to illustrate what is required through a discussion of Jeffrey Morenoff's (2003) research on birth weights in Chicago which provides an excellent example of what needs to be done. (As a note, there are other exemplary works in the field, including Ross, *et al.*, 2001). Morenoff wants to explore the relation between community effects and birth weight. The problem of birth weight offers a strategic test of neighborhood effects for various reasons (Morenoff, 2003): it is obviously an important health concern, since birth weights are associated with a range of developmental health and cognitive problems, birth weights are greatly influenced by the habits of the mother during the nine months of pregnancy, so there is a short leash on the temporal link between mothers, the neighborhood and birth weight outcomes; and there exists plenty of data to explore with over 100,000 births in Chicago in a two year span, spread over 342 identifiable and distinct neighborhoods.

Morenoff (2003) gives us a heuristic model for thinking about community effects on pregnant women that has four elements to it: 1) structural factors, such as SES composition, race, residential stability, and population density; 2) social resources, "social capital," such as one's social ties and engagement with the community; 3) sources of stress or disorder, such as urban disorder and violent crime rates; 4) and a spatial social context that is both local and bridges one's neighborhood with adjacent ones. Sources of stress or disorder in the environment are challenges to the pathways between the individual and her community. The role of a theory of mechanism in this model is to understand what mediates between, on the one hand, neighborhood structure, spatial context, and the sources of stress, and, on the other hand, individual health outcomes. In Morenoff's model, as for most of the recent literature on this the "focus . . . on the mechanisms that explain *why* neighborhoods matter . . . has been driven by interest in social capital" (Morenoff, 2003). Morenoff uses the elements of social resources to build a social capital argument on mechanism.

5.2. Social Capital as a Theory of Mechanism Linking Macro to Micro

The concept of social capital provides one of the more quantitative ways to model social ties, their density, and intensity. Although Jane Jacobs (1961) originally used the term 'social capital,' appropriately enough in a book based on a successful fight in New York against urban renewal, the French sociologist Pierre Bourdieu was the first to describe it in analytic terms. For Bourdieu (1986), social capital was one of the three fundamental ways that accumulated social energy is "inscribed in objective or subjective structures . . . that determine the [individual's] chances of success for practices." "Social capital is the aggregate of the actual or potential resources which are linked to possession of a durable network of more or less institutionalized relationships of mutual acquaintance and recognition" (1986). Bourdieu's baroque prose style and his own obsession with "cultural capital" made it possible for most U.S. based scholars and scientists to be ignorant of his description of social capital; rather, the concept entered the scholarly mainstream here through the work of two Americans, James Coleman and Robert Putnam. [Cultural capital is one's facility in high prestige aesthetic tastes and sensibilities which smooth one's way through the fields of elite education and occupations (Bourdieu, 1986)]. Coleman's (1988) definition of the concept placed the weight on social capital "as a resource that is realized through social relationships" (Morenoff, 2003); while Putnam (1993) added to the network resource aspect an emphasis on norms of trust and cooperation. Furthermore, it is of little consequence that Coleman's and Putnam's versions are reinventions of the two axis of Durkheim's model of social support from his book, *Suicide* (1951). Coleman's social ties are a reformulation of Durkheim's axis of regulation, while Putnam's norms are another way of thinking about what Durkheim called integration. Research in the social sciences frequently moves forward through a cycle of rediscovery, whereby "new ideas are always the old ones under new labels" (Abott, 2001). Our empirical knowledge can advance, even if many of our core concepts merely acquire new clothes. On balance, social capital measured as one's social ties as well as one's confidence or faith in the efficacy of those ties, provides a clean model of a mechanism that can stand between the individual and her community. It can buffer one from problems and enable one to accomplish tasks.

Morenoff's research on social capital in Chicago could capitalize on an ongoing citywide survey called the Project on Human Development in Chicago Neighborhoods (PHDCN) (2003). The survey provides information on social capital that can be articulated as two scales, an exchange scale and a voluntarism scale. "The first, reciprocated exchange, is a five-item scale measuring how often neighbors provide mutual support, exchange advice and information, and socialize with one another. . . . The second, participation in local voluntary associations, is a six-item index that measures residents' involvement" in community associations" (Morenoff, 2003). The survey's social capital scales were used by other researchers before Morenoff, so he could be confident of their validity. He found his best results came from combining the two scales into one "exchange/voluntarism" index.

To Morenoff's data on social capital resources, one of his model's four elements, he added information on the other three: structural factors, sources of stress, and spatial data. Eventually, his data enabled him to control for individual compositional effects, such as income, race, maternal health condition, and length of time in the community, to control for contextual effects from the character of the neighborhood, and to evaluate a measure of stress as the area's violent crime rate. On the fourth element, the spatial one, Morenoff was innovative. He analyzed not only spatial data at the level of the immediate neighborhood, but also at the level of adjacent neighborhoods (2003). He asked, regardless of one's neighborhood's violent crime rate or its social capital score, does it make a difference if adjacent communities have high or low crime rates, or high or low social capital scores? For example, all of the 342 neighborhoods in his study could be classified in relation to violent crime and birth weights in one of four categories: high-high, high-low, low-low, or low-high. He could code a neighborhood as being high on the crime index and being next to an area that also has a high crime rate as "high-high", or if it was high but the adjacent area was low, it would be "high-low," and so on. He found significant amounts of spatial clustering. For example, "91% of the neighborhoods that are in the significant high-high category on the violent crime map . . . are also in the significant low-low category on the birth weight map, while 77% of the significant low-low crime neighborhoods are also significant high-high clusters of birth weight" (2003).

In terms of what explains low birth weights, individual-level effects, such as poverty, and neighborhood-level measures, such as residential stability, are significant and look important until one introduces the neighborhood's violent crime rate and social capital score (2003). Morenoff tell us, "violent crime and the combined scale of reciprocal exchange and participation in voluntary associations are the two most robust neighborhood predictors of birth weight, even after controlling for the potentially confounding individual-level covariates. These neighborhood mechanisms also appear to mediate the effects of structure factors, such as poverty and residential stability" (2003). He finds some neighborhoods are disadvantaged due to violent crimes committed in the area which affect the health of pregnant women with weak social ties, producing a lower birth weight for their children. Without social capital, the stress of living in or near areas where violent crimes are believed to be common isolates pregnant women and adversely affects their own nutrition. It might help health care workers to tailor practical interventions if they mapped press coverage of violent crimes and asked at-risk pregnant women about their social support network.

5.3. Neighborhood Boundaries

Chicago is unique as the American city with the most extensive amount of systematic research devoted to it. Morenoff could tap ongoing studies of 342 intellectually and empirically well crafted neighborhoods. But what if one does not have Chicago as one's laboratory? How should one draw the geographic boundaries of one's research site? Surely, one should not define "neighborhood" by opportunistic convenience as whatever geographic area the government provides data on? In what sense are census tracts of approximately 4,000 people, or census blocks of about 1,000 people, or zip code areas with around 30,000 people in them "neighborhoods" that should have effects on the health of the individuals who compose them? How does one demarcate the boundaries of actual neighborhoods? Depending on one's research project, such as whether one poses questions on birth weights or exposure to toxic waste, one would need to draw the relevant geography differently.

For example, let us consider the problem of disparities in the community effects of industrial hazards as placed on the public agenda in the 1980s by "the release of studies by the U.S. General Accounting Office (GAO, 1983) and the United Church of Christ's Commission for Racial Justice (CRJ, 1987)" (Mennis, 2002). Those studies galvanized the environmental justice movement (EJM) as well as attempts by sociologists and others to use geographic information systems (GIS) to map the social coordinates of industrial danger. The question was whether or not corporations victimize poor minorities by releasing more toxic materials in their communities than in non-minority, affluent communities. Scientists have found that the answer varies depending on the scale of the area included in the study.

Jeremy Mennis (2002) illustrates the consequences involved in selecting one's area size for gathering data. Generally speaking, when one uses small geographic units, there does not seem to be any racial disparities in toxic venues, but when one uses large units, there are disparities. As Mennis explains, "consider the work of Glickman and colleagues . . . who used GIS to examine the demographic character of communities that host Toxic Release Inventory (TRI) facilities . . . when "communities" are defined by census block groups or tracts the percentage of minorities in the TRI-host communities is not significantly different then that in non-host communities. However, when municipalities, a generally larger unit than block groups or census tracts, form the basis for defining "community," TRI-host communities have significantly higher proportions of minorities than non-host communities" (Mennis, 2002). Mennis resolves this conundrum by showing how the relation of minorities to toxic facilities is curvilinear (2002). Hazardous facilities are disproportionately located where there are large concentrations of minorities, but usually not in a minority neighborhood. From a distance of five kilometers away from the facility, the percent of minorities and poor people goes up, peaks at 500 meters, and then goes down. "This suggests that the greatest degree of socioeconomic disadvantage is found not at the exact location of a hazardous facility, but rather in the immediately surrounding area" (Mennis, 2002). There are high concentrations of toxic facilities in areas adjacent to large numbers of minorities. While only 2 percent of the population in Mennis' study, which covered southeast Pennsylvania, lived within 2.5 kilometers of 9 hazardous sites, over 50 percent of those so exposed were racial minorities (Mennis, 2002). If one used census tracts or blocks, rather than draw one's own boundaries, one would not find signs of environmental racial disparities.

Another study that demonstrates the consequences of unit measurement choices, only this time on mortality and cancer incidence, was done by researchers at Harvard's School of Public Health (Krieger, *et al.*, 2002). Working with data from Massachusetts and Rhode Island for 1988 to 1992, they investigated the difference that geographic units make to what one's sees in the relation between neighborhood and SES, on the one hand, and mortality and cancer incidence, on the other. They used a number of carefully crafted measures of SES for individuals and with which to construct composites of geographic areas. For geographic areas, they looked at three: zip code areas; census tracts; and census blocks (Krieger, *et al.*, 2002). They found that "census block group and census tract measures performed similarly for virtually all outcomes; zip code measure, however, in some cases failed to detect gradients or detected gradients contrary to those observed with the block group and tract measures" (Krieger, *et al.*, 2002). At first glance, their conclusion seems to contradict Mennis' since they got their most powerful results from geographic measures rejected by him. They, however, were looking for the relation between low SES neighborhoods and death/cancer rates, while Mennis was looking for the distance between racial minority neighborhoods and toxic release facilities.

One's question must guide one's choice of the appropriate geographic measure. And there are many research questions where objective geographic units are irrelevant. To know how people perceive disorder or safety on their turf, one needs from survey data a cognitive map of what the person understands to be her community's boundaries. Cognitive mapping of communities is a technique that goes back at least to the 1970s (Hayden, 1997).

5.4. Integral Measures

Where one draws the perimeter of one's neighborhood does not end the list of concerns about units of measurement for community effects. What variables should count as measuring "neighborhood effects"? Multilevel statistical tools allows us to use median values of aggregated household attributes as a neighborhood-level variable, but what of variables that are "integral to the neighbourhood and only measurable at that level, such as number of recreational facilities"? (2001). Integral measures of neighborhoods that seek to capture unique features of particular urban landscapes are, unfortunately, rarely constructed, let alone used. Integral variables, nonetheless, should be valuable indications of neighborhood resources. We need research that employs integral measures, such as the per capital ratio of public space, including parks (Harnik, 2003), playgrounds, and pedestrian zones, of amenities and entertainments, such as shops and cafes, of local services, such as health facilities and public transportation systems.

There is very little systematic research showing the relationship of public space to health, an odd omission given the high quality and quantity of work we have on what makes for effective public space (Carr, *et al.*, 1992; Garvin, 1996; Lofland, 1998; Whyte, 1989). We know that public space works best when it is accessible, user friendly, and resonates with the symbolic imaginations of its users (Carr, *et al.*, 1992). And there is a strong research tradition of using field observation and video cameras to record how people actually use space in public places. William Whyte (1998) and a team of Hunter College sociology students worked for the New York City Planning Commission to empirically study and recommend ways to enhance the use of public space in New York. Zoning laws and Planning Commission decisions have set up economic incentives for the private sector to participate by trading permission to build additional floors in skyscrapers for open public space on the ground. Whyte's team enabled the Commission to know what types of chairs, greenery, and water fountains would invite the most extensive public use of that space. Now we can apply research to assess whether the quality and quantity of public space in neighborhoods contributes to the health of the community.

Another neglected integral measure of neighborhood effects concerns the physical environment. Systematic research on the size and condition of buildings and streets in an area is in its infancy (Sampson and Raduenbush, 1999; Weich, *et al.*, 2001). We know from survey research that perceptions of neighborhood disorder, including "graffiti, vandalism, noise, and abandoned buildings" (Ross, 2001) substantially undermines trust in others, one key dimension of social capital. And we have excellent survey tools for measuring the perception of disorder (Ross and Mirowsky, 1999). But we have only a few attempts to record objective measures of environmental disorder. The most ambitious effort so far to record and evaluate physical disorder in urban neighborhoods is the video recording and systemic observation of over 23 thousand street blocks in Chicago by Sampson and Raudenbush (1999). While empirical results have yet to cascade down from this project, Raudenbush and Sampson (1999) are in the forefront of developing useful measures of neighborhood landscapes. And their work has a more ambitious goal than the worthy attempt to specify integral items of urban areas, including "gang graffiti, the density of liquor stores, and abandoned cars" (Raudenbush and Sampson, 1999). Rather, they want to establish carefully tested neighborhood-level measures that are as precisely calibrated as the individual-level measures of traditional survey research. "The assessment of individual differences, building on decades of psychometric research, employs measures that have withstood rigorous evaluation" (1999); nothing of the sort has taken place with community variables. Neighborhood measures deserve their own form of psychometric verification, and Raudenbush and Sampson label that effort, "ecometrics." Ecometrics would be the science of measurement for integral and other neighborhood-level variables. This is an essential area of methodological development that is in its initial phase. Researchers, however, should not wait for an ecometrics textbook before trying out integral measures in the statistical exploration of neighborhood effects.

6.0. CONCLUSION

Space constraints do not allow us in this overview of the growing field of sociology and urban health to cover every aspect of the subject. Among important topics not even touched on, we should include mention of sociological explanations for variations between places that, although at some distance from any immediate applications as health interventions, do offer significant insights into local context. For example, there is the study by Molotch, *et al.*, (2000) on why Ventura, California was so pro-oil while Santa Barbara, California was not. Their research on the power of place overlaps with the environmental justice literature and they make a "path dependency" argument that can be applied to a wide range of local communities. In addition, this summary has not explored the critical role played by ethnographies of the sort produced by Elijah Anderson. Without the on-the-ground, local knowledge (Geertz, 1983) that ethnography provides, much of the passion that drives the field and wins broader public empathy would be lost. And researchers would not have field materials to work with when formulating models of mechanisms, such as social capital. Without the reality check ethnography provides we would not know which mechanisms make the most sense of the experience of urban people.*

What this chapter has covered, however, is how the problems of urban black communities helped to place neighborhood effects on the scholarly map. Building on the work of W.J. Wilson and others, we know that apart from the attributes of our families, the characteristics of our communities matter. And multilevel models have enabled us to empirically measure the ways communities make a difference. One central finding is that our community's stock of social capital can nurture our health or, when meager, put us at risk. But our work is far from complete. We need extensive research on integral measures of neighborhoods in relation to a range of different health effects before the field can deliver fully on its analytical as well as applied promise.

REFERENCES

Abbott, A.W. (2001). *Chaos of Disciplines.* University of Chicago Press, Chicago.

Anderson, E. (1978). *A Place on the Corner.* University of Chicago Press, Chicago.

Anderson, E. (1990). *Streetwise: Race, Class, and Change in an Urban Community.* University of Chicago Press, Chicago.

Bourdieu, P. (1985). The Social Space and the Genesis of Groups. *Theory Soc.* 14(6):723–744.

Bourdieu, P. (1986). The Forms of Capital. In: Richardson, J.G. (eds.). *Handbook of theory and research for the sociology of education.* Greenwood Press, Westport, pp. 241–258.

Boyer, P. (1978). *Urban Masses and Moral Order in America 1820-1920.* Harvard University Press, Cambridge, MA.

Bryk, A.S., and Raudenbush, S.W. (1992). *Hierarchical Linear Models: Applications and Data Analysis Methods.* Sage Press, Newbury Park.

Carr, S., Francis, M., Rivlin, L.G., and Stone, A.M. (1992). *Public Space.* Cambridge University Press, New York.

Camacho, D.E. (eds.) (1998). *Environmental Injustices, Political Struggles: Race, Class, and the Environment.* Duke University Press, Durham.

Catalano, R. (1989). Ecological Factors in Illness and Disease. In: Freeman, H.E. and Sol Levine, S. (eds.), *Handbook of Medical Sociology.* Prentice Hall, Englewood Cliffs, pp. 87–101.

Coleman, J.S. (1988). Social Capital in the Creation of Human Capital. *Am. J. Soc.* 94(Supplement):95–120.

Conley, D. (1999). *Being Black, Living in the Red.* University of California Press, Berkeley.

Diez-Roux, A. (2000). Multilevel analysis in public health research. *Annu. Rev. Public Health 2000*; 21:171-92.

Drake, S., and Cayton, H.A. (1993). *Black Metropolis: A Study of Negro Life in a Northern City.* University of Chicago Press, Chicago.

Du Bois, W.E.B. (1978). *On Sociology and the Black Community.* University of Chicago Press, Chicago.

Duncan, C., Jones, K., and Moon, G. (1998). Context, Composition, and Heterogeneity: Using Multilevel Models in Health Research. *Soc. Sci. Med.* 46(1):97–117.

Durkheim, E. (1951). *Suicide.* The Free Press, New York.

*One hopes that the new urban journal, *City & Community*, will continue to publish ethnographic work as well as historical work.

Egolf, B., Lasker, J., Wolf, S., and Potvin, L. (1992). The Roseto Effect: A 50-Year Comparison of Mortality Rates. *Am. J. Public Health* 82(8):1089–1092.

Elliott, D., Wilson, W.J., Huizinga, D., Sampson, R.J., Elliott, A., and Rankin, B. (1996). Effects of Neighborhood Disadvantage on Adolescent Development. *Journal of Research on Crime and Delinquency* 33:389–426.

Emerson, M.O., Yancey, G., and Chai, K.J. (2001). Does Race Matter in Residential Segregation? Exploring the Preferences of White Americans. *Am. Soc. Rev.* 66(6):922–935.

Erikson, K. (1994). *A New Species of Trouble: Explorations in Disaster, Trauma, and Community.* W.W. Norton & Company, New York.

Fitzpatrick, K.M., and LaGory, M. (2003). "Placing" Health in an Urban Sociology: Cities as Mosaics of Risk and Protection. *City & Community* 2(1):33–46.

Florida, R. (2002). *The Rise of the Creative Class.* Basic Books, New York.

Freedman, S.G. (2004). Still Separate, Still Unequal. *The New York Times Book Review,* Sunday, May 16, 2004, pp. 8–9.

Fullilove, M. T. (1999). *The House of Joshua: meditations on family and place.* University of Nebraska Press, Lincoln, NE.

Foreman, C.H. (1998). *The Promise and Peril of Environmental Justice.* Brookings Institution Press, Washington, D. C.

Gans, H.J. (1962). *The Urban Villagers: Group and class in the life of Italian-Americans.* The Free Press, New York.

Garvin, A. (1996). *The American City, What Works, and What Doesn't.* McGraw-Hill, New York.

Geertz, C. (1983). *Local Knowledge.* Basic Books, New York.

Goldstein, H. (1995). *Multilevel statistical models.* Edward Arnold, London.

Grant, D., and Jones, A.W. (2003). Are Subsidiaries More Prone to Pollute? New Evidence from the EPA's Toxin Release Inventory. *Soc. Sci. Q.* 84(1):162–173.

Grant, D., Jones, A.W., and Trautner, M.N. (2004). Do Facilities with Distant Headquarters Pollute More? How Civic Engagement Conditions the Environmental Performance of Plants. *Social Forces* (In press).

Hayden, D. (1997). *The Power of Place.* MIT Press, Cambridge, Massachusetts.

Harnik, P. (2003). *The Excellent City Park System.* Trust for Public Land, Washington, D.C.

Haynes, B.D. (2001). *Red Lines, Black Spaces.* Yale University Press, New Haven.

Hedstrom, P., and Swedberg, R. (1998). *Social Mechanism: an analytical approach to social theory.* Cambridge University Press, New York.

Iceland, J., Weinberg, D.H., and Steinmetz, E. (2002). *Racial and Ethnic Residential Segregation in the United States: 1980 to 2000.* U.S. Census Bureau, Washington, D.C.

Jackson, K.T. (1985). *The Crab Grass Frontier.* Oxford University Press, New York.

Jacobs, J. (1961). *The Death and Life of Great American Cities.* Random House, New York.

Jones, K., and Duncan, C. (1995). Individuals and their ecologies: analyzing the geography of chronic illness within a multilevel modeling framework. *Health Place* 1(1):27–40.

Kostof, S. (1994). His Majesty the Pick: the Aesthetics of Demolition. In: Celik, A., Favro, D., and Ingersoll, R. (eds.), *Streets: Critical Perspectives on Public Space.* University of California Press, Berkeley, pp. 9–22.

Krieger, N., Chen, J.T., Waterman, M.J.S., Subramanian, S.V., and Carson, R. (2002). Geocoding and Monitoring of US Socioeconomic inequalities in Mortality and Cancer Incidence: Does the Choice of Area-Based Measure and Geographic Level Matter? *Am. J. Epidemiol.* 156(5): 471-482.

Lofland, L. (1998). *The Public Realm: Exploring the City's Quintessential Social Territory,* Aldine De Gruyter, New York.

Longford, N.T. (1993). *Random Coefficient Models.* Oxford University Press, New York.

MacIntyre, S., and Ellaway, A. (2000). Ecological Approaches: Rediscovering the role of the Physical and Social Environment. In: Berkman, L., and Kawachi, I. (eds.), *Social Epidemiology.* Oxford University Press, New York, pp. 332–348.

Marmot, M (2004). *The Status Syndrome: How Social Standing Affects Our Health and Longevity.* New York, Time Books.

Mason, W.M., Wong, G.Y., and Entwistle, B. (1984). The multilevel model: a better way to do contextual analysis. In: Leinhardt, S. (ed.) *Sociological Methodology.* Jossey-Bass, San Francisco.

Massey, D.S., and Denton, N.A. (1993). *American Apartheid: Segregation and the Making of the Underclass.* Harvard University Press, Cambridge.

Mayer, S., and Jencks, C. (1989).Growing Up in Poor Neighborhoods: How Much Does It Matter? *Science* 243: 1441-1445.

Mennis, J. (2002).Using Geographic Information Systems to Create and Analyze Statistical Surfaces of Population and Risk for Environmental Justice Analysis. *Soc. Sci. Q.* 83(1):281–297.

Michelson, W. H. (1976). *Man and His Urban Environment: A Sociological Approach.* Addison-Wesley Publishing, Reading, Massachusetts.

Molotch, H., Freudenburg, W., and Paulsen, K.E. (2000). History Repeats Itself, but How? City Character, Urban Tradition, and the Accomplishment of Place. *American Sociological Review* 65:791–823.

Moon, G. (1995). Editorial: (Re)placing research on health and heath care. *Health Place* 1(1):1–4.

Morenoff, J.D. (2003). Neighborhood Mechanisms and the Spatial Dynamics of Birth Weight. *Am. J. Soc.* 108(5):976–1017.

Morgan, S.L., and Sorensen, A.B. (1999). Parental Networks, Social Closure, and Mathematics Learning: A Test of Coleman's Social Capital Explanation of School Effects'. *Am. Soc. Rev.* 64(October):661–681.

Nakao, K., and Treas, J. (1994). Updating Occupational Prestige and Socioeconomic Scores: How the New Measures Measure Up. *Sociol. Methodol.* 24:1–72.

O'Campo, P. (2003). Advancing Theory and Methods for Multilevel Models of Residential Neighborhoods and Health. *Am. J. Epi.* 157(1):9–13.

Oliver, M.L., and Shapiro, T.M. (1995). *Black Wealth/White Wealth.* Routledge Press, New York.

Ong, A. (2003). *Buddha Is Hiding: Refugees, Citizenship, the New America.* University of California Press, Berkeley.

Park, R. E., and Burgess, E.W. (1967). *The City.* University of Chicago Press, Chicago.

Pickett, K.E., and Pearl, M. (2001). Multilevel analyses of neighborhood socioeconomic context and health outcomes: a critical review. *J. Epidemiol. Community Health* 1(55):111–122.

Project on Human Development in Chicago Neighborhoods. (2003). Harvard School of Public Health; http://www.hms.harvard.edu/chase/projects/chicago/about.

Putnam, R. (1993). The Prosperous Community: Social Capital and Community Life. *American Prospect* 13: 35–42.

Raudenbush, S.W., and Sampson, R.J. (1999). 'Ecometrics': Toward a science of assessing ecological settings, with application to the systematic social observation of neighborhoods. *Soc. Methodol.* 29:1–41.

Robert, S.A. (1998) Community-level socioeconomic effects on adult health. *J. Health Soc. Behav.* 39:18-37.

Ross, C.E., and Mirowsky, J. (1999). Disorder and Decay: The Concept and Measurement of Perceived Neighborhood Disorder. *Urban Affairs Review* 34:412–432.

Ross, C.E., Mirowsky, J., and Pribesh, S. (2001). Powerlessness and the Amplification of Threat: Neighborhood Disadvantage, Disorder, and Mistrust. *Am. Soc. Rev.* 66(4):568–591.

Sampson, R.J., and Raudenbush, S.W. (1999). Systematic Social Observation of Public Spaces: a New Look at Disorder in Urban Neighborhoods. *Am. J. Soc.* 105(3):603–651.

Sampson, R.J., Morenoff, J.D., and Gannon-Rowley, T. (2002). Assessing "Neighborhood Effects": Social Processes and New Directions in Research. *Ann. Rev. Soc.* 28:443–478.

Sennett, R. (1993). *The Conscience of the Eye: The Design and Social Life of Cities.* Farber and Farber, Boston.

Shonkoff, J. P., and Phillips, D.A. (eds.). (2000). *From Neurons to Neighborhoods: The Science of Early Childhood Development.* National Academy Press, Washington, D.C.

Simmel, G. (1997). *Simmel on Culture.* Sage, Thousand Oaks, CA.

Singer, J.D. (1998). Using SAS PROC MIXED to Fit Multilevel Models, Hierarchical Models, and Individual Growth Models. *Journal of Educational and Behavioral Statistics* 24(4):323–355.

Skinner, Q. (eds.). (1985). *The Return of Grand Theory in the Human Sciences.* Cambridge University Press, New York.

Wakefield, S.E.L., Elliott, S.J., Cole, D.C., and Eyles, J.D. (2001). Environmental risk and (re)action: air quality, health, and civic involvement in an urban industrial neighborhood. *Health Place* 7:163–177.

Weich, S., Burton, E., Blanchard, M., Prince, M., Spronston, K., and Erens, B. (2001). Measuring the built environment: validity of a site survey instrument for use in urban settings. *Health Place* 7:283–292.

Weiss, M.J. (1988). *The Clustering of America.* Harper and Row, New York.

Whyte, W. (1989). *City: Rediscovering the Center.* Double Day, New York.

Wilkinson, R.G. (1992). National Mortality Rates: the Impact of Inequality? *Am. J. Public Health* 82(8):1082–1084.

Wilson, W.J. (1987). *The Truly Disadvantaged: the Inner City, the Underclass and Public Policy.* University of Chicago Press, Chicago.

Wilson, W.J. (1996). *When Work Disappears: the World of the New Urban Poor.* Knopf, New York.

Wilson, W. J. (1993). In: Drake, S. and Cayton, H.A. (eds.). *Black Metropolis: A Study of Negro Life in a Northern City.* Forward to the 1993 Edition. University of Chicago Press, Chicago, xlvii-lii.

Chapter 19

Bridging the Gap Between Urban Health and Urban Planning

Marlon G. Boarnet and Lois M. Takahashi

1.0. INTRODUCTION

There is an increasing recognition by health researchers and practitioners that the built environment, land use, and development patterns have a significant role to play in morbidity and mortality in communities across the U.S. While there has been an expanding number of studies by researchers in public health and urban planning that examine the relationship between health and development patterns, built form, and land use regulation, this remains a relatively under-explored topic both by urban planners and urban/public health researchers. This chapter attempts to bridge the divide between the urban health and urban planning disciplines by describing urban planning approaches to urban health, and working to develop a common language with which to approach urban health issues. We posit in this chapter that the nexus between urban health and urban planning provides an opportunity for interdisciplinary innovation to clarify the complexities characterizing urban health, and offers opportunities for developing comprehensive and multidimensional solutions to contemporary urban health issues.

In our attempts to bridge this disciplinary divide, the chapter proceeds in the following manner. First, we provide an overview of the primary urban planning approaches to urban issues, highlighting the major conceptual notions that might be relevant to urban health. Following this, we identify studies in urban planning that exemplify the interdisciplinary nature of methods and analysis. Next, we move to the methodological challenges in using urban planning approaches to study urban health, particularly in terms of accommodating distinct conceptual approaches and methodological techniques. Finally, we conclude the chapter by summarizing the major points, and pointing to ways forward in developing an urban health/urban planning research agenda.

2.0. WHAT IS URBAN PLANNING?

Urban planning, also referred to as city planning, is an applied, multi- and inter-disciplinary field that is concerned with the interaction between populations and the environments in which they live. Urban planners are employed in a variety of sectors (public, private, and nonprofit/community based), and their tasks include the preservation of historic districts in downtown areas, the development of legislation that guarantees the reduction of environmental hazards in communities of color, and the creation of strategies to reduce intergovernmental conflict among federal, state, and local government agencies. With this wide range of sectors, tasks, and objectives, the field of urban planning has had to engage conceptual approaches and analytical methods from multiple disciplines, most predominantly economics, architecture, geography, and law. What urban planners have in common across these sectors, tasks, and objectives is the notion that they "use their skills to find solutions to community problems in ways that will carry the community toward its desired long-term goals" (AICP, 2004). The "community" is broadly defined and may refer to nations, states, regions, cities, or neighborhoods. In fact, urban planners work at many of these scales to attempt to address in comprehensive ways the complex challenges that arise from urbanization, economic and population growth and decline, and increasing diversity across multiple dimensions of social life.

One way to understand urban planning from an urban health perspective is to redefine urban health using planning terminology. There are various themes that are used by planners to describe planning objectives and strategies. Five primary themes guide much of what urban planners do especially with respect to issues important to urban health: (1) economic development, (2) urban design, (3) equity and social justice, (4) governance and institutional management, and (5) sustainability (Table 1).

2.1. Economic Development Planning

The first theme that guides a great deal of urban planning is economic development. Broadly defined, this theme includes transportation, housing, and community economic development, and is primarily concerned with the economic vitality of communities, cities, counties, regions, and states. From an urban health perspective, on the one hand, an economic development strategy for investigating urban health might consist of linking urban health disparities with maldistributions of wealth and concentrations of poverty in places and populations. This is relevant for the large public health literature on health disparities that shows that poor and minority populations typically are at greater risk of morbidity and mortality (e.g. CDC, 2004). Economic development planning seeks to address the sources of disparities in income and access to resources. Urban planners have often argued that uneven distributions of wealth and poverty stem from global economic shifts. Global economic restructuring has created an expanding service sector providing a growing number of low-wage, temporary and contractual, and limited benefits jobs (Law and Wolch, 1991). The contraction in income-earning opportunities conditioned by global economic shifts has consequently led to greater competitiveness for fewer jobs and less-well-paid employment in a context of instability and uncertainty. To cope with the fallout of global economic restructuring, urban health researchers and practitioners might look to economic development strategies

Table 1. Urban Planning Approaches and Foci

Approach	Economic development	Urban design	Equity and social justice	Governance and institutional management	Sustainability
Focus	• Uneven distributions of wealth and poverty exacerbated by globalization • Generating wealth for individuals and house holds to improve urban health	• Design of buildings, parks, and streets to promote health and reduce disease • Role of locations of built form elements in steering individual and population behavior	• Socially, politically, and economically disadvantaged communities • Empowerment for greater participation in decisions about health funding, programs, and outcomes	• Impact of privatization, increasing emphasis on voluntarism and nonprofit sectors for service delivery • Cooperation, collaboration, and conflict among governmental and non-governmental agencies	• Protect and expand greenspace, parks, habitat for endangered species • Short and longer term planning for land use to effectively manage natural resources (water, forests)

coupled with health programs to develop approaches that deal with one of the presumed underlying sources of urban health disparities, that is, economic inequality. On the other hand, an economic development perspective might focus on ways to increase wealth and opportunities through economic growth and individual/household wealth generation. From this perspective, urban health initiatives might focus on human capital (education and skills building for enhancing wage earning potential), social capital (building trust and reciprocity in communities to leverage existing local tangible and intangible resources), and business development (expanding the number of small businesses and health care agencies through micro-credit and loan programs, mentoring, and tax incentives). Economic development strategies would focus on the urban health dimensions of transportation (e.g., enhancing transit and automobile access, and addressing the deleterious effects of traffic congestion), housing (e.g., working for more and better quality affordable housing), and community economic development (e.g., expanding economic opportunities in local communities experiencing marginal income earning capacity or relatively low rates of economic growth).

2.2. Urban Design

Urban design comprises an important theme that guides urban planning research and practice, linking physical structures, (what planners refer to as built form), with social environments. Urban design has become a primary emphasis for public health researchers interested in the role of land use and development patterns in obesity and rates of physical activity (Handy, *et al.*, 2002). In terms of urban health, the design of buildings, parks, and streets (e.g., sidewalks, streetscapes, bus stops), the location of these elements, and the interaction between people and these built environment elements influence, though they do not determine, the ways that individuals behave and interact with one another. Planners use urban design elements (e.g., building facades, street signage, lighting, landscaping) to encourage and facilitate economic activity (through e.g., farmers markets and street cafes), civic action (through e.g., areas for social gatherings), and physical activity (through e.g., walking paths), as well as to curb undesirable or unhealthy behaviour, such as property and violent crime (through e.g., expanded and enhanced street lighting schemes) and pedestrian/bicyclist injuries/death (through e.g., street lights, speed bumps, and street alignments), or to cope with chronic illnesses such as dementia (through e.g., room and building design). For more examples, please see Loukaitou-Sideris, (1999), and Cohen and Day, (1993).

To promote physical health, at the regional scale, some have advocated for the co-location of transit, homes, businesses, and shopping opportunities, falling under the broad rubric of "new urbanism" to encourage walking, discourage driving, and increase opportunities for social interaction (Duany and Plater-Zyberk, 1991). There has been a proliferation of studies that have examined the relationship among urban design, development patterns, and physical activity (e.g. Handy, *et al.*, 2002 or Northridge and Sclar, 2003). For example, The National Research Council recently convened a committee of transportation, land use, and public health scholars to study this topic.

At the local level, urban planners have long been interested in urban park design and location, and the influence of design and location on park use. Such studies also build on the beliefs that the built environment (its design and location) frame, though does not determine, individual, household, and community behaviour, and consequently, can motivate or constrain civic action (Jacobs, 1961). As a consequence of such beliefs, planners strive to improve, enhance, and expand public spaces and places. In a recent commentary, Banerjee (2001) recommended to planners that they advocate for parks and open space, and support grassroots initiatives, that they facilitate creative solutions by acting as mediators among public, private, and nonprofit groups, that they focus on "reinventing" deteriorating areas, including malls and downtowns, that they support the development of businesses that facilitate conviviality in public life through cultural experiences, that the design of streets and sidewalks are seen as important public spaces for interaction, and that they respond to increasing racial/ethnic diversity, including rapidly expanding immigrant populations.

A related area of longstanding interest within planning is housing – a topic that can be grouped within either urban design or economic development planning. Planning efforts to improve housing include U.S. government programs that in past decades funded the building of public housing and, more recently, subsidies made available to low income renters. At the local level, many planners work on efforts to ensure that housing is affordable for low and moderate income persons – an especially pressing issue in urban areas with high housing costs. Research has shown that there are links between the quality of the housing stock and both physical and mental health. See, e.g., Bonnefoy, *et al.*, (2003) for evidence on housing quality and physical health, and the reviews in Evans, Walls, and Moch (2003) and Evans (2003) for a discussion of the link between housing characteristics and mental health. For example, high rise living is associated with reduced psychological well being in some settings (Evans, Walls, and Hoch, 2003; Evans, 2003). Planning approaches to public housing in the generation after World War II included a large role for high-rise dwellings, with little initial attention to possible adverse mental health impacts on residents, illustrating the need for stronger links between urban health and planning.

2.3. Equity and Social Justice in Planning

Equity and social justice constitutes another primary theme that guides planning practice and urban health. In terms of urban health, an equity and social justice perspective guiding urban planning research and practice would build on the health disparities approach to prioritize improved and expanded health care services to those individuals and populations experiencing the worst health outcomes and who are least able to pay for services, for example, low-income, elderly, racial/ethnic minority, and immigrant households. Such groups often reside in central cities (with aging housing, services, and infrastructure), but many also live in older and newer suburbs (geographically isolated from health care services). From this perspective, urban planning research and practice is "applied, action oriented, problem-solving, . . . particularly concerned with socially, economically and politically disadvantaged populations" and "seeks to promote social justice through such activities as critical analyses of the distribution costs and benefits of public policies and the development of institutions that empower people at the grassroots" (UCLA Department of Urban Planning, 2004).

As with work in economic development planning, planners' efforts related to equity and social justice have much to offer urban health scholars and practitioners interested in health disparities across income groups, racial or ethnic groups, or persons with differing access to health services. Planners who seek to work in equity and social justice issues have increasingly recognized that the power relations inherent in the design and exercise of planning for decision -making must be addressed. The nature of credible and legitimate knowledge for example in defining the nature of problems and their appropriate solutions require critical self-reflection on the part of planners. Planners have advocated varying ways to accomplish this very problematic task, including code switching, participatory planning, and grassroots mobilization. (Classic works on participatory or advocacy planning include Arnstein (1969) and Davidoff (1965).) *Code switching* (or changing the codes and interpretation when moving from one language to another, or from one cultural context to another), a relatively new and innovative approach, requires that planners and urban health researchers and professionals, immerse themselves in alternative ways of thinking (e.g., non-Western knowledge bases, cultural knowledge that is recorded through oral histories) (Umemoto, 2001). A more classic approach used by planners is *participatory planning*, also referred to in urban planning as advocacy planning. This approach, drawn from 1960s critique in urban planning of modernist rational planning models and practices, may aim in its most minimal incarnation at greater input from local residents and communities and at its most empowering, the redistribution of power to disadvantaged households and communities. Such planning typically involves designing decision-making processes that incorporate residents and community stakeholders from the definition of problems through to implementation of programs. Finally, a third alternative is to *mobilize participation in grassroots actions* alongside communities fighting for better wages and health benefits, better quality housing, better schools, and better living conditions. However, this final alternative highlights the tension between the professionalization of planning practice and research (which encourages a social and spatial distance from populations and places being studied), and the need to bridge divides to authentically understand the plight and struggle of marginalized populations.

2.4. Governance and Institutional Management

The fourth prevailing theme among planners that is relevant for urban health is governance and institutional management.

2.4.1. Governance

Governance refers in general to the idea that governing in many places and at many scales has moved from predominantly public sector government policies and methods, to mechanisms that feature a greater reliance on the nonprofit/charitable sectors, on the voluntary sector, and on individuals and communities for providing and sustaining social and community programs. There has been for example in the U.S. at the local level more reliance on parents to provide time and material resources for schools, greater dependence on the nonprofit sector to develop and sustain urban health programs, and shrinking public sector funds to support what were once programs and services comprising a societal safety net (Takahashi, 1996). Such increasing privatization of health and welfare programs has impacts on families and households, as the demands of employment, family/households, and individual needs especially for low-income households mean daily trade-offs that often force individuals and communities to choose between a set of necessary needs (Roy, *et al.*, 2004). For urban planners, a governance perspective has meant a growing focus on the nonprofit/non-governmental sector, where organizations, communities, and individuals have strived to fill the gaps created by a retreating public sector, but also have increasingly become important actors in the development and enforcement of regulations. That is, non-governmental agencies, for example, health care organizations, foundations, and community-based organizations, have both experienced an expanding presence in service delivery, but also a growing influence in designing and enforcing regulations as they have become an important sector in health care design and delivery (Wolch, 1990).

These trends, referred to by urban planners as welfare state restructuring, have highlighted the political disagreements over the purpose and appropriate degree of intervention by public sector agencies. In general, the welfare state, most simply defined as the set of government agencies and institutions charged with using public resources for managing social welfare, has moved from the philosophy of striving for egalitarian social and economic conditions (through state centered programs and policies such as the New Deal) to a minimalist approach, particularly since the 1980s, promoting a minimum level of state intervention for social welfare or social programs aimed primarily at economic stability and social control (Gilbert, 1983). Welfare state restructuring, most notably initiated during the Reagan administration, consisted of narrowing eligibility requirements for using publicly funded and provided programs, shifting policy responsibility to state/local governments (called "new federalism") or more recently to non-governmental and community-based organizations (both faith-based and secular) and greater reliance on private sector mechanisms (privatization) (Palmer and Sawhill, 1982; Le Grand and Robinson, 1984).

What are the implications of welfare state restructuring for urban health? The shifting governance of the hospital system may provide clues to the future governance issues in urban health. Prior to the 20th century, hospitals were dependent on philanthropic capital, and with fluctuations in the growing industrial economy, such as economic downturns, donations correspondingly fluctuated (Bohland and Knox, 1989). Just as significant perhaps, philanthropists, because of their vital financial contributions, had important policy and governance roles in the operation of hospitals. In the 21st century, hospitals have had to cope with changing objectives to minimize treatment costs and maximize profits (McLafferty, 1989). Treatment decisions for private physical and mental health care providers are increasingly defined by the workplace, characterized by "the ability to pay for services and the need to have work-based insurance coverage" (Smith, 1989). While this is clearly a complex issue, what is important here is that the lens of governance provides a critical component to understanding urban health care systems and the obstacles and opportunities to addressing urban health.

2.4.2. *Institutional Management*

Institutional management refers to the challenges and opportunities inherent in the intra- and inter-organizational relationships that often define urban health care delivery. In the field of urban health, these would include the geographic placement of health care services and the institutional relationships within and across hospitals, clinics, and health care providers in a metropolitan area. Preventive health services, including health departments, community based advocacy and education organizations, and sewer authorities, sanitation districts, and vector control agencies are also vital parts of the urban health institutional framework. Here we discuss how urban health institutions might interact with urban planning institutions.

From an urban planning perspective, there are three primary organizational relationships that define intra- and inter-organizational relationships that apply to urban health agencies and researchers dealing with other agencies or organizations: *cooperation, collaboration, and conflict* (following Gaber, 1996). The first type of response, *cooperation,* is more reactive, and would for example occur when urban health professionals provided information when requested and insulation from urban design, economic development, or other urban planning researchers, practitioners, or policy makers. Cooperation might also be the response from urban planning agencies or researchers when approached by urban health professionals or scholars. The second type of behaviour, *collaboration,* entails a more proactive approach, for example, urban health professionals initiating conversations and then working with urban planning agencies to develop standardized procedures and data reporting methods across health and urban planning agencies and organizations, developing clear and formalized organizational connections among agencies, and outlining conflict resolution strategies. The third type of strategy, *conflict,* would also constitute a proactive stance, but opposite that of collaboration. With a conflict-centered strategy, urban health agencies would fight to maintain their autonomy and separation from decisions that steer urban design, economic development, or other perceived planning domains, and cooperate only when absolutely mandated to do so by law, regulation, or legislation. The same could be true for urban planning agencies when urban health policies or mandates breach what planners consider to be their political territory.

Though collaboration seems like the most desirable approach to take when thinking about bridging the divide between urban health and urban planning, there are also costs to consider when undertaking such a strategy. While collaboration offers the potential to leverage scarce resources, share information, and increase efficiency and effectiveness in service delivery, there are also significant challenges in designing and implementing such partnerships, including feeling of turf and territoriality, and difficulties in identifying and addressing differences in communications, organizational, and disciplinary styles and languages (Takahashi and Smutny, 2002).

2.5. Sustainability and Urban Planning

A final prevailing theme among planners is sustainability. Sustainability focuses on the whole of an urban environment, including resource usage, waste and pollution, economic conditions, the physical and mental health of residents, and the institutions, organizations, natural resources, income endowments, human capital, and social capital that influence all of those systems. Sustainability has taken on an increasingly important role as planners attempt to address the multi-faceted issues of environmental degradation and pollution, habitat regulation and protection, and environmental management in the context of economic growth/decline, urban design, equity and social justice, and governance. A sustainability approach might consist of for example encouraging reduction in water demand and the need for landfills through recycling and conservation, reducing air pollution through walking, bicycling, and use of public transit, and addressing the need for environmental justice across a myriad of environmental hazards and marginalized communities. The protection, development, and designation of greenspace, parks, and habitat for endangered species comprise primary activities within this approach. But in addition to these issues, sustainability also encompasses the development of so-called brownfields and formerly toxic sites*, the identification of uneven patterns of environmental risks and hazards that predominantly affect low-income neighbourhoods and communities of color (i.e., environmental disparities), the effective management of water and other natural resources, and the long-term planning of land development (including slow-growth and growth management policies, growth boundaries, and other strategies under the rubric of "smart growth"). What all these varied issues have in common is the keen recognition that growth and expansion cannot be sustained without a clear understanding of the environmental impacts of development, and that the conjoined relationship between development and environmental quality require that planning and, consequently urban health, require planning and program implementation that focuses on the longer term.

3.0. EXAMPLES OF URBAN PLANNING RESEARCH

In this section, we select studies by urban planners that illustrate the variety of ways that these various themes have been used. These studies by no means comprise a comprehensive literature review, but instead indicate possible means to bridge the divide between urban health and urban planning. Varying methods were used in these studies, as are used throughout planning research. In this section, we aim to highlight not only the variation in substantive focus (as organized using the themes discussed in the previous section), but also strive to show the distinct methodological approaches used to examine these urban planning issues.

3.1. Historical Approaches

In an article entitled "From Racial Zoning to Community Empowerment: The Interstate Highway System and the black Community in Birmingham, Alabama," Connerly (2002) argues that the interstate highway system in one city sustained the racial boundaries erected in a 1920s zoning law, but in addition, that these same federal programs also led to racial change as black were forced to relocate. Using the conceptual themes we outlined earlier in this chapter, this article addresses economic development, equity and social justice, and governance and institutional management. The methods used in this study primarily center on a case study approach, using historical methods (an analysis of archival documents, maps, and zoning regulations), mapping of socio-demographic and highway system characteristics, and descriptive statistics of Census data. Using this historical and qualitative approach, Connerly finds that the highway system in Birmingham designed in the late 1950s and constructed in the early 1960s negatively impacted local black neighbourhoods, and local and state agencies "manipulated the interstate highway program to perpetuate neighbourhood racial segregation". However, he also finds that

*Brownfields are older, often environmentally contaminated, land uses. These most commonly include industrial sites that pose health hazards to workers or nearby residents. More generally, brownfields refer to existing land uses that are being redeveloped – old or abandoned industrial or commercial sites, for example. While environmental contamination is not necessarily a feature of such sites, more lax environmental regulation and lower environmental awareness in decades past created circumstances that often link older land uses with contamination.

this highway program also facilitated racial change in Birmingham because the black population was "forced to relocate to other neighbourhoods", that advocates were very important in helping to protect civil rights, that grassroots mobilization was critical in efforts to lobby for services, and that these grassroots efforts exemplified a "long tradition of planning and self-determination in Birmingham's black community that took place outside of and in competition with the white-dominated traditional planning structure found in the city's planning department and housing authority". Such a study highlights the need not only to analyze the role of federal programs in local decision making processes, and the need to monitor equity outcomes in seemingly disparate policy efforts (such as transportation), but also that even within highly disadvantaged communities, there are opportunities for mobilization and political action.

This study also highlights the ways in which planning mirrors contemporary social tensions and perceptions. Though transportation planners do not often see themselves as social change agents or purveyors of social control, Connerly's study illustrates the ways in which urban planning policies and practices have direct consequences for urban health, oppression, and quality of life. As various planning scholars have argued, while urban planning as a profession has its foundation in reform movements, planning has also worked to protect private property, to maintain the status quo, and to protect existing relationships of power. For overviews on this issue, see Brooks (1988), Friedman (1987), or Beauregard (1989).

3.2. Interviews and Qualitative Approaches

Forsyth (2002), in an article entitled *Planning Lessons From Three U.S. New Towns of the 1960s and 1970s: Irvine, Columbia, and The Woodlands,* examined these three master-planned communities to determine the degree to which private sector experiments in design and development could effectively limit sprawl, support and enhance diversity, and facilitate sustainability. Using our urban planning themes, this study tackles the themes of economic development, urban design, equity and social justice, and sustainability. In this article, Forsyth uses a combination of interview data (140 interviews with developers, residents, and civic leaders, and 26 existing oral history interviews), descriptive statistics of national (census) and local (density data, existing resident surveys) datasets, and an analysis of maps and aerial photographs. She found that the three developments (Irvine, CA, Columbia, MD, and The Woodlands, TX) tended to meet smart growth goals for higher residential densities, but this higher density did not result in significantly higher use of public transit or reduced driving, that each of these communities tended to regulate the aesthetic quality of buildings and open space through the use of "architectural and land use covenants" that restrict the potential for altering or retrofitting these suburban landscapes," creating "pleasant and functional" settings, and that most residents in these developments tended to be middle class, though there is ethnic and some income mix (due in part to "government sponsored affordable housing"). She concluded that while these development types are effective at preserving habitat, improving building aesthetics, and creating areas that support a high quality of life, they have been less successful at achieving social equity and sustainability. This study makes clear that urban design is critically important in understanding quality of life, but that smart growth and new urbanist approaches (e.g., higher residential densities, pedestrian friendly streetscapes) may not result in reduced driving specifically or environmental sustainability more generally.

3.3. Quantitative Approaches

Boarnet and Crane (2001a; 2001b) used quantitative approaches to study the link between urban design and travel behaviour. They used detailed data on individual travel patterns for portions of Los Angeles, Orange, and San Diego counties in California. In various econometric models, Boarnet and Crane (2001a and 2001b) regressed the number of non-work car trips made by individuals on the individual's sociodemographic characteristics (e.g. age, number of children, gender, and income) and measures of urban design near the individual's home.*

This research combines the themes of economic development planning (as it relates to transportation), urban design, and sustainability. Boarnet and Crane's focus was on testing the idea, popularized by the New Urbanism, that dense, mixed-use developments along grid-oriented street patterns can reduce automobile travel. As part of the analysis, the authors developed measures of the grid-oriented character of the street network, population and employment densities, and proxies for land use mix, and used Geographic Information System (GIS) technology to match the values of those variables near each study subject's residence to the travel data for that subject. Using those data, and testing various econometric models, Boarnet and Crane (2001a; 2001b) found generally weak evidence that urban design elements influence the number of non-work automobile trips made by an individual.

In extensions of that work, Boarnet and Greenwald (2001) applied the same regression specification to travel data for individuals in Portland, Oregon. While the authors obtained results similar to the southern California study of Boarnet and Crane (2001a; 2001b) – namely that urban design characteristics were only weakly related to the number of non-work automobile trips – Greenwald and Boarnet (2002) found stronger evidence that urban design is associated with the number of non-work walking trips made by an individual. This research, coupled with various other studies on walking and urban form (e.g. Handy and Clifton, 2001), highlight a link between urban planning and urban health through the possible promotion of environments that encourage increased physical activity.†

3.4. Triangulation: Multiple Regression, Photographic Documentation, and Field Work/Participant Observation

An example of a study that uses multiple methods to assess a complex urban phenomenon is by Loukaitou-Sideris, *et al.*, (2002), in an article entitled *The Geography*

*The urban design measures included population and employment densities, the fraction of land characterized by mixed use zoning (commercial and residential uses allowed on the same city block), and the amount of the nearby street network that was grid-oriented (as measured by four-way intersections) as opposed to curvilinear streets with cul-de-sacs and three-way or other non-gridded intersections.

†These finding might seem inconsistent, but part of that can be explained by the change in focus from non-work automobile travel in Boarnet and Crane (2001a; 2001b) and Boarent and Greenwald (2001) to a focus on non-work walking travel in Greenwald and Boarnet (2002). One interpretation is that urban design elements are more robustly linked to walking trips than to driving trips. For a similar interpretation, see Greenwald (2003). More generally, the planning literature on urban design and travel behavior has reched differing conclusions due, in part, to differences in the way urban design is measured and variations in how travel is measured, e.g. as either number of trips, distance traveled, or choice of travel mode across automobile, transit, walking, and bicycling. See the reviews of this literature in Boarnet and Crane (2001b) and Ewing and Cervero (2001).

of Transit Crime: Documentation and Evaluation of Crime Incidence on and around the Green Line Stations in Los Angeles. The authors examined the link between the social and physical dimensions of the built environment in public transit stations (e.g. light rail and underground) and surrounding neighborhoods, and crime. The conceptual themes of interest in this study were economic development, urban design, and equity and social justice.

Multiple methods were used in this study to ascertain the built environment's role in explaining variations in crime at light rail stops. First, multiple regression is used to estimate the role of built environment elements on transit crime incidence using crime statistics, census and ridership data, and built environment attributes, such as the elements in and character of the stations (including proximity to park-and-ride lots and the existence of platforms) and surrounding neighborhoods (including land use patterns). Second, qualitative analysis in this study consisted of field work (including an environmental attribute inventory, that consisted of a standard list of physical elements that the authors have shown in previous work is associated with incidence of crime, such as fencing, visibility and lighting of station platforms, security hardware and equipment) and photographic documentation (to illustrate pictorially the types of built form elements that were associated with crime) and typology of transit station design. Finally, the study used mapping of environmental attributes to assess the spatial dimensions of crime and the built environment; this mapping included "adjoining land uses [to transit stations], the overall condition of the surrounding neighborhood, the concentration of undesirable places (e.g., bars, liquor stores, pawnshops, etc.), the visibility and lighting of platforms and park-and-rides, the flows of pedestrian and vehicular traffic, the degree of formal or informal station surveillance, the existence of fencing and security hardware and equipment at the station, the layout of the platform, and the type of linkages to the surrounding area." Linkages here refer to physical connections between the stations and nearby neighbourhoods, including, for example, street connectors or pedestrian bridges (Loudaitou-Siderias, *et al.*, 2002).

Using this multi-method approach, the authors found that in general crime rates and types (violent crimes against persons, or non-violent property based crimes) at stations were related to similar rates and types of crime in the surrounding neighbourhood. However, there were important specific connections between crime incidence at transit stations and the sociodemographic characteristics in the surrounding neighbourhood, the urban form characteristics of the surrounding neighbourhood, and transit station design. First, the regression and qualitative results indicated that "[c]rime at the [transit] platforms against people was strongly related to ridership – the busiest stations tended to concentrate the most serious crime" and that these crimes "(assaults, robberies) tended to happen primarily at the station platforms, elevators, and stairs" (Loukaitou-Sideris, *et al.*, 2002).* The multivariate regression models used census data and data from the environmental attribute survey to estimate the influence of various factors on crime rates at light rail stations along with the Green Line. The photographs were used to illustrate sta-

*Although this might seem to be a counterintuitive result, that is, that busier station platforms were related to more crime, this may be related to the low overall crive rates at these light rail stations (1.55 crime incidents per 100 riders). Like Sampson and Raudenbush (1999), the authors find that the relationship between environmental conditions and crime is not a simple direct relationship, but do argue that there are urban design factors that can reduce crime, creating a "station environment whose physical attributes contribute to its better security".

tion and neighbourhood types. Second, non-violent and property focused crimes such as vandalism were associated with neighborhoods with higher density, less than a high school education, higher proportions of youth, littered sidewalks, and buildings showing deterioration. The authors recommended a series of design and safety policies to reduce crime at transit stations, with the caveat that there were few reported crimes so these results should be treated with some caution: transit passenger safety should be broadened to include "the public environment that surrounds the station" and park-and-ride lots, designs should remove or minimize "entrapment spots and hiding places" and should increase visibility and lighting; regular security audits should be used by transit authorities to "reveal the hot spots of crime" and to "guide a targeted deployment of security personnel to the most dangerous stations during the most dangerous times". This study highlights the merit of using multiple methods to comprehensively examine complex urban issues, such as urban health. Urban design, urban problems, and health and well being are certainly intricately integrated issues, requiring that multi-method approaches and studies be considered and designed.

4.0. METHODOLOGICAL CHALLENGES IN URBAN PLANNING RESEARCH

Bridging urban health and urban planning requires an understanding of the use of methods in planning research. In this section, we describe the methods most commonly associated with each of the five planning themes identified earlier, while highlighting potential applications to health.

Urban planning is a diverse field. There is no single theory or disciplinary approach that informs planning. Similarly, planning draws on multiple methods, from many disciplines. These methods include quantitative approaches such as primary data collection surveys or secondary data analysis, with summaries drawn using descriptive statistics, and regression analysis or econometrics for inferences or hypothesis tests. The bulk of these quantitative empirical methods are informed by the traditions of economics or quantitative sociology or political science. The focus is often on testing hypotheses suggested by theory from social science disciplines related to planning, and often times linear regression models are built to allow researchers to focus on multi-variate relationships. Many variables in such regression models are included simply as controls for putative confounders, and planners often follow in the "hypothesis testing" tradition by focusing only on the coefficients on a few key variables that are specified a priori.

Keeping with the diverse nature of planning research, a large number of qualitative methods are also popular. These include case study approaches, in-depth interviews and focus groups, analysis of archival records, content analysis of media accounts, participant observation methods, and observations of the built environment. Of these, content analysis in particular can be approached from a quantitative perspective, and more generally the division between qualitative and quantitative methods is fluid, as several of the qualitative methods listed above can be approached with varying levels of numerical precision.

The methodological challenges faced by planners are, in the first measure, the challenges inherent in each method. The discussion here will focus on methodological approaches and challenges specific to linking planning and urban health. That discussion will be developed in relation to each of the five planning themes, but first we discuss a general challenge that applies to virtually all planning research. Health outcomes are rarely an intended focus of planning research. While this has begun to change in the past few years, and while there are exceptions (e.g., Conner, *et al.*, 2003; Diez Roux, 2003; Jackson, 2003; Northridge and Sclar, 2003; Takahashi, 1998; Takahashi, *et al.*, 2001), a primary challenge in linking urban planning and public health is incorporating a focus on health into planning research. This will require in part that planners use new data sources that, while common in the health community, are still rarely used within urban planning (see, e.g. Boarnet, 2004). This will include health data bases such as the Behavioral Risk Factor Surveillance System, National Health Interview Survey, and National Health and Nutrition Examination Survey. While those data sets will be useful, even more promising are other health data sets that allow researchers access to address information that provide an ability to link to characteristics of the built environment through geographic information systems. The National Longitudinal Survey of Adolescent Health and the California Health Interview Survey allow access to such detailed address information, although researchers must analyze the data at secure sites to preserve survey respondent confidentiality. For more information, see Boarnet (2004).

4.1. Economic Development

Economic development planning and associated fields such as transportation or infrastructure planning are among the most quantitative areas of planning research. The methods typically used in economic development planning are informed by economics, quantitative geography, and regional science. Regional Science is a field that combines perspectives from analytic geography and urban and regional economics. (See, for example, journals such as the *Journal of Regional Science* or *Papers in Regional Science.*) Regression analyses are common, and the focus is typically on testing hypotheses which are often derived from formal economic or geographic theory. This includes studies that have used various advanced applications in regression analysis, including panel data methods (e.g. Boarnet and Bogart, 1996), spatial econometrics (e.g. Boarnet, 1994), and simultaneous equations systems (e.g. Raphael and Rice, 2002; Wassmer and Anderson, 2001). (In health sciences, panel data are sometimes called longitudinal prospective designs. For the purposes of this chapter, panel data are data sets that tracks information on the same individual, city, state, group, or other unit of observation in each of several often regularly spaced time periods.) Simultaneous equation systems allow formal modeling of several variables that are endogenous or determined within the system. Urban health researchers might be more familiar with structural equation models, which is a similar approach.

The methodological challenges in these econometric studies fill textbooks (for example Johnston and Dinardo, 1997). Having noted that, the methodological challenges encountered and addressed in econometric research related to economic development planning typically fall into two categories: inferring causality and obtaining valid hypothesis tests.

4.1.1. *Inferring Causality*

Because the data for many planning studies are non-experimental, moving from association to inferences about causality is a key focus of many regression studies. The most common approach is to explicitly model the determinants of endogenous variables by using simultaneous equations methods. An example is the recent work of Raphael and Rice (2002), who while not planners *per se* studied a question that touches on an economic development issue within planning: does an individual's labour market experience depend on car ownership? In cities where automobiles are the dominant form of commuting, one might expect that car ownership might be linked to both the likelihood of being employed and an individual's wage. The difficulty is inferring the direction of causality. In automobile-oriented cities, owning a car can be both a determinant and a result of labour market success, since owning a car might be necessary to obtain access to geographically dispersed jobs not served by transit, while employment status also provides income to obtain a car. Raphael and Rice (2002) treat an individual's car ownership as an endogenous variable, and model the likelihood of car ownership with a separate regression that includes variables that are assumed to be exogenous to an individual's employment outcomes but that influence the likelihood that an individual owns a car. In particular, Raphael and Rice (2002) model car ownership as a function of state gasoline taxes and average state insurance premiums – both are variables that can influence an individual's decision to own a car but that are unlikely to have an effect on labour market outcomes. Raphael and Rice (2002) find that, after controlling for the effect of employment on the likelihood of owning a car, individuals who own a car are more likely to be employed. The statistical technique incorporates the two-way causality between car ownership and employment, modeling both variables within the system of equations. The results, because they control for the influence of employment on the likelihood of car ownership, give statistical point estimates that illuminate the impact of automobile ownership on the probability of being employed.* One implication is that labor market policies should be cognizant of the enabling role that car ownership plays in finding and retaining a job in the U.S.

4.1.2. Obtaining Valid Hypothesis Tests

There are several instances where ordinary least squares regression will not yield unbiased or consistent estimates of the standard errors of coefficients, and in those cases t-statistics are not valid and so hypothesis tests can be misleading (e.g., cases where regression error terms are not independent and identically distributed). A range of techniques adapts and extends regression analyses to provide valid t-statistics in cases where the classical ordinary least squares assumptions do not hold. One example is recent economic development research by Hansen, and colleagues, (2003). In that work, the authors studied whether recent graduates of Pittsburgh area universities stay in the region, to examine how that region can retain more of its highly educated workforce. The authors used a regression analysis to examine variables that are associated with a graduate's choice to stay or leave

*Note that this approach is designed to address circumstances where two variables might both cause each other but only cross-sectional data are available. The philosophical approach inherent in simultaneous equations systems does not rely strictly on temporal precedence to determine causality, because in non-experimental settings it will often not be possible to obtain data that establish temporal precedence. More importantly, given foresight on the part of behavioral actors, temporal precedence may not give a clear signal of causality. For example, persons may buy a car in anticipation of soon getting a job, but if the expectation of a future job offer was important in the decision to buy the car, employment can still be said to have caused the purchase of the automobile, even though the car purchase preceded employment. For a more detailed discussion of causal inference in the behavioral sciences, see, e.g., Cook and Campbell (1979).

the Pittsburgh metropolitan area. Because ordinary least squares modeling gives biased estimates of regression standard errors when the dependent variable is a dichotomous variable (e.g. "stay" or "leave" the Pittsburgh area), the authors used logistic regression analysis. (Other dichotomous outcome or categorical data analytic techniques include ordinal regression, polychotomous regression, and survival methods.) Hansen, and colleagues (2003) found that, among the individuals surveyed, persons with graduate degrees who were concerned about the cost of living and who valued family ties more strongly were more likely to stay in the Pittsburgh metropolitan area, while persons concerned about salary were more likely to leave the region. The college that a person attended was also a statistically significant predictor of the likelihood of staying in the Pittsburgh area, with Duquesne graduates being more likely to stay compared to University of Pittsburgh graduates, while graduates from Carnegie Mellon were more likely to leave the region, again compared to University of Pittsburgh graduates.

4.2. Urban design

Methodological approaches in planning research related to urban design have been influenced primarily by architectural thought. This includes methods that focus on normative, or non-positivist approaches, descriptive research, typologies, and attempts to measure urban design in ways that are objective and reproducible. (Non-positivist approaches do not follow classical deductive logic, and so do not test hypotheses. Non-positivist approaches can include inductive case study methods or theoretical statements of appropriate policies or plans without reference to empirical analysis.) These approaches range from those that grapple with the aesthetics of the environment, with few intentions to inform research modeled on scientific method to techniques that are self-conscious attempts to apply or mimic scientific method (attempts to measure urban design in ways that create variables for hypothesis testing).

While the non-positivist approaches might seem foreign to urban health researchers, it is important to understand that scholarship that is explicitly aesthetic and normative follows a long tradition of architectural influence in urban design. The goal in this work is often less about measurement than about developing criteria to understand, classify, and reproduce what Kevin Lynch called, in the title of his 1981 classic, "good city form". The judgments about appropriate design criteria are based on argument, theory, and persuasion, but often lack the systematic quantitative data analysis characteristic of many branches of the social sciences.

Kevin Lynch's (1981) work is a classic example of normative theory development related to urban design. Lynch (1981) examined normative theories of good city form implicit in thought and development patterns from a broad range of historical time periods and cultural settings, and then developed his own theory of city form. That theory is a deep discussion of seven criteria – vitality, sense, fit, access, control, efficiency, and justice. According to Lynch (1981), those seven criteria capture basic dimensions that can be used to judge the quality of cities. Lynch's (1981) criteria include a broad range of factors too diverse to discuss fully here. To give one a flavour of the scope of Lynch's (1981) criteria, his theory touches on the biological (the degree to which a city supports vital functions of human beings and other species), the aesthetic (the link between a city's urban form and the sensory perceptions of residents), and the economic (the cost, construed more broadly than simple monetary cost, of maintaining a city and the distribution of costs and benefits that the city confers on persons). Lynch (1981) articulates each of his seven criteria in detail, building a normative theory and explaining how that theory can be applied to judge the quality of cities.

Unlike efforts at pure theory construction, some normative work on urban design uses experts to judge the quality of particular projects or ideas. This is similar to the use of juries in architecture, where experts judge the quality of a particular project. Juries are a common way to choose design teams for buildings, large developments, and major public projects. The use of a jury as part of the selection of the team to lead the reconstruction of the World Trade Center is a well known recent example (see, e.g., Ouroussof, 2002, for a description of the designs selected by the initial part of that jury process). The concept of judging urban design by either expert evaluation or based on theory and aesthetics extends into planning research that advocates particular design styles. Examples of such advocacy include the writings of the New Urbanists such as Duany and Plater-Zyberk (1991) and Talen and Ellis (2002). In this school of thought, the goal is not to gather data, make measurements, and test hypotheses, but to critique designs based on theory or aesthetics and to articulate criteria for recognizing preferred urban designs.

Given the normative focus in urban design, it is not surprising that when urban design research is more data oriented, the use of data is often descriptive. When planners who study urban design systematically measured the built environment, some of the earliest attempts included typologies to classify types of built environments and types of interactions with the built environment. More recently, planners have developed typologies to measure and characterize urban sprawl (e.g. Ewing, *et al.*, 2002, or for related work in public health, see, e.g., Dannenberg, 2003, or Jackson, 2003).

Following on the research that describes and categorizes the built environment, a growing literature has studied ways to measure urban design characteristics. Much of this research attempts to systematically measure the built environment in ways that allow researchers to test hypotheses about the built environment. Examples include Loukaitou-Sideris (1999), who studied how urban design characteristics are linked to crime near bus stops in Los Angeles, and whose work was also discussed earlier in this chapter. This style of research applies the traditional hypothesis testing and scientific method focus familiar to public health research in ways that incorporate urban design. If the built environment is an object of hypothesis testing, then the built environment must be measured in ways that are objective and can be reproduced. Fields related to urban health have contributed to advancing the measurement of the built environment in recent years. Some public health researchers who study physical activity have developed audit methods to measure the built environment by having teams of observers answer questions about urban design on a block-by-block basis (e.g. Pikora, *et al.*, 2002). Other research projects, currently underway, seek to extend that work (e.g. current research funded by the Robert Wood Johnson Foundation, 2004). As part of this work, the measurement focus typical of public health research is being adapted to the study of urban design. In particular, some studies have examined issues such as inter-rater reliability in the use of audit instruments (Pikora, *et al.*, 2002).

The studies that attempt to systematically measure the built environment are of most immediate utility in linking urban health and planning. Several studies have attempted to link travel patterns, including active travel such as walking or bicycling, to characteristics of the built environment (e.g. Handy and Clifton, 2001; Greenwald and Boarnet, 2002). Such studies include, by necessity, measures of the built environment, and the recent round of built environment audit instruments (e.g. Pikora, 2002 or the ongoing studies described at Active Living Research, 2004) are intended to provide methods for measuring the built environment in ways that can support urban health research.

4.2.1. Equity and Social Justice

Like research into urban design, planning research in the area of equity and social justice falls into two categories – normative and positive. (Here we adopt language typical of economics, and positive is distinct from the discussion of non-positivist research methods described earlier. Normative and positive research approaches, in this context, are defined below.)

The normative research, like its counter-part in urban design, articulates theories about power relationships, economic structures, and interprets those ideas while advocating for changes that the authors argue will lead to more just arrangements. Such work often critiques government policies that lie at the intersection of the economy and the welfare state. Examples include the work of Castells (1979), and Davis (1990).While compelling work, especially in its examination of the political economy of modern cities, the links to empirically based urban health research are not as direct as the empirical (or positive) research that follows similar themes.

Positive research on equity and social justice has burgeoned in recent years. Much of this work in planning has leveraged Geographic Information System (GIS) technology to track the geographic nature of patterns of inequality in urban areas. This includes access or proximity to transportation infrastructure and, through that access, job opportunities (e.g. Shen, 2001), spatial patterns of inequality (e.g. Rey, 2004), and the geographic pattern of proximity to environmental hazards (e.g., Forkenbrock and Schweitzer, 1999; Lejano and Iseki, 2001).

One particularly rapidly growing area of empirical urban planning research related to social justice is commonly called "environmental justice." Research on environmental justice has been motivated by the observation that environmental hazards often are clustered near low income or minority populations, exposing those less politically powerful groups to larger than average environmental risks (Bryant, 1995; Mohai and Bryant, 1992). Advances in GIS technology have made it possible to map the spatial pattern of environmental risk. This research has a clear link to health, and that link could be made stronger by combining planning's focus on the spatial distribution of environmental hazards with research on health outcomes.

4.2.2. Governance and Institutional Management

Research on governance and institutional management includes both quantitative and case study approaches. Quantitative approaches include statistical or econometric studies of particular types of government behaviour. This includes studies that examine how local government support for public housing relates to characteristics of that government (e.g. Basolo, 1999) and a large literature in economics that examines the determinants of government tax and spending patterns (e.g. Boarnet and Glazer, 2002; Case, *et al.*, 1993). Yet most planning research in the area of governance relates to questions about non-governmental sectors and institutional management. Research in this area includes a strong case study component.

The case study methodology uses an in-depth examination of particular cities, policies, or organizations. The research approach is often informed by qualitative methods (e.g. Feldman, 1995), even when the methods include quantitative approaches. As opposed to the deductive, hypothesis testing framework typical of much research on economic development topics within planning, case study methods in this area are inductive in nature. Conclusions are drawn from deep knowledge, rather than random samples, and generalization is often not to a larger population but to theories.

4.2.3. *Sustainability*

The methods used in sustainability research draw broadly from the techniques outlined above. Much sustainability research is linked to environmental issues, and so sustainability studies often draw on tools and methods that are common in planning research related to environmental topics. This includes the use of GIS data, attention to spatial detail, and quantitative approaches. Some examples of sustainability research use regression analysis to test hypotheses. Other examples use case study approaches or detailed evaluations of plans and archival documents (e.g. Berke and Conroy, 2000).

The methodological challenges in linking this work to health include challenges inherent in measuring complex systems. The concept of sustainability is inherently ecological, seeking to model the interaction of a large number of systems. The challenges in this research include difficulties in theorizing, modeling, and measuring the interaction of complex environmental and social systems that are imperfectly understood. This includes difficulties that range from the interface of particular systems to the challenge inherent in studying the full scope of the entire urban system.

As an example of sustainability research, problems of urban runoff lie at the interface of complex systems related to planning and urban health. As the developed, and hence paved, footprint of metropolitan areas grows, storm water runoff that previously filtered through wetlands or aquifers increasingly travels unobstructed to rivers, lakes or oceans (see, e.g., the U.S. Environmental Protection Agency, 2004) washes pollutants into water sources. Designing policy approaches that better manage this problem requires understanding the links between hydrology, water-borne pollutant transfer, and urban development (U.S. Environmental Protection Agency, 2002). The health impacts of storm-water runoff are discussed in, e.g., Gaffield, *et al.*, (2003).

A similarly complex sustainability challenge is the problem of urban heat islands. Urban areas retain daytime heat more efficiently than do rural areas and thus cities have average temperatures that are higher than non-urbanized areas in the same climate. Stone (2004) notes that in the context of debates about climate change, localized temperature changes due to metropolitan development patterns can have implications for air quality. Combining traits of sustainability studies and urban design measurement (via GIS), Stone and Rodgers (2001) assess the link between urban form and the heat island effect.

5.0. FUTURE DIRECTIONS

Urban planning has strong potential links to the study of urban health, yet those links have until recently largely been unnoticed by both planners and urban health specialists. This is in some ways ironic, given that the fields of urban planning and urban health have common roots in concerns about health conditions in overcrowded tenements at the turn of the 19th Century. At that time, the link between cities as objects of planning, urban design, and governance and health problems related to communicable diseases, nutrition, housing and workplace conditions, and mental well-being seemed obvious. Now, a century later, attention is again focused on the link between planning's focus on the health of cities and urban health's focus on the well-being of city residents.

We highlighted several links between the objects of planning study and urban health. To recap, we note again examples from each of the five planning themes discussed in this chapter. Economic development planners study topics that relate to employment opportunities and hence the distribution of wealth, poverty, and access to transportation, public services, and housing in urban areas. All have implications for physical and mental health. Urban design – a field sometimes dominated by a study of aesthetics – has links to a host of environmental and health impacts. A growing body of research now analyzes the link between the design of neighbourhoods and physical activity and obesity, water shed quality (through, for example, urban runoff), and air quality (through driving patterns and heat island effects). For an example, see the special issue of the *American Journal of Public Health*, September 2003, devoted to health and planning. The December 2003 issue of the *Journal of Urban Health* also includes a series of articles on the links between health and planning.

The theme of equity and social justice has links to health outcomes, especially as that theme relates to access to public services or environmental risks. Research on environmental justice often explicitly examines the link between exposure to health risk and settlement patterns in urban areas. Planning research related to governance and institutional management often studies implementation issues related to the practice of solving problems at the intersection of urban health and urban planning. Sustainability, with its focus on the interaction of environmental, economic, social, and governance systems, might be viewed as an attempt to understand the broad "urban ecology" that ties together many of the other themes discussed here.

Building a more direct link between planning and urban health research will require some attention to methodological and research issues. The most important issue is incorporating health as an outcome in planning studies. Planners often focus on problems that touch on human health, but planning research typically stops short of measuring health as an outcome. Instead, planners have assumed that the health implications of their work will be addressed by other fields. Urban health research, in turn, often does not make an explicit link to the elements of urban planning that are, in part, underlying cause or potential solution to the health problems under study. To solidify the link between urban planning and urban health research, researchers from both fields should work to include both health outcomes and the objects of planning practice in the same studies.

This will require, in some cases, the use of spatially coded health outcome data. Tools such as GIS and spatial statistics will be useful in handling geographic characteristics of health data. To link health outcomes to the built environment, planners and public health researchers should continue to refine methods to objectively measure urban design.

Beyond measurement and methodological issues, planning and urban health researchers will need to learn to bridge the gap in their empirical research approaches. Quantitative planning studies typically focus on hypothesis testing, with less emphasis on questions of relative risk, and hence magnitude, that are common on public health. Planners often use case studies and other inductive techniques, since such approaches are necessary for the topics that planners study. Planning's use of secondary data has led to a tradition where questions of data and measurement – including the validity and reliability of measures – are not examined as commonly as in public health. In planning research, secondary data are often obtained from large surveys (such as the U.S. census), and individual researchers have little input into the form of the questionnaires. These and other differences between the fields will lead to some need to communicate across methodological gaps, but those gaps are already being closed in some of the studies discussed in this chapter.

A century ago, the links between urban health and the built environment gave birth to the fields of public health and urban planning. After having drifted apart, researchers from both fields are now working to bridge the gap between the two fields. Much can be learned from integrating public health and planning research. This chapter has outlined some recent advances in linking urban health and planning scholarship, while pointing the way toward future progress.

REFERENCES

Active Living Research Web Site, 2004, San Diego, CA (June 11, 2004); http://www.activelivingresearch.org.

AICP (American Planning Association, American Institute of Certified Planners website), 2004, Washington D.C., (May 22, 2004); www.planning.org/aicp.

Arnstein, S.R. (1969). A Ladder of Citizen Participation. *J. Am. Inst. Plann.* 35:216–244.

Banerjee, T. (2001). The Future of Public Space: Beyond Invented Streets and Reinvented Places. *J. Am. Plann. Assoc.* 67(1):9–24.

Basolo, M.V. (1999). The Impacts of Intercity Competition and Intergovernmental Factors on Local Affordable Housing Expenditures. *Housing Policy Debate* 10(3):659–688.

Beauregard, R. A. (1989). Between Modernity and Postmodernity: The Ambiguous Position of U.S. Planning. *Environment and Planning D: Society and Space* 7:381–395.

Berke, P., and Conroy, M.M. (2000). Are We Planning for Sustainable Development? An Evaluation of 30 Comprehensive Plans. *J. Am. Plann. Assoc.* 66(1):21–33.

Boarnet, M.G. (1994). The Monocentric Model and Employment Location. *Journal of Urban Economics* 36(1): 79-97.

Boarnet, M. G. (2004). The Built Environment and Physical Activity: Empirical Methods and Data Resources. Paper prepared for the Transportation Research Board and the Institute of Medicine Committee on Physical Activity, Health, Transportation, and Land Use. In press.

Boarnet, M.G., and Bogart, W.T. (1996). Enterprise Zones and Employment: Evidence From New Jersey. *J. Urb. Econ.* 40(2):198–215.

Boarnet, M.G., and Amihai, G. (2002). Federal Grants and Yardstick Competition. *J. Urb. Econ.* 52(1):53–64.

Boarnet, M.G., and Crane, R. (2001a). The Influence of Land Use on Travel Behavior: Empirical Strategies. *Transportation Research* 35A(9):823–845.

Boarnet, M.G., and Crane, R. (2001b). *Travel by Design: The Influence of Urban Form on Travel.* Oxford University Press, Oxford, England.

Boarnet, M.G., and Greenwald, M. (2001). Land Use, Urban Design, and Non-Work Travel: Reproducing for Portland, Oregon Empirical Tests from Other Urban Areas. *Transportation Research Record* 1722:27–37.

Bohland, J., and Paul L.K. (1989). Growth of Proprietary Hospitals in the United States: A Historical Geographic Perspective. In: Scarpaci, J.L., (ed.), *Health Services Privatization in Industrial Societies.* Rutgers University Press, New Brunswick, NJ, pp. 27–64.

Bonnefoy, X.R., Braubach, M., Moissonnier, B., Monolbaev, K., and Robbel, N. (2003). Housing and Health in Europe: Preliminary Results of a Pan-European Study 93(9):1559–1563.

Brooks, M.P. (1988). Four Critical Junctures in the History of the Urban Planning Profession. *J. Am. Plann. Assoc.* 54:241–248.

Bryant, B. (1995). *Environmental Justice: Issues, Policies, and Solutions.* Island Press, Washington D.C.

Case, A.C., Hines, J.R., and Rosen, H.S. (1993). Budget spillovers and fiscal policy interdependence-evidence from the states. *Journal of Public Economics* 52:285–307.

Castells, M. (1979). *The Urban Question: A Marxist Approach.* MIT Press, Cambridge, MA.

CDC, 2004, Atlanta, GA, (September 10, 2004); http://www.cdc.gov/health/disparities.htm.

Cohen, U., and Day, K. (1993). *Contemporary environments for people with dementia.* Johns Hopkins University Press, Baltimore, MD.

Conner, R.F., Tanjasiri, S.P., Dempsey, C., Robles, G., Davidson, M., and Easterling, D. (2003). The Colorado Healthy Communities Initiative: Communities Defining and Addressing Health. In: Easterling, D., Gallagher, K., and Lodwick, D., (eds.), *Promoting Health at the Community Level.* Sage Publications, Thousand Oaks, CA.

Connerly, C. E. (2002). From Racial Zoning to Community Empowerment: The Interstate Highway System and the African American Community in Birmingham, Alabama. *Journal of Planning Education and Research* 22:99–114.

Cook, T.D., and Campbell, D.T. (1979). *Quasi-experimentation: Design and analysis issues for field settings.* Houghton-Mifflin Company, Boston, MA.

Dannenberg, A.L., 2003, Impacts of Sprawl and Community Design on Public Health. Presentation Archive, http://www.uic.edu/sph/cade/asph2003/morning.htm.

Davidoff, P. (1965). Advocacy and Pluralism in Planning. *J. Am. Inst. Plann.* 31:596–615.

Davis, M. (1990). *City of Quartz: Excavating the Future in Los Angeles.* Verso, New York, NY.

Diez-Roux, A.V. (2003). Residential Environments and Cardiovascular Risk. *J. Urban Health* 80(4): 569–589.

Duany, A., and Plater-Zyberk, E. (1991). *Towns and Town-Making Principles.* Rizzoli, New York, NY.

Evans, G.W. (2003). The Built Environment and Cardiovascular Risk. *J. Urban Health* 80(4):569–589.

Evans, G.W., Wells, N.M., and Moch, A. (2003). Housing and Mental Health: A Review of the Evidence and a Methodological and Conceptual Critique. *J. Soc. Iss.* 59:475–500.

Ewing, R., Pendall, R., and Chen, D. (2002). *Measuring Sprawl and Its Impact.* Smart Growth America, Washington D.C.

Ewing, R., and Cervero, R. (2001). Travel and the Built Environment: A Synthesis. *Transportation Research Record.* 1780:87–113.

Feldman, M. S. (1995). *Strategies for Interpreting Qualitative Data.* Sage, Newbury.

Forkenbrock, D., and Schweitzer, L. (1999). Environmental Justice and Transportation Planning. *J. Am. Plann. Assoc.* 65(1):96–111.

Forsyth, A. (2002). Planning lessons from Three U.S. New Towns of the 1960s and 1970s: Irvine, Columbia, and The Woodlands. *J. Am. Plann. Assoc.* 68(4):387–415.

Friedmann, J. (1987). *Planning in the Public Domain: From Knowledge to Action.* Princeton University Press, Princeton, NJ.

Gaber, S.L. (1996). From NIMBY to Fair Share: The Development of New York City's Municipal Shelter Siting Policies, 1980-1990. *Urban Geogr.* 17:294–316.

Gaffield, S.J., Goo, R.L., Richards, L.A., and Jackson, R.J. (2003). Public Health Effects of Inadequately Managed Stormwater Runoff. *Am. J. Public Health* 93(9):1527–1533.

Gilbert, N. (1983). *Capitalism and the Welfare State: Dilemmas of Social Benevolence.* Yale University Press, New Haven, CT.

Greenwald, M. J. (2003). The Road Less Traveled: New Urbanist Inducements to Travel Mode Substitution for Nonwork Trips. *Journal of Planning Education and Research* 23(1): 39–57.

Greenwald, M., and Boarnet, M.G. (2002). The Built Environment as a Determinant of Walking Behavior: Analyzing Non-Work Pedestrian Travel in Portland, Oregon. *Transportation Research Record* 1780:33–42.

Handy, S.L., Boarnet, M.G., Ewing, R., and Killingsworth, R.E. (2002). How the built environment affects physical activity: views from urban planning. *Am. J. Prev. Med.* 23:64-73.

Handy, S., and Clifton, K. (2001). Local Shopping as a Strategy for Reducing Automobile Travel. *Transportation* 28(4):317–346.

Hansen, S. B., Ban, C., and Huggins, L. (2003). Explaining the "Brain Drain" from Older Industrial Cities: The Pittsburgh Region. *Economic Development Quarterly* 17(2):132–147.

Jackson, R. J. (2003). The Impact of the Built Environment on Health: An Emerging Field. *Am. J. Public Health* 93(9):1382–1384.

Jacobs, J. (1961). *The death and life of great American cities.* Random House, New York, NY.

Johnston, J., and DiNardo, J. (1997). *Econometric Methods.* McGraw-Hill, New York, NY.

Kennedy, P. (1985). *A guide to econometrics.* MIT Press, Cambridge, MA.

Law, R., and Wolch, J.R. (1991). Homelessness and Economic Restructuring. *Urban Geogr.* 12(2):105–136.

Le Grand, J., and Robinson, R. (1984). *Privatization and the Welfare State.* George Allen & Unwin, London, England, pp. 1–24.

Lejano, R., and Iseki, H. (2001). Environmental Justice: Spatial Distribution of Hazardous Waste Treatment, Storage, and Distribution Facilities in Los Angeles. *Journal of Urban Planning and Development* 127(2):51–62.

Loukaitou-Sideris, A. (1999). Hot Spot of Bus Stop Crime: The Importance of Environmental Attributes. *J. Am. Plann. Assoc.* 65(4):395–411.

Loukaitou-Sideris, A., Liggett, R., and Iseki, H. (2002). The Geography of Transit Crime: Documentation and Evaluation of Crime Incidence on and around the Green Line Stations in Los Angeles. *Journal of Planning Education and Research* 22:135–151.

Lynch, K. (1981). *A theory of good city form.* MIT Press, Cambridge, MA.

McLafferty, S.L. (1989). The Politics of Privatization: State and Local Politics and the Restructuring of Hospitals in New York City. In: Scarpaci, J.L., (ed.), *Health Services Privatization in Industrial Societies.* Rutgers University Press, New Brunswick, NJ, pp.130–151.

Mohai, P., and Bryant, B. (1992). Race, Poverty, and the Environment. *EPA Journal* 18(1):6–8.

National Academy Council, Committee on Physical Activity, Health, Transportation, and Land Use, Project, 2004, Identification Number: SAIS-P-02-04-A, (May 20, 2004); http://www4.nas.edu/webcr.nsf.

Northridge, M. E., and Sclar, E. (2003). A Joint Planning and Public Health Framework: Contributions to Health Impact Assessment. *Am. J. Public Health* 93(1):118–121.

Ouroussoff, N. (2002). At Last, Designs that Will Stand the Test of Time. *Los Angeles Times* December 19, 2002, pp. A40 and A41.

Palmer, J.L., and Sawhill, I.V. (1982). Perspectives on the Reagan Experiment. In: Palmer, J.L. and Sawhill, I.V, (eds.), *The Reagan Experiment.* The Urban Institute, Washington D.C., pp.1–30.

Pikora, T. J., Fiona, C.L., Bull, K.J., Knuiman, M., Giles-Corti, B., and Donovan, R.J. (2002). Developing a Reliable Audit Instrument to Measure the Physical Environment for Physical Activity. *Am. J. Prev. Med.* 23(3):187–194.

Raphael, S., and Lorien R. (2002). Car Ownership, Employment, and Earnings. *J. Urban Economics* 52:109–130.

Rey, S. J. (2004). Spatial Analysis of Regional Economic Growth, Inequality, and Change. In: Goodchild, M.F., and Janelle, D.G., (eds.), *Spatially Integrated Social Sciences.* Oxford University Press, Oxford, England.

Robert Wood Johnson Foundation, 2004, Princeton, NJ, (October 12, 2004); http://www.activelivingresearch.org/index. php/Measurement%20Studies/166.

Roy, K.M., Tubbs, C.Y., and Burton, L.M. (2004). Don't Have No Time: Daily Rhythms and the Organization of Time for Low Income Families. *Family Relations* 53(2):168–178.

Sampson, R. J., and Raudenbush, S.W. (1999). Systematic Social Observation of Public Spaces: A New Look at Disorder in Urban Neighborhoods. *Am. J. Soc.* 105(3):603–651.

Shen, Q. (2001). A Spatial Analysis of Job Openings and Access in a U.S. Metropolitan Area. *J. Am. Plann. Assoc.* 67(1):53–68.

Smith, C. J. (1989). The Restructuring of Mental Health Care in the United States. In: Scarpaci, J.L., (ed.), *Health Services Privatization in Industrial Societies.* University Press, New Brunswick, NJ, pp. 155–181.

Stone, B. Jr. (2004). Urban heat and Air Pollution: An Emerging Role for Planners in the Climate Change Debate. *J. Am. Plann. Assoc.* In press.

Stone, B. Jr., and Rodgers, M.O. (2001). Urban Form and Thermal Efficiency: How the Design of Cities Influences the Urban Heat Island Effect. *J. Am. Plann. Assoc.* 67(2):186-198.

Takahashi, L.M. (1996). A Decade of Understanding Homelessness: From Characterization to Representation. *Progress in Human Geography* 29(3):291–310.

Takahashi, L.M. (1998). *Homelessness, AIDS, and Stigmatization: The NIMBY Syndrome at the End of the Twentieth Century.* Oxford University Press, Oxford, England.

Takahashi, L.M., Wiebe, D., and Rodriguez, R. (2001). Navigating the Time-Space Context of HIV and AIDS: Daily Routines and Access to Care. *Soc. Sci. Med.* 53:845–863.

Takahashi, L.M., and Smutny, G. (2002). Collaborative Windows and Organizational Governance: Exploring the Formation and Demise of Social Service Partnerships. *Nonprofit and Voluntary Sector Quarterly* 31(2):165–185.

Talen, E. (1998). Visualizing Fairness: Equity Maps for Planners. *J. Am. Plann. Assoc.* 64(1):22–38.

Talen, E., and Ellis, C. (2002). Beyond Relativism: Reclaiming the Search for Good City Form. *Journal of Planning Education and Research* 22: 36-49.

UCLA Department of Urban Planning, 2004, Los Angelos, CA, (May 22, 2004); http://www.sppsr.ucla.edu/dup.

Umemoto, K. (2001). Walking in Another's Shoes: Epistemological Challenges in Participatory Planning. *Journal of Planning Education and Research* 21:17–31.

U.S. Environmental Protection Agency, 2004, Washington D.C., (October11, 2004); http://www.epa.gov/OWOW/NPS/facts/point7.htm

U.S. Environmental Protection Agency, 2002, Washington D.C, (June, 3, 2002); http://www.epa.gov/owow/nps.

Wassmer, R.W., and Anderson, J.E. (2001). Bidding for Business: New Evidence on the Effect of Locally Offered Economic Development Incentives in a Metropolitan Area. *Economic Development Quarterly* 15(2):132–148.

Wolch J. (1990). *The Shadow State: Government and Voluntary Sector in Transition.* The Foundation Center, New York, NY.

Chapter 20

Environmental Health Studies

Environmental Health Methods for Urban Health

Jonathan M. Samet and Joseph H. Abraham

1.0. INTRODUCTION

The potential for environmental exposures in cities to affect human health adversely is well documented; the examples range from devastating disasters, such as the London Fog of 1952, to far more subtle but equally tragic exposures, such as lead exposures of children in urban settings. Environmental agents contribute measurably to society's burden of acute and chronic diseases and to diminished quality of life. The adverse effects of environmental agents have long been a focus of societal concern and research, and regulatory and non-regulatory approaches are in place throughout the world to protect the public from environmental pollutants. While many diseases are multi-factorial in etiology, with etiologic factors including not only environmental agents but susceptibility-determining genes, the environmental contribution to the disease burden is potentially subject to control and environmental polluters threaten a common good: the public's health.

For people living in urban environments, there is particular and justifiable concern about the environment and health (Table 1). A confluence of factors increases the potential for exposure to environmental agents, and sources of pollution are often visible and inescapable. Additionally, in conceptualizing "the environment," the boundaries are broad, taking in not only pollutants, but the characteristics of work, housing, and leisure locations, and the nature of the food and water supplies. Within the field of environmental health, the focus has long been on specific pollutants which contaminate the three media – air, water, and soil – and also on radiation. However, for urban as for other environments, a broader framework is needed that sets out the interactions of people with these media, as activity patterns are determined by the physical and social contexts (Figure 1). For example, urban dwellers may have access only to areas for exercise that are adjacent to sources of pollution, such as roads or factories, and they may not be able to improve the quality of air in a rented apartment. Research on the health consequences of environmental

Table 1. Examples of Environmental Contaminants Found in the Urban Environment

Media	Source	Agents	Effects
Outdoor air	Automobile/Truck Exhaust	Polycyclic aromatic Hydrocarbons	Carcinogenic Respiratory/Cardiovascular
		Particulate matter	Neuro-cognitive Respiratory
		Nitrogen oxides Particulate matter	Respiratory/Cardiovascular
	Power Generation	Volatile organic Compounds Lead	Neuro-cognitive
Indoor air	Environmental Tobacco Smoke	Polycyclic Aromatic Hydrocarbons Particulate Matter	Respiratory
			Respiratory
	Pests	Cockroach Allergen Rodent Allergen	Respiratory
Dust/Soil	Manufacturing, Industrial Processing	Methylmercury	Neuro-cognitive
Water	Disinfection of drinking water	Trihalomethane	Carcinogenic
	Manufacturing, industrial processing	Methylmercury	Neuro-cognitive

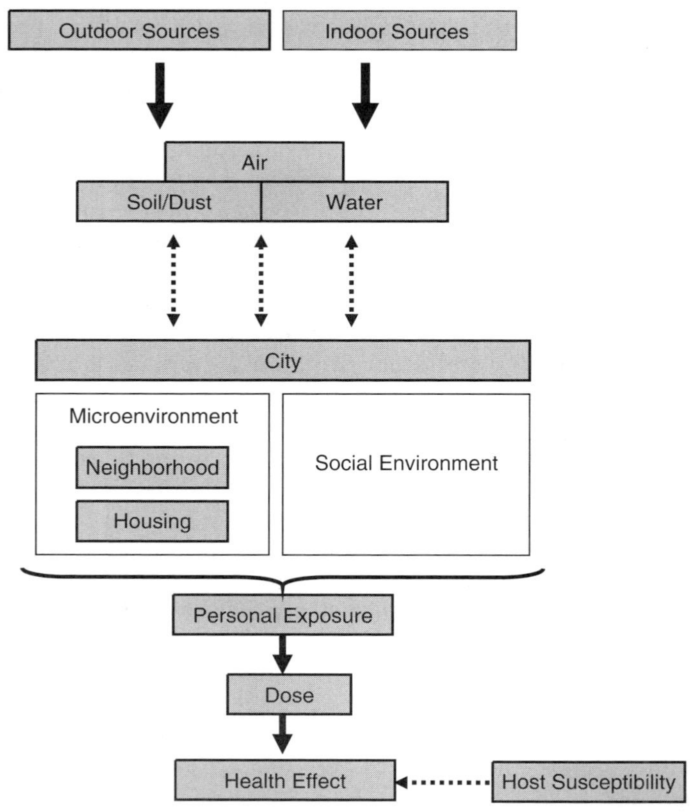

Figure 1. Conceptual Framework.

agents needs to acknowledge and incorporate these interactions and is thus inherently multidisciplinary and integrative.

In recent decades, substantial emphasis has been given to the overlay of environmental exposures, particularly within urban areas, and the socioeconomic characteristics of the population. In many settings, an unfortunate pattern has been demonstrated with socioeconomically disadvantaged persons sustaining the greatest burden of environmental exposures in reflection of the distribution of traffic, industry, and inadequate housing. This recognition led to the emergence of the "environmental justice" movement and a research agenda on the consequences of the additional jeopardy arising from the confluence of adverse environmental exposures on the disadvantaged (American Lung Association, 2001) The investigation of social and economic factors leading to exposure is now recognized as a key component of environmental health research.

This chapter addresses environmental health methods developed to identify and characterize the impact of environmental exposures on human health, with a focus on applications to urban health. In this chapter, we will provide a general framework for conceptualizing exposures to environmental agents and a description of methodologies used to assess their impacts on human health. We will consider the application of environmental health methods to the study of urban health in substantive areas defined by the primary media through which urban environmental hazards are conveyed for human exposure. Specific methodologies are covered, along with their limitations. We offer several examples, including the problem of asthma in inner-city children, now widely referred to as "inner-city asthma;" particulate air pollution in the air of cities; and exposures of urban children to carcinogens.

We also introduce readers to the scientific disciplines that are relevant to urban environmental health. Although environmental health science is considered an academic discipline in and of itself, gaining an understanding the relationship between a toxic agent and the health of the population is a multidisciplinary process involving toxicologists, exposure assessors, epidemiologists, and risk assessors. Toxicologists use controlled exposures to identify whether agents have toxicity in bioassays and also to identify mechanisms of action. Modern toxicology explores the uptake, distribution, and metabolism of environmental agents and characterizes mechanisms of injury, often at the molecular level. This mechanistic information is critical to the extrapolation of findings from bioassay systems to people. Exposure assessors evaluate the distribution and determinants of exposure in the population. Their tools include questionnaires, pollution monitors, and biomarkers to be used in studying exposures of individuals and models for projecting the exposures of populations. Epidemiologists also address patterns of population exposures and characterize the risks associated with these exposures. Increasingly, epidemiologic research incorporates biomarkers of dose, outcome, and susceptibility in an attempt to enhance the sensitivity of epidemiological studies. Risk assessors use qualitative and quantitative risk assessment methods to characterize the scope of environmental health and other problems as a basis for setting priorities and for guiding interventions, whether through regulatory or other means. We have already commented on the need for engagement of other disciplines in urban environmental health research, including the social and behavioral sciences.

Environmental health scientists often use terminology, definitions, and concepts which differ from their colleagues in other fields. An additional aim of this chapter is to sort through relevant terminology used by environmental health scientists in different fields. The success of future environmental health research in urban settings will depend on the continued collaboration between these different sub-areas of expertise. In addition, environmental health researchers must continually expand their partnerships to include other scientific disciplines, stake-holders and service providers in urban communities. The chapter will conclude with examples of such partnering and suggestions for future collaboration.

2.0. FRAMEWORKS FOR EXPOSURE ASSESSMENT

2.1. Concepts and Models of Human Exposure

The concept of personal exposure is fundamental to addressing urban environmental health problems. Exposure refers to contact of an individual with a pollutant; its units are concentration x time. Exposure is distinct from dose, which represents the amount of material entering into an exposed person; dose may be further classified as the biologically effective dose, that portion of the total dose that reaches the site of action within the body.

A 1991 report of the National Research Council offers a useful framework for considering the linkages from pollution sources to exposures to doses and subsequent human health effects (NRC, 1991). In general, pollutant sources are linked to human exposure through the three principal environmental media: air, water, and food. Pollutants may contaminate food directly or through transport of the toxic agent by an environmental medium. Food sources often concentrate toxic environmental agents across the food chain, as with the example of methylmercury in fish. In addition to these three media, some agents reach people through direct physical contact, which is how ionizing and non-ionizing radiation, for example, exert their effects. In urban environments, water may be contaminated centrally at treatment facilities or at buildings through aged or contaminated pipes, which may contain potentially toxic materials, such as lead.

Another relevant framework for considering environmental exposures in the urban context is offered by the microenvironmental model for total personal exposure (Duan, 1982; Klepeis, 1999a). A microenvironment can be thought of as a spatial compartment where one's time is spent and, for purposes of estimating exposure, has a reasonably uniform concentration of the pollutant during the time that is spent there. People pass through a series of microenvironments across the day (e.g., home → vehicle → work → restaurant → home) and the pollutant concentrations in these environments determine exposure. A microenvironment-specific exposure $\bar{E}_m$ can be expressed as $\bar{E}_m = \bar{c}_m \times t_m$, where $\bar{c}_m$ is an estimate of the average concentration for the microenvironment and t_m is the time spent by the individual in the microenvironment. In this conceptual model, total personal exposure, E_p, is estimated by the sum of the pollutant exposures in each microenvironment, $E_p = \sum_{m=1}^{M} \bar{E}_m$. To apply the microenvironmental model, information is needed on time-activity patterns and also on pollutant concentrations within the microenvironments. The time spent by individuals in given microenvironments has been assessed on a study-by-study basis using diaries (Schwab, *et al.*, 1990), or questionnaires (Quackenboss, *et al.*, 1986), or estimated using data from large-scale assessments of time-activity patterns such as the National Human Activity Pattern Survey (NHAPS) (Chapin, Jr., 1974; Klepeis, *et al.*, 2001; Reid and Watson, 1988). An average time-activity pattern for an adult latino is shown in Table 2, adapted from NHAPS (Klepeis, *et al.*, 2001). Time-activity patterns of

Table 2. Time-Activity Data for an Individual in NHAPS

Activity	Start time	End time	Time spent (min)
At night club	0:00	1:45	105
Traveling home after night club	1:45	2:00	15
Sleeping or napping	2:00	11:00	540
Brushing teeth	11:00	11:05	5
Preparing meals or snacks	11:05	11:15	10
Eating meals or snacks	11:15	11:25	10
Dressing or personal grooming	11:25	11:30	5
Traveling to play football	11:30	11:37	7
Playing flag football	11:37	13:37	120
Traveling home	13:37	13:44	7
Preparing meals or snacks	13:44	13:54	10
Traveling to bar	13:54	13:57	3
At bar	13:57	15:30	93
Traveling from bar	15:30	15:33	3
Watching TV	15:33	16:30	57
Bathing or showering	16:30	17:00	30
Watching TV	17:00	19:00	120
Traveling to shopping	19:00	19:10	10
Shopping for food	19:10	19:25	15
Travel related to shopping for food	19:25	19:35	10
Watching TV	19:35	21:00	85
Studying	21:00	24:00	180

Source: Adapted from Table 4 (Klepeis, *et al.*, 1999).

urban dwellers are likely to differ from those of people living in suburban and rural locations, although we could not identify recent data confirming this hypothesis.

Time-activity data from throughout the U.S. show that most time is spent at home, with the workplace and schools being the second most frequent microenvironments for adults and children, respectively. Concentrations of airborne pollutants within a given microenvironment may reflect both sources in that microenvironment and the penetration of pollutants in air brought in from outside of the particular microenvironment.

The microenvironmental model provides a conceptual basis for considering how exposures in urban environments could differ from those in suburban and rural environments: concentrations in microenvironments could differ in urban and other locations and urban settings could offer unique microenvironments. Particular urban microenvironments may not be found in other locations, such as the "hot spots" of air pollution at busy intersections or adjacent to bus or truck terminals. Residences in urban environments are often multi-story and relatively small, older, and poorly maintained in comparison with newer, suburban housing. Additionally, some key microenvironments in urban locations, including city streets, the home, schools, and transportation environments, may have particularly high concentrations of some pollutants. Inner-city apartments, for example, may have high concentrations of allergens, reflecting rodent and cockroach infestation and high humidity levels. Studies of profiles of air pollution on city streets show "hot spots," places where the combination of high-volume and slow-moving vehicle traffic produce high concentrations of pollutants emitted by vehicles. For example, Levy and colleagues (Levy, *et al.*, 2001) measured concentrations of fine particulate matter and polycyclic aromatic hydrocarbons in inner-city Boston. The measurements had high spatial and temporal detail and showed concentration profiles that closely mirrored traffic.

The microenvironmental model is useful for designing research in urban environments; it should bring focus to those microenvironments that may be particularly relevant to the research question under investigation and it can guide exposure assessment strategies. Research findings interpreted in the context of the microenvironmental model may be used to apportion the burden of risk and to target pollution sources that contribute to observed risks.

2.2. Approaches to Exposure Assessment

The exposures of urban populations to pollutants may be measured with the goal of characterizing the distribution of exposures and determining those factors that lead to exposure, particularly those exposures above limits of acceptability. They may also be measured in support of epidemiological studies. Depending on the purpose, approaches range in intensity from making detailed and sometimes sophisticated measurements to characterize individual exposures to classifying exposures of large populations using questionnaires, routine monitoring data, or models. Biomarkers of exposure or dose are another useful assessment tool.

Questionnaires used for exposure assessment generally cover sources of exposure, e.g., presence of cigarette smoking or pets, and time-activity; in general, people cannot accurately classify the intensity of an exposure. Information on concentrations at which exposures are taking place can be gained with use of personal monitors for airborne contaminants or of microenvironmental modeling. Concentrations of contaminants in water supplies can be directly measured and combined with information on quantities consumed to estimate dose.

Biomarkers of exposure or dose measured in biological materials are available for some pollutants (Table 3). In general, the term biomarker refers to a measurement of an indicator of susceptibility, exposure, dose, or response that is made in a biological material—blood, saliva, cells, tissues, or urine, for example (Committee on Advances in Assessing Human Exposure to Airborne Pollutants and National Research Council (NRC, 1991). For exposure or dose, biomarkers have been developed with the expectation of obtaining indicators that may provide a more accurate

Table 3. Biomarkers of Human Exposure

Exposure	Biomarker	Biological material
Nicotine in cigarette smoke (ETS)	Cotinine	Body fluids
Lead in the environment DDT*	Lead	Body fluids and tissues
	DDE**	Adipose tissue
Benz[a]pyrene, PAHs	DNA adducts	White blood cells
1,3-butadiene (BD)	Hemoglobin Adducts	Red Blood Cells
Allergens	Allergen-specific Immuoglobulin E IgE	Serum
Contemporary-use pesticides (e.g., organophosphates)	Dialkylphosphate, Cholinesterase Enzymes Activity	Urine, Serum
Diesel Exhaust	1-hydroxypyrene	Urine

*DDT: dichlorodiphenyletrichlorethylene
**DDE: dichlorodiphenyldichloraethylene

assessment of risk and that will not be subject to the error that frequently affects estimates made using standard epidemiological approaches.

A biomarker of exposure is an exogenous substance or its metabolite; it is the product of an interaction between xenobiotic agent and a target molecule in the body which can be measured in some compartment of the human body including tissues, cells, fluids, or expired air (National Research Council (NRC, 1989). There is a full continuum of biomarkers from indicators of exposure to sensitive indicators of the earliest phases of adverse health effects. Biomarkers are surrogates for exposure or dose; the relationship of the biomarker to exposure may be physiologically complex and variable among individuals. Many well-know examples of biomarkers of exposure are now proving useful not only for research purposes but for tracking exposures of population or worker groups. For lead exposure, concentrations have been measured in blood, bone, and teeth; each of these biomarkers provides an indication of typical exposure across a time domain reflecting the kinetics for the medium in which the measurement is made. For involuntary exposure of nonsmokers to cigarette smoke, levels of nicotine or cotinine can be measured in body fluids, providing a highly specific and valid marker of exposure (Benowitz, 1999) (Samet and Wang, 2000). Adducts of carcinogens bound to DNA in white blood cells can also be measured; adducts of the polycyclic aromatic hydrocarbon carcinogen, benzo-(a)-pyrene, have been associated with exposure to outdoor air pollution (Perera, *et al.*, 1992) and to cigarette smoke (Crawford, *et al.*, 1994).

For air contaminants, exposure assessment approaches can be divided broadly into direct and indirect assessment methods; this same broad scheme has general applicability. In direct assessments of exposure, a measurement is made for each individual. For example, for measuring exposure to an air pollutant, each individual carries a personal monitor which registers the encountered concentrations continuously or integrated over a given time-period. Small, light-weight instrumentation that can measure particle concentrations and multiple gaseous pollutants is now available for this purpose; the instruments can be placed in a small backpack and worn throughout the day across all microenvironments where time is spent. Measurement of a biomarker would also constitute a direct measure of exposure. In indirect assessment, exposure for individuals is estimated using the microenvironmental model by capturing the time spent in relevant microenvironments and measuring or estimating pollutant concentrations in these microenvironments. This approach is feasible for use in large epidemiological studies or for estimating population exposures for the purpose of risk characterization. In an epidemiological study, direct and indirect approaches may be combined with the direct assessment providing a standard for validation of the indirect approach.

For some environmental contaminants, e.g., lead, exposures may occur through multiple environmental media. Polycylic aromatic hydrocarbons, carcinogens produced by combustion, offer an additional example. Exposures to polycyclic aromatic hydrocarbons may result from contact with air contaminated by vehicle emissions or industrial point sources, such as steel mills or power plants, and from ingestion of cooked foods. The relative contributions of sources and media to total personal exposure depend on the strengths of the sources and individual behavior, including patterns of food cooking and consumption and time activity (Butler, *et al.*, 1993; Lioy, *et al.*, 1988). In a study of 10 homes in one industrial U.S. town, food ingestion was found to be the predominant pathway for exposure to benzo(a)pyrene (BaP), even though industrial sources of emissions were present (Butler, *et al.*, 1993). During a two-week interval, both outdoor and indoor air samples were collected over a 24-hour period for two weeks. Food samples were collected from family meals each day, and two samples of water and one sample of soil were taken for analysis for BaP. In addition, one person within each household completed daily questionnaires on time spent on various activities (Lioy and Waldman, 1990). Water and soil were found to be minor pathways for exposure to BaP, while air and food were the most significant sources of exposure. A comparison of the levels of BaP in air and in food pointed to food ingestion as the predominant exposure source. These findings imply that a study directed at airborne exposures from an industrial source may need to estimate background exposures from other sources.

3.0. STUDY DESIGNS FOR HUMAN RESEARCH

3.1. Overview

Studies of people in urban environments pose specific challenges, but the relevant study designs are those that would be used in addressing health problems of any population: the cross-sectional study or survey, the cohort study, and the case-control study, as well as the more recently developed nested designs. Ecological studies, that is studies carried out with groups, e.g., cities, as the unit of observation have also been used to address urban health issues, but evidence from such studies has long been viewed as seriously constrained by the "ecological fallacy", a term used generally for potential bias arising in extending results from group-level observations to individuals. However, there is a growing recognition that the factors affecting health operate at individual and broader levels of societal organization and increasingly, multi-level designs are used that reflect the tiers of factors that determine health and well-being and incorporate features of both individual-level and ecological designs. Such designs when applied to urban health issues might incorporate data at the individual, neighborhood, and city levels.

Experimental designs have been used infrequently in environmental health generally, although investigations directed at "natural experiments" of changing exposures have been carried out, as have trials of exposure reduction measures and of preventive agents to reduce adverse effects of environmental agents. For air pollution, the concept of "accountability" has been recently advanced; that is, research to characterize the consequences of regulations that are intended to reduce risks of exposures to the population (Health Effects Institute, 2003).

3.2. Ecological Studies

Ecological studies have long been cast as useful for "hypothesis generation" and not for hypothesis testing. Nonetheless, studies of the ecological design have been widely used for testing hypotheses concerning the risks of environmental agents and, in fact, the risks of some environmental exposures, which are relatively uniform across communities, may only be addressed using ecological designs. Ecological studies involve groups, defined typically by geographic location and time and demographic characteristics, as the unit of analysis. Exposures are inferred for groups of individuals and health characteristics of the group are assessed in relation to the inferred exposures. For example, rates of lung cancer mortality have been compared across urban and rural areas to assess urban air pollution as a risk factor for lung cancer (Samet and Cohen, 1999) and associations of mortality rates from various causes have been examined with county-level mortality and air pollution data. The feasibility of this design is enhanced by use of data collected routinely for administrative or regulatory purposes, such as air pollution, water quality, and mortality data. An inherent limitation, often referred to as the "ecologic fallacy," is the assumption that exposure-outcome relationships observed at the group level hold at the individual level. Additionally, confounding may be difficult to control because group-level data on potential confounders are not available and ecological regression models cannot fully adjust for the potential confounders (Robins and Greenland, 1989).

For some environmental exposures, e.g., air pollution, the routinely collected monitoring data provide exposure estimates at the population level, although it may be possible to use additional information from supplemental monitoring or questionnaires to develop estimates for specific individuals. Properly, studies using group-level exposure information for individuals should reflect this structure in their design, using a multi-level formulation of the study. Newer, hierarchical designs that incorporate individual-level information on potential confounding and modifying factors and group-level information on environmental exposures offer the possibility of both controlling confounding and exploring effect modification (Diez-Roux, 2000). For example, Peters and colleagues (Peters *et al.*, 1999a; Peters, *et al.*, 1999b) are assessing the effects of air pollution exposure on respiratory health of children in the Los Angeles area. Twelve communities were selected to provide a gradient of exposure to the air pollutants of interest, particularly ozone. Exposure for individuals is inferred based on measurements made at schools in the communities; these estimates will be refined using information based on individual-level time-activity information. In a recent report (Gauderman, *et al.*, 2004), these investigators showed that air pollution exposure during adolescence reduces the rate of lung growth; the analytic outcome was community-level rate of lung growth adjusted for potential confounders, using information at the individual level.

Air pollution has long been a major focus of environmental health research in cities. Time-series analysis, a population-level design, has long been used to assess whether variation in air pollution levels is associated with variation in health outcome measures, including daily counts of deaths, hospitalizations, or outpatient clinic visits (Bell *et al.*, 2004). Dramatic air pollution episodes, such as the London Fog of 1952, showed that air pollution can acutely elevate mortality and morbidity. At air pollution levels in today's urban areas in developed countries, the levels are far lower and sophisticated modeling approaches are used to find a far weaker signal of air pollution effects. The general approach is to control for potential temporal confounders, such as season or epidemic influenza, using appropriate smoothing so that shorter-term associations of air pollution with mortality can be evaluated (Kelsall, *et al.*, 1997). In such time-series designs, confounding at the individual-level may be of little concern, because personal characteristics do not vary on the time-frame of the analysis and confounding at the ecological-level by time-varying factors, e.g., season, can be handled in the analysis. Flexible modeling approaches, such as generalized additive models (GAM) and generalized linear models (GLM) can be used to control for potential temporal confounding by season or other factors; these models can also handle complex and correlated data structures that may have led to uncontrollable bias with prior modeling approaches (Bell, *et al.*, 2004).

The time-series approach has now been refined and strengthened by its extension to incorporate multiple locations into a common analysis, whether through meta-analysis or pooled analysis. The APHEA (Air Pollution and Health: A European Approach) Study applies a common analytic approach to European data on morbidity and mortality from multiple cities and then combines the city-specific estimates of the effect of air pollution using meta-analysis (Katsouyanni, *et al.*, 1997). Dominici and colleagues (Dominici, *et al.*, 2000; Dominici, *et al.*, 2003) have developed a Bayesian hierarchical modeling approach for combining evidence on the health effects of air pollution across locations. In the National Morbidity, Mortality, and Air Pollution Study (NMMAPS) carried out in the U.S., evidence on the health effects of air pollution has been combined from the largest 90 cities (Figure 2). Using these methods, it is also possible to explore the factors responsible

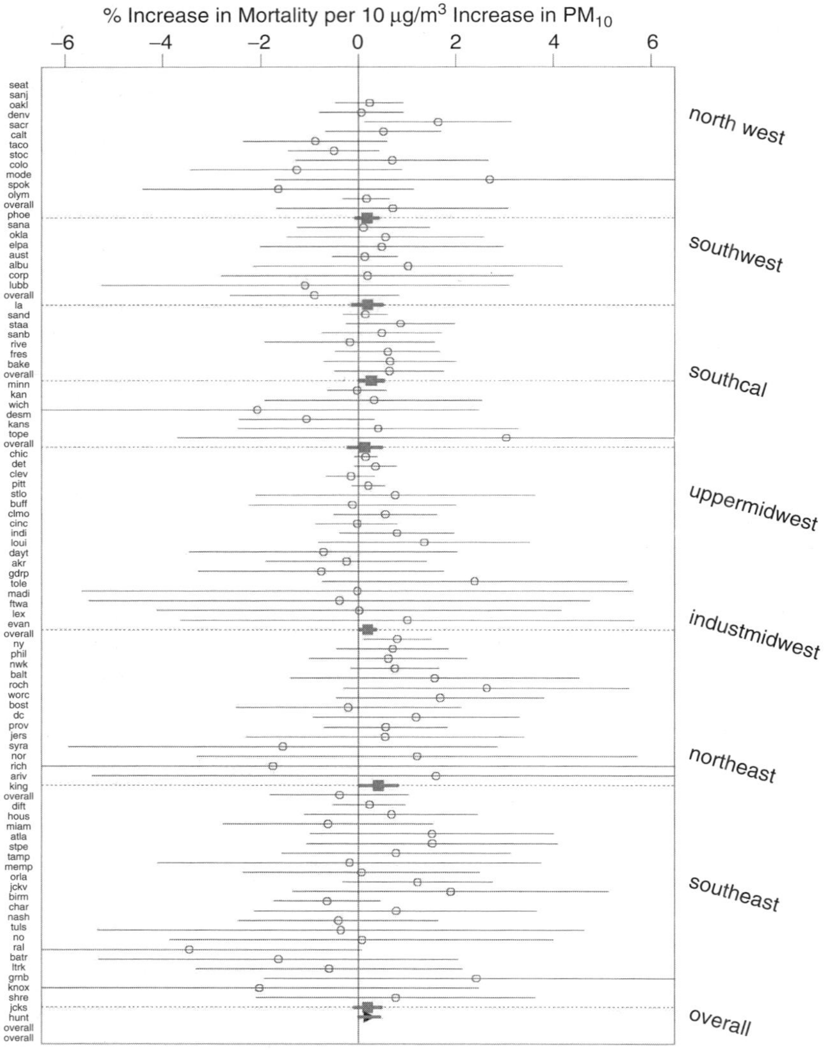

Figure 2. Effects of PM10 on total mortality and 95% Confidence Intervals on 90 Cities, Grouped by Region (*Source:* Samet *et al.*, 2000).

for any heterogeneity of the effect of air pollution across locations. The general approach should have abundant application to other types of environmental agents of concern in urban locations that have informative patterns of variation spatially and temporally.

Small-area analysis, using data from small geographic areas across which exposures can be reasonably assumed to be uniform, has also been applied to air pollution and other environmental agents (Elliott, *et al.*, 1992b). This approach is useful for research on urban environmental problems if exposures can be estimated for small geographical units and outcome data are available at the same geographical scale. In using this design, analyses should account for spatial autocorrelation, that is, the non-independence of data for geographical units that are likely to have correlated exposures. As an example of this approach, Elliott and colleagues (Elliott, *et al.*, 1992a) explored the risk of lung and larynx cancers associated with exposure to emissions from waste incinerators, using circular areas around 10 incinerator sites as indicators of exposure levels. For each site, two circular geographic bands were defined around the incinerator, with the inner band being 0-3 km in radius from the incinerator and the outer band being 3-10 km from the site. For their main analysis, Elliott and colleagues pooled together the observed and expected numbers of cancers from the ten incinerator sites, combining information from the inner and outer bands. Smaller increments of bands within the 10 km were used to analyze for decreasing trend in cancer risk with increasing distance from the sites. Despite having adequate power through pooling of data from multiple sites, no statistically significant excesses in lung and larynx cancers were found either near (0-3 km) or distant from (3-10 km) the incinerators.

3.3. Cross-Sectional Studies

The survey remains a widely used, although inherently limited design, for investigating risks of environmental agents in urban settings. The design of a survey is usually straightforward, feasibility is generally not a barrier, and costs are typically not high. In a survey, observations concerning exposure and outcome are made at one point in time, although an attempt may be made to capture past exposures and to relate prior exposures to current disease status or other measures. Interpretation of cross-sectional data for causality is consequently limited, as the temporal relationship between exposure and outcome may be uncertain, and only persons with prevalent disease can be accessed for investigation.

Cross-sectional designs can be used to investigate the risks to communities or neighborhoods from specific sources, e.g., emissions from trucks at a depot in an urban neighborhood. In this context, feasibility remains a key rationale for using this approach, and a cross-sectional study can be completed on a sufficiently rapid timeframe to address immediate concerns. Thus, cross-sectional studies have been conducted to investigate the effects of secondhand smoke on lung function (Schwartz, *et al.*, 2000), of the frequency of allergic and respiratory diseases in children in the former eastern and western parts of Germany (Von Mutius, *et al.*, 1994), and more recently of urban social context on health (Lochner, *et al.*, 2003).

Cross-sectional studies have the potential to be informative if valid gradients of exposure can be established. This goal may be met by selecting communities or neighborhoods that offer a range of exposure, based on available monitoring information, and making comparisons across communities, or by establishing gradients of exposure within communities. For example, the 24-Cities Study was conducted by investigators at Harvard to address the health effects of acidic air pollution on the health of children (Cunningham *et al.*, 1996). The communities were selected based on prior monitoring data to provide a gradient of exposure to acid aerosols. While the outcome data were collected for each child, this design approach is now recognized as hierarchical and may be referred to as "semi-ecologic" (Kunzli and Tager, 1997). While data on outcome and potential confounding and modifying factors have been collected at the individual level, exposure has been estimated at the community level. In a study of school children in 12 Southern California communities (Peters, *et al.*, 1999b), lung function as well as demographic and environmental factors were assessed at the individual level, while air pollution exposures were assessed at the community level using ambient air monitors. The communities were selected to represent a range of air pollution levels and profiles

3.4. Cohort Studies

The cohort design, involving follow-up of individuals with ascertainment of outcome over time, has a central role in investigating the risks of environmental agents, regardless of setting. The design affords the opportunity to prospectively assess exposures so that misclassification can be minimized and the temporal relationship between exposure and outcome is not ambiguous. The cohort design can be applied either retrospectively, if available data are sufficient for cohort selection, exposure assessment and outcome characterization, or prospectively, if resources are sufficient for follow-up of a population of adequate size, exposure assessment over time, and outcome tracking. If carried out retrospectively, the design gains in feasibility and efficiency because events that have already taken place are the focus of investigation and, if carried out prospectively, the design affords the opportunity to characterize exposures using the optimal, affordable strategy. The retrospective design has been predominantly used for occupational cohorts with historical data available and it has had limited application to urban environmental health problems. Nested designs, the nested case-control and case-cohort studies, offer efficient approaches for carrying out cohort studies, particularly if exposure characterization is resource intensive (Samet and Muñoz, 1998).

The prospective cohort design has also been extensively used for studies of environmental agents. By virtue of being carried out prospectively, many aspects of the design can be made optimal. The investigators can implement exposure and outcome assessment strategies that will be as comprehensive as resources will permit; validation studies can be nested within the full cohort study; and potential confounding and modifying factors can be characterized. These strengths have given the prospective cohort study the greatest credibility among the epidemiological study designs, but a modern cohort study of an environmental agent may require substantial resources and funding, as well as sufficient observation time. The informativeness of the cohort design has also been advanced by new methods for longitudinal analysis that can flexibly model time-varying relationships in the data and accommodate correlated observations over time (Diggle, *et al.*, 1994).

The cohort design may be used on either short or long timeframes in investigating environmental agents. For environmental exposures, particularly, air pollution, short-term cohort studies, often termed "panel" studies, may be used to track variation in physiological measures and symptoms in relation to variation in exposure. Potentially susceptible groups are often investigated with the goals of enhancing the sensitivity of the investigation to detecting effects and of obtaining evidence relevant to protecting their health. For example, panel studies of air pollution often involve persons with asthma or chronic obstructive pulmonary disease (COPD). Ostro and friends (Ostro, *et al.*, 1994) included adults with asthma in two panel studies on respiratory morbidity and indoor and outdoor air pollution. Exposure to indoor air pollution (i.e., combustion from gas or wood stoves and fireplaces and environmental tobacco smoke) was assessed from daily diary recordings by the panel of 164 asthmatics, as well as the occurrence of several respiratory symptoms (Ostro, *et al.*, 1994). In a study on outdoor air pollution, 138 subjects in central Los Angeles recorded respiratory symptoms in a daily diary, while exposure data were obtained from air monitoring for daily levels of several ambient air pollutants, including ozone, fine particulates, and nitrates (Ostro, *et al.*, 2001).

Longer-term prospective cohort studies may be needed to address chronic effects of the urban environment on health status and disease risk. Such studies have been carried out, for example, to address the effect of air pollution on mortality (Dockery, *et al.*, 1993), lead exposure on neuropsychological development (Needleman and Gatsonis, 1990), and endotoxin exposure on respiratory symptoms (Litonjua, *et al.*, 2002; Park, *et al.*, 2001).

The Port Pirie study of lead-exposed children illustrates the strength of the design with its incorporation of repeated measures of blood lead, the exposure measure, and of neuropsychological functioning, the outcome measure (Tong, *et al.*, 1998). The Port Pirie cohort consisted of 537 children born to women living near a lead smelter. Maternal blood lead levels were measured antenatally and at delivery, while children's blood lead levels were measured at delivery from the umbilical cord, at six and 15 months, and then annually from age 2 through 7 years (McMichael, *et al.*, 1988; Tong, *et al.*, 1998). Additional factors and qualitative measures of outcomes were assessed through interviews of the mother at the time of each blood sample collection. Neuropsychological development of the children was quantitatively evaluated using a number of behavioral and cognitive assessments, including intelligence tests, at various ages. The most recent assessment of this cohort at ages 11-13 years showed increased frequency of behavioral and emotional problems associated with higher lifetime blood lead exposure.

The prospective cohort design may be strengthened and made more efficient by using an intermediate marker of the outcome of interest, rather than waiting for the final outcome itself (Muñoz and Gange, 1998). For example, rate of decline of lung function may be measured as the primary outcome measure, rather than awaiting for the development of clinically evident lung disease or death from lung disease. The rate of decline of lung function could be determined in a prospective cohort study by repetitively measuring lung function and estimating its change over follow-up. Studies of such intermediate markers are most properly carried out with the prospective cohort approach, as in the example of the Children's Health Study in Southern California (Gauderman, *et al.*, 2004).

3.5. Case-Control Studies

The case-control design has been used extensively to characterize occupational and environmental causes of cancer, but much less frequently for other diseases, and it has had limited application specifically to urban environmental health problems. The design has proved particularly useful for cancer, as there is often a lengthy period from the time of first exposure until excess risk is manifest. The cases and controls themselves are the principal source of information on exposure. Some exposure misclassification is unavoidable as a result, as study participants may be asked to supply a profile of environmental and occupational exposures across their lifetimes. For some exposures, such as urban air pollution, it may be possible to only obtain information on surrogates, such as place of residence, and some exposures, such as diet, are unavoidably reported with misclassification.

Hybrid approaches, the nested case-control and case-cohort studies, have features of the case-control and cohort designs. In a nested case-control study, the cases constitute those persons within the full cohort developing the outcome of interest during follow-up; the controls are selected, typically with matching, from those persons at risk when the cases developed the outcome. This design is often used if exposure assessment is resource intensive or based in biomarker measurement; efficiency is gained because exposures are not calculated for the full cohort. With sampling of a sufficient number of controls, estimates of effect from a nested case-control study and a full cohort study are comparable (Breslow, *et al.*, 1982). In the case-cohort design, a sample of the cohort is drawn at the start of follow-up and exposures are characterized for these persons and those cohort members who subsequently develop disease (Prentice, 1986). This design has not yet had widespread application to environmental and occupational exposures.

The case-crossover design is a recently proposed approach useful for studying acute events associated with brief exposures (Maclure, 1991). It is a variant of the case-control study involving cases only and comparison of exposures during the biologically-relevant time period for the outcome and a comparison time period. In effect, the case-crossover design enhances study efficiency by having each case serve as his or her own control, thereby eliminating potential confounding by such personal characteristics as age, gender and socioeconomic status. Analysis is generally self-matched using conditional logistic regression modeling.

The design has application to time-varying environmental exposures in urban environments, such as air pollution, temperature, and noise (Basu and Samet, 2002; Neas, *et al.*, 1999). A representative application is to investigate the short-term association of air pollution with mortality; relevant case exposures are postulated to occur shortly before the time of death and control exposures can be estimated at times just prior to or even after time of death. In one study of this design in Philadelphia by Neas and colleagues (Neas, *et al.*, 1999), the case exposures occurred in the "48-hour period ending at midnight on the day of death" and the control exposures occurred 1, 2 and 3 weeks before and after the case exposure period. The Philadelphia study confirmed the results of earlier Poisson regression analysis of the same data, showing a positive association between total suspended particulates and daily mortality.

3.6. Intervention Studies

In intervention studies, the investigator controls the exposure status of study participants. The randomized clinical trial, which has the central elements of randomization to control and comparison arms, is generally used to evaluate the efficacy of therapeutic regimens, including drug therapies. A key strength of the randomized clinical trial is control of selection bias and confounding through randomization. The design has potential application to occupational and environmental exposures in evaluating interventions to reduce disease risk, although few such trials have been carried out. The use of randomized trials is distinct from studies based around regulatory and programmatic interventions to reduce exposures, which may afford an opportunity to evaluate the consequences of reducing exposures.

Randomized controlled trials have been carried out to evaluate the effects of reduced pollution exposures and also the effects of chemopreventive agents hypothesized to reduce the effect of exposure to occupational and environmental agents. For example, Romieu and colleagues (Romieu, *et al.*, 1998) used a randomized trial combined with a cross-over design to examine the effect of antioxidant supplementation on respiratory function of street workers in Mexico City, who have chronically high exposures to ambient ozone. Participants were randomly assigned to take daily supplements of vitamins E and C and beta-carotene, all anti-oxidants, or a placebo. Results showed significant differences between the two groups in terms of pulmonary function tests. The placebo group had decreased pulmonary function with increasing ozone levels, while the supplement group did not show the same inverse association with ozone levels. After the crossover, when the placebo group began taking the supplement and the supplement group began taking the placebo, there appeared to be a residual effect of the antioxidants. In this second phase of the study, Romieu, *et al.* found that the placebo group had decreases in pulmonary function that were less pronounced that the decrements found before the cross-over (Romieu, *et al.*, 1998).

Intervention studies have also been carried out to assess the consequences of reducing urban environmental exposures. For example, the Inner-City Asthma Study evaluated the benefits of reducing exposures of children with asthma to indoor allergens and secondhand smoke (Morgan, *et al.*, 2004). The intervention arm received education as well as several measures intended to reduce exposures, while the control arm participants had a visit for measurement purposes only. The intervention reduced allergen exposures and the participants in the intervention arm had fewer days with symptoms compared with those in the control arm. The Inner-City Asthma Study illustrates the feasibility of carrying out large-scale intervention trials in urban areas. The study was of large size (N=937), and recruitment was possible and retention satisfactory. The experimental approach is relevant to those environmental factors for which intervention is possible at the individual level.

4.0. CASE STUDIES

4.1. Airborne Particles and Morbidity and Mortality

We offer the topical example of the adverse health effects of airborne particles to illustrate the multidisciplinary approach to urban environmental health problems and collaboration with communities in carrying out research that is directly relevant to the health of community members. In urban environments, particles have diverse sources indoors and outdoors and particles from outdoor sources may penetrate indoors as air is exchanged or infiltrates into buildings. In urban environments, key sources of particles in outdoor air include motor vehicles and industries, along with particles from regional sources; indoor sources include tobacco smoking, cooking, and space heating devices, along with sources of biological materials, including pets, rodents, and cockroaches. The particles to which people are exposed in urban environments represent a complex mixture that will vary in characteristics from microenvironment to microenvironment. Analytical studies show that much of the particle mass exists in the small size fraction that can penetrate to the upper airways and lungs, where deposited particles can cause both local and systemic injury. A substantial proportion of the population is considered to be at increased risk from inhaled particles, including infants and children whose lungs are still developing, children and adults with asthma whose lungs have increased responsiveness to environmental stimuli, adults with chronic heart and lung diseases, and the elderly.

In the U.S., the concentration of particles in outdoor air is regulated under the Clean Air Act by an evidence-based standard, referred to as a National Ambient Air Quality Standard (NAAQS) (US Environmental Protection Agency (EPA) and Office of Air Quality Planning and Standards, 1996). Since the early 1990s, there has been persistent controversy concerning the threat posed to public health by the fine particles which reach the lungs. In an unanticipated finding at the time, time-series studies reported in the early 1990s showed that daily mortality counts in a number of U.S. and European cities were positively associated with levels of airborne particles on the same or recent days. This type of study had been made feasible by advances in hardware and statistical software and methods for longitudinal analysis and the data (mortality counts, air pollution concentrations, and meteorological data) are available from public sources. Consequently, many further, confirmatory time-series studies were quickly reported. One complexity in interpreting the time-series studies is the extent to which the observed short-term associations translate into life-shortening. Cohort studies of mortality over the long-term also showed positive associations, suggesting that urban particulate air pollution does significantly reduce lifespan. The new epidemiological evidence motivated a tightening of the NAAQS for particulate matter in 1997 (US Environmental Protection Agency (EPA), 1997).

Because of the sweeping consequences of the new standard and the potential costs of its implementation, the certainty of the underlying scientific evidence was questioned and a substantial national research agenda was initiated with guidance from a committee of the National Research Council (National Research Council (NRC) and Committee on Research Priorities for Airborne Particulate Matter, 1998). Because diverse microenvironments contribute to exposure to airborne particles, the contribution of outdoor sources to total personal exposure to particles was addressed in a number of locations. In these studies, participants wore particle monitors and noted their time-activity, and particle measurements were made in a number of key microenvironments. Some of the studies targeted those groups considered to be at increased risk from particle exposure. Overall, the studies showed that outdoor air pollution is a significant determinant of particle exposures, particularly for persons who do not smoke or live with smokers.

A further uncertainty was the limited understanding of the mechanisms by which seemingly low-dose exposures to particles could cause adverse health effects. Approaches to this gap reflect the interdisciplinary nature of environmental health research. One study design uses a particle concentrator, which increases particle concentration by up to 10-fold or more so that brief exposures of human volunteers or toxicologic assays of exposures to actual urban air particles can be carried out. In studies underway in Southern California, rodents are transported daily to roadside locations and exposed concentrated ambient particles (Kleinman, *et al.*, 2003). Epidemiological studies are in progress in some of the same locations so that coherence can be sought between results of human and animal exposures to the same complex mixture. Assays are also in development that characterize the potential of particles to cause injury; approaches that assay the particles for ability to oxidant-mediated injury and microarray methods are also being used to assess gene activation by particles, so-called "toxicogenomics."

Increasingly sophisticated epidemiological designs are also being used to assess the effect of exposure to particles and other urban air pollutants. Multi-level designs have now been used for addressing urban air pollution in several paradigmatic studies. For epidemiological research, exposure estimates are generally based in routine, regulatory monitoring of pollutant concentrations. The monitoring data capture variation in concentrations across cities, but not within cities. Consequently, epidemiological studies have now incorporated multiple locations to gain heterogeneity of exposures by using multiple sites. Data are analyzed in a multi-level fashion, first estimating effects within locations and then combining across locations at the regional and even the national levels. In the National Morbidity, Mortality, and Air Pollution Study (NMMAPS), for example, time-series analyses were carried out within each of 90 individual cities and then the risk estimates were combined at the regional and national levels using a Bayesian hierarchical model (Figure 2) (Samet, *et al.*, 2000). Similar approaches have been used in studies at the individual level. The Children's Health Study (Peters, *et al.*, 1999a; Peters, *et al.*, 1999b), carried out in Southern California, includes 12 locations selected initially to provide contrasting concentration profiles for ozone and particulate air pollution. A recent report on air pollution and rate of lung function growth in adolescents exemplified the multi-level approach. In each of the 12 communities, the lung function growth of children was tracked and for each community a confounder-adjusted rate of lung growth was estimated. These estimates were then regressed on air pollution concentrations for the communities, with the finding that a set of vehicle-related pollutants were associated with lower lung function growth. In an extension of this study (Gauderman, *et al.*, 2004), the investigators are now developing exposure estimates for the study participants that reflect within-community variation in exposure. For this purpose, they are using models in combination with information on residence location, time-activity, and indoor sources.

Urban communities are often concerned by visible sources of particle emissions on their streets—diesel and other vehicles—and by facilities that lead to large amounts of traffic—bus depots and trucking terminals, for example. Academic-community partnerships have been successfully formed to characterize profiles of exposure to particulate matter. In New York City, two academic institutions partnered with a community organization, West Harlem Environmental Action (WE-ACT), in a study that made measurements of fine particulate matter on sidewalks in Harlem; the findings pointed to the importance of local diesel sources (Kinney, *et al.*, 2000). In Boston, a similar partnership resulted in monitoring of concentrations of fine particulate matter and polycyclic aromatic hydrocarbons in Roxbury (Levy, *et al.*, 2001).

4.2. Inner City Asthma

Inner city asthma, a pressing public health concern, illustrates the complexity of developing research evidence to reduce morbidity and mortality for a disease that is affected by a broad range of urban microenvironments. The prevalence and severity of childhood asthma have increased in the last 20 years, and the greatest increase has been seen among children and young adults living in U.S. inner cities (Crain, *et al.*, 1994; Eggleston, *et al.*, 1999). Despite deepening insight into the pathophysiology of asthma and a better understanding of chronic management of the disease, asthma remains the leading cause of chronic illness among children. According to the US National Health Interview Survey, nine million U.S. children under 18 years of age (12%) have ever been diagnosed with asthma. More than 4 million children (6%) had an asthma attack in the previous year (Dey, *et al.*, 2004). Children in poor families (16%) were more likely to have ever been diagnosed with asthma than children in families that were not poor (11%) (Dey, *et al.*, 2004). Among poor inner-city children, asthma is more severe and less likely to be appropriately managed relative to asthma in more affluent communities. In addition to having the highest asthma prevalence, inner-city children have the highest asthma hospitalization rates in the country (Centers for Disease Control and Prevention (CDC), 1997). Asthmatic children living in urban environments have a higher frequency of attacks and more severe attacks relative to their suburban and rural dwelling counterparts (Graham, 2004). The burden of asthma is particularly prominent among minority children. Among black and latino children living in the inner city, as many as 25% suffer from asthma (Webber, *et al.*, 2002). As a consequence of the greater burden of asthma, increased severity, and poor management, mortality from asthma is as much as three times higher in minorities (Perera, *et al.*, 2002; Weiss, *et al.*, 1993).

As researchers have approached inner-city asthma, they have faced numerous challenging questions: What are the environmental and genetic determinants of susceptibility to asthma? What environmental agents cause asthma among those who are susceptible? For asthmatics, what agents exacerbate the disease and provoke attacks and where do exposures to these agents take place? What are their sources and what social and neighborhood factors determine exposure? What social-environmental factors mediate access to health care and compliance with disease management strategies? What interventions are effective in modifying the burden of disease in urban populations? These questions have set an extensive research agenda that has now been pursued for over a decade, through both specific initiatives such as the *Inner City Asthma Studies* and through investigator-initiated studies (Gergen, *et al.*, 1999; Mitchell, *et al.*, 1997; Wade, *et al.*, 1997). The full spectrum of designs has been used for investigating inner-city asthma.

Environmental exposures to allergens and air pollutants affect a susceptible child, resulting in respiratory morbidity. In addition to, and perhaps interacting with, genetic susceptibility factors are characteristics of urban life that increase vulnerability to disease, including psychosocial stress, high smoking rates, inappropriate medication use, inadequate resources, and poor access to quality health care.

The microenvironmental model sets a useful framework for considering both research and intervention. For children with asthma, the home is likely the single most important environment for assessing exposure; as school-age children spend most of their time indoors at home (68%). School is the next most important microenvironment, at 15% of time on average. Inner city children spend greater time in their homes than their non-urban dwelling counterparts (Chapin, Jr., 1974). Many environmental factors have been associated with exacerbation of asthma and some may also hasten the onset of asthma. Table 4 summarizes some of the many biological and chemical agents found in homes that may cause or exacerbate asthma. In urban environments, secondhand smoke, biological agents, and combustion emissions are prevalent and often at high concentrations.

Table 4. Indoor Biological and Chemical Agents That May Cause or Exacerbate Asthma

Biological Agent		Chemical Agent
Sufficient Evidence of a Causal Relationship		
Cause	*Exacerbate*	*Cause*
House Dust Mite*	Cat Cockroach* House Dust Mite*	ETS (in preschool-aged children)*
Sufficient Evidence of an Association		
Biological Agent		
Cause	*Exacerbate*	
	Dog Fungi or molds* Rhinovirus	
Limited or Suggestive Evidence of an Association		
Cause	*Exacerbate*	
Respiratory Syncytial Virus (RSV) Cockroach (in preschool-aged children)*	Domestic birds *Mycoplasma pneumoniae* *Chlamydia pneumoniae* Respiratory Syncytial Virus (RSV)	
Inadequate or Insufficient Evidence to Determine Whether an Association Exists		
Cause	*Exacerbate*	
Cat Dog Domestic birds Rodents* Cockroach (except in preschool-aged children)* Endotoxins Fungi or molds* *Chlamydia pneumoniae* *Chlamydia trachomatis* *Mycoplasma pneumoniae* Houseplants Pollen	Rodents* *Chlamydia trachomatis* Endotoxins Houseplants Pollen exposure indoors e Insects other than cockroaches	
Limited or Suggestive Evidence of No Association		
Cause		
Rhinovirus		

*Indicates particular relevance to the indoor environment. *Source:* Institute of Medicine, 2000.

4.2.1. Secondhand Smoke

Among indoor pollutants, secondhand smoke (SHS) is closely linked with increased childhood asthma morbidity (Ehrlich, *et al.*, 1992). There are various methods for assessing SHS exposure in the home microenvironment, each with their advantages and disadvantages (Jaakkola and Jaakkola, 2002). Most commonly, exposure is estimated indirectly, employing time-activity information with questionnaire data (Leaderer, 1990) (Klepeis, 1999a; Klepeis, 1999b; Klepeis, *et al.*, 2001). Parents/caregivers are asked to report smoking habits of persons living in the child's home. This approach can potentially capture long-term average indoor SHS patterns, at least on a relative basis. For example, in a study to evaluate asthma management among inner city asthmatics living in the Baltimore, MD/Washington, D.C. area, Morkjaroenpong and colleagues queried childcare providers regarding smoking patterns using a questionnaire administered over the telephone (Morkjaroenpong, *et al.*, 2002). Thirty-nine percent of care providers smoked and 66% of those smoked inside the home, thus labeling one quarter of all homes as SHS positive. The authors found an association between exposure to higher levels of SHS and increased frequency of nocturnal symptoms. Reports of smoking habits are easily and inexpensively obtained. However, questionnaire-based self-reports generally do not directly ascertain childhood SHS exposure, but rather the potential for exposure to SHS. As such, estimates of exposure derived from these methods may not precisely reflect true exposure. Also respondents may mis-report exposure to cigarette smoke. A limitation of questionnaire-based assessment is the potential for differential reporting of smoking patterns, although whether individuals under-report or over-report their exposure may depend on their psychosocial environment, their health status, and the health status of their children.

Direct methods for assessing child SHS exposure are also employed. A number of biomarkers have been proposed (e.g., nicotine, cotinine) that can provide unbiased estimates of exposure. Cotinine, measured in blood, saliva, or urine, appears to be the most specific and the most sensitive biomarker in use (Benowitz, 1999). However, assaying for biomarkers on a population scale is time-consuming, resource intensive, and potentially burdensome to study subjects. Thus, biomarker assessments are often used to validate more efficient methods of exposure ascertainment, like self-report combined with microenvironmental modeling. Willers and colleagues has assessed SHS exposure both via questionnaire and by quantifying cotinine in body fluids in an urban population of Swedish children (Willers, *et al.*, 2000). The children's' cotinine levels in plasma (Spearman correlation, $r = 0.59$), saliva ($r = 0.70$) and urine ($r = 0.74$) were correlated with the number of cigarettes smoked by the mother at home. These results validate the use of the questionnaire methodology, which can be implemented more broadly.

Personal monitoring, such as sampling of air in subjects' breathing zone, provides yet another direct assessment methodology for SHS exposure (Infante-Rivard, 1993; Jenkins, *et al.*, 1996). Other novel exposure assessments of home SHS include measuring nicotine in house dust (Willers, *et al.*, 2000), and cigarette "butt" collection (Stepans and Fuller, 1999).

4.2.2. Allergens

Exposure to indoor allergens induces airway inflammation and has been identified as a source of respiratory morbidity, particularly for asthmatics (Institute of Medicine and Committee on the Assessment of Asthma and Indoor Air, 2000). Between 70% and 90% of children and young adults with asthma have one or more positive skin tests to aeroallergen; the frequency is similar in asthmatic patients in urban clinics, although the pattern of specific allergen sensitivity differs from that in the general population, with a higher frequency of sensitivity to cockroach and molds and less frequent sensitivity to cats, dogs, and house dust mites. Household exposure is most commonly estimated indirectly by assaying for allergens in dust samples (Chew, *et al.*, 1999; Finn, *et al.*, 2000; Leaderer, *et al.*, 2002). Typically, dust is vacuumed from various microenvironments within the home (e.g., living room, bedroom, mattress) using a standardized protocol. House dust is thought to serve not only as a source of allergen, but also as a sink or reservoir for airborne allergens, offering investigators the ability to quantify cumulative exposure. Home allergens can be assessed efficiently by questionnaire, although these assessments have severe limitations. Chew and colleagues, investigating home allergen exposure in Boston,

MA, found that allergen is often present, as assessed by dust sampling, even when no signs (e.g., cockroach presence) are reported (Chew, *et al.*, 1998).

4.2.3. Diesel Exhaust

Exposure to diesel exhaust is of concern to those living in urban areas. Diesel exhaust is a complex mixture of gases, vapors, and fine particles. At least 40 components are listed by the Air Resources Board as toxic air contaminants. In 1989, the International Agency for Research on Cancer identified exhaust emissions from diesel engines as a probable human carcinogen Need Reference. Exposure to the components of diesel exhaust has also been associated with decrements in lung function and increased asthma morbidity (Holgate, *et al.*, 2003). Microenvironmental exposures of significant concern include in-vehicle exposures (e.g. school buses and cars), and in "urban canyons."

A study conducted in Harlem by Northridge and colleagues found that diesel exhaust biomarker 1-hydroxypyrene could be detected among most (76%) of the 26 adolescents sampled (Northridge, *et al.*, 1999). In a follow-on study, Kinney *et al.*, (Kinney, *et al.*, 2000) reported elemental carbon concentrations, an index of diesel particles, from personal monitors worn by study staff on sidewalks at four Harlem intersections. Concentrations were found to be associated with diesel bus and truck counts.

As part of an ongoing research partnership between Columbia University and a community-based organization, the West Harlem Environmental Action, Inc. (WE-ACT), Northridge and colleagues assessed diesel exhaust exposure in Harlem school children by measuring an exposure biomarker 1-hydroxypyrene in urine samples (Northridge, *et al.*, 1999). Over three-quarters of the students had detectable levels of the diesel biomarker. The same group in New York City studied the relationship between particulate matter less than 2.5 microns in aerodynamic diameter ($PM_{2.5}$) and elemental carbon, a marker of diesel exhaust, on sidewalks adjacent to city streets (Kinney, *et al.*, 2000). Three monitoring sites were selected for simultaneous air sampling and traffic counting, based on community concerns regarding high traffic volume and vehicle emissions. A fourth monitoring site in a comparatively quite residential neighborhood was selected as a control site. The investigators found little spatial variation and comparatively large temporal variation in the level of $PM_{2.5}$. In contrast, elemental carbon concentrations, displayed strong spatial variation, likely reflecting the importance of local diesel sources.

4.3. PAHs and Cancer

Polycyclic aromatic hydrocarbons (PAHs), a family of organic compounds, are the products of incomplete combustion and pyrolysis of organic material (e.g., burning of garbage). PAHs are found in air, water and soil, and remain in the environment for months or even years. Many PAHs are ranked as probable human carcinogens by the US EPA. Although hundreds of PAHs exist, among the most common are benzo(a)pyrene and naphthalene. Relatively economically disadvantaged populations in urban settings may be at higher risk of PAH effects, either because of higher exposure or to heightened susceptibility. Levels of PAHs in urban air are estimated to be as much as 10 times greater than those found in rural areas. In urban environments, PAH exposure is driven by proximity to motor vehicle emissions and by exposure to secondhand smoke.

Microenvironmental modeling of PAH exposure has been conducted in urban environments. Sisovic and colleagues assessed PAH levels inside and outside of homes, at work and in transport of 15 study participants (Sisovic, *et al.*, 1996). Taking into account time spent in the various microenvironments, they developed a model to indirectly estimate personal exposure. They also directly measured personal exposure. Comparing the two, they found that the calculated inhalation exposure often deviated substantially from the directly measured exposure. This was attributed to gaps in their microenvironmental model. However, they noted that on average, there were no statistically significant differences between the directly and indirectly assessed PAH exposures. This suggests that the microenvironmental approach is suitable for assessing average inhalation exposure but not for individual assessments.

Indeed, monitoring of airborne PAHs at the individual level is considered preferable to assessment of PAH in ambient air, because differences in personal activity likely affect the potential for exposure. Personal sampling integrates PAH exposure across multiple times and locations. Other examples of personal PAH monitoring include a study by Tonne and colleagues which assessed PAH exposure in non-smoking, pregnant minority women using personal samplers (Tonne *et al.*, 2004) and Perera *et al.* (Perera, *et al.*, 2003), who assessed associations between PAH exposure and birth outcomes. Both studies were conducted in New York City.

Despite its strengths relative to microenvironmental modeling of PAH exposure, personal sampling can be burdensome to study subjects, as it requires study subjects to carry a personal monitor, usually contained in a small backpack. Recently, studies involving PAH biomarkers have reached investigations in the urban environment. Genotoxic damage derived from exposure to PAHs can be measured in healthy adults or children by specific assays as PAH-DNA adducts. These DNA lesions are an indicator of DNA damage, and likely represent a critical step in exposure driven carcinogenesis. As such, DNA adducts offer a sensitive and specific biomarker of exposure and are also likely a biomarker of early biological effect (Perera, *et al.*, 1992). Perera and colleagues have assessed presence of adducts between the PAH benzo(a)pyrene and DNA among mothers living in New York City and their newborns, finding detectable adducts in 42% of mothers and 45% of newborns (Perera, *et al.*, 2004). Moreover, an association between PAH-DNA adducts and cancer risk has been demonstrated in several studies (Veglia, *et al.*, 2003). There are several different methods to assay for DNA adducts, including ^{32}P-postlabeling, ELISA, and HPLC-fluorescence, and the methods differ with respect to specificity for exposure. Also, the presence of adducts often does not correlate well with exposure measured by microenvironmental or personal sampling. This is perhaps because adduct formation, as a measure of early biological effects, reflects both exposure and susceptibility (Perera, *et al.*, 2004).

5.0. RISK ASSESSMENT

Urban environmental health problems are addressed through regulatory and nonregulatory approaches. For some problems that reflect the consequences of sources at the local, regional, and even national levels, only regulatory approaches may prove satisfactory to cover multiple pollution sources that contribute to a single public health problem, as in the example of particulate air pollution. However, local problems also require solution, and evidence of the magnitude of the public health threat is often needed to force action, whether through regulation, litigation, or other means.

Risk assessment, both qualitative and quantitative, has proved effective for integrating information on exposure and risk for the purpose of policy formulation. As set out in a landmark report of the U.S. National Research Council in 1983 (National Research Council (NRC) and Committee on the Institutional Means for Assessment of Risks to Public Health, 1983), often referred to as the "Red Book," risk assessment has four components: 1) Hazard identification: is there a risk to health from the agent? 2) Exposure assessment: what is the distribution of exposure in the population? 3) Dose-response assessment: what is the relationship between dose of the agent received and risk? And 4) Risk characterization: what is the burden of risk posed to the population? This approach can be applied to an environmental contaminant in general, e.g., fine particulate air pollution, or to a specific source of the pollutant, diesel particles associated with a bus depot. In characterizing the risks of an environmental agent, the methods of a quantitative risk assessment should make clear what is know for each component of the process and indicate where assumptions have been made to bridge gaps in knowledge.

6.0. CONCLUSION

The urban environment has long posed difficult challenges for controlling threats to public health. Nonetheless, evidence-based strategies can be developed to advance the health of urban dwellers. This chapter sets a general context for researchers who carry out studies to develop the needed evidence. The examples cited make clear that informative studies can be completed, in spite of the challenges faced in carrying out research in urban settings.

REFERENCES

American Lung Association. (2001). Urban air pollution and health inequities: a workshop report. *Environ. Health Perspect.* 109:357–374.

Basu, R., and Samet, J.M. (2002). Relation between elevated ambient temperature and mortality: a review of the epidemiologic evidence. *Epidemiol. Rev.* 24:190–202.

Bell, M.L., Samet, J.M., and Dominici, F. (2004). Time-series studies of particulate matter. *Annu. Rev. Public Health* 25:247–280.

Benowitz, N.L. (1999). Biomarkers of environmental tobacco smoke. *Environ. Health Perspect.* 107:349–355.

Breslow, N.E., Lubin, J.H., and Marek, P. (1982). Multiplicative models and the analysis of cohort data, 50. U. S. National Institutes of Health, Bethesda, MD.

Butler, J.P., Post, G.B., Lioy, P.J., Waldman, J.M., and Greenberg, A. (1993). Assessment of carcinogenic risk from personal exposure to benzo(a)pyrene in the Total Human Environmental Exposure Study (THEES). *J. Air Waste Manage. Assoc.* 43:970–977.

Centers for Disease Control and Prevention (CDC). (1997). National Health Interview Survey. National Center for Health Statistics, Atlanta, GA.

Chapin, F.S., Jr. (1974). *Human activity patterns in the city.* A Wiley-Interscience Publication, New York, NY.

Chew, G.L., Burge, H.A., Dockery, D.W., Muilenberg, M.L., Weiss, S.T., and Gold, D.R. (1998). Limitations of a home characteristics questionnaire as a predictor of indoor allergen levels. *Am. J. Respir. Crit Care Med.* 157:1536–1541.

Chew, G.L., Higgins, K.M., Gold, D.R., Muilenberg, M.L., and Burge, H.A. (1999). Monthly measurements of indoor allergens and the influence of housing type in a northeastern US city. *Allergy* 54:1058–1066.

Committee on Advances in Assessing Human Exposure to Airborne Pollutants and National Research Council (NRC). (1991). *Human exposure assessment for airborne pollutants: advances and opportunities.* National Academy Press, Washington D.C.

Crain, E.F., Weiss, K.B., Bijur, P.E., Hersh, M., Westbrook, L., and Stein, R.E. (1994). An estimate of the prevalence of asthma and wheezing among inner-city children. *Pediatrics* 94:356– 362.

Crawford, F.G., Mayer, J., Santella, R.M., Cooper, T.B., Ottman, R., Tsai, W.Y., Simon-Cereijido, G., Wang, M., Tang, D., and Perera, F.P. (1994). Biomarkers of environmental tobacco smoke in preschool children and their mothers. *J. Natl. Cancer Inst.* 86:1398–1402.

Cunningham, J., O'Connor, G.T., Dockery, D.W., and Speizer, F.E. (1996). Environmental Tobacco Smoke, Wheezing, and Asthma in Children in 24 Communities. *Resp. Crit. Care Med.* 153:218– 224.

Dey, A., Schiller, J., and Tai, D. (2004). Summary health statistics for U.S. children: National Health Interview Survey 2002. *Vital Health Stat* 10(22).

Diez-Roux, A.V. (2000). Multilevel analysis in public health research. *Annu. Rev. Public Health* 21:171–192.

Diggle, P.J., Liang, K.Y., and Zeger, S.L. (1994). *Analysis of longitudinal data.* Oxford University Press, New York, NY.

Dockery, D.W., Pope, C.A., III, Xu, X., Spengler, J.D., Ware, J.H., Fay, M.E., Ferris, B.G. Jr, and Speizer, F.E. (1993). An association between air pollution and mortality in six U.S. cities. *N. Engl. J. Med.* 329:1753–1759.

Dominici, F., McDermott, A., Zeger, S.L., and Samet, J.M. (2003). National maps of the effects of particulate matter on mortality: exploring geographical variation. *Environ. Health Perspect.* 111:39–44.

Dominici, F., Samet, J., and Zeger, S.L. (2000). Combining evidence on air pollution and daily mortality from the largest 20 U.S. cities: a hierarchical modeling strategy (with Discussion). *J. Royal Stat. Soc. Series A* 163:263–302.

Duan, N. (1982). Microenvironmental types: a model for human exposure to air pollution. *Environ Int* 8:305–309.

Eggleston, P.A., Buckley, T.J., Breysse, P.N., Wills-Karp, M., Kleeberger, S.R., and Jaakkola, J.J. (1999). The environment and asthma in U.S. inner cities. *Environ. Health Perspect.* 107 (Suppl 3):439–450.

Ehrlich, R., Kattan, M., Godbold, J., Saltzberg, D.S., Grimm, K.T., Landrigan, P.J., and Lilienfeld, D.E. (1992). Childhood asthma and passive smoking. Urinary cotinine as a biomarker of exposure. *Am. Rev. Respir. Dis.* 145:594–599.

Elliott, P., Hills, M., Beresford, J., Kleinschmidt, I., Jolley, D., Pattenden, S., Rodrigues, L., Westlake, A., and Rose, G. (1992a). Incidence of cancers of the larynx and lung near incinerators of waste solvents and oils in Great Britain. *Lancet* 339:854–858.

Elliott, P., Kleinschmidt, I., and Westlake, A.J. (1992b). Use of Routine Data in Studies of Point Sources of Environmental Pollution. In: Elliott, P., Cuzick, J., English, D., and Stern, R. (eds.), *Geographical and Environmental Epidemiology: Methods for Small-Area Studies.* Oxford University Press, Oxford, England.

Finn, P.W., Boudreau, J.O., He, H., Wang, Y., Chapman, M.D., Vincent, C., Burge, H.A., Weiss, S.T., Perkins, D.L., and Gold, D.R. (2000). Children at risk for asthma: home allergen levels, lymphocyte proliferation, and wheeze. *J. Allergy Clin. Immunol.* 105:933–942.

Gauderman, W.J., Avol, E., Gilliland, F., Vora, H., Thomas, D., Berhane, K., McConnell, R., Kuenzli, N., Lurmann, F., Rappaport, E., Margolis, H., Bates, D., and Peters, J. (2004). The effect of air pollution on lung development from 10 to 18 years of age. *N. Engl. J. Med.* 351:1057–1067.

Gergen, P.J., Mortimer, K.M., Eggleston, P.A., Rosenstreich, D., Mitchell, H., Ownby, D., Kattan, M., Baker, D., Wright, E.C., Slavin, R., and Malveaux, F. (1999). Results of the National Cooperative Inner-City Asthma Study (NCICAS) environmental intervention to reduce cockroach allergen exposure in inner-city homes. *J. Allergy Clin. Immunol.* 103:501–506.

Graham, L.M. (2004). All I need is the air that I breath: outdoor air quality and asthma. *Paediatr. Respir. Rev.* 5(Suppl A):S59-S64.

Health Effects Institute. (2003). Assessing Health Impact of Air Quality Regulations: Concepts and Methods for Accountability Research. HEI Communication 11. HEI Accountability Working Group, Boston, MA.

Holgate, S.T., Sandstrom, T., Frew, A.J., Stenfors, N., Nordenhall, C., Salvi, S., Blomberg, A., Helleday, R., and Soderberg, M. (2003). Health effects of acute exposure to air pollution. Part I: Healthy and asthmatic subjects exposed to diesel exhaust. *Res. Rep. Health Eff. Inst.* 1–30.

Infante-Rivard, C. (1993). Childhood asthma and indoor environmental risk factors. *Am. J. Epidemiol.* 137:834– 844.

Institute of Medicine and Committee on the Assessment of Asthma and Indoor Air (2000). *Clearing the air: asthma and indoor air exposures.* National Academy Press, Washington, D.C.

Jaakkola, J.J. and Jaakkola, M.S. (2002). Effects of environmental tobacco smoke on the respiratory health of children. *Scand. J. Work Environ. Health* 28(Suppl 2):71–83.

Jenkins, R.A., Palausky, A., Counts, R.W., Bayne, C.K., Dindal, A.B., and Guerin, M.R. (1996). Exposure to environmental tobacco smoke in sixteen cities in the United States as determined by personal breathing zone air sampling. *J. Expo. Anal. Environ. Epidemiol.* 6:473–502.

Katsouyanni, K., Touloumi, G., Spix, C., Schwartz, J., Balducci, F., Medina, S., Rossi, G., Wojtyniak, B., Sunyer, J., Bacharova, L., Schouten, J.P., Ponka, A., and Anderson, H.R. (1997). Short-term effects of ambient sulphur dioxide and particulate matter on mortality in 12 European cities: results from the APHEA project. *Br. Med. J.* 314:1658–1663.

Kelsall, J.E., Samet, J.M., Zeger, S.L., and Xu, J. (1997). Air pollution and mortality in Philadelphia, 1974-1988. *Am. J. Epidemiol* 146:750–762.

Kinney, P.L., Aggarwal, M., Northridge, M.E., Janssen, N.A., and Shepard, P. (2000). Airborne concentrations of PM(2.5) and diesel exhaust particles on Harlem sidewalks: a community-based pilot study. *Environ. Health Perspect.* 108:213–218.

Kleinman, M.T., Hyde, D.M., Bufalino, C., Basbaum, C., Bhalla, D.K., and Mautz, W.J. (2003). Toxicity of chemical components of fine particles inhaled by aged rats: effects of concentration. *J. Air Waste Manag. Assoc.* 53:1080–1087.

Klepeis, N.E. (1999a). An introduction to the indirect exposure assessment approach: modeling human exposure using microenvironmental measurements and the recent National Human Activity Pattern Survey. *Environ. Health. Perspect.* 107:365–374.

Klepeis, N.E. (1999b).Validity of the uniform mixing assumption: determining human exposure to environmental tobacco smoke. *Environ. Health. Perspect.* 107:357–363.

Klepeis, N.E., Nelson, W.C., Ott, W.R., Robinson, J.P., Tsang, A.M., Switzer, P., Behar, J.V., Hern, S.C., and Engelmann, W.H. (2001). The National Human Activity Pattern Survey (NHAPS): a resource for assessing exposure to environmental pollutants. *J. Expo. Anal. Environ. Epidemiol.* 11:231–252.

Kunzli, N., and Tager, I.B. (1997). The semi-individual study in air pollution epidemiology: a valid design as compared to ecologic studies. *Environ. Health. Perspect.* 105:1078– 1083.

Lave, L.B., and Seskin, E.P. (1977). *Air Pollution and Human Health.* Johns Hopkins University Press, Baltimore, MD.

Leaderer, B.P. (1990). Assessing exposures to environmental tobacco smoke. *Risk Anal.* 10:19–26.

Leaderer, B.P., Belanger, K., Triche, E., Holford, T., Gold, D.R., Kim, Y., Jankun, T., Ren, P., McSharry, J.E., Platts-Mills, T.A., Chapman, M.D., and Bracken, M.B. (2002). Dust mite, cockroach, cat, and dog allergen concentrations in homes of asthmatic children in the northeastern United States: impact of socioeconomic factors and population density. *Environ. Health Perspect.* 110:419–425.

Levy, J.I., Houseman, E.A., Spengler, J.D., Loh, P., and Ryan, L. (2001). Fine particulate matter and polycyclic aromatic hydrocarbon concentration patterns in Roxbury, Massachusetts: a community-based GIS analysis. *Environ. Health Perspect.* 109:341–347.

Lioy, P.J., and Waldman, J.M. (1990). The personal, indoor and outdoor concentrations of PM-10 measured in an industrial community during the winter. *Atmos. Environ.* 24B:57–66.

Lioy, P.L., Waldman, J.M., Greenberg, A., Harkov, R., and Pietarinen, C. (1988). The Total Human Environmental Exposure Study (THEES) to benzo(a)pyrene: comparison of the inhalation and food pathways. *Arch. Environ. Health* 43:304–312.

Litonjua, A.A., Milton, D.K., Celedon, J.C., Ryan, L., Weiss, S.T., and Gold, D.R. (2002). A longitudinal analysis of wheezing in young children: the independent effects of early life exposure to house dust endotoxin, allergens, and pets. *J. Allergy Clin. Immunol.* 110:736–742.

Lochner, K.A., Kawachi, I., Brennan, R.T., and Buka, S.L. (2003). Social capital and neighborhood mortality rates in Chicago. *Soc. Sci. Med.* 56:1797–1805.

Maclure, M. (1991). The case-crossover design: A method for studying the transient effects of risk of acute events. *Am. J. Epidemiol* 133:144–153.

McMichael, A.J., Baghurst, P.A., Wigg, N.R., Vimpani, G.V., Robertson, E.F., and Roberts, R.J. (1988). Port Pirie Cohort Study: environmental exposure to lead and children's abilities at the age of four years. *N. Eng.l J. Med.* 88:468–475.

Mitchell, H., Senturia, Y., Gergen, P., Baker, D., Joseph, C., McNiff-Mortimer, K., Wedner, H.J., Crain, E., Eggleston, P., Evans, R., 3rd, Kattan, M., Kercsmar, C., Leickly, F., Malveaux, F., Smartt, E., and Weiss, K.. (1997). Design and methods of the National Cooperative Inner-City Asthma Study. *Pediatr. Pulmonol.* 24:237–252.

Morgan, W.J., Crain, E.F., Gruchalla, R.S., O'Connor, G.T., Kattan, M., Evans, R., III, Stout, J., Malindzak, G., Smartt, E., Plaut, M., Walter, M., Vaughn, B., Mitchell, H., and Inner-City Asthma Study Group.

(2004). Results of a home-based environmental intervention among urban children with asthma. *N. Engl. J. Med.* 351:1068–1080.

Morkjaroenpong, V., Rand, C.S., Butz, A.M., Huss, K., Eggleston, P., Malveaux, F.J., and Bartlett, S.J. (2002). Environmental tobacco smoke exposure and nocturnal symptoms among inner-city children with asthma. *J. Allergy Clin. Immunol.* 110:147–153.

Muñoz, A., and Gange, S.J. (1998). Methodological issues for biomarkers and intermediate outcomes in cohort studies. *Epidemiol. Rev.* 20:29–42.

National Research Council (NRC). (1989). Biologic Markers in Pulmonary Toxicology. National Academy Press, Washington, D.C.

National Research Council (NRC). (1991). Human Exposure Assessment for Airborne Pollutants: Advances and Opportunities. Board on Environmental Studies and Toxicology and Committee on Advances in Assessing Human Exposure to Airborne Pollutants, National Academy of Sciences, Washington.

National Research Council (NRC) and Committee on Research Priorities for Airborne Particulate Matter. (1998). Research Priorities for Airborne Particulate Matter: No. 1. Immediate priorities and a long-range research portfolio. National Academy Press, Washington, D.C.

National Research Council (NRC) and Committee on the Institutional Means for Assessment of Risks to Public Health. (1983). Risk Assessment in the Federal Government: Managing the Process. National Academy Press, Washington, D.C.

Neas, L.M., Schwartz, J., and Dockery, D. (1999). A case-crossover analysis of air pollution and mortality in Philadelphia. *Environ. Health Perspect.* 107:629–631.

Needleman, H.L., and Gatsonis, C.A. (1990). Low-level lead exposure and the IQ of children. A meta-analysis of modern studies. *JAMA* 263:673–678.

Northridge, M.E., Yankura, J., Kinney, P.L., Santella, R.M., Shepard, P., Riojas, Y., Aggarwal, M., and Strickland, P. (1999). Diesel exhaust exposure among adolescents in Harlem: a community-driven study. *Am. J. Public Health* 89:998–1002.

Ostro, B., Lipsett, M., Mann, J., Braxton-Owens, H., and White, M. (2001). Air pollution and exacerbation of asthma in African-American children in Los Angeles. *Epidemiol.* 12:200–208.

Ostro, B.D., Lipsett, M.J., Mann, J.K., Wiener, M.B., and Selner, J. (1994). Indoor air pollution and asthma. Results from a panel study. *Am. J. Resp. Crit. Care Med.* 149:1400– 1406.

Park, J.H., Gold, D.R., Spiegelman, D.L., Burge, H.A., and Milton, D.K. (2001). House dust endotoxin and wheeze in the first year of life. *Am. J. Respir. Crit Care Med.* 163:322– 328.

Perera, F., Brenner, D., Jeffrey, A., Mayer, J., Tang, D., Warburton, D., Young, T.I., Wazneh, L., Latriano, L., and Motykiewicz, G. (1992). DNA adducts and related biomarkers in populations exposed to environmental carcinogens. *Environ. Health Perspect.* 98:133–137.

Perera, F.P., Illman, S.M., Kinney, P.L., Whyatt, R.M., Kelvin, E.A., Shepard, P., Evans, D., Fullilove, M., Ford, J., Miller, R.L., Meyer, I.H., and Rauh, V.A. (2002). The challenge of preventing environmentally related disease in young children: community-based research in New York City. *Environ. Health Perspect.* 110:197–204.

Perera, F.P., Rauh, V., Tsai, W.Y., Kinney, P., Camann, D., Barr, D., Bernert, T., Garfinkel, R., Tu, Y.H., Diaz, D., Dietrich, J., and Whyatt, R.M. (2003). Effects of transplacental exposure to environmental pollutants on birth outcomes in a multiethnic population. *Environ. Health Perspect.* 111:201–205.

Perera, F.P., Tang, D., Tu,Y.H., Cruz, L.A., Borjas, M., Bernert, T., and Whyatt, R.M. (2004). Biomarkers in maternal and newborn blood indicate heightened fetal susceptibility to procarcinogenic DNA damage. *Environ. Health Perspect.* 112:1133–1136.

Peters, J.M., Avol, E., Gauderman, W.J., Linn, W.S., Navidi, W., London, S.J., Margolis, H., Rappaport, E., Vora, H., Gong, H., Jr., and Thomas, D.C. (1999a). A study of twelve Southern California communities with differing levels and types of air pollution. II. Effects on pulmonary function. *Am. J. Resp. Crit. Care Med.* 159:768–775.

Peters, J.M., Avol, E., Navidi, W., London, S.J., Gauderman, W.J., Lurmann, F., Linn, W.S., Margolis, H., Rappaport, E., Gong, H., and Thomas, D.C. (1999b). A study of twelve Southern California communities with differing levels and types of air pollution. I. Prevalence of respiratory morbidity. *Am. J. Resp. Crit. Care Med.* 159:760–767.

Prentice, R.L. (1986). A case-cohort design for epidemiologic cohort studies and disease prevention trials. *Biometrika* 73:1–11.

Quackenboss, J.J., Spengler, J.D., Kanarek, M.S., Letz, R., and Duffy, C.P. (1986). Personal exposure to nitrogen dioxide: Relationship to indoor/outdoor air quality and activity patterns. *Environ. Sci. Technol.* 20:775–783.

Reid, D., and Watson, K. (1988). Assessment of human exposure to air pollution. In *Air pollution, the automobile, and the public health.* National Academies Press, Washington, D.C., pp. 207–238.

Robins, J.M., and Greenland, S. (1989). Estimability and estimation of excess and etiologic fractions. *Stat. Med.* 8:845–859.

Romieu, I., Meneses, F., Ramirez, M., Ruiz, S., Perez, P.R., Sienra, J.J., Gerber, M., Grievink, L., Dekker, R., Walda, I., and Brunekreef, B. (1998). Antioxidant supplementation and respiratory functions among workers exposed to high levels of ozone. *Am. J. Respir. Crit. Care Med.* 158:226–232.

Samet, J.M., and Cohen, A.J. (1999). Air pollution and lung cancer. In: Holgate, S.T., Samet, J.M., Koren, H.S., and Maynard, R.L. (eds), *Air Pollution and Health.* Academic Press, San Diego, CA, pp. 841–864.

Samet, J.M. and Muñoz, A. (1998). Evolution of the Cohort Study. *Epidemiol. Rev.* 20:1–14.

Samet, J.M., and Wang, S.S. (2000). Environmental Tobacco Smoke. In: Lippmann, M. (ed.), *Environmental Toxicants: Human Exposures and Their Health Effects.* Van Nostrand Reinhold Company, Inc., New York, pp. 319-375.

Samet, J.M., Zeger, S., Dominici, F., Curriero, F., Coursac, I., and Dockery, D. (2000). The National Morbidity, Mortality, and Air Pollution Study (NMMAPS); Part 2. Morbidity and mortality from air pollution in the United States, Report no 94.Baltimore, MD.

Schwab, M., Colome, S.D., Spengler, J.D., Ryan, P.B., and Billick, I.H. (1990). Activity patterns applied to exposure assessment: data from a personal monitoring study in Los Angeles. *Toxicol. Ind. Health* 6:517–532.

Schwartz, J., Levin, R., and Goldstein, R. (2000). Drinking water turbidity and gastrointestinal illness in the elderly of Philadelphia. *J. Epidemiol. Community Health* 54:45–51.

Sisovic, Fugas, M., and Sega, K. (1996). Assessment of human inhalation exposure to polycyclic aromatic hydrocarbons. *J. Expo. Anal. Environ. Epidemiol.* 6:439–447.

Stepans, M.B., and Fuller, S.G. (1999). Measuring infant exposure to environmental tobacco smoke. *Clin. Nurs. Res.* 8:198– 218.

Thomas, D. (1998). New techniques for the analysis of cohort studies. *Epidemiol. Rev.* 20:122–134.

Tong, S., Baghurst, P.A., Sawyer, M.G., Burns, J., and McMichael, A.J. (1998). Declining blood lead levels and changes in cognitive function during childhood. The Port Pirie Study. *JAMA* 280:1915–1919.

Tonne, C.C., Whyatt, R.M., Camann, D.E., Perera, F.P., and Kinney, P.L. (2004). Predictors of personal polycyclic aromatic hydrocarbon exposures among pregnant minority women in New York City. *Environ. Health Perspect.* 112:754–759.

US Environmental Protection Agency (EPA). (1997). National Ambient Air Quality Standards for Particulate Matter; Part KK. *Fed. Reg.* 62:138.

US Environmental Protection Agency (EPA) and Office of Air Quality Planning and Standards. (1996). Review of the National Ambient Air Quality Standards for Particulate Matter: Policy Assessment of Scientific and Technical Information. OAQPS Staff Paper, Report no EPA-452\R-96-013. U.S. Government Printing Office, Research Triangle Park, North Carolina.

Veglia, F., Matullo, G., and Vineis, P. (2003). Bulky DNA adducts and risk of cancer: a meta-analysis. *Cancer Epidemiol. Biomarkers Prev.* 12:157–160.

Von Mutius, E., Martinez, F.D., Fritzsch, C., Nicolai, T., Roell, G., and Thiemann, H.H. (1994). Prevalence of asthma and atopy in two areas of West and East Germany. *Am. J. Resp. Crit. Care Med.* 149:358–364.

Wade, S., Weil, C., Holden, G., Mitchell, H., Evans, R.,III, Kruszon-Moran, D., Bauman, L., Crain, E., Eggleston, P., Kattan, M., Kercsmar, C., Leickly, F., Malveaux, F., and Wedner, H.J. (1997). Psychosocial characteristics of inner-city children with asthma: a description of the NCICAS psychosocial protocol. National Cooperative Inner-City Asthma Study. *Pediatr. Pulmonol.* 24:263–276.

Webber, M.P., Carpiniello, K.E., Oruwariye, T., and Appel, D.K. (2002). Prevalence of asthma and asthma-like symptoms in inner-city elementary schoolchildren. *Pediatr. Pulmonol.* 34:105– 111.

Weiss, K.B., Gergen, P.J., and Wagener, D.K. (1993). Breathing better or wheezing worse? The changing epidemiology of asthma morbidity and mortality. In: Omenn, G.S. and Lave, L.B. (eds), *Annual Review of Public Health.* Annual Reviews Inc., Palo Alto, pp. 491–513.

Willers, S., Axmon, A., Feyerabend, C., Nielsen, J., Skarping, G., and Skerfving, S. (2000). Assessment of environmental tobacco smoke exposure in children with asthmatic symptoms by questionnaire and cotinine concentrations in plasma, saliva, and urine. *J. Clin. Epidemiol.* 53:715–721.

Chapter 21

Cost-Effectiveness Analysis for Urban Health Research

Ahmed M. Bayoumi

1.0. INTRODUCTION

A frequently voiced concern of urban health researchers and practitioners relates to whether their program is "cost effective." An assertion in favor of cost effectiveness may be viewed as a strong rhetorical argument for a program's application, reflecting a practical recognition that multiple policies are competing for scarce dollars (particularly when they are publicly financed). Alternatively, critics of cost effectiveness analysis may argue that such considerations hamper social justice objectives by constraining policy decisions to arbitrary economic criteria. Regardless of which position one adopts, an understanding of the language and approach of cost effectiveness is essential for policy relevant research conducted in a setting of enhanced consciousness of costs and concerns about debt. A decision maker allocating resources to an intervention must consider the associated monetary costs, health effects, and the relationship between costs and effects. Cost-effectiveness analysis (CEA) is a formal method of analyzing the relationship of costs to health effects that can inform health care policy decision in meaningful ways (Gold, *et al.*, 1996; Detsky and Naglie, 1990).

This chapter is structured as follows. First, we introduce the urban health perspective used in this chapter and an example of a cost effectiveness analysis. Second, we review some conceptual issues and relevant definitions in cost effectiveness analysis. Third, we discuss the elements of a cost effectiveness analysis, including defining strategies, measuring both direct and indirect costs of an illness, discounting of future costs and effects, estimating life duration, and incorporating quality of life considerations. Fourth, we examine the data sources used by analysts, including the role of modeling and extrapolation. Fifth, we present methods used to analyze cost effectiveness analyses. Finally, we conclude by exploring the application of cost effectiveness analysis to urban health by posing several controversial questions. Recent publications have made considerable strides towards establishing standards for cost effectiveness analysis and are worthwhile sources of reference material (Canadian Coordinating Office for Health Technology Assessment, 1997; International Society for Pharmacoeconimics and Outcomes Research, 2004).

1.1. An Urban Health Perspective: Focus on the Disadvantaged

Urban health research and cost effectiveness analysis are both broad academic disciplines that incorporate diverse theories and disciplines. Throughout this chapter, we adopt a perspective that is concerned with the health of urban dwelling individuals and focus on those who experience ill health as a consequence of social disadvantage. While the determinants of health of urban populations are broad, cities have special characteristics that are strongly linked to health. For example, the recent history of urbanization is, strikingly, one of increasing concentration of poverty (Davis, 2004). Other health problems are not uniquely urban, but the conditions or their determinants are more prevalent in cities. For example, the human immunodeficiency virus (HIV) epidemic in North America is closely linked to the urban concentration of gay men, injection drug users, and sex trade workers. Internationally, the HIV epidemic has devastated several cities and remains an overwhelming challenge for many public health departments. This chapter will use an HIV-specific example to illustrate some issues in cost effectiveness analysis. More generally, this chapter assumes that the goal of economic analyses in urban health is to improve efficiency in resource allocation against a backdrop of social disadvantage and inequity.

To illustrate how cost effectiveness analysis can inform urban health (particularly when focused on the disadvantaged), this chapter will conclude by reviewing three questions relevant to this interaction. First, does cost effectiveness analysis discriminate against the disadvantaged? Second, are cost effectiveness analyses transferable from one urban center to another? Third, how can other considerations, particularly those relating to health equity, be combined with cost effectiveness analysis by decision makers?

1.1.1. An Example: HIV Screening in Pregnant Women

Throughout this chapter, the following health care program will serve to illustrate some of the advantages and limitations of cost effectiveness analysis, which will be referred to as the "pregnant women" example. Screening pregnant women for HIV infection offers opportunities to initiate prenatal antiretroviral therapy, a medical intervention proven to decrease the rates of HIV transmission from mothers to infants. Additionally, identifying women early in their infection provides opportunities for counseling about breast feeding and safe sex. The newborn baby also benefits from early identification and appropriate therapy for HIV infection. However, recent studies estimate about 25% of HIV-seropositive individuals are unaware of their status (Fleming, *et al.*, 2000). Furthermore, a significant proportion of women are still not tested during pregnancy or in labor (Bulterys, *et al.*, 2004; Lansky, *et al.*, 2001; Aynalem, *et al.*, 2004). As an alternative to testing women (with consent), some legislators have proposed routine mandatory testing of newborns for HIV infection (in which case consent is not required). Others have objected to such programs on civil libertarian grounds (Powderly, 2001). Note that this objection focuses solely on the issue of testing newborns for HIV and not on other related but similarly complex issues such as mandatory testing of pregnant women or the optimal choice or cost-effectiveness of antiretroviral therapy for expectant mothers (de Zulueta, 2000; Phillips, *et al.*, 2003; Clark, 2003; Lallemant, *et al.*, 2004).

From an economic perspective, one might question whether programs of mandatory testing of newborns are an efficient use of resources, and how questions of efficiency relate to local prevalence patterns. A published cost effectiveness analysis suggests that a program to increase voluntary screening has a "cost effectiveness ratio" of $8,900 U.S. per life year gained (Zaric, *et al.*, 2000). Furthermore, routine newborn HIV screening has a cost effectiveness ratio of $7,000 U.S. per life year gained compared to the status quo condition and $10,600 U.S. per life year gained if implemented after enhanced voluntary screening was implemented. The article concludes that such programs are cost effective. Throughout this chapter, we will return to this analysis to see how the analysts calculated the program's cost effectiveness ratio, how they estimated the program's costs and benefits, and how these findings should be interpreted to assist decision makers in policy making.

2.0. CONCEPTS, TERMS, AND DEFINITIONS

2.1. Cost Effectiveness Analysis

Cost effectiveness analysis typically expresses the tradeoff between the costs of an intervention to the non-financial outcomes as a ratio. Cost effectiveness analysis is concerned with what is happening at the margins – that is, an accounting of the additional, or incremental, costs and effects of an intervention. Cost effectiveness analysis can inform health care decision making by indicating which of several alternative demands for health care spending can improve health the most. For example, consider a city public health official who must decide between expanding one of three programs – smoking cessation, safe sex counseling, or food inspection – within a fixed budget. CEA can indicate which of the three programs will be associated with the greatest improvement in health effects. These health effects could be measured as life years gained, hospitalizations averted, improvements in quality of life scores, or many other metrics. Real world decision making can highlight the complexities involved in making such decisions. For example, the gains from smoking cessation therapy may only be realized many years after the program is instituted. Accordingly, the estimation of this program's costs and health outcomes may be based on more extrapolations and assumptions than those related to food safety. As well, smoking cessation and safe sex counseling may save many more lives than food inspections, although the latter may have important quality of life effects that are widely distributed over a population. Furthermore, a full economic analysis might consider not merely the funding of alternative public health programs, but also whether other non-health programs are a more efficient use of resources. We return to these issues below when we consider some of the limitations of cost effectiveness analysis.

2.2. A Note on Terminology

It is important to realize that the health economics literature, and more generally the field of health services research, tends to use the term "cost effectiveness" analysis in two distinct ways. The first terminology defines CEA as any analysis that calculates the incremental costs relative to a measure of incremental health effects, without consideration of the units with which the effects are measured. For example, this approach would include studies that calculate the cost to avert a case of HIV infection, the costs associated with housing a currently homeless person, or the cost per life year gained for a medical intervention. The second terminology restricts CEA to those analysis that use "life years gained" as the outcome measure. In keeping with the more common and general approach, we adopt the first convention. Thus, cost utility analysis, which is sometimes considered a distinct alternative, will be treated here as a form of cost effectiveness analysis. In this approach, the outcomes are life years which have been "adjusted" by quality of life weights to yield Quality Adjusted Life Years (QALYs), which are discussed further below.

2.2.1. *Quality Adjusted Life Years (QALYs)*

QALYs are calculated by dividing the expected survival into discrete life states, assigning a quality of life weight to each health state, multiplying the quality of life weight of each state by the duration of time spent in the state, and summing across all health states (Zaric, *et al.*, 2000; Carr-Hill, 1989). Consider a hypothetical 35-year-old HIV-positive woman who is projected to live for 12 years before developing acquired immune deficiency syndrome (AIDS) and 5 years afterwards. Although her life expectancy is 17 years (12+5), these years will be spent in suboptimal health. The quality adjusted life year (QALY) model "adjusts" this survival estimate by applying quality weights to this patient's life expectancy (Figure). If the health states our patient experiences before and after AIDS are assigned quality adjustment weights of 0.80 and 0.42, respectively 11, the quality adjusted life expectancy will be 11.7 QALYs (12×0.80 + 5×0.42). A major reason for the QALY model's popularity is its incorporation of both survival and quality of life effects into a single outcome measure. Alternative models, including the Disability Adjusted Life Year (DALY) and

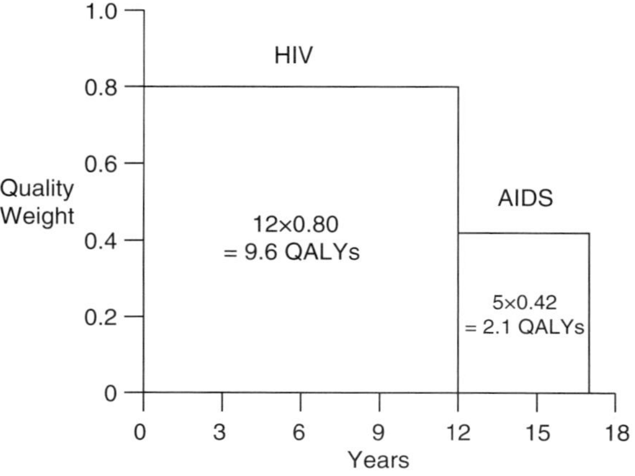

Note: The projected life expectancy (17 years) of a person with HIV is illustrated. To calculate his projected QALYs, four steps are followed: 1) his projected life course is divided into discrete intervals defined by changes in health status (HIV and AIDS); 2) each interval is assigned a quality weight (0.80 and 0.42); 3) a quality adjusted survival for each interval is calculated by multiplying together the quality weight and duration (9.6 and 2.1); and 4) the quality adjusted survivals for all intervals are summed to yield a quality adjusted life expectancy. Thus, the QALY model asserts that our patient's remaining 17 years of life in suboptimal health are equivalent to 11.7 (9.6+2.1) years of life in best possible health.

Figure 1. Calculation of Quality Adjusted Life Years.

Healthy Year Equivalent, have proved less popular or tractable for modeling (Carr-Hill, 1989, Arnesen and Nord, 1999; Gold, *et al.*, 2002; Fryback, 1993; Ried, 1998; Mehrez and Gafni, 1989; Mehrez and Gafni, 1993).

2.2.2. *Discounting*

Discounting is an economic concept that reflects that people value future costs and health effects less than those that occur in the immediate future (Redelmeier and Heller, 1993). The rationale for discounting comes from the recognition that money invested today will be worth more in the future; similarly, money borrowed today will be paid back at a higher value because of interest charged on the loan. For cost effectiveness analyses, where the tradeoff between money and health is being investigated, it makes sense to use the same discount rate for costs as for health effects. In the pregnant woman example, the estimated average gain in life expectancy for a newborn whose HIV infection was averted was 66.9 years. After applying a 3% annual discount rate, this gain was valued at 22.1 years.

2.2.3. *The Incremental Cost-Effectiveness Ratio (ICER)*

The results of a cost effectiveness analysis are typically expressed as an incremental cost effectiveness ratio (ICER). Mathematically, the incremental cost effectiveness of a program, designated B, relative to another program, designated A, is calculated as:

$$\frac{cost_B - cost_A}{effect_B - effect_A}$$

Note that the costs and effects are net values; that is, they reflect both expenditures and savings in the cases of costs and gains and losses in the case of health effects. Thus, the ICER is the cost of obtaining one extra unit of health effect*.

2.2.4. *Dominance*

An intervention which results in lower net costs and enhanced health effects than an alternative strategy is deemed to dominate the alternative. However, the number of dominant interventions are relatively few (examples include prenatal care for pregnant women and some immunizations) (Tengs, *et al.*, 1995). For non-dominant intervention, the decision maker must decide whether the incremental cost is low or high relative to the health effect; that is, whether the intervention represents good value for the money needed to implement the program.

*CEAs generally assume that there is a constant return to scale. That is, the ratio of costs to effects is constant regardless of the scale under which the intervention under evaluation is implemented. Such assumptions are usually not problematic for large scale assessments, but may be problematic when translating national CEA results to a smaller urban setting. Additionally, the assumption of a constant return to scale may not hold for interventions where a threshold exists after which additional marginal benefits are negligible. For example, the additional benefit for mass immunization campaigns likely declines after a large proportion of the population has been immunized.

3.0. THE CONCEPT OF ECONOMIC ANALYSIS IN HEALTH CARE

A tenet of economics is that resources are scarce relative to wants (Drummond, *et al.*, 1987). That is, there will never be enough money available to pay for everything. Accordingly, decision makers require some guidance in how to optimally allocate resources in order to maximize well-being. Consider, for example, two different antiretroviral regimens to prevent transmission of HIV from pregnant women to their fetuses. If the regimens are equally effective but differ in costs, a rational decision maker would clearly choose the less costly option. Unfortunately, decisions are rarely this easy. Consider a third antiretroviral regimen that is slightly more effective than the currently preferred regimen but a great deal more expensive. In this situation, the decision about which regimen to use intrinsically incorporates a trade off between spending more money and averting more infections. Furthermore, money spent in this setting necessarily means that the money will be unavailable for other potential uses.

By posing the question "How much money must be spent to obtain a certain improvement in health?" CEAs directly assess the efficiency, from a cost perspective, of health care expenditures. CEAs can be complex, because to fully assess the intervention might require incorporating disparate outcomes into the costs or health effects, including medication toxicities, the potential for antiretroviral resistance for mothers and infants, productivity losses related to death and illness, and the societal cost of caring for orphans. The impact of such issues may be unknown for some issues and may be context-specific (different in urban vs. rural environments or resource-rich vs. resource-poor countries, for example). Although the methodology of cost-effectiveness continues to evolve, the techniques have obtained popularity as a quantitative method of technology assessment and an aid to policy making. When a health benefit can only be obtained at a relatively large cost, policy makers may judge the health care program to be an unwise use of limited resources, although concerns about justice and equity may mean that decision makers are sometimes willing to trade-off some efficiency to promote other societal goals (See "9.4. How can other considerations, particularly those relating to health equity, be combined with Cost Effectiveness Analysis by decision makers?" below). Internationally, cost effectiveness considerations are now used in many jurisdictions when deciding about which medications to add to formularies and which health services to cover under social insurance programs (Gold, *et al.*, 1996; Canadian Coordinatoring Office for Health Technology Assessment, 1997; International Society for Pharmacoeconomics and Outcomes Research, 2004). For example, at least 32 countries require a pharmacoeconomic component in submissions for drug reimbursement for publicly funded formularies (International Society for Pharmacoeconomics and Outcomes Research, 2004). Similarly, the United Kingdom's National Institute for Clinical Excellence issues technology appraisals to guide public health insurance decisions, in which cost effectiveness analysis plays a central role (Wailoo, *et al.*, 2004).

Returning to the pregnant women example, the authors of the article estimated that enhanced prenatal screening would be associated with an additional annual cost in 1997 of $50.83 million U.S. dollars (related to testing, counseling, infant formula and HIV treatment) while saving $21.48 million U.S. dollars (because of averted HIV infections), for a net cost of $29.35 (50.83-21.48) million U.S. dollars. They further quantified the effectiveness by estimating how many HIV infections would be averted with enhanced prenatal screening (150). Thus, one measure of cost effectiveness is the marginal cost to avert one HIV infection; in this study, the amount is $195,700 ($29.35 million ÷ 150). For comparison, the cost per HIV infection averted for a needle exchange program in 1996 was estimated at about $20,900 (Laufer, 2001). Alternative measures might include the cost per life year gained for infants, for mothers, or for infants and mothers combined.

3.1. Perspective in CEA

CEA can be performed from a number of perspectives. Considering the pregnant women example, the decision maker might be women paying for all or part of prenatal services directly, decision makers at an urban health clinic where she receives prenatal care, state or provincial health officials responsible for hospital financing where the baby will be born and may be tested, or federal financing authorities responsible for funding and administering health care programs. The perspective of a cost effectiveness analysis indicates the point of view from which the analysis is conducted.

Defining the perspective is important because this determination will establish which costs should be included in the analysis. For example, analyses conducted from the perspective of the pregnant woman may include only those costs borne by her (such as co-payments or lost wages due to time away from work) but would not include costs covered by her insurer. Alternatively, a CEA conducted from the perspective of the community health clinic would address those costs incurred by the clinic but not those paid for at the regional or federal level. Most guidelines recommend that the optimal perspective for a CEA is the societal one, which comprehensively covers all of the costs, direct and indirect, included in treating individual patients (Gold, *et al.*, 1996). To provide another example, a recent study estimated the societal costs associated with drug abuse include health care costs (including drug services and medical complications of drug use), productivity losses dues to premature death and illness as well as losses due to criminal activity, and costs related to the administration of the criminal justice and social welfare systems relating to drug use (Cartwright, 1999). In this estimation, health care costs accounted for only 4.5% of total societal costs, illustrating the importance of a comprehensive cost accounting when using a societal perspective.

4.0. ELEMENTS OF A COST-EFFECTIVENESS ANALYSIS

The components of a CEA include a clear description of the alternative strategies under consideration, an estimate of the costs associated with each strategy, and an estimate of the corresponding health effects including survival and often, quality of life.

4.1. Strategies

It is important that CEAs adequately specify the strategies under consideration. Typically, one strategy under consideration is the "status quo" condition; in some instances, this may be doing nothing at all. In other situations, doing nothing may be ethically objectionable and adding this strategy yields little additional information. The strategies should be realistic and comprehensive. When more than two strategies are compared, the comparisons between strategies should be reasonable and, when appropriate, combinations of non-mutually exclusive strategies should also be compared.

In the pregnant women example, the "status quo" condition reflects the current level of voluntary HIV testing; it does not reflect a condition of no testing since such a condition does not exist and would not be a reasonable policy to purse. Furthermore, comparing interventions to a strategy of "no testing" would make them seem more attractive than they really are. The authors compared two strategies – enhanced voluntary testing and mandatory screening of newborns – each to the status quo condition. Importantly, they also analyzed a strategy of mandatory screening of newborns and enhanced voluntary screening to a strategy of enhanced voluntary screening alone, after demonstrating that voluntary screening was associated with a favorable cost effectiveness ratio.

4.2. Costs

The costs associated with a health care intervention include the cost of the intervention itself, changes in the use of health care resources as a result of the intervention, changes in the use of non-health care resources, changes in the use of informal caregiver time, and changes in the use of patient time for treatment (Luce, *et al.*, 1996). For example, a pregnant HIV-positive woman might incur costs related to the medication (the intervention), physician and nursing costs associated with her treatment (health care costs), costs associated with traveling to the clinic (non-health care costs), costs associated with her partner and friends taking time from work (informal caregiver time), and costs related to not being able to work while attending the clinic (patient time costs). An additional source of potential costs comes from decreased productivity related to her HIV status and to caring for her infant if the newborn is infected with HIV; U.S. guidelines on the conduct of cost effectiveness analyses recommended that these productivity losses be treated as health outcomes rather than costs (Gold, *et al.*, 1996). Because CEAs are incremental in their analysis (they are interested in an intervention's extra, rather than total, costs), costs that can be shown or safely assumed to be equivalent between strategies need not be explicitly valued. Similarly, it is often not worthwhile to estimate costs that are small relative to the overall costs of a program, viewed from a societal perspective. Some modeling assumptions (such as the exclusion of certain costs) may be controversial; their potential impact can be assessed by performing sensitivity analyses, in which the value of certain parameters are varied across a reasonable range, even if the true value for a parameter is unknown. If the results are robust to changing values, the analyst can have some assurance that the conclusions are not sensitive to the incorporated assumptions (See "7.1 Uncertainty in Cost Effectiveness Analysis" below).

Costing studies can be performed at the "micro" level, in which each resource used is identified, measured, and valued, or at the "gross" level, in which average costs from a large area are used (Luce, *et al.*, 1996; Diehr, *et al.*, 1999). For example, micro-costing an HIV test includes costing the materials used and the labor to perform the test, while gross-costing a physician visit include counting the number of visits and assigning each an "average" cost based on reimbursement rates or other studies. Many analyses combine both micro and gross approaches.

In the cost effectiveness analyses of testing for HIV in pregnant women and their newborns, the researchers included the costs of HIV testing, counseling before and after an HIV test, infant formula, antiretroviral therapy, and future lifetime healthcare costs. The analysis did not explicitly incorporate costs related to informal caregiver time or patient time for treatment, although some of these costs by be capture in the estimate of future costs and others may be negligible if, for example, the incremental patient time costs are small relative to the counseling and treatment costs.

4.3. Life Duration

Perhaps the most common health effect measure used in cost effectiveness analysis is survival. Although survival is virtually always an important outcome measure, there are several caveats associated with its use in an analysis. First, the available data for estimating cost effectiveness may be of limited duration. Hence, incorporating survival into the model necessitates extrapolations from intermediate outcomes and assumptions about future therapies, both of which may have considerable associated uncertainty. In the pregnant woman example, the investigators based their life expectancy assumptions on the best currently available therapy. Second, an intervention may have life-extending effects beyond those received by the person being treated. In the pregnant woman example, the effects on both the mother and her newborn baby are important to consider. A more extensive analysis may also have looked at the health benefits of diagnosing early HIV infection with the potential for decreasing HIV transmission. Third, interventions may have important quality of life effects that are not captured by focusing solely on survival. For example, an intervention may improve quality of life but have no effect on survival, or may even have divergent effects on quality of life and survival. For this reason, U.S. guidelines recommend the quality adjusted life year (QALY) as the preferred method of measuring health benefits, although this assertion remains controversial (McGregor, 2003; Carr-Hill, 1989; Freemantle, 2000; Loomes and McKenzie, 1989; Williams, 1991).

4.4. Quality of Life Weights

Quality of life weights are usually derived from utilities, which are values that summarize preferences for health states in a single number (Torrance, 1987; Froberg and Kane, 1989a). Utility elicitation methods are based on decision science theory. Formally, utilities are numbers that describes an individual's strength of preference for outcomes under conditions of uncertainty (Torrance, 1987; Froberg and Kane, 1989b; Torrance 1986). The rationale for using utilities as quality of life weights in cost effectiveness analysis is that both the need for health interventions and the benefit from the intervention are usually unknown; as such, preference weights from the field of decision sciences, which focuses on judgments under conditions of uncertainty, are appealing.

In health care, the utility scale is typically anchored at 0, representing death, and 1, representing best possible health. Several methods are commonly used for measuring utilities, which typically involve asking individuals to choose between hypothetical alternative and calculating their utilities from their responses. Although the methods are widely used, several observations can lead investigators to approach their use cautiously. First, alternative methods for measuring utility for health states often differ, sometimes greatly (Bayoumi and Redelmeier, 1999; Dolan, *et al.*, 1996; Hornberger, *et al.*, 1992, Read, *et al.*, 1984; Stiggelbout, *et al.*,

1994; Bombardier, 1982; Martin, *et al.*, 2000, Torrance, 1976). Second, the assessment tasks can be cognitively demanding (Hershey, *et al.*, 1988; Bleichrodt, 2002; Llewellyn-Thomas, *et al.*, 1984). Third, some individuals may object to the form of the task and refuse to answer (for example, religious people sometimes object to the notion that they could shorten or extend their life). Fourth, the methods can be internally inconsistent (Llewellyn-Thomas, *et al.*, 1982).

U.S. guidelines recommend that community preferences (from representatives of the general population) be surveyed when conducting cost effectiveness analyses from a societal perspective, since these will most accurately reflect "societal" values (Gold, *et al.*, 1996). However, there are some situations in which it may be difficult for community members to adequately characterize a health condition. As well, it may be difficult to find an appropriate proxy to evaluate health states for some health states (like dementia) or stages of life (like infancy). In the pregnant women example, the authors did not measure utilities or incorporate quality of life weights as their main outcome measure was the health effects of children and mothers combined. Thus, even if quality of life weights for infants could have been applied, the authors would have faced the additional formidable problem of ascertaining that these weights were measured on the same scale as that used for mothers. More generally, CEAs incompletely capture some benefits, including the benefit obtained by others from an individual's well-being, both directly (for example, the benefit to children from saving the life of a parent) and indirectly expressed as altruism (for example, the well-being felt by men from the existence of a program of screening for cervical cancer among low income women).

5.0. DATA SOURCES

CEA generally integrate data from a number of sources. Primary data collection has been used to conduct economic analyses parallel to randomized controlled trials or observational studies. Additionally, many studies have used primary data collection to measure utilities. Systematic reviews of the medical literature are an effective method of synthesizing large amounts of data to answer specific clinical questions. Secondary analyses of either primary research data or administrative databases have also proven invaluable. Finally, when no data is available, CEA have made use of expert consensus opinion.

5.1. The Role of Modeling

Although analysts can estimate effectiveness from empiric estimations, the time frame of CEAs often exceeds that of clinical trials or observational databases. Additionally, CEAs may address questions or include populations that are more general than those included in traditional studies of effectiveness. Accordingly, CEAs are usually integrative studies that combine data from several sources into a mathematical model to simulate the natural history of a condition. While models necessarily simplify representations of complex processes, the selection of an appropriate model is not always straightforward (Sculpher, *et al.*, 2000). Salient points to consider include the complexity of the populations and disease under consideration, the importance of including individual or population level outcomes, and the degree of uncertainty associated with the outcome. Quantifying the latter concern can help prioritize future research. How results from different models differ is a largely unexplored area.

6.0. ANALYZING THE RESULTS

The incremental cost effectiveness ratio (ICER) will estimate the amount needed for a gain in one unit of health effect. But what constitutes an attractive ICER? No consensus exists on the appropriate threshold at which an intervention stops being cost effective, although many decision makers consider interventions with a cost-effectiveness ratio of greater than $50,000 to $100,000 per quality adjusted life year (QALY) to be economically unattractive for interventions when analyzed from the societal perspective (Owens, 1998; Laupacis, et al., 1993). Analyses performed in different urban settings, countries (particularly resource poor states) or from other perspectives may adopt alternative thresholds. Some analysts have criticized the threshold approach to designating interventions as cost effective, arguing that such an approach does not offer decision makers an effective means to control budgetary expenditures.

7.0. TECHNICAL AND ALLOCATIVE EFFICIENCY

The ICER is a measure of efficiency. It is useful to consider two types of efficiency: technical and allocative (Oliver, *et al.*, 2002). Technical (also called productive) efficiency is the comparison of costs to outcomes, whether as a ratio (in cost-consequence and cost-utility analyses) or as a difference (in cost benefit analyses). An intervention is technically efficient when, for the same amount of money, no additional health benefits can be achieved. In the pregnant woman example, implementing 71% of the routine newborn screening strategy would yield the same costs (about $29 million U.S.) as the enhanced prenatal screening strategy but would avert 41 additional HIV infections. Hence, from a technical efficiency perspective, a strategy of enhanced prenatal screening is not preferred.

Now consider the combination of enhanced screening and routine screening of newborns. Such a program would result in additional costs ($32 million U.S.) and 135 additional HIV infections averted. Would an alternative use of this $32 million U.S. result in better health outcomes?* Because other interventions likely will not measure outcomes as the number of HIV infections averted, it is not possible to compares these alternative financial allocations directly. Thus, assessing this type of efficiency, known as allocative efficiency, necessitates a common outcome measure for economic analyses. The strong preference for the QALY by official agencies is in part because it is not specific to any one health condition (or even to life-extending conditions) and therefore can be used to assess both technical and allocative decisions within the health sector.

Allocative efficiency asks whether there is a net gain in health by assigning resources from one intervention to another. Assuming that budgets are fixed, there will necessarily be some losses in health effects for a group whose intervention is deprived of funds. Although decision makers may rationally want information about allocative efficiency to make their decisions, few economic analyses present their results in this way. Furthermore, because non-health interventions are typically not measured using QALYs, allocative efficiency between health and other sectors cannot be readily assessed with the QALY model.

*Economists refer to the "opportunity cost" of a decision – the cost of the next best alternative which is foregone as a result of the decision made.

7.1. Uncertainty in Cost Effectiveness Analysis

Several aspects of a cost effectiveness analyses are often uncertain. For example, the precise values of some of the parameters in the analysis may be uncertain. Many models incorporate assumptions and extrapolations. U.S. guidelines recommend looking at three types of uncertainty (Gold, *et al.*, 1996). Parameter uncertainty refers to examining how model results vary when parameter values are changed. Parameter uncertainty is best examined by performing sensitivity analysis, in which changing one or two parameters at a time can yield important insights into which model parameters most influence the model results while sophisticated methods of varying multiple model parameters simultaneously are often the best method of assessing overall model uncertainty. Model structural uncertainty refers to changing the model structure to examine the robustness of the model to modeling assumptions. Model process uncertainty refers to examining results from different models to see if divergent approaches yield consistent results.

Although the analysis of uncertainly around an ICER, a ratio statistic without a defined distribution, has historically been difficult, recent advances have used transformations, graphical representations, and re-sampling methods (Fenwick, *et al.*, 2001). These advances now enable analysts to derive reasonable confidence intervals for cost effectiveness statistics. Nevertheless, some have argued that the reason to assess uncertainty in the ICER is not to preclude decision making, but rather to point to areas in which additional research is needed for more definitive conclusions (Claxton, 1999).

8.0. ALTERNATIVES TO COST EFFECTIVENESS ANALYSIS

Cost effectiveness analysis has been endorsed as the preferred method of economic analysis by several national technology assessment authorities. Several alternatives to cost effectiveness analysis have been proposed, of which the most common are summarized below (Gold, *et al.*, 1996):

- *Cost minimization analysis* is a form of analysis in which the effectiveness of the interventions under consideration are assumed to be equivalent. Thus, the goal of the analysis is to find the strategy that minimizes costs. Because it is rarely the case that effectiveness is truly equivalent across strategies, cost minimization analysis is not commonly used.
- *Cost consequence analysis* is a form of analysis in which costs and consequences of the interventions being considered are presented in a disaggregated form. The advantage of such an approach is that the consequences that can be considered are comprehensive and there is no attempt to combine divergent outcomes, as in the QALY model.
- *Cost benefit analysis* is closely related to cost effectiveness analysis, except that the health effects are valued in dollar amounts (McIntosh, *et al.*, 1999; O'Brien and Gafni, 1996; Klose, 1999; Diener, *et al.*, 1998; Olsen and Smith, 2001). Although cost benefit analysis has been considerably less popular in health services research than cost effectiveness analysis, there are some clear advantages for the former approach. For example, it is easy to compare allocative efficiency across different programs or even across sectors and it is also straightforward to include non-health benefits in the analysis. The greatest limitation of cost benefit analysis is the requirement for health

effects to be expressed in dollar amounts. This raises measurement problems as well as ethical ones. For example, health problems of the rich may be valued more highly than the poor simply because they can afford to pay more to address them. For some features of cost benefit analysis, there are both advantages and drawbacks. For example, cost benefit analysis is directly grounded in welfare economic theory, which appeals to economists working from this perspective but may be objectionable to others (see below). Because of the concerns about cost benefit analysis, U.S. guidelines have endorsed cost effectiveness analysis as the preferred method for economic analysis in health care (Gold, *et al.*, 1996).

9.0. CONTROVERSIES IN COST EFFECTIVENESS ANALYSIS AND URBAN HEALTH

9.1. Does Cost Effectiveness Analysis Discriminate against the Disadvantaged?

To the extent that urban health researchers and decision makers are focused on helping the urban disadvantaged, they may be particularly interested whether there are aspects of CEA that may be discriminatory. Briefly, there are five main considerations: (1) The use of community ratings of quality of life may further disempower the disadvantaged and introduce biases due to stigmatization; (2) The cognitive and experiential requirements of utility surveys may be disadvantageous for populations with these limitations; (3) The use of QALYs as a health outcome may introduce biases against the elderly and disabled; (4) The reliance on welfare economic theory may favor resource distribution to the rich; (5) Cost effectiveness analysis is silent about the status quo distribution of resources. Each of these are presented in turn.

9.1.1. Community Ratings of Quality of Life

Who should provide quality of life weights for use in cost effectiveness analyses? From an urban health perspective, the recommendation that community ratings be used raises two significant concerns. First, some health situations may be insufficiently familiar to members of the general population (Froberg and Kane, 1989a). Thus, editing and misinformation biases may result in respondents not truly evaluating the intervention of interest, but rather their (mis)interpretation thereof. For example, urban health researchers may be concerned that few members of the population would have sufficient experience to rate conditions associated with homelessness, such as scabies. More broadly, the use of community references raises questions of agency; that is, ought members of the general population be judging the health conditions of a disadvantaged minority? This intensely political question may trouble community health researchers who are unwilling to cede such judgments to external evaluators, with the accompanying concerns about power and control.

Another concern with community ratings relates to biased responses that reflect how respondents feel about the potential beneficiaries of an intervention rather than how they rate the health state, particularly if the beneficiaries are stigmatized. For example, respondents may rate a health condition highly if the potential respondents are newborn babies out of a desire to appear gracious.

Alternatively, respondents may rate a health condition too harshly if the potential beneficiaries are stigmatized. For example, respondents may provide low ratings for health conditions associated with hepatitis C if they harbor discriminatory feelings against injection drug users. For such reasons, the use of community ratings, and the attendant potential for introducing biases, should be carefully considered in each valuation study.

9.1.2. *Cognitive and Experiential Requirements of Utility Surveys*

For some outcome measures, providing utility ratings may be cognitively or emotionally challenging. The utility elicitation methods with the strongest theoretical bases require individuals to consider scenarios in which they must trade off a chance of death or future survival. Individuals who have a hard time understanding such scenarios, or find them too psychologically disturbing, may give responses that are systematically too high (reflecting an unwillingness to accept the trade off, for example). Similarly, religiosity – which is associated with ethnicity – may influence individual ratings (Tsevat, *et al.*, 1996). The result of such a valuation would be that these ratings, if taken at face value, would indicate that individuals with such characteristics these are not experiencing adverse quality of life and hence, may be less deserving of funding priorities. Thus, utility elicitation studies should carefully assess the role of biases related to cognition, emotion, and religiosity when reporting their results.

9.1.3. *QALYs and Discrimination*

Another concern relating to the disadvantaged stems from the use of QALYs to measure health effects and individuals' potential for increasing quality of life or survival. Consider three individuals who are being considered for a given treatment. One is 40 years old and otherwise healthy, another is 30 years old with HIV infection with AIDS complications, and the third is 70 years old with some mild chronic medical problems. Although all may benefit from the treatment, the 40 year old has the greatest potential QALY improvement since his potential for improvement and life prolongation is not limited by comorbidity (such as AIDS) or advanced age. Indeed, ethicists have criticized resource allocation decisions that aim to only maximize QALYs (without considering other patient characteristics) as being inherently discriminatory against the disabled and elderly (Harris, 1987; Singer, *et al.*, 1995) a point to which we return below when discussing equity considerations in resource allocation decisions.

9.1.4. *Welfare Economic Theory*

Other critics have raised questions about welfare economic theory as a basis for cost effectiveness analysis. While a full review of theory is available elsewhere, I restrict my comments here to considerations that are important for applying CEA to urban health. Welfare theory is a branch of economics that examines the desirability of alternative allocation of resources (Garber and Phelps, 1997; Brouwer and Koopmanschap, 2000). (It is not at all about "welfare", financial assistance to disadvantaged individuals, as social policy). The underlying assumption of welfare economics is that each individual in a society, acting as rational agents, would use the resources available to him or her to maximize their own welfare, or well-being. The way in which these resources are combined are determined at the individual level, according to each person's preference (or utility) function. For example, some individuals would spend their money on cars while others would spend it on housing, but all would maximize their utility (happiness) by allocating their personal resources appropriately. Welfare economic theory asserts that the overall welfare of a society is determined through aggregating individual welfare.

Under welfare economics, the optimal allocation of resources is obtained when each individual's welfare is maximized. When such conditions are met, some individuals may have worse health than others, but if this distribution reflects individual differences in preferences for health, then the inequality in health is unimportant. That is, what welfare economics seeks to maximize is aggregate utility not aggregate health. This approach accepts that individual preferences for health often vary. For example, some people may have decided to accept some other benefit (such as more money) while trading off health, but this combination of characteristics maximizes their happiness. Welfare economics uses a hypothetical "compensation test" to ascertain if the allocation of resources is truly optimal. This test assumes that with the introduction of an intervention there will be winners (for example, those who benefit from the intervention) and losers (for example, those who pay for the intervention but do not benefit). The compensation test asserts that if the amount the winners are willing to pay exceeds the amount the losers demand for compensation, then the reallocation of resources is worthwhile.

Three salient criticisms of welfare theory are notable. First, the compensation test as a basis for resource allocation is controversial, since resources are often allocated in such a way that the winners benefit but the losers are not compensated, or insufficiently so. As such, the compensation test has been criticized as a basis for resource allocation since there is no assurance that resource allocation will meet this internal standard of fairness (Weinstein and Stason, 1977). Of course, decision makers may want even more rigorous standards to be considered. An additional concern about the compensation test is that it may actually lead to less aggregate health, particularly if the losers are giving up more health than the winners are buying. If the losers are poor and the winners are rich, then society may have maximized individual preferences but worsened overall health and exacerbated class differences in health.

A second criticism of welfare theory is that there is unlikely to be any acceptable means of aggregating utilities across individuals, even if good methods of measuring utilities were available. Third, some have argued that health is a "primary social good" that should be treated differently than other commodities. That is, we may be happy as a society to let individuals determine what basket of consumer goods maximizes individual utility, but we may be unwilling to let individuals trade off health to improve wealth. Proponents of this view argue that health is different from other goods, since good health is frequently a precondition for enjoyment of other aspects of life. Accordingly, health is a good that everyone should be entitled to, regardless of their willingness to pay. This last view, which has been termed "extra-welfarist" seeks to maximize health, rather than utility, when allocating societal resources (Birch and Donalson, 2003; Wagstaff, 1991).

To illustrate this difference, consider society's response to the question of individuals interested in selling their body organs for money. An extra-welfarist perspective might agree to ban this sale, since the goal of resource allocation is to maximize health. Accordingly, individuals who voluntarily sacrifice some element of their health would be acting contrary to society's best interest. In contrast, the welfarist perspective might argue that, assuming the seller has full information of the inherent risk, such a sale might result in a net increase in personal, and hence societal, utility and is unobjectionable.

Why should urban health researchers care about the tension between the welfarist and extra-welfarist viewpoints? It is important to recognize that this discrepancy should not be interpreted as a rejection of CEA as a method as a health technology assessment tool. Rather, the debate informs how QALYs are interpreted and how cost-effectiveness analyses are used for resource allocation decisions. Adopting an extra-welfarist orientation leads to the conclusion that the goal of cost-effectiveness analysis is to maximize health, not utility. While health maximization does not imply that QALYs are a good measure of health, analysts who adopt this perspective will be considerably less concerned about whether the QALYs are themselves utilities or whether the QALY model violates the tenets of welfare economic theory (Bleichrodt, 1997). Accordingly, this approach views CEA less as an overarching theory of resource allocation and more as a guide to decision making, to be incorporated with other pertinent information (Brouwer and Koopmanschap, 2000).

9.1.5. Cost Effectiveness Analysis and Social Justice

As discussed above, cost effectiveness analysis will be most helpful to decision makers when addressing allocative efficiency – that is, are the health gains from reallocating resources from one group to another efficient in maximizing health (or utility)? Importantly, such analyses do not question the underlying distribution of financial resources. That is, the "winners" in a resource allocation decision are chosen based on their potential for health improvement. Even when analysts have considered applying equity considerations to cost effectiveness decision making (see below), the concern has been for health equity; that is, reducing inequalities in health need, access, or status. The application of cost effectiveness analysis to address issues of societal equity – that is, to examine social justice issues – is almost certainly beyond such analyses' capabilities.

9.2. Are Cost Effectiveness Analyses Transferable from One Urban Center to Another?

The application of the results of cost effectiveness analysis conducted in one location to another is not automatic (Owens and Nease, 1997). Urban health researchers considering applying a cost effectiveness analysis conducted in another situation to their own should consider the following questions:

9.2.1. Is the Perspective of the Analysis Similar?

Although the societal perspective is preferred for societal level decision making, it may not be the most relevant perspective when applying decisions in a specific context. For example, urban public health departments may want to adopt a narrower perspective when deciding on policy implications. Of note, many analyses that assume a "payer" (public insurer) perspective adopt that of a state, provincial, or federal and much less commonly, an urban perspective. Although it is common to assume that an intervention can be easily scaled up or down without changing the results, it is worthwhile to explicitly interrogate this assumption before applying analyses conducted at a large-scale level to a more local environment. For example, consider a local public health department considering a program of directly observed therapy for people infected with tuberculosis. From the perspective of the urban health department, some costs may be excluded in a particular local situation (for example, if travel costs were not paid for directly by the local health department). Furthermore, the startup costs related establishing such an infrastructure may vary considerably between locations. As a result, simply scaling down national cost effectiveness estimates can be misleading.

9.2.2. Which Parameters Need to Be Adapted to the Local Level?

Many parameters in a cost effectiveness analysis may need to be adapted to a local situation. In the pregnant women example, the prevalence of HIV infection and the rate of maternal to infant transmission is a key determinant of cost effectiveness. In the tuberculosis example cited above, the health effects may depend on the prevalence of multi-drug resistant tuberculosis and medication non-adherence. Accordingly, the application of this analysis would require careful customization of the results to local situations. Similarly, local costs may differ considerably from those in an analysis. If the analysis incorporates community ratings of quality of life, it is worthwhile to ask if local ratings would be similar to those in an analysis. Finally, risk adjustment to local considerations may be important. In the pregnant women example, if the distribution of prognostic factors is different in a local population than in that described in the analysis, the projected life expectancies may also vary. An analysis of model uncertainty can often be helpful if the parameter values examined in sensitivity analysis are similar to those of the local setting.

Apart from model parameters, two other considerations are noteworthy when applying CEAs to the local level, particularly when approaching such issues from a global perspective. First, the approach to the analysis, particularly if based on a model, should be carefully examined. Are the interventions described feasible to implement at a local level? Is the description of the health care provided in the analysis different enough to warrant changes in the model structure? Second, is the cost effectiveness threshold similar across settings? That is, the cost per incremental health gain may be very different in an economically well off country and one that is resource poor. Thus, even if the analysis is accepted without major changes, the interpretation of the results requires careful attention.

9.2.3. What Are the Budgetary and Allocative Implications of the Decisions?

Most cost effectiveness analyses only report an incremental cost effectiveness ratio (ICER). Decision makers will ordinarily require at least two additional pieces of information before making a decision about allocating resources to the intervention under consideration. First, they will need to ascertain the budgetary implications of such a decision. Recall that two interventions can have the same ICER although one's incremental costs and effects are small and the others are large. Decision makers will need to know the intervention's cost as well as its cost effectiveness.

In addition, and related to the above, decision makers will likely want to know where the resources allocated to this decision are coming from. That is, are other programs being cut to fund the new allocation? Are taxes being raised or bonds being generated? If so, are the losses that some individuals will incur offset by the gains in the new program?

9.4. How Can Other Considerations, Particularly Those Relating to Health Equity, Be Combined with Cost Effectiveness Analysis by Decision Makers?

Most applications of cost effectiveness analysis focus only on efficiency and neglect equity implications associated with the distribution of changes in health and wealth. That is, there is no attention paid to how widely the health effects are distributed. While "what gain?" matters, "who gains?" may matter as much or more (Culyer, 2001; Ubel, *et al.*, 1996; Holm, 1998; Culyer and Wagstaff, 1993).

To illustrate, consider three interventions (A, B, and C), each associated with an increase of 200 QALYs (Table). Intervention A yields an average of 1 QALY gain for 200 individuals, whereas intervention B yields 2 QALYs for 100 individuals and intervention C yields 0.5 QALYs for 400 individuals. A simple application of the QALY model, without consideration of the number of people who are benefiting, may lead decision makers to conclude that these interventions are equivalent. However, empirical evidence shows that members of the general public, ethicists, and decision scientists place a value on how wide the benefits are shared. For example, individuals who prefer intervention C over A would be willing to trade off smaller individual gains (0.5 vs. 1 QALY) to gain a wider distribution of benefits (400 people helped instead of 200).

In addition to considerations about how gains are distributed across individuals, reporting outcomes as incremental QALY gains can obscure two other factors that may be important for decision makers making resource allocation decisions. First, focusing on QALYs may obscure the fact that some interventions extend (or save) more lives than others. For example, our hypothetical intervention C is associated with no increase in survival, although it does increase quality of life. In contrast, interventions A and B are both associated with an increased survival of two years. Decision makers may wish to place a higher priority on life-saving interventions.

A second feature that is not apparent when focusing on QALYs arises from the focus of cost utility analysis on incremental QALY gains. In our example, a patient

Table 1. Gains with Three Hypothetical Interventions

	A	B	C
Gains per individual			
Life expectancy before intervention (years)	10	20	20
Life expectancy after intervention (years)	12	22	20
Gain in life years	2	2	0
QALYs before intervention*	5	16	19
QALYs after intervention	6	18	19.5
Gain in QALYs	1	2	0.5
Gains across individuals			
Number of people affected	200	100	400
Total QALY gain	200	200	200

*QALY denotes quality-adjusted life year.

receiving intervention A gains half as many QALYs as a patient receiving intervention B; however, the quality adjusted life expectancy of a patient in group A, even with the intervention, is only one-third that of a patient in group B. Decision makers may wish to allocate financial resources preferentially to the sickest patients.

Because cost effectiveness analysis as commonly reported seeks to maximize the health effect (such as QALYs) without consideration for the benefits, some have criticized the approach as utilitarian. To address concerns about distributional concerns, several recent approaches have investigated the relationship between efficiency (as measured by cost effectiveness analysis) and equity (Olsen, 1997). The assumption in many such analyses is that decision makers may be willing to accept a somewhat less efficient allocation of resources if the decision meets equity criteria. The health economics literature largely focuses on an equitable distribution of resources, rather than equity in other areas relevant to public health (such as access to care).

Several approaches have been put forward to capture equity weights in CEA. One has attempted to apply "equity weights" to the measure of health effect. For example, equity-weighted QALYs may give greater weight to QALYs gained by individuals whom decision makers wish to single out for treatment. Another approach has been to use alternative outcome measures that incorporate some element of equity measurement (Ubel, 2000; Nord, 1992). For example, the Person Trade-off method directly elicits preferences for distribution among divergent groups as the weight for health effects, rather than preferences for health states (Nord, 1995). A third approach uses standard outcome measures, but uses different cost effectiveness thresholds for distinct groups (Hoch and Bayoumi, 2003). Yet another approach compares the distributional implications of a resource allocation decision based on a CEA against the optimal distribution of resources as determined by societal preferences for inequity (termed a "social welfare" function) (Wagstaff, 1991). Because each of these approaches have both limitations in theory and practice (particularly related to measurement issues), none consensus has emerged to the optimal method. Nevertheless, many agree that such approaches offer important methods to extend the analysis of CEA to provide additional important information to decision makers.

Besides equity, other considerations that may be important for decision makers are not well captured by CEA (Deber and Goel, 1990). For example, there may be benefits to individuals that are not captured in the health effects measured. Additionally there may be other ethical or political concerns that guide decision making. In the pregnant women example, additional benefits may include decreased transmission of HIV to other sex partners and potentially prolonged survival for the mother, which may be important for the emotional well-being of all of her children. Additional concerns may include ethical and legal concerns about the possible infringement on civil liberties associated with mandatory testing of newborns or political concerns associated with not testing infants for a potentially treatable disease.

10.0. CONCLUSION

Cost effectiveness analysis is the principal method for examining the efficiency of health interventions, with both widespread acceptance and official sanction from a number of governmental agencies. Although some have criticized such analyses as a means on which to base decisions, three important caveats to the use of CEA are necessary. First, such analyses are models that attempt to estimate efficiency, but the application of such analyses should always question the models assumptions to ascertain if they are applicable in a particular urban setting. Second, users and analysts of CEA should carefully assess the uncertainty in the analysis. Too often, the base case analysis receives the bulk of attention in an attempt to classify an intervention as "cost effective" or not. Appropriate attention to the assessment of uncertainty is important for identifying questions that are important for making better decisions. Finally, CEA – even if accepted as a good measure of efficiency – is only one attribute that decision makers should consider when making resource allocation decisions. CEA can be an important input to such decisions, but so are considerations of politics, law, ethics and justice. Resource allocation decisions will remain complicated without simple technical solutions.

REFERENCES

Arnesen, T., and Nord, E. (1999). The value of DALY life: Problems with ethics and validity of disability adjusted life years. *BMJ.* 319:1423–5.

Aynalem, G., Mendoza, P., Frederick, T., and Mascola, L. (2004). Who and why? HIV-testing refusal during pregnancy: implication for pediatric HIV epidemic disparity. *AIDS Behav.* 8:25–31.

Bayoumi, A.M., and Redelmeier, D.A. (1999). Economic methods for measuring the quality of life associated with HIV infection. *Qual. Life Res.* 8:471–80.

Birch, S., and Donaldson, C. (2003). Valuing the benefits and costs of health care programmes: where's the `extra' in extra-welfarism? *Soc. Sci. Med.* 56:1121–1133.

Bleichrodt, H. (2002). A new explanation for the difference between time trade-off utilities and standard gamble utilities. *Health Econ.* 11:447–56.

Bleichrodt, H., and Johannesson, M. (1997). The validity of QALYs: An experimental test of constant proportional tradeoff and utility independence. *Med. Decis. Making* 17:21–32.

Bombardier, C., Wolfson, A.D., Sinclair, A.J., and McGeer, A. (1982). Comparison of three preference measurement methodologies in the evaluation of a function status index. In: Deber, R.B. and Thompson, C.G. (eds.), *Choices in health care: decision-making and evaluation of effectiveness.* Toronto, pp. 145–159.

Briggs, A.H., Goeree, R., Blackhouse, G., and O'Brien, B.J. (2002). Probabilistic analysis of cost-effectiveness models: choosing between treatment strategies for gastroesophageal reflux disease. *Med. Decis. Making* 22:290–308.

Briggs, A.H., O'Brien, B.J., and Blackhouse, G. (2002). Thinking outside the box: recent advances in the analysis and presentation of uncertainty in cost-effectiveness studies. *Annu. Rev. Public Health* 23:377–401.

Briggs, A.H., Wonderling, D.E., and Mooney, C.Z. (1997). Pulling cost-effectiveness analysis up by its bootstraps: a non-parametric approach to confidence interval estimation. *Health Econ.* 6:327–340.

Brouwer, W.B., and Koopmanschap, M.A. (2000). On the economic foundations of CEA. Ladies and gentlemen, take your positions! *J. Health Econ.* 19:439–59.

Bulterys, M., Jamieson, D.J., O'Sullivan, M.J., Cohen, M.H., Maupin, R., Nesheim, S., Webber, M.P., Van Dyke, R., Wiener, J., and Branson, B.M. (Mother-Infant Rapid Intervention At Delivery (MIRIAD) Study Group). (2004). Rapid HIV-1 testing during labor: a multicenter study. *JAMA.* 292(2):219-23

Canadian Coordinating Office for Health Technology Assessment (1997). *Guidelines for economic evaluation of pharmaceuticals: Canada. 2nd ed.* Canadian Coordinating Office for Health Technology Assessment (CCOHTA), Ottawa.

Carr-Hill, R.A. (1989). Assumptions of the QALY procedure. *Soc. Sci. Med.* 29:469–77.

Cartwright, W.S. (1999). Costs of drug abuse to society. *J Ment. Health Policy Econ.* 2:133–134.

Clark, P.A. (2003). The ethics of mandatory HIV testing of all pregnant women. *Linacre. Q.* 70:2–17.

Claxton, K. (1999). The irrelevance of inference: a decision-making approach to the stochastic evaluation of health care technologies. *J. Health Econ.* 18:341–364.

Culyer, A.J. (2001). Equity -some theory and its policy implications. *J. Med. Ethics* 27:275–83.

Culyer, A.J., and Wagstaff, A. (1993). Equity and equality in health and health care. *J. Health Econ.* 12:431–57.

Davis, M. (2004). Planet of Slums. *New Left Review* 26:5–34.

Deber, R.B., and Goel, V. (1990). Using explicit decision rules to manage issues of justice, risk, and ethics in decision analysis: when is it not rational to maximize expected utility? *Med. Decis. Making* 10:181–94.

Detsky, A.S., and Naglie, I.G. (1990). A clinician's guide to cost-effectiveness analysis. *Ann. Intern. Med.* 113:147–54.

de Zulueta, P. (2000). The ethics of anonymized HIV testing of pregnant women: a reappraisal. *J. Med. Ethics* 26:16–21.

Diehr, P., Yanez, D., Ash, A., Hornbrook, M., and Lin, D.Y. (1999). Methods for analyzing health care utilization and costs. *Annu. Rev. Public Health* 20:125–44.

Diener, A., O'Brien, B., and Gafni, A. (1998). Health care contingent valuation studies: a review and classification of the literature. *Health Econ.* 7:313–26.

Dolan, P., Gudex, C., Kind, P., and Williams, A. (1996). Valuing health states: A comparison of methods. *J. Health Econ.* 15:209–31.

Drummond, M.F., Stoddart, G.L., and Torrance, G.W. (1987). *Methods for the economic evaluation of health care programmes.* Oxford University Press, Oxford.

Fleming, P.L., Byers, R.H., Sweeney, P.A., Daniels, D., Karon, J.M., and Janssen, R.S., 2000, HIV Prevalence in the United States, *9th Conference on Retroviruses and Opportunistic Infections,* Seattle, WA (September 16, 2004); http://www.retroconference.org/2002/Abstract/13996.htm.

Freemantle, N. (2000). Valuing the effects of sildenafil in erectile dysfunction. Strong assumptions are required to generate a QALY value. *BMJ.* 320:1156–1157.

Fenwick, E., Claxton, K., and Sculpher, M. (2001). Representing uncertainty: the role of cost-effectiveness acceptable curves. *Health Econ.*

Froberg, D.G., and Kane, R.L. (1989a). Methodology for measuring health-state preferences–I: Measurement strategies. *J. Clin. Epidemiol.* 42:345–54.

Froberg, D.G., and Kane, R.L. (1989b). Methodology for measuring health-state preferences–III: Population and context effects. *J. Clin. Epidemiol.* 42:585–92.

Fryback, D.G. (1993). QALYs, HYEs, and the loss of innocence. *Med. Decis. Making* 13:271–2.

Gafni, A., and Birch, S. (1993). Guidelines for the adoption of new technologies: A prescription for uncontrolled growth in expenditures and how to avoid the problem. *CMA.* 148:913–7.

Garber, A.M., and Phelps, C.E. (1997). Economic foundations of cost-effectiveness analysis. *J. Health Econ.* 16:1– 31.

Garber, A.M., Weinstein, M.C., Torrance, G.W., and Kamlet, M.S. (1996). Theoretical foundations of cost-effectiveness analysis. In: Gold, M.R., Seigel, J.E., Russell, L.B., and Weinstein, M.C. (eds.) (1996). *Cost-effectiveness in health and medicine.* Oxford University Press, New York, NY.

Gold, M.R., Seigel, J.E., Russell, L.B., and Weinstein, M.C. (eds.) (1996). *Cost-effectiveness in health and medicine.* Oxford University Press, New York, NY.

Gold, M.R., Stevenson, D., and Fryback, D.G. (2002). HALYS and QALYS and DALYS, Oh My: similarities and differences in summary measures of population health. *Annu. Rev. Public Health* 23:115–134.

Graham, J.D. (1995). Five-hundred life-saving interventions and their cost-effectiveness. *Risk Anal.* 15:369–90.

Harris, J. (1987). QALYfying the value of life. *J. Med. Ethics* 13:117–23.

Hershey, J.C., Kunreuther, H.C., and Schoemaker, P.J.H. (1988). Sources of bias in assessment procedures for utility functions. In: Bell, D.E., Raiffa, H. and Tversky, A. (eds.), *Decision making: Descriptive, normative, and prescriptive interactions.* Cambridge University Press, Cambridge; New York and Melbourne, pp. 422–42.

Hoch, J., and Bayoumi, A. (2003). Mary had a little lambda: incorporating group-specific values into cost-effectiveness analysis using the net benefit regression framework. *25th Annual Meeting of the Society for Medical Decision Making,* Chicago, IL (Abstract).

Hoch, J.S., Briggs, A.H., and Willan, A.R. (2002). Something old, something new, something borrowed, something blue: a framework for the marriage of health econometrics and cost-effectiveness analysis. *Health. Econ.* 11:415–430.

Holm, S. (1998). The second phase of priority setting. Goodbye to the simple solutions: The second phase of priority setting in health care. *BMJ.* 317:1000–2.

Hornberger, J.C., Redelmeier, D.A., and Petersen, J. (1992). Variability among methods to assess patients' well-being and consequent effect on a cost-effectiveness analysis. *J. Clin. Epidemiol.* 45:505–12.

International Society for Pharmacoeconomics and Outcomes Research, 2004, Pharmacoeconomic Guidelines Around The World. (September 15, 2004); http://www.ispor.org/PEguidelines/ index.asp.

Klose, T., (1999). The contingent valuation method in health care. *Health Policy* 47:97–123.

Laupacis, A., Feeny, D., Detsky, A.S., and Tugwell, P.X. (1993). Tentative guidelines for using clinical and economic evaluations revisited. *CMAJ.* 148:927–9.

Lallemant, M., Jourdain, G., Le Coeur, S., Mary, J.Y., Ngo-Giang-Huong, N., Koetsawang, S., Kanshana, S., McIntosh, K., and Thaineua, V. (2004). Single-dose perinatal nevirapine plus standard zidovudine to prevent mother-to-child transmission of HIV-1 in Thailand. *N. Engl. J. Med.* 351:217–228.

Lansky, A., Jones, J.L., Frey, R.L., and Lindegren, M.L. (2001). Trends in HIV testing among pregnant women: United States, 1994-1999. *Am. J. Public Health* 91:1291–1293.

Laufer, F.N. (2001). Cost-effectiveness of syringe exchange as an HIV prevention strategy. *J Acquir. Immune. Defic. Syndr.* 28:273–278.

Llewellyn-Thomas, H., Sutherland, H.J., Tibshirani, R., Ciampi, A., Till, J.E., and Boyd, N.F. (1984). Describing health states. Methodologic issues in obtaining values for health states. *Med. Care* 22:543–52.

Llewellyn-Thomas, H., Sutherland, H.J., Tibshirani, R., Ciampi, A., Till, J.E., and Boyd, N.F. (1982). The measurement of patients' values in medicine. *Med. Decis. Making* 2:449–62.

Loomes, G., and McKenzie, L. (1989). The use of QALYs in health care decision making. *Soc. Sci. Med.* 28:299–308.

Luce, B.R., Manning, W., Siegel, J.E., and Lipscomb, J. (1996). Estimating costs in cost-effectiveness analysis. In: Gold, M.R., Seigel, J.E., Russell, L.B. and Weinstein, M.C. (eds.), *Cost-effectiveness in health and medicine.* Oxford University Press, New York, pp. 176–213.

Martin, A.J., Glasziou, P.P., Simes, R.J., and Lumley, T. (2000). A comparison of standard gamble, time trade-off, and adjusted time trade-off scores. *Int. J. Technol. Assess. Health Care* 16:137–47.

McGregor, M. (2003). Cost-utility analysis: use QALYs only with great caution. *CMAJ* 168:433–4.

Mehrez, A., and Gafni, A. (1989). Quality-adjusted life years, utility theory, and healthy-years equivalents. *Med. Decis. Making* 9:142–9.

Mehrez, A., and Gafni, A. (1993). Healthy-years equivalents versus quality-adjusted life years: In pursuit of progress. *Med. Decis. Making* 13:287–92.

McIntosh, E., Donaldson, C., and Ryan, M. (1999). Recent advances in the methods of cost-benefit analysis in healthcare. Matching the art to the science. *Pharmacoeconomics* 15:357– 67.

Nord, E. (1992). An alternative to QALYs: the saved young life equivalent (SAVE). *BMJ.* 305(6865):1365–6.

Nord, E. (1995). The person-trade-off approach to valuing health care programs. *Med. Decis. Making* 15:201–8.

Oliver, A., Healey, A., and Donaldson, C. (2002). Choosing the method to match the perspective: economic assessment and its implications for health-services efficiency. *Lancet* 359:1771–4.

Owens, D.K. (1998). Interpretation of cost-effectiveness analyses. *J. Gen. Intern. Med.* 13;716–7.

Owens, D.K., and Nease, R.F. (1997). A normative analytic framework for development of practice guidelines for specific clinical populations. *Med. Decis. Making* 17:409–426.

O'Brien, B., and Gafni, A. (1996). When do the "dollars" make sense? Toward a conceptual framework for contingent valuation studies in health care. *Med. Decis. Making* 16:288–99.

Olsen, J.A., and Smith, R.D. (2001). Theory versus practice: a review of `willingness-to-pay' in health and health care. *Health Econ.* 10:39–52.

Phillips, K.A., Bayer, R., and Chen, J.L. (2003). New Centers for Disease Control and Prevention's guidelines on HIV counseling and testing for the general population and pregnant women. *J. Acquir. Immune. Defic. Syndr.* 32:182–191.

Powderly, K. (2001). Ethical and legal issues in perinatal HIV. *Clin. Obstet. Gynecol.* 44:300–311.

Read, J.L., Quinn, R.J., Berwick, D.M., Fineberg, H.V., and Weinstein, M.C. (1984). Preferences for health outcomes. Comparison of assessment methods. *Med. Decis. Making* 4:315–29.

Redelmeier, D.A., and Heller, D.N. (1993). Time preference in medical decision making and cost-effectiveness analysis. *Med. Decis. Making* 13:212–7.

Ried, W. (1998). QALYs versus HYEs–What's right and what's wrong. A review of the controversy. *J. Health Econ.* 17:607–25.

Sculpher, M., Fenwick, E., and Claxton, K. (2000). Assessing quality in decision analytic cost-effectiveness models. A suggested framework and example of application. *Pharmacoeconomics* 17:461–477.

Singer, P., McKie, J., Kuhse, H., and Richardson, J. (1995). Double jeopardy and the use of QALYs in health care allocation. *J. Med. Ethics* 21:144–50.

Stiggelbout, A.M., Kiebert, G.M., Kievit, J., Leer, J.W., Stoter, G., and De Haes, J.C. (1994). Utility assessment in cancer patients: adjustment of time tradeoff scores for the utility of life years and comparison with standard gamble scores. *Med. Decis. Making* 14:82–90.

Stinnett, A.A., and Paltiel, A.D. (1997). Estimating CE ratios under second-order uncertainty: the mean ratio versus the ratio of means. *Med. Decis. Making* 17:483–489.

Tengs, T.O., Adams, M.E., Pliskin, J.S., Safran, D.G., Siegel, J.E., Weinstein, M.C., and Graham, J.D. (1995). Five-hundred life-saving interventions and their cost-effectiveness. *Risk Anal.* 15(3):369-90.

Torrance, G.W. (1976). Social preferences for health states: an empirical evaluation of three measurement techniques. *Socio-Econ Planning Sci.* 10:129–136.

Torrance, G.W. (1987). Utility approach to measuring health-related quality of life. *J. Chronic Dis.* 40:593–603.

Torrance, G.W. (1986). Measurement of health state utilities for economic appraisal. *J. Health Econ.* 5:1–30.

Tsevat, J., Solzan, J., Kuntz, K., Ragland, J., Currier, J., Sell, R., and Weinstein, M. (1996). Health values of patients infected with Human Immunodeficiency Virus: relationship to mental health and physical functioning. *Med. Care* 34:44–57.

Ubel, P.A., DeKay, M.L., Baron, J., and Asch, D.A. (1996). Cost-effectiveness analysis in a setting of budget constraints– Is it equitable? *N. Engl. J. Med.* 334:1174–7.

Ubel, P.A., Nord, E., Gold, M., Menzel, P., Prades, J.L., and Richardson, J. (2000). Improving value measurement in cost-effectiveness analysis. *Med. Care* 38:892–901.

Wagstaff, A. (1991). QALYs and the equity-efficiency trade-off. *J. Health Econ.* 10:21–41.

Wade, N.A., Zielinski, M.A., Butsashvili, M., McNutt, L.A., Warren, B.L., Glaros, R., Cheku, B., Pulver, W., Pass, K., Fox, K., Novello, A.C., and Birkhead, G.S. (2004). Decline in Perinatal HIV Transmission in New York State (1997-2000). *J Acquir. Immune. Defic. Syndr.* 36:1075–1082.

Wailoo, A., Roberts, J., Brazier, J., and McCabe, C. (2004). Efficiency, equity, and NICE clinical guidelines. *BMJ.* 328:536–537.

Webber, M.P., Van Dyke, R., Wiener, J., and Branson, B.M. (2004). Rapid HIV-1 testing during labor: a multicenter study. *JAMA.* 292:219–223.

Weinstein, M.C. (ed.), *Cost-effectiveness in health and medicine.* Oxford University Press, New York, pp. 25–53.

Weinstein, M.C., and Stason, W.B. (1977). Foundations of cost-effectiveness analysis for health and medical practices. *N. Engl. J. Med.* 296:716–21.

Williams, A. (1991). Is the QALY a technical solution to a political problem? Of course not! *Int. J. Health Serv.* 21:365–9.

Zaric, G.S., Bayoumi, A.M., Brandeau, M.L., and Owens, D.K. (2000). The cost effectiveness of voluntary prenatal and routine newborn HIV screening in the United States. *J Acquir. Immune. Defic. Syndr.* 25:403–16.

Chapter 22

Integrative Chapter

Multi-Disciplinary Work and the Study of Urban Health

The Editors

The preceding nine chapters are probably the most diverse chapters in the book. Each chapter is contributed by authors from different disciplines and these disciplinary perspectives clearly color the chapter content and offer different perspectives on the methods that may be applied to the study of the health of urban populations. However, we suggest that despite these obvious differences, three themes emerge from most, if not all, chapters and point us towards next steps as we consider how best to move beyond this book.

There appears to be an emerging consensus regarding the need for both multilevel and cross-disciplinary analysis when considering how cities may shape the health of populations. This is brought home clearly and forcefully in the chapter that considers the contribution that demography can make to the study of urban health with a particular focus on health in cities of developing countries. The authors make the case that there has been a surprising paucity of research about the contribution of factors at multiple levels to the health of populations in developing world cities, and that this shortcoming of the existing research hampers efforts to develop effective interventions that can improve health in the most rapidly urbanizing regions of the world. Several authors consider the need for multilevel analysis as self-evident within the context of urban health inquiry, although as we discuss in our summary of the role of epidemiology, multilevel analysis, at least as applied to intra-urban analyses, is merely one (and a relatively new) empiric approach to studying the health of urban populations. Importantly, as each chapter considers the potential role of multilevel analyses, it quickly becomes evident that different disciplines have particular and distinct skills to contribute to these analyses. For example, anthropology and sociology bring perspectives that are clearly essential complements to the statistical considerations inherent in considerations of group-level factors that may affect the health of persons living in cities.

The second key theme that emerges from these chapters is, simply stated, that the relationship between cities, characteristics of cities, and the health of persons in cities is complicated and that as such it requires recourse to methods from different disciplines and the development of new methods (and theories), beyond our current capabilities, to push this understanding forward. For example, the different elements of urban planning that may be brought to bear on determining city form that in turn affects health readily suggest some of the complexities that await those who aim to understand how cities shape population health, and perhaps even more so, who are working to implement interventions that aim to improve health in cities. The addition of cost effectiveness perspectives to the equation provides, we suggest, an important counterpoint to the tendency that those of us interested in public health might otherwise have to try to "just make everything better". Clearly, understanding, and improving the elements of cities that may affect health is not easy and these methodologic chapters read very much like pieces of a puzzle that is slowly, ever so slowly, coming together.

Importantly, it is the fact that there is indeed one puzzle that we suggest is the third theme to emerge from these chapters. Several authors discuss the role of personal characteristics, spatial groupings, the passage of time, and characteristics of place as all contributing to urban health. However, these elements of city living are not disembodied elements that should, or even could, be studied in isolation. Indeed, as we see in the chapter considering the role of health service research in understanding urban health, an appreciation of how urban health services have changed over time is essential to understanding current snapshots of urban population health. Clearly, some disciplines offer methods more effective at understanding pieces of the puzzle than those offered by other disciplines. It seems to us that the task at hand is to effectively and systematically parse the problems in urban health in such a way that we can apply the appropriate methods in concert, and perhaps in certain cases, such as the derivation of multi-level power calculations by statisticians, in isolation.

Our suggestion that a fuller understanding of urban health will require a cross-disciplinary perspective perhaps is easier said than done. It is one thing to suggest, as we do in chapter 12, that we might do well to consider urban populations as a whole, and quite another thing altogether to suggest that we need to integrate methods from across disciplines. Methods tend to be understood from disciplinary perspectives and are largely a reflection of training of professionals in different disciplines. A real extension of methods across disciplines to questions that may be vital to urban health may well require researchers and practitioners who understand, and are able to apply, these methods. The next section offers some suggestions about how such persons can be trained and what these interventions, using insights from across disciplines, may look like.

Part III

Practice

Chapter 23

Building Healthy Cities

A Focus on Interventions

Jan C. Semenza

1.0. INTRODUCTION

Healthy cities do not exist, rather they must be created. As a result, healthy cities are characterized by a constant stream of interventions that strive to improve the social, environmental, occupational and economic conditions of their residents. These interventions augment city health and should never cease.

Cities of the 19th century were plagued by pollution, pathogens, and over-population and suffered from smells, dirt and noise. These living conditions were dangerous to peoples' health. A review of historic public health regulations and interventions in cities and towns illustrates the process of progressive improvements in urbanites' health. The design and layout of urban sewage lines and trash incineration, public water collection, and distribution systems extended longevity and reduced morbidity. Besides sanitration and hygiene, housing occupancy restrictions helped to prevent the spread of infectious diseases such as tuberculosis, building and fire codes, and workplace regulations helped to improve environmental and occupational health. Public health is a far reaching discipline that not only aims to meet basic human needs such as safe water, food, shelter, work and safety but also to create environments that support a healthy way of life. For example, single land use zoning laws were designed to create physical environments that separated industrial emissions from residential areas to prevent toxic exposures. Segregated land use created the modern American cities with remote suburban subdivisions separated from commercial and industrial areas connected by a vast expansion of highway networks. The rise of the suburbs is also linked to the decline of the inner cities, with resources being diverted to support the construction of a costly dispersed infrastructure. In turn, some urban centers have become desolate, unappealing, and anonymous. The rectangular grid layout of American cities with long monotonous city blocks is not conducive to community life which is torn apart by speeding traffic. This development has resulted in a number of public health problems that need to be addressed with targeted interventions for healthier cities.

The extent of decline of the urban core, varies from city to city and while not ubiquitous is nevertheless sufficiently widespread to be of concern; it manifests itself in abandoned downtowns that lack vitality, as well as degraded infrastructure, damaged homes, trash accumulation, and graffiti, which negatively affects mental and physical health over and above personal risk factors. Dilapidated physical environments of inner cities have been associated with poor vaccine coverage and high infectious disease rates, including measles and AIDS (CDC, 1998; Wallace, *et al.*, 1990; Kenyon, *et al.*, 1998). Inner city neighborhoods have also been associated with chronic diseases such as cardiovascular diseases, diabetes and asthma (Shewry, *et al.*, 1992; Rosenstreich, *et al.*, 1997; Diez-Roux, *et al.*, 1999). An epidemic of obesity that cuts across all demographic groups is sweeping the U.S and has been increasing over time nationwide (Mokdad, *et al.*, 2001; Ogden, *et al.*, 2002; Flegal, *et al.*, 2002; Wolf-Maier, *et al.*, 2003). Obesity is a serious health hazard also responsible for sleep apnea, hypertension, low self-esteem, and depression. Neighborhood of residence is associated with elevated body mass index, even after adjusting for age, sex, class, smoking, and material deprivation (Ellaway, *et al.*, 1997), and it is proposed that the built environment affects physical activity (Poston and Foreyt, 1999; King, *et al.*, 2000; Handy, *et al.*, 2002). While the obesity epidemic has disproportionally affected low density sprawl developments it is also associated with multiethnic, low income, inner city neighborhoods (O'Louhlin, *et al.*, 1998). Thus, neighborhoods that encourage physical activity may help to control the obesity epidemic (Goran, *et al.*, 2000).

Neighborhood stressors can trigger depression and decrease physical functioning in the elderly (Aneshensel and Sucoff, 1996; Balfour and Kaplan, 2002; Latkin and Curry, 2003; Kingsley, 2003). The diagnosis of depressive disorders increased across ethnic groups in the U.S. with prescription for antidepressants escalating three-fold between 1988 and 1998 (Skaer, 2000). Urban blight has been associated with negative emotions and a sense of hopelessness (Greenberg and Schneider, 1996; Fitzpatrick and LaGory, 2000). A direct link between the environment and mental health has been established in a variety of urban settings (Stiffman, *et al.*, 1999; Black and Krishnakumar 1998; Marsella, 1998; Dalgard and Tambs, 1997; Frumkin, 2002). Environmental features such as public gathering places and worthwhile destinations for pedestrians that facilitate social contacts and support can improve mental health (Halpern, 1995; Dalgard and Tambs, 1997). More recently, an experimental study that randomized subjects to different living environments found neighborhood effects on mental health both in adults and children (Leventhal and Brooks-Gunn, 2003). Social disorder such as crime, public drinking and drug use, also negatively affect well-being and neighborhood satisfaction (Dembo, *et al.*, 1985; Wallace 1990; Sampson, *et al.*, 1997).

The most prevalent risk factor for chronic diseases such as obesity, hypertension, cardiovascular disease and depression is physical inactivity and even moderate physical activity has a beneficial health benefit (Pate, *et al.*, 1995). What urban features encourage active living? Some neighborhood designs are more conducive to walking, social interactions and social networks and community involvement have distinct mental and physical health benefits (House, *et al.*, 1988; Berkman and Kawachi, 2000; Kawachi and Berkman, 2001). Moreover, cities are engines of art, civic life, and economic activity and enrich the human experience with religious, cultural, and racial/ethnic diversity. Urbanicity has the quality to generate collective amenities such as libraries, theaters, and hospitals that serve the common good. These characteristics of certain urban settings can be health promoting and thus be beneficial to public health. This chapter describes an urban intervention to enhance these characteristics by retrofitting the urban setting. The approach was developed by a non-profit organization entitled "The City Repair Project" in Portland, Oregon. City Repair works with hundreds of volunteers and activists committed to making urban communities better places to live. The intervention described here aims to revive the existing urban city layout with novel urban features and amenities that help to create healthy urban environments that foster healthy social environments. The following section describes the problem at hand of building healthy cities and the implications for urban community organizing. The next section explains the specific steps of the "intersection repair" strategy, followed by a case study. This intervention strategy has been applied to a number of settings in different cities with the original prototype "intersection repair" projects in Portland.

2.0. FRAMING THE PROBLEM

2.1. Life in the Grid City

Most American towns and cities have been laid out with a grid pattern comprised of streets and side streets crossing at right angles (Figure 1). Such a simple network of orthogonal streets that intersect in a regular manner creates rectangular or square city blocks. The rationale of city planning to shape the urban environment with this pattern of vertical and horizontal streets lies in increased connectivity: the possible routes between any given two points is maximized. Short of diagonal connections (which are missing in a rigid grid layout) the distance between the starting point and the destination is minimized, diversifying the transportation options and

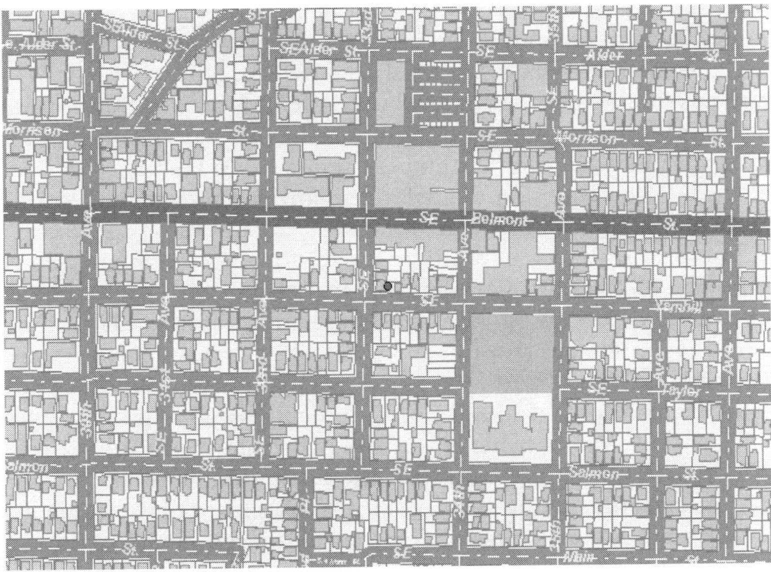

Figure 1. The Grid City with a Predetermined Rectilinear Layout, Portland OR. (Reproduced with permission, City of Portland)

improving the transportation system. In contrast, with the hierarchical traffic pattern found in more recent development such as urban sprawl, trip lengths increase because the residential streets with few connections feed into arterial streets that move traffic out of the neighborhood. In this model, a trip across the neighborhood is very difficult, while a trip around the neighborhood is very easy and fast. Thus, the grid is the geometric form of choice for a planned network with high connectivity for efficient movement of goods and services.

The origin of the gridiron has its roots in ancient settlements since biblical times. Modular grid patterns were used 3000 B.C. in Assyria and Babylonia for military camps and city designs and the temple complex of Zoser at Sakkara in Egypt was laid out orthogonally in 2650 B.C. (Kostof, 1985). The discipline of rational city planning has been attributed to the architect Hippodamus of Miletus (498-408 BC). He is credited with designing orthogonal towns including Olynthus, Priene, and Miletus; for example, he designed the Mediterranean harbor town Miletus in such a way that the sea and mountain winds could freely breeze through the city blocks and bring relief during the hot summer months. The orthogonal design was used by the Greeks for solar architecture to fully capture the sun rays during the winter but to escape the full solar impact during the summer, when the angle of the sun has shifted. These ancient methods to fight the urban heat island effect are remarkable in light of persistently high heat-related mortality and morbidity in urban centers today, that are entirely preventable. (Semenza, *et al.*, 1996; Semenza, *et al.*, 1999). The Greeks also invented the Phalanx, a rectangular arrangement of soldiers, and exported the grid city to their colonies as a tool of military control.

The Romans imposed a rigid quadrilateral structure over the conquered land and allocated square subdivisions to war veterans; they introduced the castrum to urban planning in their colonies, a fortified legionary camp with a predetermined grid pattern. At the heart of the ancient Roman city planning is the crossing of the two main streets, the east-west oriented decumanus and the perpendicular north-south cardus. At the center of the castrum was an institutional building or temple with the two mayor perpendicular crossroads extending through the fortification into the landscape. The forum in the center was thus able to control the traffic passing through the gates of the walled rectangular castrum.

European settlement of North America was characterized by towns with a concentric layout with a common meeting house in the center and public squares. Population growth and immigration necessitated more land acquisitions and the rectangular grid plan was adapted as the organizing theme. For example, New Haven, Connecticut or Savannah, Georgia, were laid out on the grid with a central public square for the church or a public square for the community. The National Land Ordinance of 1785 dictated that the westward expansion from the existing colonies be divided by a rectangular grid pattern, which was also applied to the planning of cities and towns (Kostof, 1985). Such a subdivision assured an efficient way to effectively plan and sell new acquisitions (Maholy-Nagy, 1968). Furthermore, the uniform distance between sections and blocks facilitated transport of people and goods. Inherent in the principle of the classic grid design applied to the city is the uniform distribution of traffic circulation: there are no major arterial roads that are at the top of the hierarchy of high volume traffic and conversely there are no residential streets that are spared the high volume travel of cars. Residential neighborhoods can therefore fall victim to a constant stream of through traffic which negatively impact the quality of urban life (APHA, 1948). Unlike the cities in the east such as, New Haven and Savannah, the National Land

Ordinance did not provide for public centers, parks, or open landscapes since it carved the land into squares of private property and virtually omitted the public realm, except streets. The monotony of the rectangular pattern did not consider topography or the natural curvilinear layout of the land and was imposed over the undeveloped landscape to neutralize the environment. The lack of open space deprived the urban population of recreational sites with fresh air and abundant light, and fostered monotonous housing standards. Furthermore, the omission of public squares, ceremonial places, and public structures as nodes of community life was a serious limitation of the relentless grid design; it could potentially be the source of social isolation and alienation in urban centers. The grid layout fulfilled a number of technocratic goals, but fell short to take into account a number of human qualities. Aristotle criticized the Hippodamian approach to city planning stating that every city core should have a haphazard arrangement and he stressed the importance of tradition and habit in making city residents orderly and law-abiding. Indeed, cultural identity may be stronger in an organically evolved city plan with historic and artistic landmarks.

The intervention described here aims to retrofit the layout of the grid city by integrating public gathering places into the public realm. These gathering places aim to reinstate the town commons that historically had been the geographic glue of community stewardship. These restorative public places with interactive art installations are intended to inspire a sense of belonging and identity, trigger conversations among strangers, spark creativity, cultivate civic capacity, and even stimulate local economic vitality. These commons are essential parts of the democratic process to facilitate collective responsibility and tolerance. The approach has been implemented by the local non-profit organization The City Repair Project, and has been field-tested and evaluated at numerous sites.

3.0. COMMUNITY ORGANIZING IN URBAN NEIGHBORHOODS

This particular intervention has been designed to enhance the urban core of American grid cities which tend to have been planned without any provisions of significant public gathering places. Community organizing in urban neighborhoods can reverse alienation and foster a sense of responsibility that counteracts urban blight; it encourages residents to take initiative against social disorder and physical deterioration (Wilson, 1996). Neighborhood stewardship manifested in physical improvements of the urban environment is a direct consequence of the community organizing capacity; this capacity that can directly be translated into concrete action such as physical improvements to solve local problems (Perkins, *et al.*, 1990). Often residents have little control over the demographic composition of their neighborhood nor over transient populations that may be involved in drug trafficking and crime; however, residents can revitalize their built urban environment. Factors that determine participation in such community efforts to reverse urban decay are sense of social connectedness and sense of community (Crenson, 1978; Florin and Wandersman, 1984; McMillan and Chavis, 1986; Taylor, 1988). Once a more inviting place has been created that is aesthetically pleasing, friendly and safe, such as the public squares described here, social interactions are facilitated which in turn increases the sense of community and participation in community efforts.

Community organizing relies on social capital which refers to the potential and resources inherent in social networks or social cohesion (Putnam, *et al.*, 1995) and comprises a web of social relationships and their characteristics (Berkman and Glass, 2000). Social network ties have been associated with decreased rates of mortality among adults and increased sense of well-being (Seeman, *et al.*, 1988; Oxman, *et al.*, 1992). Social capital relies on such networks for cooperation between residents of dilapidated urban environments to initiate collective problem solving. Social capital can be seen as a by-product of social relations that promote trust and mutual cooperation and is therefore not a characteristic of one particular individual, but rather a collective characteristic. As such, social capital can facilitate remedial action in an urban setting and promote specific steps necessary for local problem solving.

There are two components to social capital: localized and bridging capital. Localized capital, inherent in existing social or religious groups, is necessary but not sufficient for community problem solving, because it may produce redundant information not pertinent to improving inner-city neighborhoods (Granovetter, 1973). In contrast, bridging social capital connects various groups and can reveal new information for local problem solving and create new opportunities. Therefore, a public health intervention that sequentially builds social networks to augment localized social capital and facilitates bridging capital should result in collective efficacy that would engage residents in direct social action (Sampson, *et al.*, 1999). This intervention aims to realize community projects in the grid city that build community capacity and governance skills for consensus decision-making and community stewardship.

Although building social networks and social capital to solve community problems has merit on its own, it can also indirectly promote public health: social support and friendship ties reduce mortality and morbidity (House, *et al.*, 1988; Semenza, *et al.*, 1996, Semenza, *et al.*, 1999); lack of trust between neighborhood residents is associated with increased risk of death from cardiovascular diseases (Kawachi, *et al.*, 1997) and in U.S. states with lower levels of social capital, self-reported health is poorer, controlling for individual risk factors (Lochner, *et al.*, 1999; Kawachi, *et al.*, 1999). Social capital has also been related to mental health in adolescents (Aneshensel and Sucoff, 1996), adolescent birth rates (Denner, *et al.*, 2001), and firearm deaths (Kennedy, *et al.*, 1998).

It has been recognized that voluntary involvement in organizations and institutions is crucial for local problem solving (Bellah, *et al.*, 1996), disease prevention (Green, 1990) and mental health (Naparstek, *et al.*, 1982); however, it has proven challenging to realize such programs (Sieler-Wells , 1989). The procedure described here has been institutionalized and builds both localized and bridging social capital, through an ecologic intervention. The intervention encourages residents to improve the urban "grid-scape" physically (streets and public squares) in order to stimulate walking; it supports neighbors to build worthwhile destinations for pedestrians in the public realm that are inviting socially in order to improve social networks and cohesion and it engages participants to beautify the neighborhood symbolically thereby to creating a sense of belonging and pride.

4.0. THE STRATEGY: INTERSECTION REPAIR

4.1. An Urban Intervention

The process of creating healthy cities involves the political support of a wide range of governmental agencies that are willing to engage in trans-disciplinary integration and community involvement. The success of such interventions depends on the political commitment and leadership that can lead to institutional change. While these strategies are important for the long-term planning process of new urban developments, the question remains how current urban features can be retrofitted to improve public health.

A successful intervention within the city limits of Portland, Oregon has been conceived by The City Repair Project, initiated by community members and supported by City officials. The intervention aims to retrofit the urban orthogonal grid to create public gathering places for human interactions. This approach illustrates both the importance of public participation in neighborhood design but also the relevance of urban amenities and art to improve the qualities of urbanity.

The objective of this health-promoting neighborhood intervention is to engage residents in neighborhood stewardship in the interest of public health. It is an urban revitalization strategy that directly engages communities in urban design, a field that has traditionally been dominated by professional planners, architects, and developers. The community-initiated neighborhood-enhancement project is intended to dynamically connect individuals by involving them in the planning and implementation of creative and attractive urban places. These interactive communities intentionally design vibrant places that are restorative to mental and physical health. This health-promoting neighborhood intervention creates sustainable communities by creating gathering places with environmentally conscious construction that benefit both the livability of the neighborhood and the well-being of its residents. Improvements in the physical environment have positive ripple effects across social indicators, such as changes in the social fabric of the community and expansion of social networks after the intervention. Working together on ecological construction, particularly working with cob (a natural building material), which relies on collective physical labor, stimulates social interactions and increases physical activity. Other activities, such as community organizing and design workshops contribute to expanding social ties as well.

4.2. Community Outreach

A step by step description of the health-promoting neighborhood intervention is described here. Community organizers are hired who are responsible for outreach to neighborhoods with significant urban problems (Figure 2; step 1). Particular attention is placed on involving underrepresented populations such as groups of different socioeconomic status, race, ethnicity, age, sexual-orientation, etc. To begin the process of site selection the organizers communicate with a wide range of residents and collect information about potential sites (Figure 2; step 2). Informal meetings are held at a residence close to any site where an intervention project is anticipated to be implemented (Figure 2; step 3). At the initial meeting, residents socialize with each other and social networks are initiated in a process of building localized social capital. In subsequent meetings, information is provided about mechanisms for improving the built urban environment and staff from City Repair holds a slide presentation about projects that have been created in the past. This step sparks discussions and questions and an open forum is held to allow different points of views to be expressed. The community organizers track these discussions and create contact sheets, including names, addresses, phone, and e-mail contact information of engaged residents. The community organizing staff assures that all residents within a two block radius are included (or informed) in this process, since these individuals need to sign off on the final project (see below). Thus it is important to canvass systematically from door to

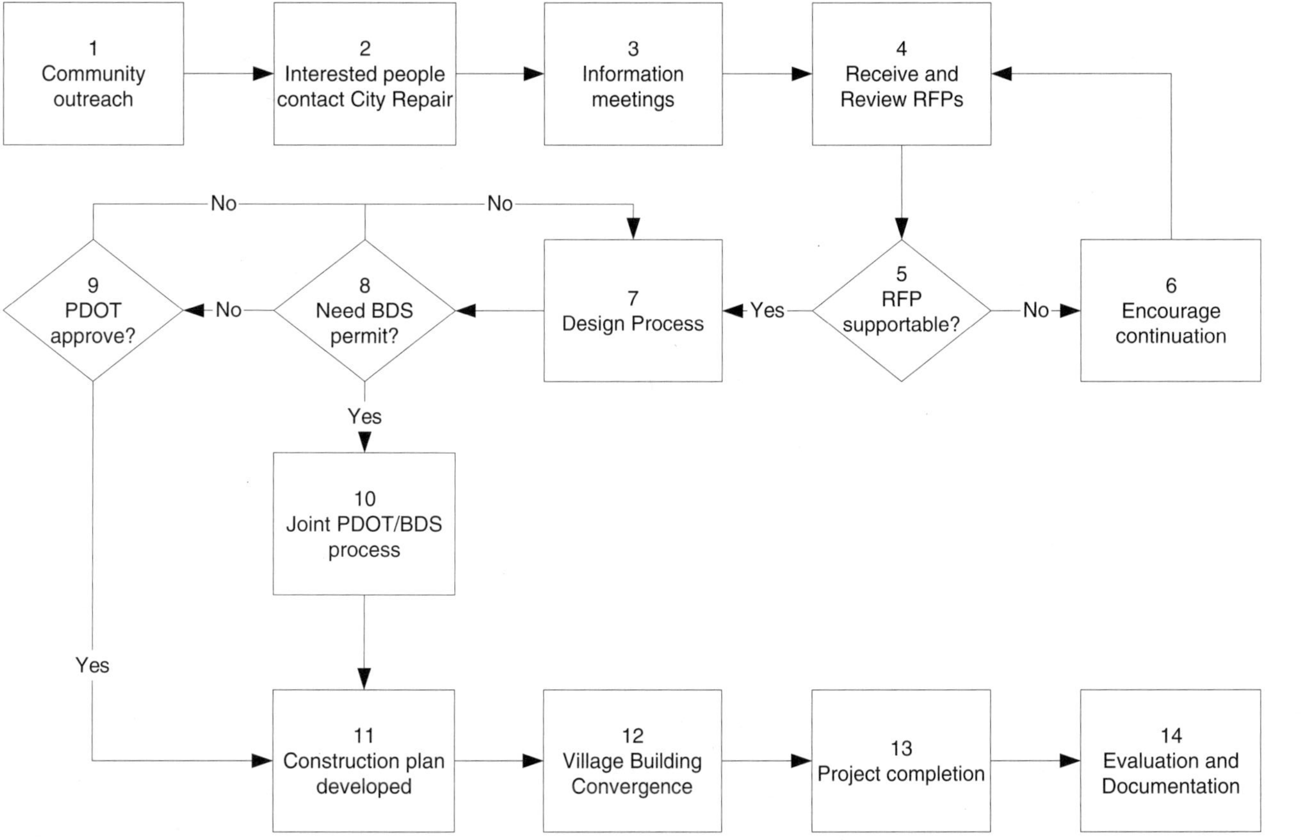

Figure 2. Flow-diagram: A Health Promoting Neighborhood Intervention. See text for details; PDOT: Portland Department of Transportation; BDS: Bureau of Development Services; RFP: Request for Proposals. (*Source:* Adapted with permission from Cowan, S., Lakeman, M., Leis, J., Lerch, D., and Semenza, J.C. The City Repair Project. Belltown Paradise/Making Their Own Plans. Bloom, B., and Broomberg, A. [eds.] White Walls, Inc., Chicago, Il).

door to inform interested residents beyond the two block radius. Beyond personal outreach, flyers, phone banks, email listservs, and information bulletin boards are used to disseminate information about meeting time and location. Representatives from Neighborhood Associations also participate in this process since they are local advocates for neighborhood issues and represent a voice to the larger City government. Representatives from City Bureaus are also informed about the process and community members are encouraged to work with the City to discuss different project ideas; this step builds bridging social capital.

4.3. Design Process

Following these meetings, interested neighborhood groups receive a "request for proposals" (Figure 2; RFP; step 4) and are asked to provide information about their motivation to initiate such a project, the depth of neighborhood participation, and their vision. From the pool of these applications, sites are selected (Figure 2; step 5) for formal development. As a result of the community outreach, a core group of residents is formed in these neighborhoods. The neighborhood core group serves as leaders that organize planning meetings and encourage participation in the design process from residents within a two block radius. The neighborhood core group also determines the schedule for community involvement, organizational structure, design workshops, installation dates, and plans for maintenance and future development of the project. The group ensures that all voices are heard, that the decision-making process is accessible, and that there is a process to address concerns, such as consensus decision making. The neighborhood core group is also responsible for regularly communicating with their neighborhood associations and with affected neighbors. Neighbors are provided with information about the project, results of recent meetings, next steps, how to get involved and/or respond. This process involves: door to door outreach, flyers, listservs or websites, activating neighborhood phone trees, posting information either in a temporary "communication station" at the intersection or in someone's front yard, hosting small gatherings, etc.

In collaboration with trained facilitators and design professionals, a base map of each of these sites is developed with critical landscape features and architectural structures. Suggestions for worthwhile destinations for pedestrians and other improvements is discussed and incorporated into preliminary drawings. Designs for the public place reflects the local culture and public art and may incorporate features such as seating areas, lighting, signage, paths, landmarks, water fountains, and information centers/information kiosks. These design workshops involves a series of steps with feedback loops, where ideas are turned into designs, moving from the general to the specific (Figure 2; step 7). Neighborhood skills are assessed and supported by architects and design professionals. Design concepts are disseminated by the core group as part of the outreach activities, and feedback is incorporated into technical drawings for permitting and building. At least two design workshops per neighborhood are held to develop artistic destinations for pedestrians and other features and structures. The design workshops are the focus of the public participation process. In these workshops neighbors share ideas and concerns and together produce both the design and process for creating the project. Workshops are as accessible as possible, including choice of time and location, and providing translation, childcare, food, etc. A workshop design team assists in the development of technical drawings. The team is composed of design professionals, trained facilitators, and providers of technical assistance in the areas of natural building, permaculture design, and relevant forms of public art. The workshop design team is charged with guiding the design process. The final plan is presented at an informal community gathering and routed for signature within a two block radius of the project, as required by City Ordinance (see below) prior to obtaining permits and approval. The Neighborhood Core Group and volunteers from the City Repair Project present the proposal to City traffic engineers for evaluation and authorization, in a process of building bridging social capital.

This design process is the basis for the development of plans for structures that foster walking activity, social interactions and cultural development. Furthermore, the actual process of collectively constructing a feature in the public right of way empowers communities and builds social networks.

4.4. Permitting Process

The City of Portland allows street painting and construction in the right of way, according to City Ordinance #172207 (September 19, 2001), which regulates the implementation of such activities. The Portland Department of Transportation (PDOT) has established a precedent for these projects by granting revocable permits (Figure 2; step 10) for ongoing intersection modifications, if the two streets can be classified as Local Service Streets and carry less than 2,500 vehicles on an average day. A petition of support is required by the city; the petition has signatures from each of the adjacent residents and at least 80% of the residents on the project street frontage(s) within two standard city blocks of the proposed project. The City Traffic Engineer has the authority to modify the petition boundaries when considered appropriate. The residents provide a written description of the proposed changes, including diagrams depicting how the intersection will look when completed. The residents have to demonstrate how the project will improve, or at least maintain, traffic safety and the safety of individuals at or in the vicinity of the intersection. Issues of concern may be as follows.

4.4.1. Pedestrian, Bicyclist and Automobile Safety

Concerns for safety are incorporated into all designs, as outlined by PDOT requirements and the technical expertise of the design professionals involved. Concerns may also be addressed by reviewing statistics for car-to-person collisions at the sites, inviting representatives of existing sites to speak at neighborhood meetings to discuss pedestrian safety issues.

4.4.2. Vandalism and Crime

Social disorder tends to be a problem at the intersection repair sites prior to the intervention. Reported offenses within a two block radius of one site have decreased statistically compared to two unimproved sites.

4.4.3. Disability Accommodation

Concerns for disability accommodation is incorporated into all designs, as outlined by PDOT and ADA requirements and technical expertise of design professionals involved. Concerns may also be addressed by inviting a representative from Independent Living Resources to the neighborhood organization to discuss disability issues and how to develop a space that is safe and inclusive for people with disabilities.

4.4.5. Maintenance

The Neighborhood Core Group at each site is committed to overseeing the long-term responsibility, maintenance and development of the intersection repair project.

The City of Portland, OR has provided political support to institutionalize the intersection repair process and has collaborated with neighborhood associations, non-profit organizations and residents to implement the projects.

4.5. Construction Workshop

An organizing committee is formed of volunteers, neighbors, students, professionals, builders, designers, activists and artists for project implementation and coordination of all project aspects (Figure 2; step 11). Implementation of projects provides many opportunities for individuals and organizations to contribute their resources, expertise and vision. The media are used to alert the public to the upcoming event and how to get involved; information is disseminated through web sites, neighborhood newsletters and newspapers, Community Radio, and nonprofit organization networks. The organizing committee helps the neighborhoods to mobilize and to build the community public places that they have envisioned, designed, and funded (at least in part) for themselves. These physical places will be created by the communities in order to facilitate public gatherings. While all of these projects build community in similar ways, they vary according to each neighborhood's expression of their local culture. Most projects are located in or adjacent to the public right of way in prominent locations.

In order to assist communities with the implementation of their construction plans, a building workshop (Village Building Convergence) is held (Figure 2; step 12). Through a synchronized effort multiple projects in a range of different neighborhoods are realized simultaneously. This approach allows for more efficiency by sharing resources. The workshop is coordinated by a spokecouncil that is comprised of representatives of committee members in charge of different tasks, such as publicity, fund raising, design, etc.

This process is called "Intersection Repair", and is outlined in City Ordinance # 172207 (see above). It, has been implemented in the past in response to the high level of interest among Neighborhood Associations to increase communication between neighbors, actively involve new people in the neighborhood association, host successful community events, build relationships with local organizations, and activate public spaces; these findings are reported by the Healthy Neighborhood Project Neighborhood Association Questionnaires, Neighbor Surveys and various neighborhood meetings. Natural and ecologic builders assist in the construction of artistic destinations for pedestrians, developed by the communities (for examples, see Table 1). Proactive neighborhood groups revitalize their own streets by working together over a time span of several months to create a common vision for their neighborhood. In the past several thousand neighbors, volunteers, and visitors have participated in the building of physical elements in the public realm as a showcase of neighborhood improvement.

Table 1. Examples of Work Completed at Nine Sites during the Village Building Convergence 2003, Portland, OR

1. Two neighborhood kiosks, benches and garden, in conjunction with local day laborers, Citybikes Cooperative, KBOO Community Radio and many local businesses and volunteers.
2. A neighborhood kiosk, herb spiral, two benches and a painted mural in the intersection.
3. Three trellises arching over the sidewalk, a mosaic garden wall, re-painted sunflower street mural and a gigantic sunflower-shaped dome over the sidewalk and fountain.
4. A poetry garden including lantern and make-a-poem/take-a-poem station.
5. An earthen floor and earth plaster on an existing straw bale studio.
6. Two benches (with Portland Parks and Recreation), and six planter boxes in the street.
7. Two benches, a 24-hour chalk station, re-painted mural on the street intersection.
8. Two benches at a community store.
9. A community sanctuary at a school.

5.0. A CASE STUDY: THE SUNNYSIDE PIAZZA

5.1. The Setting

In 2000, the Sunnyside Neighborhood in Portland, OR was plagued by a variety of problems, including a large transient population, social disorder, street litter, noise, and parking violations. The neighborhood, laid out on the grid network (Figure 1), was composed of 65% renters, low to moderate income, and predominantly white residents. A local church offered free dinners on Wednesdays and Fridays to the homeless population of Portland. The neighborhood was exposed to an onslaught of individuals seeking these services. Unfortunately, the Wednesday and Friday events were accompanied by an escalation of undesirable public behaviors such as excessive public alcohol drinking, and drug use that had a detrimental effect on the community living in close proximity to the church. Numerous storefronts were vandalized, continuing a history of graffiti incidents in the neighborhood.

Automobile traffic was unduly heavy and often exceeded the residential speed limit, creating numerous safety problems in this neighborhood. Another problem arouse late at night when the local taverns and liquor store closed and the customers drove home. The speed limits and traffic regulations were rarely respected, and many drivers were clearly under the influence of alcohol as evidenced by numerous DUI arrests. Families with children were particularly concerned about safety issues, although all pedestrians and drivers were at risk from these conditions.

This neighborhood had an unusually high frequency of pedestrians due to the vicinity of grocery stores and cafes and restaurants within two blocks of the intersection. While a litter-fighting organization supplied and serviced small trash cans at a few locations, these often overflowed into the street. There were no means of disposing of litter in the public realm. As a result there was a considerable amount of littering in this neighborhood, and since the presence of trash on the street invited more trash, the situation tended to spiral out of control. Many neighbors experienced and complained about the detrimental effects of excess noise from reckless driving, individuals under the influence of alcohol, and street fights. On several occasions, the police were involved in resolving such conflicts.

5.2. Placemaking

As a result of these neighborhood problems, a group of residents around a prominent intersection started to organize ways to improve the livability and sense of community in this grid neighborhood. Informal meetings began in January 2001, and the group quickly grew to consist of 20 to 30 neighbors who met regularly to discuss strategies to build neighborhood cohesion. The goal was to create a sense of place, and constructively address the local problems in the neighborhood by building a sense of community and providing an urban model for integrating art, neighborhood gathering spaces, and improving the quality of life in a mixed-use neighborhood.

During nine months of meetings, discussions, workshops, designs plans, outreach and block parties the community conceived and implemented a neighborhood enhancement project in collaboration with The City Repair Project, City officials, and the Neighborhood Association. Plans were drawn up for a three-phase implementation of various design features that would convert a regular street intersection into a pedestrian-friendly public square (Figure 3). The plan called for a large street mural, trellises in the four corners, planter boxes in the street, an art wall and an information kiosk to exchange local news. Over 100 households within two square blocks of the intersection signed a petition in support of the project in 2001, including residents of the immediately adjacent houses.

In September 2001, traffic was blocked off during a block party, and in a joint effort residents painted a giant sunflower motif (the symbol of the neighborhood; Figure 4) in the middle of the intersection that symbolizes the organization of the seeds of a mature sunflower. With the intention to incorporate educational opportunities in urban design, the natural geometry of the sunflower was used: the pattern resembles two opposing spirals, and mathematically represents a Fibonacci series. Irrespective of size of the seed head the numbers of the two spirals are always a pair in the series: 0, 1, 1, 2, 3, 5, 8, 13, 21, 34, 55, 89, 144, etc (the sum of the two previous numbers add up to the next number). For example in a small sunflower 34 spirals can be counted in one direction and 55 in the other direction, while in a bigger one there may be 89 spirals in one direction and 149 in the other. The sunflower mural spans 40 feet across and extends up onto the sidewalk with 12 foot long petals. By connecting the sidewalks and drawing people into the center, the "piazza" creates a focal point for community events. While automobile traffic still crosses the intersection the mural draws attention to pedestrians and circuitously slows traffic speed. With the sunflower being the unifying theme all houses in close proximity displayed a colorful sunflower on their porch.

In May 2002, during a natural building workshop organized by the City Repair Project hundreds of residents, workshop participants and ecological builders constructed a new neighborhood information kiosk on-site with cob, a building material similar to adobe. The kiosk featured a living roof, and a solar-powered battery light for nighttime illumination. Residents created a colorful stained class mosaic art wall with a solar powered fountain with rain water catchments.

The next year, as part of the Village Building Convergence the community erected a metal dome, towering 13 feet over the Sunnyside Piazza. A local artist created the artwork for the dome sculpture and trellises and coordinated the construction. The dome sculpture was designed according to the scheme of a sunflower: iron rods spiral out from the center with 5 spirals in one direction and 8 in the other, according to the Fibonacci Series. The structure was welded together in a nearby driveway and carried to the Piazza. As part of a dome raising ceremony

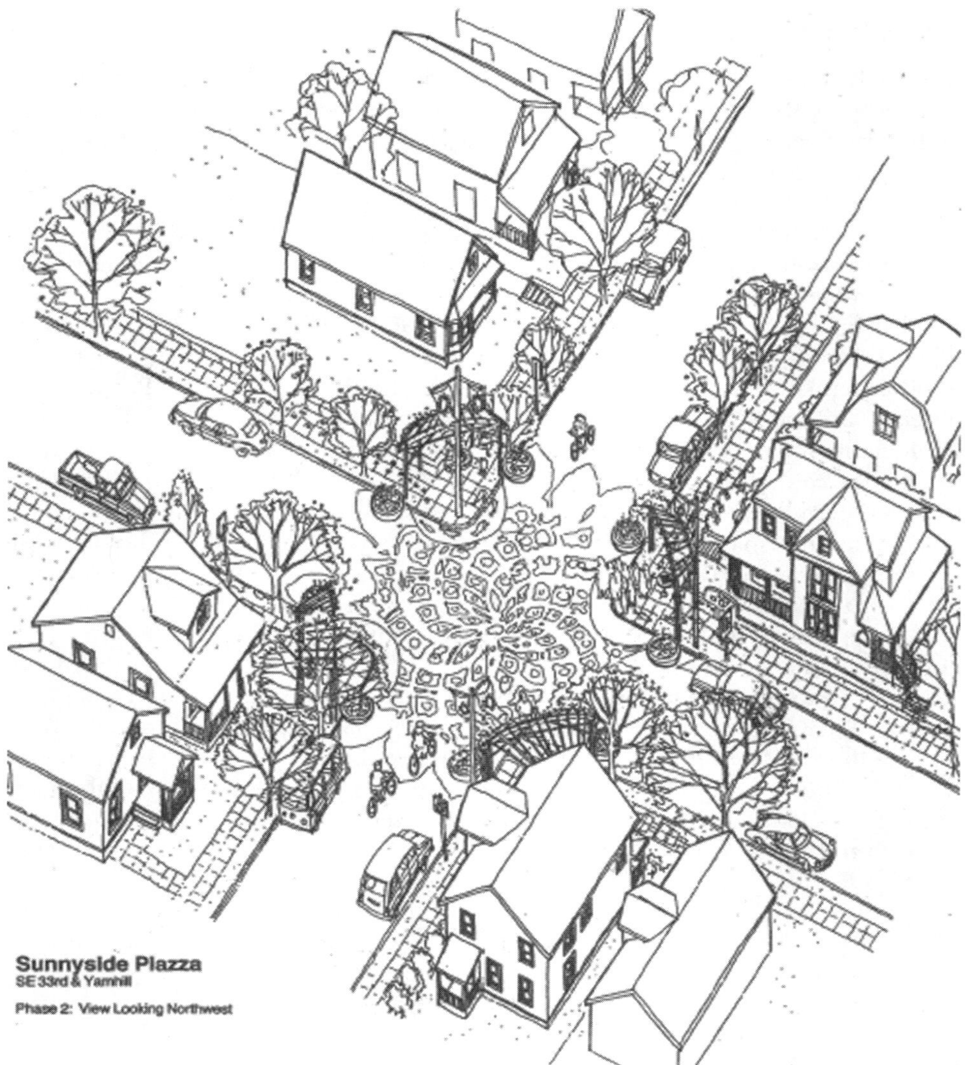

Figure 3. Plan for an Intersection Repair Project, Sunnyside Piazza, Portland, OR. (*Source*: Reproduced with permission. Semenza, J.C. (2003). The Intersection of Urban Planning, Art, and Public Health: The Sunnyside Piazza. *Am. J. Public Health* 93(9): 1439-1441.)

(analogous to an Amish barn raising ceremony) the 300-pound dome that mimics the sunflower design painted in the middle of the intersection, was raised onto wooden pillars over one of the corners; three wooden trellises were installed in the other corners of the intersection. Over 100 residents, friends of the Sunnyside Piazza and workshop participants of the Village Building Convergence joined forces to lift the structure onto its new home. In this metaphorical act, the large dome was raised onto ladders and installed over the sidewalk, secured to the hatches and bolted to the footings. Written comments were collected from participants: "I have never seen so many active, creative, awesome people from one community gathering together and having so much fun making their home such a wonderful place."

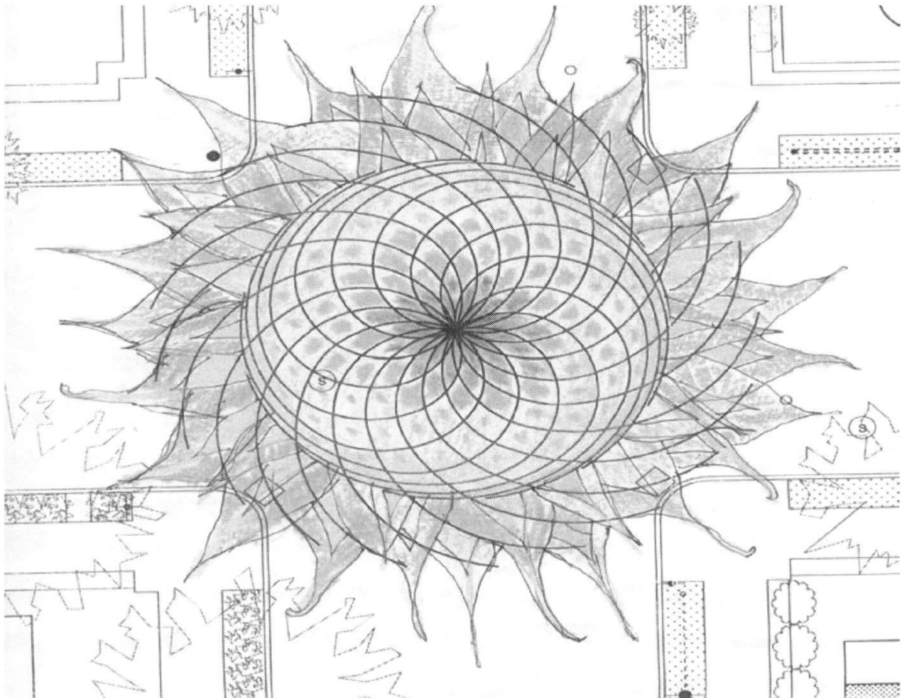

Figure 4. Sunflower Motif of Large Street Mural.

"It is not only aesthetically pleasing but it clearly demonstrates the community involvement and dedication to a united and sustainable future." "I love seeing so many of my neighbors getting together, taking pride in their community. The intersection is a place of beauty, and I am glad to have it in my neighborhood."

During block parties, the neighbors got together to plant and maintain hanging gardens on trellises on the other three corners and installed eight planters in the parking lanes within 15 feet of the intersection in order to enforce no-parking zone that will prevent parked cars from blocking vision clearance for on-coming traffic. In response to a community need, the neighbors helped to beautify the neighborhood with flowers and other plants in these planters. Recently, several benches were placed in the right of way next to the intersection, inviting by-passers to interact with each other and enjoy the giant sunflower, newly constructed cob structures and solar-powered fountain.

These activities allowed the neighbors to build social capital and to create a public square where neighbors and by-passers can interact to get to know each other. By building social relationships and mutual cooperation around collective problem solving, they embarked on an urban experiment to modify the physical design of an intersection in the grid city, as a manifestation of reclaiming the neighborhood. These new features were designed for everybody to enjoy the richness of the urban experience at the Sunnyside Piazza. The community art projects sparked conversations among strangers and pedestrians were observed to interact with the new urban features (see below).

However, support of the modification of the built urban environment was not unanimous; objections by a number or residents were addressed by accommodating their concerns and incorporating their suggestions into the design. Initially, the petition for the intersection repair project had been rejected on the grounds that the traffic frequency was too high at the particular intersection. This hurdle was eventually overcome by taking the initiative to City Council.

The homeless participated in all community activities such as the street painting and as a result took pride and ownership in the neighborhood; the homeless helped to clean up litter and waste and have donated materials that were incorporated into the structures. Burglary, assault, vehicle theft, robbery, etc have declined significantly ($P<0.001$), and call for service has diminished as well, compared to two unimproved control sites. Drug abuse and trafficking has been reduced, based on subjective assessments, but no official data exist to verify this trend. Similarly, traffic speed has been reduced but official measurements have not been conducted. Furthermore, many of the low/moderate income neighbors have been strong participants of these activities and have built previously non-existing relationships. University students and high school students have been brought to the intersection on field trips to learn the concept of mathematical relationships in nature (e.g. Fibonacci series, golden mean, etc). The site has become a destination for community residents, as well as visitors from within Portland and beyond. On a regular basis, residents hold potluck parties with outdoor movie screenings and groups of tourists and conference attendees come to the site and enjoy the Sunnyside Piazza.

5.3. Evaluation

Pedestrians passing by the Sunnyside Piazza were compared to pedestrians at an unimproved, adjacent intersection and it was observed that 32% interacted in some way with the art projects by either addressing a stranger about the mural, reading the signs, taking photographs, playing with the water fountain, etc while only 7% ($P<0.01$) of pedestrians at the adjacent control intersection interacted in any way with the urban environment or another pedestrian (Semenza, 2003). Residents at the intervention site were compared to residents at two unimproved, nearby intersections; of 97 Sunnyside Piazza residents surveyed within a two block radius of the intersection the majority (65%, n=63) of respondents classified their neighborhood as an excellent place to live, compared to 35% at the control sites. Residents at the Sunnyside Piazza scored better with other social indicators as well and indicated better general health compared to the two unimproved control sites ($P<0.01$). The administration of a detailed 11-point depression scale indicated also better mental health among residents of the Sunnyside Piazza ($P<0.01$).

However, these data are limited by their ability to differentiate between the contribution of the demographic composition of the population at the comparison sites and the environmental context. It is possible that the observed differences between the Sunnyside Piazza, compared to the two control intersections can be attributed to demographic discrepancies between the sites rather than physical improvements of the urban landscape. This distinction between contextual and compositional sources of variation is essential in the examination of neighborhood effects on health. In order to address this potential limitation of the above evaluation we have recently conducted a number of prospective longitudinal studies before and after intersection repair interventions at different sites. By doing so, the study population is maintained the same, while the built urban environment is modified. Each study subject is

Table 2. Outcome Measures of Evaluation Tool: Numbers of Questions per Category and One Sample Question

- Neighborhood (4):
  How would you rate your *present* neighborhood as a place to live?
- Sense of community (6):
  My neighborhood is a good place for kids to grow up.
- Neighborhood social interaction (4):
  Have you asked one of your neighbors for help?
- Perceived control at the neighborhood level (5):
  I can influence decisions that affect my neighborhood.
- Neighborhood participation (4):
  Most people in the neighborhood are active in groups outside of the local area.
- Mental health (11)
  I felt that everything I did was an effort.
- General health (1)
  In general, would you say your health is:

his or her own control and within subject variation is recorded. Two consecutive cross-sectional surveys were conducted to evaluate the impact of intersection repair interventions. Residents within a two-block radius of the sites were systematically sampled by going from door to door and survey data were collected before and after the intervention from the same study subjects. Subjects were blinded to the purpose of the study and no reference was made to the upcoming workshop in order to prevent the Hawthorne effect. Demographic and general health information, as well as personal identifiers for the follow-up survey, was recorded.

The subjects' perception of their own general health on a five point rating scale was collected as well as mental health with 11 survey items pertaining to depression (Table 2). Four other variables were assessed from multiple questions on the survey, sense of community, neighborhood social interaction, perceived control at the neighborhood level, and neighborhood participation. Preliminary analysis of the data indicated a beneficial effect of these community activities on public health (Semenza, March, and Bontempo, unpublished observations): a correlation matrix revealed that these four variables displayed a positive direct bivariate relationship with each other, indicating that these four variables are all related to each other and are a measure of social capital. The strongest relationships were between perceived control, neighborhood participation and sense of community. All three correlations exceeded 0.4 indicating that these three aspects are at the heart of social capital. Depression was negatively correlated with these social measures, and general health was positively correlated, suggesting a beneficial effect of the social fabric on mental health and well-being. Statistically significant improvements were documented for sense of community, social interactions, mental health and social capital while the improvements in the other variables were positive but not statistically significant. This ecologic intervention demonstrates the benefit to health promotion through community participation in local neighborhood projects.

6.0. CONCLUSION

Through community organizing this approach has proven to build both localized and bridging social capital that has manifested itself through physical improvements of urban environments. Over its eight years of existence The City Repair Project has created over 30 public gathering places and events in Portland, OR that engage people to connect with the community and place around them. Intersection Repair projects outside the Portland area have been implemented or are in the process of being implemented in Olympia, WA, Ottawa, Ontario, Ashland, NC, Minneapolis, MN, and Ithaca, NY. They all have a core group of people committed to making their neighborhoods better places to live and have strategically organized their community. The goal is to help people physically change their neighborhoods to be more community-oriented, ecologically sustainable, and simply more beautiful. This work is inspired by the idea that localization of decision-making, culture, and economy is a necessary foundation for healthy cities.

ACKNOWLEDGEMENTS: Funding for this intervention study was obtained from the Community Initiatives Small Grant Program from the Bureau of Housing and Community Development at the City of Portland; a faculty enhancement award; and scholarly and creative activity grants for undergraduates (to Andrea Thompson, Eva Rippetau, and Troy Hayes) from Portland State University. Project funding also was obtained in part from local fundraising, businesses, and in-kind donations, particularly from The Laughing Planet Café.

I am grateful to the members The City Repair Project who are dedicated to create community-oriented places, in particular Mark Lakeman, Daniel Lerch, Charla Chamberlain, Saskia Dresler, Jordan Fink, Jenny Leis, Eva Miller, Diane Beck, Greg Raisman, and many others; City of Portland traffic engineers Robert Burchfield and Elizabeth Papadopoulos; and local artists Matt Cartwright, Brian Borello, and Sukita Crimmel. Thanks to Dr. Lisa Weasel from PSU for critical feedback on the manuscript.

REFERENCES

APHA, American Public Health Association. (1948). *Planning the Neighborhood.* American Public Health Association, Committee on the Hygiene of Housing. Chicago: Public Administration Service.

Aneshensel, C.S., and Sucoff, C.A. (1996). The neighborhood context of adolescent mental health. *J. Health and Soc. Behav.* 37(4):293–310.

Balfour, J.L.,and Kaplan, G.A. (2002). Neighborhood environment and loss of physical function in older adults: evidence from the Alameda County Study. *Am. J. Epidemiol.* 155(6):507–15.

Bellah, R.N., Madsen, R., Sullivan, W.M., Swidler, A., and Tipton, S.M. (1996). *Habits of the heart: Individualism and commitment in American life.* University of California Press, Berkeley.

Berkman, L., and Glass, T. (2000). Social integration, social networks, social support, and health. In:

Berkman, L.F., Glass, T. Brissette, I., and Seeman, T,E. (eds.), From social integration to health: Durkheim in the new millennium. *Soc. Sci Med.* 51(6):843-57.

Berkman, LF, and Kawachi, I. (eds.). (2000). *Social Epidemiology.* Oxford U. Press, New York, NY, pp. 137–173.

Black, M.M., and Krishnakumar, A. (1998). Children in low-income, urban settings. Interventions to promote mental health and well-being. *Am. Psychol.* 53(6):635–46.

CDC. (1998.)Vaccination coverage by race/ethnicity and poverty level among children aged 19-35 months-United States, 1997. *MMWR* 47:956–59.

Crenson, M.A. (1978). Social networks and political processes in urban neighborhoods. *Am. J. Polit. Sci.* 22:578–594.

Dalgard, O.S., and Tambs, K. (1997). Urban environment and mental health. A longitudinal study. *Br. J. Psychiatry.* 171:530–6.

Dembo, R., Schmeidler, J., Burgos, W., and Taylor, R. (1985). Environmental setting and early drug involvement among inner-city junior high school youths. *Int. J. Addict.* 20(8):1239-55.

Denner, J., Kirby, D., Coyle, K., and Brindis, C. 2001). The protective role of social capital and cultural norms in Latino communities: a study of adolescent births. *Hispanic J Behav. Sci.* 23(1):3–22.

Diez-Roux, A.V., Northridge, M.E., Morabia, A., Bassett, M.T., and Shea, S. (1999). Prevalence and social correlates of cardiovascular disease risk factors in Harlem. *Am. J. Public Health* 89:302–307.

Ellaway, A., Anderson, A., and Macintyre, S. (1997). Does area of residence affect body size and shape? International Journal of Obesity & Related Metabolic Disorders: *J. Int. Assoc. Study of Obesity.* 21(4):304–8.

Fitzpatrick, K., and LaGory, M. (2000). *Unhealthy Places.* Routledge, New York.

Flegal, K.M., Carroll, M.D., Ogden, C.L., and Johnson, C.L. (2002). Prevalence and trends in obesity among US adults, 1999-2000. *JAMA.* 288(14):1723–7.

Florin, P., and Wandersman, A. (1984). Cognitive social learning and participation in community development. A comparison of standard and cognitive social learning variables. *Am. J. Community Psychol.* 12:689–708.

Frumkin, H. (2002). Urban sprawl and public health. *Public Health Rep.* 117(3):201–17.

Goran, M.I., and Weinsier, R.L. (2000). Role of environmental vs. metabolic factors in the etiology of obesity: time to focus on the environment. *Obesity Res.* 8(5):407–9.

Granovetter, M. (1973). The strength of weak ties. *Am. J. Sociol* 78:1360–1380.

Green, L.W. (1990). The theory of participation: a qualitative analysis of its expression in national and international health policies. In: Patton, R., and Cissell, W. (eds.), *Community organization: Traditional principles and modern applications.* Latchpins Press, Johnson City, TN.

Greenberg, M., and Schneider, D. (1996). *Environmentally Devastated Neighborhoods: Perceptions, Policies, and Realities.* Rutgers University Press, New Brunswick, NJ.

Halpern, D. (1995). *Mental health and the built environment: more than bricks and mortar?* Taylor and Francis, London.

Handy, S.L., Boarnet, M.G., Ewing, R., and Killingsworth, R.E. (2002). How the built environment affects physical activity: views from urban planning. *Am. J. Prev. Med.* 23(2 Suppl):64–73,

House, J.S., Landis, K.R., and Umberson, D. (1988). Social relationships and health. *Science.* 241(4865):540-5.

The City Repair Project, 2004, Portland, OR, (September 1, 2004); http://www.cityrepair.org

Kawachi, I., and Berkman, L.F. (2001). Social ties and mental health. *J. Urban Health* 78(3):458–67.

Kawachi, I., Kennedy, B.P., and Glass, R. (1999). Social capital and self-rated health: a contextual analysis. *Am. J. Public Health* 89(8):1187–93.

Kawachi, I., Kennedy, B.P., Lochner, K., and Prothrow-Stith, D. (1997). Social capital, income inequality, and mortality. *Am. J. Public Health.* 87(9):1491-8.

Kennedy, B.P, Kawachi, I., Prothrow-Stith, D., Lochner, K., and Gupta, K. (1998). Social capital, income inequality, and firearm violent crime. *Soc. Sci. Med.* 47(1):7–17.

Kenyon, T.A., Matuck, M.A., and Stroh, G. (1998). Persistent low immunization coverage among inner-city preschool children despite access to free vaccine. *Pediatrics* 101:612–616.

King, A.C., Castro, C., Wilcox, S., Eyler, A.A., Sallis, J.F., and Brownson, R.C. (2000). Personal and environmental factors associated with physical inactivity among different racial-ethnic groups of U.S. middle-aged and older-aged women. *Health Psychol.* 19(4):354–64.

Kingsley, G.T. (2003). Housing, health, and the neighborhood context. *Am. J. Prev. Med.* 24(3 Suppl):6–7.

Kostof, S., (1985). *A History of Architecture, Settings and Rituals.* Oxford University Press, Oxford, England.

Latkin, C.A., and Curry, A.D. (2003). Stressful neighborhoods and depression: a prospective study of the impact of neighborhood disorder. *J. Health Soc. Behav.* 44(1):34–44.

Leventhal, T., and Brooks-Gunn, J. (2003). Moving to opportunity: an experimental study of neighborhood effects on mental health. *Am. J. Public Health* 93(9):1576–82.

Lochner, K., Kawachi, I., and Kennedy, B.P. (1999). Social Capital: a guide to its measurement. *Health Place* 5:259– 270.

Maholy-Nagy, S. (1968). M*atrix of man: An illustrated history of urban environment.* Pall Mall Publishers, London, England.

Marsella, A.J. (1998). Urbanization, mental health, and social deviancy. A review of issues and research. *Am. Psychol.* 53(6):624–34.

McMillan, D.W., and Chavis, D.M. (1986). Sense of community: A definition and theory. *J. Comm. Psychol.* 14:6–23.

Mokdad, A.H., Ford, E.S., Bowman, B.A., Dietz, W.H., Vinicor, F., Bales, V.S., and Marks, J.S. (2003). Prevalence of obesity, diabetes, and obesity-related health risk factors, 2001. *JAMA.* 289(1):76–9.

Naparstek, A.J., Biegal, D.E., and Spiro, H.R. (1982). *Neighborhood networks for human mental health care.* Plenum Press, New York, NY.

O'Louhlin, J., Paradis, G., Renauld, L., Meshefedjian, G., and Gray-Donald, K. (1998). Prevalence and correlates of overweight among elementary school children in multiethnic, low income, inner-city neighborhoods in Montreal, Canada. *Ann. Epidemiol.* 8:422–432.

Ogden, C.L., Flegal, K.M., Carroll, M.D., and Johnson, C.L. (2002). Prevalence and trends in overweight among US children and adolescents, 1999-2000. *JAMA*. 288(14):1728–32.

Oxman, T.E., Berkman, L.F., Kasl, S. Jr, Freeman, D.H., and Barrett, J. (1992). Social support and depressive symptoms in the elderly. *Am. J. Epidemiol.* 135:356–68.

Pate, R.R., Pratt, M. Blair, S.N., Haskell, W.L., Macera, C.A., Bouchard, C., Buchner, D., Ettinger, W., Heath, G.W., and King, A.C. (1995). Physical activity and public health. A recommendation from the Centers for Disease Control and Prevention and the American College of Sports Medicine. *JAMA*. 273(5):402–7.

Perkins, D.D., Florin, P., Rich, R.C., Wandersman, A., and Chavis, D.M. (1990). Participation and the social and physical environment of residential blocks: Crime and community context. *Am. J. Comm. Psychol.* 18(1):83–115.

Poston, W.S. 2nd., and Foreyt, J.P. (1999). Obesity is an environmental issue. *Atherosclerosis.* 146(2):201–9.

Putnam, R. (1995). Bowling alone: America's declining social capital. *J. Democracy* 6:65–78.

Rosenstreich, D.L., Eggleston, P., Kattan, M., Baker, D., Slavin, R.G., Gergen, P., Mitchell, H., McNiff-Mortimer, K., Lynn, H., Ownby, D., and Malveaux, F. (1997). The role of cockroach allergy and exposure to cockroach allergen in causing morbidity among inner-city children with asthma. *N. Engl. J. Med.* 336(19):1356–1363.

Sampson, R.J., Morenoff, J., and Earls, F. (1999). Beyond social capital: Spatial dynamics of collective efficacy for children. *Am. Sociol. Rev.* 64:633–660.

Sampson, R.J., Raudenbush, S.W., and Earls, F. (1997). Neighborhoods and violent crime: a multilevel study of collective efficacy. *Science* 277(5328):918–24.

Seeman, T.E., Kaplan, G., Knudsen, L., Cohen, R., and Guralnik, J. (1988). Social network ties and mortality among the elderly in the Alameda County Study. *Am. J. Epidemiol.*, 126:714–23.

Semenza, J.C., Rubin, C.H., Falter, K.H., Selanikio, J.D., Flanders, W.D., Howe, H.L., and Wilhelm, J.L. (1996). Heat-related deaths during the July 1995 heat wave in Chicago. *N. Engl. J. Med.* 335(2):84–90.

Semenza, J.C. (2003). The Intersection of Urban Planning, Art, and Public Health: The Sunnyside Piazza. *Am. J. Public Health* 93(9):1439–1441.

Semenza, J.C., McCullough, J., Flanders, D.W., McGeehin M.A., and Lumpkin JR. (1999). Excess hospital admissions during the 1995 heat wave in Chicago. *Am. J. Prev. Med.* 16(4):269—277.

Shewry, M.C., Woodward, M., and Tinstall-Pedoe, H. (1992). Bariation in coronary risk factors by social status: results from the Scottish Heart Health Study. *Br. J. Gen. Prect.* 42:406–410.

Sieler-Wells, G.L. (1989). Challenges of the Gordian knot: Community health in Canada. In *International symposium on community participation and empowerment strategies in health promotion.* Center for Interdisciplinary Studies, University of Bielefeld, Bielefeld, Germany.

Skaer, T.L., Sclar, D.A., Robison, L.M., and Galin, R.S. (2000). Trends in the rate of depressive illness and use of antidepressant pharmacotherapy by ethnicity/race: an assessment of office-based visits in the United States, 1992-1997. *Clinical Therapeutics.* 22(12):1575–89.

Stiffman, A.R., Hadley-Ives, E., Elze. D., Johnson, S., and Dore P. (1999). Impact of environment on adolescent mental health and behavior: structural equation modeling. *Am. J. Orthopsychiatry.* 69(1):73–86.

Taylor, R.B. (1988). Human Territorial Functioning: An Empircal Evolutionary Perspective on Individual and Small Group Territorial Cognitions, Behaviors and Consequences. Cambridge University Press, New York, NY.

Wallace, R. (1990). Urban desertification, public health and public order: `planned shrinkage', violent death, substance abuse and AIDS in the Bronx. *Soc. Sci. Med.* 31(7):801–13.

Wilson, W.J. (1996). When work disappears: The world of the new urban poor. Vintage Press, New York, NY.

Wolf-Maier, K., Cooper, R.S., Banegas, J.R., Giampaoli, S., Hense, H.W., Joffres, M., Kastarinen, M., Poulter, N., Primatesta, P., Rodriguez-Artalejo, F., Stegmayr, B., Thamm, M., Tuomilehto, J., Vanuzzo, D., and Vescio, F. (2003). Hypertension prevalence and blood pressure levels in 6 European countries, Canada, and the United States. *JAMA*. 289(18):2363–9.

Chapter 24

Building Healthy Cities

The World Health Organization Perspective

Roderick J. Lawrence

1.0. INTRODUCTION

A city is a human construct *par excellence* because the "natural world" does not provide urban or domestic space. Cities and all their buildings and services must be conceptualized before they are constructed (Lawrence, 1995). The foundation and the construction of cities implies that geographical space and environmental resources are cultivated by people to serve their daily basic requirements and sustain human societies over time. Human sustenance is dependant on the availability of basic resources and the quality of living conditions both within and beyond the geographical boundaries of cities (Boyden, 1987). The construction of cities can be interpreted in relation to those collective decisions, lifestyles and adaptive responses that individuals and groups make in relation to the local environmental conditions of their habitat, their available resources and knowledge. Traditionally, shared lifestyles, conventions, and meanings about the ordering of society have also been used implicitly and explicitly in the construction of cities (Lawrence, 2000a).

The historical development of specific cities has been widely documented and clearly shows that sustaining health in cities is not straightforward. During the last 8 or 9 millennia many cities have flourished, whereas others have struggled for survival and some have collapsed (Bairoch, 1988). Today, Alexandria, Delos, Jericho, Ur and Venice still exist but only as fragments of ancient civilizations and seats of authority that previously had jurisdiction over vast geographical regions extending far beyond the boundaries of these cities. These examples of the prosperity and decline of cities illustrate that the sustenance of human settlements should not be taken for granted.

Data, statistics, and reports of events in many cities around the world highlight a range of contemporary problems (Hardoy, *et al.*, 1994; Lawrence, 2000b). These problems include environmental conditions; for example, an increasing incidence of summer and winter smog, which can affect health as discussed by Schwela (2000). They also include social inequalities and economic deprivation that lead to relatively high levels of homelessness and unemployment which can affect health as discussed by Lawrence (2002). In addition there can be social, cultural and political problems leading to incivilities, riots and warfare as shown by recent events in many cities in Africa and the Balkan region.

There are no simple answers to these kinds of urban problems which have both direct and indirect impacts on health and the quality of life of urban populations (Galea and Vlahov, 2004; Satterthwaite, 1993) . It should be acknowledged that policy makers and professional practitioners have often identified and isolated these kinds of problems too narrowly. This means that some problems and the interrelations between them have not been foreseen (Lawrence, 1996). Consequently, negative impacts on health and quality of life have usually been addressed by piecemeal, remedial measures. Today, there is a growing consensus that these reactive approaches need to be replaced by broader, proactive ones that strategically place health promotion and quality of life as a societal goal. This kind of approach is a key component of the World Health Organization Healthy Cities project.

In 1987, 11 cities became the founding members of the Healthy Cities project co-ordinated by the WHO Regional Office for Europe (Tsouros, 1990). A decade later there are more than 30 national and regional networks in Europe involving about 600 municipalities, now complemented by many hundreds more in each of the regions of the world (Goldstein, 2000; Tsouros and Farrington, 2003; Werna, *et al.*, 1998). The Health For All strategy provides the strategic framework for this project. The Healthy Cities project in the WHO European region includes four main components. First, designated cities that are committed to a comprehensive approach to achieving the goals of the project. Second, national and sub-national networks together with EURONET that facilitate co-operation between partners. Third, multi-city action plans (MCAPs) implemented by networks of cities collaborating on specific issues of common interest. And, fourth, special (model) projects in central and eastern Europe.

The Healthy Cities project involves intersectoral collaboration by formulating a "City Health Plan" that identifies the interrelations between living conditions in urban areas and the health of the residents (Green, *et al.*, 2003). It is argued that health can be improved by addressing the physical environment, and the social and economic determinants of health in all situations (such as the home, the school, the workplace). This broad interpretation has meant that equity and social inequalities are identified as key factors in cities that need to be addressed. In particular, the plight of vulnerable social groups (including the handicapped, homeless, unemployed, single mothers and street children) are ranked as a high priority for interventions. This approach is meant to focus not only on specific groups but also particular geographical areas in cities where there are concentrations of vulnerable people with relatively high health risks.

This chapter argues that it is necessary to reconsider the construction of cities and urban development in a broad environmental, economic, social and political context that *explicitly* accounts for health and well-being. It begins with a presentation of some key concepts, definitions and interpretations of health and cities. Then it presents the eleven key principles that the World Health Organization has presented as being the main constituents of healthy cities. It also discusses those prerequisites that are necessary in order to apply these principles in practice in order to achieve the goal of constructing healthy cities. A review of common approaches during the 20th century clearly shows that it is not an easy feat to apply the eleven principles in practice. Prior to the conclusion, this chapter suggests and illustrates a few innovative approaches that have been applied successfully. Hopefully, these kinds of contributions will serve as a catalyst for many more innovative projects in the near future.

2.0. CONCEPTS, DEFINITIONS, AND INTERPRETATIONS

2.1. Health

Health is a word derived from the old English word *hal* which meant whole, healed and sound. In this chapter health is defined as a condition or state of human beings resulting from the interrelations between humans and their biological, chemical, economic, physical and social environment. All these components of urban environments should be compatible with basic human needs and full functional activity including biological reproduction over a long period (Lawrence, 1999). Health is the result of both the direct pathological effects of chemicals, some biological agents and radiation, and the influence of physical, psychological and social dimensions of daily life including housing, transport and other characteristics of metropolitan areas. For example, improved access to medical services is a common characteristic of urban neighborhoods that is rare in rural areas.

In the field of health promotion, health is not considered an abstract condition, but as the ability of an individual to achieve her/his potential and to respond positively to the challenges of daily life. From this perspective, health is an asset or a resource for everyday life, rather than a standard or goal that ought to be achieved. This definition implies that the capacity of the health sector to deal with the health and well-being of populations is limited and that close collaboration with other sectors would be beneficial.

2.2. Healthy City

According to Hancock and Duhl (1988), "a healthy city is one that is continually creating and improving those physical and social environments and expanding those community resources which enable people to support each other in performing all the functions of life and in developing themselves to their maximum potential."

This definition of a healthy city implies that health is determined by both short- and long-term processes. A healthy city is not only a quantified outcome, such as the measurement of health status of the population. The long term goals of the WHO Healthy Cities project are to integrate health in the agenda of policy decision-makers in cities, to create a strong partnership for health promotion between groups in the public and private sectors, and to apply a local, participatory approach when implementing projects (Werna, *et al.*, 1998; Werner, *et al.*, 1999; World Health Organization, 2000c).

2.3. Building as Product and Process

In order to direct the debate between scientists, practitioners and policy decision makers about building health cities, some conceptual clarification is required (Lawrence, 1993). First, it is necessary to distinguish between *building as a product* (that is the analysis of the built environment as the physical outcome of decisions about how to accommodate human life in cities) and *building as process* (by referring to the multiple sets of processes that occur in cities and between cities and their hinterlands). It is common to adopt only one of these interpretations of building, whereas this chapter argues that both should be applied simultaneously in order to deal with the complexity of constructing healthy cities. When this integrated interpretation is applied, then the term building can denote the ordering of resources, people and their activities, as well as a set of goals, priorities and actions that are meant to achieve desired ends.

In essence, building a healthy city is intentional, not haphazard. It always occurs in a human context which defines and is mutually defined by a wide range of cultural, societal and individual human factors. Building involves choosing between a range of options in order to achieve objectives that may or may not give a high priority to health and quality of life. The complexity of building cities raises some critical questions including: What parameters are pertinent for a specific building task, such as the construction of a new residential neighborhood? Whose values, goals and intentions will be taken into consideration? How and when will these goals and intentions be achieved? What will be the monetary and non-monetary costs and benefits of specific options?

In order to answer these kinds of questions it is necessary to recall those inherent characteristics of cities that can influence health status. Although the definition of a city varies from country to country, the United Nations uses national definitions that are commonly based on population size (Vlahov and Galea, 2002). Other definitions are based on the administrative or political authority of municipalities, especially the degree of autonomy in relation to the national or regional administration. Some definitions include the socioeconomic status of the resident population, especially their livelihood (such as the proportion of all employed people with non-agricultural occupations). A combination of these characteristics could be used to interpret rural and urban areas, but this has been rare, especially in recent published research on the determinants of health in urban environments. In order to distinguish cities from other kinds of human settlements, notably suburban areas and rural towns, it is important to identify the distinguishing characteristics of cities.

The first characteristic of cities is *centralization*. The choice of a specific site, and the definition of the administrative and political boundaries of a city distinguish it from the hinterlands. Studies in urban history and geography confirm that many factors have been involved in the location of cities (Bairoch, 1988). For example, coastal sites for ports like New York, Cape Town, or Sydney can be contrasted with sites on inland trade routes such as Geneva or Vienna. It is important to note that modern economic rationality has an interpretation of the World and human societies which has rarely accounted for the climatic, geological and biological characteristics of specific localities. This has meant that urban populations have been confronted with unforeseen natural and human-made disasters including earthquakes, floods, and landslides (Mitchell, 1999).

The expansion of the built-up area, the construction of roads, water reservoirs and drains together with land clearance and deforestation can effect drastic changes to landscapes and ecosystems which lead to negative impacts on health. Rapid urban development has been associated with new diseases (McMichael, 1993; 2000). Natural foci for disease vectors may become entrapped within the peri-urban extension and new ecological habitats for the animal reservoirs may be created. Within urban agglomerations, disease vectors may adapt to new habitats and introduce new infections to spread among the urban population. For instance, in India, where the vector of lymphatic filariasis is a peridomestic mosquito, there has been a rapid increase in the incidence of the disease and in the vector population associated with the steady increase in the growth of human populations in these endemic areas. Anopheline mosquitoes generally shun polluted water yet A Stephensi, the principal vector for urban malaria, is also reported in India and the Eastern Mediterranean region to have adapted to survive in the urban environment (World Health Organization, 1992).

The second characteristic of cities is *verticality*. During the 8000–9000 year history of cities, societies have constructed buildings of several floors. Bairoch (1988) noted that Jericho included buildings of seven floors. This characteristic underlies the compact or dense built environment of cities in contrast to the dispersed character of rural towns. The height of buildings in cities increased dramatically from the late 19th century with the construction of skyscrapers, first in Chicago, then other cities around the World. The relations between high-rise housing conditions and health status are not easy to decipher owing to the vast number of confounding factors (Fuller-Thomson, *et al.*, 2000). However, there is empirical evidence that those residents who do not choose where they live, especially households with young children who are allocated housing units in high-rise buildings, may suffer from stressors that impact negatively on their health (Halpern, 1995; Lawrence, 1993).

Concentration is the third characteristic of cities that is directly related to the two preceding ones. Urbanization is dependent on the availability of natural resources and the exportation of waste products in order to sustain their populations. Cities import energy, fuels, materials and water which are transformed into goods and services. The high concentrations of activities, objects and people in cities, and the flows between rural and urban areas, mean that city authorities must manage the supply of food and water as well as the disposal of solid and liquid wastes in a sustainable way. Urban history confirms that cities are localities that favor the rapid spread of infectious diseases, fires, social unrest and warfare (Bairoch, 1988).

In terms of questions related to public health, concentration can be quantified in terms of activities, building density, and population density. Surveys of empirical studies show that the number of persons per meter of habitable floor area is related to the propagation of infectious diseases such as tuberculosis and cholera (Gray, 2001; Rosen, 1993; UNCHS, 1998). Concentration also implies relatively easy access to all community services, including primary health care, and social welfare.

Diversity is a refining characteristic of cities that can be used effectively to promote ecological, economic and social well-being. Diversity is known to be an important characteristic of natural ecosystems because it enables adaptations to unforeseen (external) conditions and processes that may impact negatively and even threaten survival (Laughlin and Brady, 1978). In the same way, we have learnt from history that those cities with a diverse local economy have been able to cope much better with economic recessions and globalization. This was not the case for Detroit, Glasgow, or cities of the mid-West in North America. Therefore, diversity – be it economic, ecological or cultural – is an important principle that enables human settlements to adapt to unforeseen factors that can impact on their sustenance.

Social, economic and material diversity are inherent characteristics of cities (Lawrence, 2002). The heterogeneity of urban populations can be considered in terms of age, ethnicity, income, and socio-professional status. These kinds of distinctions are often reflected and reinforced by education, housing conditions, employment status, property ownership and material wealth. Data and statistics show that in specific cities different neighborhoods are the locus of ethnic, political, monetary, and professional differentiation between "us and them" and "here and there". When these dimensions of human differentiation become acute they are often reflected and reinforced by spatial segregation and social exclusion in urban agglomerations (OECD, 1986). In recent decades, there have been several empirical studies which show how these characteristics of urban neighborhoods, especially acute socio-economic inequalities and lack of social cohesion, are linked to morbidity and mortality (Landon, 1996; Marmot and Wilkinson, 1999).

The fifth characteristic is *information and communication*. Cities have always been centers for the development and exchange of ideas, information and inventions (Castells, 1991). It is well known that targeted information is crucial for effective preventive measures in public campaigns about risk behaviors including tobacco smoking, alcohol consumption, drug abuse and safe sexual intercourse. City authorities can play a crucial role in health prevention and promotion by communicating information in innovative ways. There is much to be learnt from successful marketing strategies by private enterprises if public health campaigns about risk behaviors are to become more successful than they have been. Health education is a key factor in increasing the responsible behavior of individuals, social groups and communities (Wallerstein, 1992).

Mechanization is the sixth characteristic. Cities have depended on machines to import supplies, to treat waste products and to efficiently use their built environment. Contemporary cities are heavily dependent on machinery for a wide range of functions and services that guarantee sanitary living conditions. Mechanical and technological characteristics of cities that directly or indirectly affect health include industrial production, transportation, the processing of mass-produced foods and the increasing use of synthetic materials in the built environment. In particular, the incidence of accidents in urban areas is a major challenge for public health (Mancieux and Romer, 1986). For example, in 1998, injuries caused by motor vehicle accidents were ranked 10th among leading causes of mortality worldwide and 9th among the leading causes of disability. Today, children and young adults in all regions of the World bear a disproportionate burden of these accidents, and the burden is significantly higher in urban areas compared with rural areas, and also in developing countries compared with developed countries (World Bank, 2001).

The last characteristic is *political authority*. The city was the *polis* in ancient Greece, meaning it had a specific political status which is still the case today in the form of municipal government. During the 1990s, much attention has been given to urban governance rather than municipal government. Governance can be defined as "the sum of the ways through which individuals and institutions (public and private) plan and manage their common affairs. It is a continuing process that may either lead to conflict or to mutually beneficial co-operative action. It includes formal institutions and informal arrangements, as well as the social capital of citizens" (UNCHS, 2001, p. 90). Governance is based on the effective co-ordination of three main components: market-based strategies for the private sector, hierarchical strategies articulated by the public sector and networking in civil society. The goal of governance should be to develop synergies between these partners so there is a better capacity to deal with the most urgent priorities. These priorities can be developed by "city health profiles" which provide the empirical evidence for strategic action for health planning (Webster, 2003). City health profiles are crucial components of the WHO Healthy Cities project agenda for implementation, because local authorities must deal with a wide range of management questions concerning the environmental, economic, technological, and social hazards that collectively challenge the health and well-being of citizens.

Last but not least, politicians and professionals make crucial decisions about the allocation of financial and other kinds of resources to promote living conditions, the local economy and public health. Therefore, the ethical conduct of politicians, public administrators and professionals in the private sector can exacerbate or counteract the social inequalities between citizens. These kinds of differences are maintained by social control, asymmetries of power, and the hierarchical order of urban affairs (Wallerstein, 1992).

3.0. ELEVEN PRINCIPLES OF THE WHO HEALTH CITIES PROJECT

The following section considers those basic principles underlying the building of healthy cities. It briefly presents the eleven principles that the World Health Organization has repeatedly presented in documentation about the WHO Healthy Cities project to characterise healthy cities (Goldstein, 2000; Tsouros, 1990). Each paragraph explains how these principles can be interpreted to construct healthy cities. The 11 principles of a healthy city are shown in Table 1.

1. *The meeting of basic needs (for food, water shelter, income, safety and work) for all the city's people.* During the 8000 to 9000 year history of cities, the health of urban populations has been closely related to the management of diverse kinds of natural and human-made hazards which can be a cause of serious injury, illness or premature death. A major task of public authorities is to sustain the supply of basic resources (especially safe water and uncontaminated food), and to ensure the disposal of all kinds of solid and liquid wastes.

Rapid urbanisation during the last century has induced stress on natural ecosystems (Boyden, 1987; McMichael, 1993; Giradet, 1999). This has meant that it is increasingly difficult to guarantee the supply of unpolluted water, uncontaminated fresh foods, sanitary housing and efficient community services and facilities. For example, the large majority of urban populations in the world are totally dependent on imported foods from far beyond the hinterland of their city. In 2000, only an estimated 15% to 20% of all food in the world was produced in urban areas.

Table 1. Eleven Principles of the WHO Healthy Cities Project

1. The meeting of basic needs (for food, water, shelter, income, safety, and work) for all the city's people
2. A clean, safe physical environment of high quality, including housing quality.
3. An ecosystem that is stable now and sustainable in the long-term.
4. A diverse, vital and innovative economy
5. A strong, mutually supportive and non-exploitive community
6. A high degree of participation and control by the public over the decisions affecting their lives, health, and well-being.
7. The encouragement of connectedness with the past, with the cultural and biological heritage of city-dwellers and with other groups and individuals.
8. Access to a wide variety of experiences and resources with the chance for a wide variety of contact, interaction, and communications.
9. A form that is compatible with and enhances the preceding characteristics.
10. An optimum level of appropriate public health and sick care services accessible to all.
11. High health status (high levels of positive health and low levels of disease).

Source: World Health Organization, in diverse publications; refer to (Goldstein, 2000).

In 2000, the World Health Organization estimated that more than 30% of the world population suffered from one or more of the numerous kinds of malnutrition, and that urban populations were disproportionately at risk. Malnutrition is more common among refugees and displaced populations concerning an estimated 21.5 million people in 1999 (WHO, 2000b). The health implications of malnutrition range from stunted growth during childhood, development of brain damage, risks of other illness and mortality from non-communicable diseases.

An integrated approach to food production and consumption, environmental quality, sustainable resource use and health can be achieved by policies that promote the local production of fresh foods. This innovative approach to urban agriculture can address deficiencies in the nutrition of citizens and reduce the risk of food-borne and non-communicable diseases while simultaneously promoting food security. Food security means that all people continually have "physical and economic access to enough food for an active, healthy life." This concept implies that food production and consumption are sustainable, governed by principles of equity and that "the food is nutritionally adequate and personally and culturally acceptable; and that food is obtained (and consumed) in a matter that upholds basic human dignity." (Pederson, *et al.*, 2000).

2. *A clean, safe physical environment of high quality, including housing quality.* Urban environments are known to be an important determinant of quality of life and well-being following the results of numerous studies in a range of disciplines cited in other chapters of this Handbook. The multiple components of private and public buildings, infrastructure and services, as well as public outdoor space ought to be considered in terms of their potential and effective contribution to physical, social and mental well-being. It has been common for the World Health Organization to refer to the following eight main components of urban environments.

First, the characteristics of the site, in ensuring safety from "natural" disasters including earthquakes, landslides, flooding and fires; and protection from any potential source of natural radon (World Health Organization, 1997a). Second, the built environment as a shelter for the inhabitants from the extremes of outdoor temperature, as a protector against dust, insects and rodents, and as a provider of security from unwanted persons, and as an insulator against noise (World Health Organization, 1990). Third, effective provision of a safe and continuous supply of water that meets standards for human consumption, and the maintenance of sewage and solid waste disposal (World Health Organization, 1992). Forth, ambient atmospheric conditions in the residential neighbourhood and indoor air quality. Both of these sets of conditions are related to emissions from industrial production in urban areas, as well as transportation, fuels used for domestic cooking and heating, and the local climate and ventilation inside and around buildings (Schwela, 2000). Fifth, occupancy conditions in buildings (notably population density in residential buildings), which can influence the transmission of airborne infections including pneumonia and tuberculosis, and the incidence of injury from domestic accidents (Gray, 2001; Landon, 1996). Sixth, accessibility to community facilities and services (for commerce, education, employment, leisure and primary health care) that are affordable and available to all individuals and groups irrespective of age, socio-economic status, ethnicity or religion (World Health Organization, 2000a). Seventh, food safety, including the provision of uncontaminated fresh foods and water that can be stored with protection against spoilage (World Health Organization, 1997b). Eighth, the control of vectors and hosts of disease outdoors and inside buildings which can propagate in the building structure, the use of non-toxic materials and finishes for building construction, the use and storage of hazardous substances or equipment in the urban environment (World Health Organization, 1990).

Research in environmental psychology during the 1990s confirms that the relations between urban environments and health are not limited to the above eight components. In addition, the urban environment, especially residential neighborhoods, ought to be considered in terms of its capacity to nurture and sustain social and psychological processes (Gabe and Williams, 1993; Halpern, 1995; Ludermir and Harpham, 1998). For example, the capacity of the resident in her/his home environment to alleviate stress accumulated at school or in the workplace, and whether this capacity is mediated by views of nature or being in natural surroundings such as urban parks. The multiple dimensions of residential environments that circumscribe the resident's capacity to use her/his domestic setting to promote well-being is a subject that has been studied by a limited number of scholars during the last decade (Ekblad, 1993; Halpern, 1995). Studies in several industrialized countries show that more than half of all non-sleep activities of employed people between 18 and 64 years of age occur inside housing units. Children, the aged and housewives spend even more time indoors. Consequently, their prolonged exposure to shortcomings in the indoor residential environment may have a strong impact on their health and well being (World Health Organization, 1990).

3. *An ecosystem that is stable now and sustainable in the long term.* The construction of new cities or urban neighborhoods should be considered after a careful appraisal of the constituents of the local environment. Explicit land use guidelines and policies should avoid flood plains, seismic faults and dangers from landslides, while preserving wildlife habitat and agricultural fields in the hinterlands (Girardet, 1999). The site chosen for future urban development can be identified by establishing that it will incur the least ecological, economic and social costs. Consequently, new cities and urban neighborhoods can be developed in a way that preserves the ecological infrastructure underlying the human settlement, especially genetic diversity, soil fertility, mineral reserves, and water catchment areas.

Data and statistics show that many informal housing areas are located on sites that are at risk from natural or human-made hazards. For example, on 17th January 1995, an earthquake in the Kobe-Osaka urban region killed over 6000 people, and ten times that number were injured. In 1999, the cyclone that hit Orissa, India caused the destruction of 742,143 housing units (Mitchell, 1999). After an earthquake in Turkey that year about 1 million people were recorded as homeless including 70% of the population of Izmit.

During the period 1990-1999 more than 186 million people lost their homes due to a natural or a human-made disasters. Armed conflict contributed to about 100 million homeless people. Technological disasters were less significant in the 1990s resulting in about 164'200 homeless people following accidental chemical pollution, explosions and fires in or near industrial plants (UNCHS, 2001). What is also notable in these cases of natural disasters is that injury and death are disproportionately high among low-income groups who live on sloping sites prone to landslides, or in residential buildings least able to withstand the tremors (Mitchell, 1999; UNCHS, 1996). During the 20th century, social development and urban policies in many countries were dominated by issues related to economic and population growth, the accumulation and distribution of capital and material goods, as well as managing the interrelations between public and private interests. This means that the health and well-being of current and future generations, as well as the ecological impacts of urbanization have not been a high priority.

4. *A diverse, vital and innovative economy.* Urbanization is a process that has been considered in relation to the economic growth of national economies and more recently the global economy (Duffy, 1995; Lo and Yeung, 1998). In some countries, cities are locations for about two-thirds of Gross Domestic Product (GDP). The Bangkok Metropolitan Area, for example, accounts for 74% of manufacturing even though it includes only 10% of Thailand's population. Likewise, Manila comprises 15% of the total population of the Philippines but it produces a third of GDP and it includes about two-thirds of all manufacturing plants (Fuchs, *et al.*, 1994).

Economic, health and other social policies share a goal of improving the livelihood of the inhabitants. Nonetheless, not all cities, nor the inhabitants of a specific city, benefit equally. Economic, health and other social policies raise complex questions that do not have simple answers (Lawrence, 1995). The implementation of these kinds of policies may have outcomes that are neither symmetrical, predictable, nor equitable. During the last three decades, those countries in the South that urbanized most rapidly also had the highest levels of economic growth (UNCHS, 1996). Nonetheless, these trends have also led to relatively high levels of urban poverty and limited achievements in improving environmental conditions including a sufficient volume of potable water, and effective site drainage, and sewage and solid waste disposal. These consequences can have direct, negative impacts on health (Lee, 1999). They have been one reason why urbanization has often been interpreted negatively. In recent years, urban development has received a growing amount of attention leading up to and following the United Nations Summit on Human Settlements (HABITAT II) held in Istanbul in 1996.

It is important to consider all feasible development options and their environmental, economic, health and other social impacts *before* any decisions are made (Lawrence, 1995). For example, economic incentives to promote local employment by constructing new factories in a city may be successful in creating jobs, while simultaneously permitting emissions that have negative impacts on the quality of air and local water supplies in that locality and adjoining areas. This example shows that what is positive for the local economy may not be positive for some constituents of the local environment and that there can be negative impacts on the health of the population. It also shows that the capacity of the health sector to deal with the health and well-being of populations is limited and that close collaboration with other sectors would be beneficial.

5. *A strong, mutually supportive and non-exploitive community.* Equity is a key concept of the WHO Healthy Cities project (Goldstein, 2000; Tsouros and Farrington, 2003). Equity refers to a set of legal principles founded on justice and fair conduct that counteract unjustifiable acts or deeds. It implies fairness in the relationship between an individual and other persons, and between an individual, groups and the state. These relationships include a just distribution of the benefits and services in a society with respect to a universal standard or values such as human rights. For example, no individual or institution should act in a way to damage, compromise or limit the freedom and rights of others. Equity is an important component of the division of capital, as well as access to and distribution of information, resources and services including education, health care and social welfare (Lawrence, 2002).

The distinction between equality and equity is important because equality means equal circumstances, treatment and outcomes for all, whereas equity recognizes social differences and seeks to establish whether these differences are fair and just.

Inequalities of professional status, income, housing and work conditions are reflected in and reinforced by inequalities of health and well-being (Dahlgren and Whitehead, 1992; Townsend, *et al.*, 1992). Although the economic, social and physical characteristics of urban neighborhoods can be correlated with rates of morbidity and mortality, the lifestyle of groups and individuals cannot be ignored (Marmot and Wilkinson, 1999). Residents in deprived urban areas commonly have diets that contain relatively high levels of sugar, starch and fats, because foods high in protein, minerals and vitamins are relatively expensive. Smoking is also more prevalent, especially among women (Wilkinson, 1996). In essence when poverty is interpreted as a compound index of deprivation including lack of income and lack of access to education, employment, housing and social support, it is a significant indicator of urban morbidity and mortality.

6. *A high degree of participation and control by the public over the decisions affecting their lives, health and well-being.* The WHO Healthy Cities project includes a strong commitment to public participation, which is considered to be a prerequisite for a healthy city (World Health Organization, 2002).

The term participation has a wide range of meanings because it can be interpreted as a means of achieving a goal or objective, and as a dynamic process that is not quantifiable or predictable. In the health sector, Wallerstein and Bernstein (1994) concluded from a literature review that there is no consensus about participation, which can refer to a process, a program, a technique or a methodology. Participation can be interpreted as a broad term that refers to dialogue between policy institutions and civic society in order to formulate goals, projects and the allocation of resources in order to achieve desired outcomes. A wide range of techniques and methods can be used including civic forums, focus groups, citizen's juries, surveys, role playing and gaming. These methods can be applied using aids or tools such as maps, plans, photographs, small- or large-scale simulation models and computed aided design kits (Marans and Stokols, 1993).

In the late 1970s, citizen participation was considered for the first time in relation to primary health care in the Declaration of Primary Health Care at Alma Ata in 1977. Since then, participation has become an established component of definitions of health and as a means of promoting health in communities (Eklund, 1999). Participatory approaches have also been widely applied for housing construction, urban planning, and environmental conservation policies by municipal governments and non-governmental organizations (NGOs) on the understanding that complex issues should *not* be interpreted in democratic societies by one set of criteria or values (Gibbons, *et al*, 1994). In 1992, this trend was endorsed by Agenda 21, which advocates citizen participation in decision-making (United Nations, 1992).

An interest in the concept and practice of empowerment has developed since the 1970s in a number of fields of enquiry including social psychology, community studies and urban planning (Chavis and Wandersman, 1990). In the 1990s, empowerment was explicitly linked to citizen control in health education, primacy health care and housing. Today, there is no shared definition of empowerment. Some argue that is not normative because it is only defined in terms of its societal context. Nonetheless, the core of empowerment includes the concepts of authority and power. These enable a process by which individuals and communities assume power and then act effectively in changing their lives and their local environment. In the field of public health, Wallerstein (1992) states, "Empowerment is a multi-level construct that involves people assuming control and mastery over their lives in the context of their social and political environment; they gain sense of control and purposefulness to exert political power as they participate in the democratic life of their community for social change."

This interpretation indicates that it is necessary to distinguish between empowerment of individuals and groups or communities in relation to health promotion policies and programs.

7. *The encouragement of connectedness with the past, with the cultural and biological heritage of city-dwellers and with other groups and individuals.* The natural heritage of cities is commonly associated with the biological and ecological components of their site location, such as Cape Town, Rio de Janeiro, San Francisco and Sydney. The cultural heritage of cities is often considered in relation to human-made monuments, public buildings and cultural festivals. However, in addition to these, urban history can be used creatively as a warehouse of knowledge, including the achievements and shortcomings of specific urban development projects, in order to build healthier cities. In terms of shortcomings, it is important to recognise the legacy of urban renewal programs and projects in many cities around the World after the Second World War. From 1945, land-use and housing policies were enacted to address the housing shortage that accumulated during the previous decade. At the same time decisions were taken to demolish the historic quarters of inner cities by vast programs of urban renewal or reconstruction. Today these so called "model housing estates" are the locus of compound architectural, economic, social and technical problems which negatively affect the health and well-being of residents (Lawrence, 1993).

One positive lesson from urban history could be learned from the public health reform movement that began in Britain in the mid-19th century following rapid urban population growth, industrialization, the concentration of poverty in cities, and the propagation of infectious diseases (Rosen, 1993). The public health problems of unsanitary housing, lack of a supply of safe water, ineffective sewage and solid waste disposal were related to health inequalities that were tackled by devolving responsibility and authority to local municipalities in Britain in 1866. The important role of local public administrations should be remembered at the beginning of the 21st century when neo-liberalism seems to have replaced state initiatives in many countries. It is appropriate to stress the need for public health interventions including solid waste disposal, sewage and water services, and affordable health service and medical care. In many countries today, including those in the former Soviet Union, local public administrations lack the human and financial resources to counteract conditions in cities that have negative impacts on health and well-being.

8. *Access to a wide variety of experiences and resources with the chance for a wide variety of contact, interaction and communications.* It is necessary to reconsider the city as the focal point of creativity and culture; of conviviality and as places for sedentary living. Today, cities are too frequently interpreted as centers for the mobilization of people, goods and services. Consequently land use planning has adopted zoning laws to locate precise kinds of activities in specific urban areas. This approach has led to the demarcation and separation of land for housing, retailing, industry and leisure activities. Proximity and accessibility were two key characteristics of cities that have

been challenged by urban sprawl in the 20th century, including the construction of retailing malls on the outskirts of cities, coupled with inefficient public transport. In contrast, the long-standing custom of mixed activities -still found in Manhattan, and some inner quarters of Paris -provides vitality, and social amenity accessible on foot. Traditionally, these mixed activities enabled interaction between different population groups. Cities of the 21st century should not only be important motors for national economic development but also functionally rich, having a sense of security and being people-friendly.

Social development is a key component of the WHO Healthy Cities project which challenges quantified, economic growth at the expense of sustained qualitative development (Tsouros and Farrington, 2003). Consequently a healthy city should foster an ecologically sound and secure local environment, a diverse and equitable local economy, and a reduction in inequalities leading to the social integration of diverse groups.

Individual and community awareness, and responsibility are prerequisites for a strong commitment by policy decision makers and practitioners to the redefinition of goals and values that promote health and well-being in cities (World Health Organization, 1995). Without this commitment, based on a sound knowledge base and shared goals and values, recent requests for more public participation cannot redefine policy formulation and implementation in meaningful ways. Public participation and empowerment alone are not panaceas for current urban and broader environmental problems, but they can serve as vehicles for identifying what local residents consider as key issues concerning the promotion of health and well-being (Eklund, 1993; Wallerstein, 1992). Before individuals and community groups can effectively participate with scientists, professionals and politicians in policy formulation and implementation there are long-standing institutional and social barriers that need to be dismantled as Lawrence (1995) has argued.

9. *A form that is compatible with and enhances the preceding characteristics.* Urbanization during the 20th century was characterized by a growth in the number, population size, and total surface area of cities on a scale previously unknown, and this trend is expected to continue (Galea and Vlahov, 2004). Urbanization in the last century has transformed the physical, psychological and social dimensions of daily life including housing, transport and other characteristics of metropolitan areas. For example, improved access to medical services is a common characteristic of urban neighborhoods that is rare in rural areas. Urban life has other important health benefits including easy access to job markets, education, cultural and leisure activities (Lawrence, 1999).

There are many types of human settlement layouts, including linear and nodal, compact and dispersed. The concentration of many kinds of human activities, the built environment and the resident population have many ecological and economic advantages compared with a more dispersed form of human settlement. In essence, a compact form of human settlement uses less arable land, which is a precious non-renewable resource for the sustenance of all ecosystems (Wackernagel and Rees, 1996). In addition, compact human settlement has a lower unit cost for most kinds of infrastructure and services such as roads, drainage, piped water and sanitation.

One of the most significant changes in the layout and growth of cities during the 20th century was the trend for the development of dispersed suburbs, rather than compact neighborhoods. For example, the resident population of New York has increased by only 5% in the last 25 years, whereas the surface area of its built environment has increased by 61% (Girardet, 1999). This kind of urban and suburban sprawl has many negative impacts, including the increased loss of fertile agricultural lands, the destruction of forests, and irreversible damage to wetlands and coastal ecosystems. The dispersed form of urban development has larger ecological, economic and social costs than the compact city and some of these costs can have negative impacts on health and well-being (Barton and Tsourou, 2000). Therefore, trends that have dominated urban development during the 20th century should be regulated more strictly by land-use controls in order to make urban living less dependent on the ecological resource base. Architects and urban planners can promote ecological efficiency in existing urban neighborhoods by not accepting to design new out of town shopping malls or housing estates that are not accessible using public transport (Dubé, 2000; Kenworthy, 2000). These kinds of peripheral developments on the outskirts of cities converts productive agricultural land and forests into new suburban sprawl that destroys both the ecological and the social fabric of human settlements. They also frequently create dependence on automobiles, thus isolating those who do not drive motor cars, notably children, the handicapped, the aged, and the poor.

10. *An optimum level of appropriate public health and sick care services accessible to all.* National and local governments, sometimes with the private sector, are responsible for the institutions, organizations and resources that are devoted to promote, sustain or restore health. A health system has important functions including the provision of services and the human, monetary and physical resources that make the delivery of these services possible (World Health Organization, 2000a). These resources can include any contribution whether in informal personal health care, or public or private professional health and medical services. The primary purpose of all services is to improve health by preventive or curative measures. A health system should not only strive to attain the highest average level of the health status of the population, but also simultaneously strive to reduce the differences between the health of individuals and groups. Health care systems have the important responsibility to ensure that people are treated equitably, in an affordable manner and in accordance with human rights.

Today, national governments have less influence on housing, urban planning and the local urban economy than they did two decades ago, when the majority of decisions about urban development were made at the national level. Decentralization (or devolution) has been common in the 1990s, applying the principle of subsidiarity that was endorsed by the United Nations Conference on Environment and Development in Rio de Janeiro in 1992. Decentralization can only be effective if the new roles and responsibilities of local authorities and municipal services are financially supported by the transfer of appropriate resources from the national to the local level (Green, 1998).

Poor municipal management has not relieved the inadequacy of the quantity or quality of water supplied to populations in urban areas. For example, the joint WHO/UNICEF monitoring program estimates that in Asia and the Pacific region less than 65% have water supplied and less than 40% of all households in urban agglomerations have a sewage connection (WHO/UNICEF, 2000). These deficiencies can be compounded by poor environmental management such as the conversion of water catchment areas, deforestation in the hinterlands around cities, pollution from industrial production and land-fill dumps for the disposal of solid wastes. According to available information 85% of India's urban population has access to drinking water but only 20% of the available drinking water meets health and safety standards.

11. *High health status (high levels of positive health and low levels of disease).* One hundred years ago, about 80% of the World's population lived in rural areas, whereas in the year 2001 about a half of the global population live in cities. At the beginning of the 21st century, urban health can be characterized by relatively high levels of tuberculosis, respiratory and cardiovascular diseases, cancers, adult obesity, and malnutrition, tobacco smoking, mental ill health, alcohol consumption and drug abuse, sexually transmitted diseases (including AIDS), as well as fear of crime, homicides, violence and accidental injury and deaths (Galea and Vlahov, 2004). It is noteworthy that in the 1990s mental ill health was integrated into the etiology of urban health, and that the promotion of both physical and mental health were accepted as a complementary goal for national and local policy makers and professionals (Parry Jones and Quelquoz, 1991).

Unfortunately, during the 1990s, a number of negative trends related to the provision of basic infrastructure and services have been recorded by UNCHS Habitat and other organizations. In particular, per capita investment in basic urban services is declining for a number of reasons including urban population growth, especially on the outskirts of cities; in addition, lack of security of tenure offers little incentive for residents to invest in services themselves (UNCHS, 2001). These recent trends in investments in basic infrastructure and services need to be highlighted and challenged by all those who promote public health because they present a major obstacle to the building of healthier cities.

4.0. PREREQUISITES FOR APPLYING PRINCIPLE IN PRACTICE

Data and statistics from numerous sources both in and outside the health sector show that the health status of urban populations is the result of numerous factors (Lawrence 2000b). The promotion of health and the prevention of illness relies on the contribution of actors working in many sectors. There is no doubt that their contributions should be co-ordinated. There are several prerequisites that are essential for the building of healthy cities based on the application of the preceding principles. If these prerequisites are *not* guaranteed over the long term then it is meaningless to discuss a set of principles that are not effectively applied. According to the author of this chapter, the following prerequisites are necessary for the effective application of the eleven principles.

1. *Proactive policies and programs with sufficient monetary and non-monetary resources over the long term should complement remedial measures.* The formulation and implementation of traditional approaches in urban affairs has not led to optimal results. Incremental improvements (in sectors such as employment, housing or transport) are often achieved in tandem with unintended consequences, which may include negative impacts on the environmental conditions in cities, the economy, and the health of citizens (Lawrence, 1996). These unforeseen outcomes are due to the number and complexity of all those factors that policy decision-makers need to consider.

Although city authorities have used conventional urban planning to apply reactive approaches to correct or remove inadequate housing and working conditions, today we know that infectious diseases stemming from unsanitary conditions are not the leading cause of morbidity and mortality in many countries north of the Equator (Murray and Lopez, 1996). Instead, non-communicable illnesses having multiple causes are the main challenge for public health at the beginning of the 21st century. Therefore, urban planning in these countries could shift from using reactive to proactive approaches. Urban planning should not only deal with reducing negative health impacts but also actively promote well-being (Dubé, 2000; Barton and Tsourou, 2000; World Health Organization, 1997c; 2000d).

One example of an innovative approach would reconsider urban planning and transportation from a broader ecological perspective (Lawrence, 2002). This approach would imply a shift from dealing with piecemeal approaches to road transport, car parking and traffic safety. It would reinterpret accessibility and mobility in and between urban areas not only in terms of public and private modes of transport but also air and noise pollution, consumption of non-renewable resources, monetary costs and public investments, active and sedentary lifestyles, as well as health and well-being. This broader perspective not only raises questions about the high priority attributed to private motor cars during the 20th century. It also shows that investments in efficient public transport systems and pedestrian precincts can be considered as investments to promote environmental quality, reduce energy consumption and air pollution while also promoting health and well-being.

During the last two decades, governments in many countries introduced policies to reduce public spending, repay debts and apply "new public management" principles to make public authorities more effective. Consequently, many municipal authorities have reduced expenditure on housing and urban infrastructure and cut allowances for welfare, health, and community care even thought there has been an increasing number of citizens who rely on social support (OECD, 1986). These trends ought to be questioned because the primary purpose of these kinds of public services is to improve health by preventive or curative measures. A health system should not only strive to attain the highest average level of the health status of the population, but also simultaneously strive to reduce the differences between the health of individuals and groups (World Health Organization, 2000a). Therefore, the way that health systems are designed, managed and financed does effect peoples lives, can contribute to or reduce inequalities in health, and also influence how the situation of the underprivileged can be improved. All groups of the population, especially the underprivileged, need protection against health risks (Marmot and Wilkinson, 1999).

2. *Intersectoral collaboration between scientists, professionals, policy-decision makers and representatives of community groups.* This is a more effective way to deal with the complexity and diversity of urban health than traditional sectoral approaches. According to the World Health Organization intersectoral action is necessary to deal with complex health and environmental problems. Intersectoral action can be defined as a recognized relationship between part or parts of the health sector with part or parts of another sector which has been formed to take action on an issue to achieve health outcomes (or intermediate health outcomes) in a way that is more effective, efficient or sustainable than could be achieved by the health sector acting alone: "Intersectoral action is needed to address the driving forces (for example of economic development) which ultimately influence health and environmental conditions (through policy development and implementation), the pressures placed on the environment (for example through adequate housing and service provision, cleaner production methods and emissions reduction), the state (quality) of the environment (through pollution control devices for example), human exposures (through legislation, behavior modification, personal protection), and the resultant health effects (through medical care of those who become ill)" (World Health Organization, 1997b).

Intersectoral action should occur at each administrative level ranging from the local city level, to the national level as well as trans-national, regional and international levels. Consequently, co-ordinated strategies and plans at each level need to be developed in order to apply systemic approaches to deal with complex, multidimensional problems. In order to be effective the roles and responsibilities of actors in each sector need to be clearly defined.

3. *A shared definition of goals, priorities and resources allocation in order to achieve desired outcomes.* Partnerships involving the private and public sectors as well as community associations are advocated as a means to define goals, order priorities and allocate resources in cities which can be characterized by populations with increasingly diverse sets of values. The word partnership has been used to refer to either formal or informal collaboration using alliances, or networks that are meant to provide synergy to reach shared goals. The general goal of partnerships in the health sector is to provide better results in the treatment of illness as well as health prevention and promotion.

Partnerships should be formed not just within but also beyond the health sector. Intersectoral partnerships are a key component of the WHO Healthy Cities project (Tsouros and Farrington, 2003). Partnerships enable the duplication of roles and responsibilities to be identified and eliminated, they can promote better co-ordination, and they can clarify whether lack of consensus can be resolved by conflict negotiation.

4. *Systematic monitoring and feedback in order to develop a coordinated database and information about the specific characteristics of cities including the health and well-being of the population.* Evidence on the determinants of health of urban populations increased during the 1990s especially in relation to the ambient environmental conditions and the socio-economic inequalities of people living in urban areas. There is sufficient evidence from statistics and field studies to show that a narrow focus on the individual determinants of health cannot deal effectively with the social and economic determinants of health status in urban neighborhoods. A geographical and community based approach is essential if the health if people in urban areas is to be dealt with in terms of inequalities and equity (Curtis, 2004). Fortunately, the WHO Healthy Cities Project has provided a set of indicators to monitor determinants of health and health (Sanderson and Webster, 2003). Nonetheless, too little attention has been given to assessing the effectiveness of interventions to change these determinants in specific localities and monitor the outcomes on health. If these evaluations are not available, then policy decision making is handicapped. More research is required to evaluate different kinds of interventions that improve the built environment in urban areas in order to identify impacts on health and well-being by the collection of time series data.

Today, policy makers in most countries still have great difficulty in measuring, describing, and explaining constancy, change and differences in health, housing, and environmental conditions in cities. Part of the difficulty has been the lack of systematic data collection. A dynamic set covering several sectors is required across a range of administrative levels and geographical scales. Alone, official statistics based on national census returns do not provide comprehensive accounts of the quantity and quality of the housing stock, urban infrastructure and services in rapidly developing urban areas and they ignore illegal buildings in informal settlements. Today, there are several kinds of innovative techniques and tools that can be used to monitor and analyze the spatial distribution, dynamics and interrelated nature of environmental, housing, demographic and health profiles in urban areas (World

Health Organization, 1996). For example, several types of remote sensing and data analysis were used to identify and monitor human settlements, animal and vector habitats, and natural resources including forests, water catchment areas and rivers. The propagation of vector-borne diseases and their transfer between rural and urban areas can be monitored using remote sensing methods which can be used as an early warning system to identify environmental health hazards and the assessment of disasters (such as flooding, landslides or earthquakes). Early warnings enable the timely, safe and environmentally sound use of interventions to reduce injury, death or the spread of infectious diseases. For example, the Rotterdam Local Health Information System, which has its origins in the WHO Healthy Cities project, is an extremely useful database that enables professionals and policy decision makers to monitor living conditions and health status in urban neighbourhoods (Swart, *et al.*, 2002).

5.0. A NEW AGENDA FOR RESEARCHERS, PRACTITIONERS, AND POLICY MAKERS

The eleven principles about building healthy cities in specific localities need to be understood and applied using innovative empirical research and professional practice. This stems from the fact that many contributions that are meant to address health promotion and prevention have not been wholly successful, even though many urban planners, public health officers and medical practitioners are convinced they have the "right answers". There is an urgent need for innovative approaches in many situations, such as the blatant failure of the wealthiest countries of the world to provide all citizens with secure employment, affordable housing and appropriate health care that meet at least minimal requirements. The failure of so-called "model" housing estates and urban planning projects constructed in the 1960s and 1970s in numerous cities around the World clearly shows that new ideas, working methods, objectives and criteria are needed (Lawrence, 1993).

Our incapacity to deal with the above-mentioned problems is related to the complexity of dealing with urban health, to the compartmentalization of scientific and professional knowledge about urban ecosystems, to the bureaucratic division of responsibilities in cities, and to the increasing diversity of living conditions between various cities and within specific cities. In addition, the lack of effective collaboration between scientists, professionals and policy decision-makers has led to the "applicability gap" in sectors that deal with urban planning, public health and many other sectors concerned with the construction and maintenance of cities. These shortcomings of mainstream scientific research and professional practice are not necessarily the result of the lack of political commitment, or financial resources, or viable propositions. They are, above all, the logical outcome of the narrow vision of so-called experts who do not address fundamental issues but only topics isolated from their urban context. In order to deal with these limitations, at least three sets of obstacles need to be overcome. First, conceptual frameworks that do not recognize the pertinence of an ecological interpretation of urban health and living conditions; second, methodological contributions that value rational, quantified interpretations of illness and disease at the expense of qualitative interpretations of health and well-being, use and management of human and natural ecosystems, and third, the segmentation and bureaucratization of professional knowledge and expertise often at the expense of the experience of lay-people.

The health status of populations in specific urban areas is not only the result of many material and immaterial constituents but also the relationships between them. Hence, several concepts and methods need to be examined to understand the constituents and the relationships between them. For example, a constituent should not be isolated from the context in which it occurs. Instead, ecological approaches ought to be applied to understand both the constituents and the relationships between them (Lawrence, 2001).

The distinction between biomedical models and ecological interpretations of health is fundamental for urban health (Lawrence, 1999). The germ theory, for example, is an incomplete explanation of human illness and disease because it ignores the contribution of numerous physical and social dimensions of the environment that can affect health. Ecological interpretations maintain that the presence of a germ is a necessary but not a sufficient condition for an individual to become ill. They accept that some individuals become more susceptible to certain illnesses because of their differential exposure to numerous environmental, economic and social factors that can promote or be harmful to health and well-being. This interpretation does not ignore the influence of genetics, individual behavior or primary health care. However, it maintains that, alone, these do not address possible relations between social problems and illness (e.g. inequalities) or positive social dimensions and health promotion (e.g. public education). The distinction between potential and actual health status can be the foundation for a new interpretation of urban health which includes the way ecological, economic, social, political and psychological factors transgress traditional disciplinary boundaries in order to address specific issues that may only be pertinent in precise situations.

Today it is necessary to carefully reconsider the relationships between the social, economic and health inequalities (and other kinds of problems) in urban agglomerations. The interrelations between housing, urban planning, health, social and environmental policies have been poorly articulated until now (World Health Organization, 1997b; 2000c; 2000d). However, it is crucial to acknowledge the important role of cities as localities for the management of resources, as places for accommodating diverse ways of life and as forums for inventions of all kinds. Although housing and land use policies have rarely been a high priority in the manifestos of governments, or political parties, these trends imply that health, social, housing and urban policies should become important components of domestic agendas in order to promote social cohesion and the quality of life in cities and towns. This is an important challenge for both current and future generations.

6.0. CONCLUSION

The biological, environmental, economic, and other social determinants of the health of citizens have become an increasingly important priority for scientists, professionals, and policy makers during the last two decades (Lawrence, 1999). Urban health has been integrated into public health by a limited number of professionals (Marmot and Wilkinson, 1999; McMichael, 1993; Murray and Lopez, 1996). During the 1990s, a decade of rapid economic, technological and political change, it was increasingly recognized that other factors including industrial-agricultural food products, global climate change, and globalization are also important determinants of health of urban populations (World Bank 2000; 2001). Recent trends provide new opportunities and challenges for improving the health of citizens in the 21st century by applying a broad ecological perspective (Lawrence, 2001).

History shows that human health and quality of urban life are closely related to the sustenance or decline of urban and natural ecosystems. Health and these types of ecosystems are multidimensional. Hence these subjects are not structured within traditional disciplinary and professional boundaries. Therefore, urban health ought to be considered in terms of the multiple factors that influence humans and their living conditions as well as the interrelations between them (Lawrence 1999). An ecological perspective recognizes that behavioral, biological, cultural, economic, social, physical and political factors need to be considered in order to provide a comprehensive understanding of urban health.

Today, many cities are confronted with serious environmental, economic and social problems -high unemployment, social and spatial segregation, social exclusion, economic instability, crime, the general quality of life, negative impacts on health and pressures on natural and historic assets. In addition, cities are handling wider global and societal changes due to the globalization of the economy and financial exchange, changes in household demographics and family structure, and new technological innovations.

Healthy living environments have been a goal or a societal objective since the dawn of urban civilizations between 8000 and 9000 years ago. Some cities and towns have existed for thousands of years, whereas others were founded, grew, then declined and were abandoned. Both the sustainability of cities and towns and the health and quality of life of citizens should not be taken for granted. The WHO Healthy Cities project does promote understanding and provide examples of good practice for the building of healthier cities and towns.

ACKNOWLEDGEMENTS: The author of this chapter was appointed Chair of the Evaluation Advisory Committee of the Healthy Cities project in the WHO European region for the third phase of this project from 1999 to 2003. The content of this chapter is a personal statement that does not represent the official point of view of the World Health Organization or other institutions quoted or referenced in the text. The author wishes to thank Sandro Galea and David Vlahov for the invitation to contribute to this Handbook, and for their advice and constructive comments during the preparation of this manuscript.

REFERENCES

Bairoch, P. (1988). *Cities and Economic Development: From the dawn of history to the present.* Mansell, London.

Barton, H., and Tsourou, C. (2000). *Healthy Urban Planning.* E & FN Spon, London.

Boyden, S. (1987). *Western Civilisation in Biological Perspective: Patterns in biohistory.* Oxford University Press, Oxford.

Burridge, R., and Ormandy, D. (eds.). (1993). *Unhealthy Housing: Research, remedy and reform.* E & FN Spon, London.

Castells, M. (1991). *Informational City: Economic restructuring and urban development.* Blackwell Publishing, Oxford.

Chavis, D., and Wandersman, A. (1990). Sense of community in the urban environment: A catalyst for participation and community development. *Am. J. Comm. Psychol.* 18(1):55–81.

Curtis, S. (2004). *Health and Inequality: Geographical Perspectives.* Sage Publications, London.

Dahlgren, G., and Whitehead, M. (1992). *Policies and strategies to promote equity in health.* World Health Organization Regional Office for Europe, Copenhagen.

Dubé, P. (2000). Urban health: An urban planning perspective. *Reviews on Environmental Health* 15(1-2): 249–265.

Duffy, H. (1995). *Competitive Cities: Succeeding in a global economy.* E & FN Spon, London.

Ekblad, S. (1993). Stressful environments and their effects on quality of life in Third World cities. *Environ. Urban.* 5(2):25–134.

Eklund, L. (1999). *From Citizen Participation Towards Community Empowerment.* University of Tampere, (Doctoral dissertation) Tampere.

Fuchs, R., Brennan, E., Chamie, J., Lo Fu-Chen, and Juha U. (eds) (1994). *Mega-City Growth and The Future, Second Edition.* United Nations University Press, Tokyo.

Fuller-Thomson, E., Hulchanski, D., and Wang, S. (2000). The health-housing relationship. What do we know? *Reviews on Environmental Health* 15(1-2):109–134.

Gabe, J., and Williams, P. (1993). Women, crowding and mental health. In: Burridge, R., and Ormandy, D. (eds.), *Unhealthy housing: Research, remedy and reform.* E & FN Spon, London, pp. 191–208.

Galea, S., and Vlahov, D. (2005). Urban Health: Evidence, Challenges, and Directions. *Ann. Rev. Public Health* 26:341–365.

Gibbons, M., Limoges, C., Nowotny, H., Schwartzman, S., Scott, P., and Trow, M. (1994). *The New Production of Knowledge.* Sage, London.

Girardet, H. (1999). *Creating Sustainable Cities. Schumacher Briefings No.2.* Green Books, Dartington UK.

Goldstein, G. (2000). Healthy cities: Overview of a WHO international program. *Rev. Environ Health* 15(1-2):207–214.

Gray, A. (2001). Definitions of crowding and the effects of crowding on health: A literature review. The Ministry of Social Policy, Research Series Report 1. Wellington, New Zealand.

Green, G. (1998). Health and Governance in European Cities: A compendium of trends and responsibilities for public health in 46 member states of the WHO European Region. European Hospital Management Journal Limited, London.

Green G., Acres, F., and Price, C. (2003). City health development planning. In: Tsouros, A., and Farrington, J. (eds.). *WHO Healthy Cities in Europe: A compilation of papers on progress and achievements.* World Health Organization European Office for Europe, Copenhagen, pp. 103–133.

Hancock, T., and Duhl, L. (1988). *Promoting Health in the Urban Context.* FADL Publishers, Copenhagen.

Halpern, D. (1995). *Mental Health and the Built Environment.* Taylor and Francis, London.

Hardoy, J., Mitlin, D., and Satterthwaite, D. (2001). *Environmental Problems in an Urbanizing World.* Earthscan, London.

Harpham, T. (1994). Urbanization and mental health in developing countries: A research role for social scientists, public health professionals and social psychiatrists. *Soc. Sci. Med.* 39(2):233–245.

Kenworthy, J. (2000). Building more liveable cities by overcoming automobile dependence: An international comparative review. In: Lawrence, R. (ed.), *Sustaining Human Settlement: A challenge for the new millennium.* Urban International Press, Newcastle-upon-Tyne UK, pp. 271–314.

Landon, M. (1996). Intra-urban health differentials in London – urban health indicators and policy implications. *Environ. Urban* 8(2):119–128.

Laughlin, C., and Brady, I. (eds.). (1978). *Extinction and survival in human populations.* Columbia University Press, New York.

Lawrence, R. (1993). An ecological blueprint for healthy housing. In: Burridge, R., and Ormandy, D. (eds.), *Unhealthy housing: Research, remedy and reform.* E & FN Spon, London, pp. 338–360.

Lawrence, R. (1995). Meeting the challenge: Barriers to integrate cross-sectoral urban policies. In: Rolén, M. (ed.), *Urban Policies for an Environmentally Sustainable World.* The OECD-Sweden seminar on the ecological city, 1–3 June 1994. Swedish Council for Planning and Co-ordination of Research, Stockholm, pp.9–37.

Lawrence, R. (1996). Urban environment, health and the economy: Cues for conceptual clarification and more effective policy implementation. In: Price, C., and Tsouros, A. (eds.), *Our Cities, Our Future: Policies and action plans for health and sustainable development.* World Health Organization European Office for Europe, Copenhagen, pp. 38–64.

Lawrence, R. (1999). Urban health: An ecological perspective. *Rev. Environ. Health* 14(1):1–10.

Lawrence, R. (ed.). (2000a). *Sustaining Human Settlement: A challenge for the new millennium.* Urban International Press, Newcastle-upon-Tyne, UK.

Lawrence, R. (ed.). (2000b). Urban health: A new research agenda? *Rev. Environ. Health* 15(editorial, special issue):1–11.

Lawrence, R. (2001). Human Ecology. In: Tolba, M.K., (ed.). *Our Fragile World: Challenges and Opportunities for Sustainable Development, Volume 1.* Eolss Publishers, Oxford, pp. 675–693.

Lawrence, R. (2002). Inequalities in urban areas: innovative approaches to complex issues. *Scand. J. Public Health* 59(Suppl):34–40.

Lee, K. (1999). Globalisation and the need for strong public health response. *Eur. J. Public Health* 9(4):249–250.

Lo, Fu-chen, and Yeung, Yue-man (eds.). (1998). *Globalization and the World of Large Cities.* United Nations University Press, Tokyo.

Ludermir, A., and Harpham, T. (1998). Urbanization and mental health in Brazil: Social and economic dimensions. *Health Place* 4(3):223–232.

Manciaux, M., and Romer, C. (1986). Accidents in children, adolescents and young adults: A major public health problem. *World Health Statistics Quarterly* 39(3):227–231.

Marans, R., and Stokols, D. (eds.). (1993). *Environmental Simulation: Research and policy issues.* Plenum Press, New York.

Marmot, M., and Wilkinson, R., (eds.). (1999). *Social Determinants of Health.* Oxford University Press, Oxford.

McMichael, A. (1993). *Planetary overload: Global environmental change and the health of the human species.* Cambridge University Press, Cambridge.

McMichael, A. (2000). The urban environment and health in a world of increasing globalization: Issues for developing countries. *Bulletin of World Health Organization* 78(9): 1117–1126.

Mitchell, J. (ed.). (1999). *Crucibles of hazards: Mega-cities and disasters in transition.* United Nations University Press, Tokyo.

Murray, C., and Lopez, A. (eds.). (1996). *The Global Burden of Disease: A comprehensive assessment of mortality and disability from diseases, injuries and risk factors in 1990 and projected to 2020.* Harvard University Press, Cambridge, MA.

Organization for Economic Co-operation and Development, (OECD). (1986). Strategies for housing and social integration in cities. Organization for Economic Co-operation and Development, Paris.

Parry-Jones, W., and Quelquoz, N. (eds.). (1991). Mental health and deviance in inner cities. Report no. WHO/MNH/PSF/91.1 World Health Organization, Geneva.

Pederson, R., Robertson, A., and de Zeeuw, H. (2000). Food, health and the urban environment. *Rev. Envir. Health* 15(1-2): 231–247.

Rosen, G. (1993). *A History of Public Health.* John Hopkins University Press, Baltimore.

Rossi-Espagnet, A., Goldstein, G., and Tabibzadeh, I. (1991) Urbanization and health in developing countries: A challenge for health for all. *World Health Statistics Quarterly* 44(4): 186-247.

Sanderson, D., and Webster, P. (2003). Healthy City Indicators. In: Tsouros, A., and Farrington, J. (eds.), WHO Healthy Cities in Europe: A compilation of papers on progress and achievements. World Health Organization European Office for Europe, Copenhagen, pp.63–87.

Satterthwaite, D. (1993) The impact on health of urban environments. *Environ. Urban.* 5(2): pp. 87–111.

Schwela, D. (2000) Air pollution and health in urban areas. *Rev Envir Health* 15(1-2):13–42.

Swart, W., Bleeker, J., and de Haes, W. (2002). The Rotterdam Local health Information System 1987-2000: from Rebus and the health barometer to the health monitor. *Scand. J. Public Health* Supplement 59:63–71.

Townsend, P., Davidson, N., and Whitehead, M. (1992). *Inequalities in Health, Second edition.* Penguin, London

Tsouros, A. (1990). *WHO Healthy Cities Project: A project becomes a movement.* FADL Publishers, Copenhagen.

Tsouros, A., and Farrington, J. (eds.). (2003). WHO Healthy Cities in Europe: A compilation of papers on progress and achievements. World Health Organization European Office for Europe, Copenhagen.

United Nations Commission on Human Settlements, (UNCHS). (1996). An Urbanizing World: Global report on human settlements 1996. Oxford University Press, Oxford.

United Nations. (1992). Agenda 21: Programme of Action for Sustainable Development. United Nations Publications, New York.

United Nations Commission on Human Settlements, (UNCHS). (1998). Crowding and Health in Low-income Settlements. United Nations Commission on Human Settlements (UNCHS-Habitat), Nairobi.

United Nations Commission on Human Settlements, (UNCHS) (2001). The State of the World's Cities, Report no. HS/619/01[E]. United Nations Commission on Human Settlements (UNCHS Habitat), Nairobi.

Vlahov, D., and Galea, S. (2002) Urbanization, urbanicity, and health. *J. Urban Health* 79(4 Suppl 1):S1–S12.

Wackernagel, M., and Rees, W. (1996). *Our Ecological Footprint: Reducing human impact on earth.* New Society Publishers, Gabriola Island Canada.

Wallerstein, N. (1992). Powerlessness, empowerment, and health: implications for heath promotion programs. *American Journal of Health Promotion* 6:197–205.

Wallerstein, N., and Bernstein, E. (1994). Introduction to community empowerment, participatory education, and health. *Health Ed. Q.* 21(2):141–148.

Webster, P. (2003). Healthy City Profiles. In: Tsouros, A., and Farrington, J. (eds.), WHO Healthy Cities in Europe: A compilation of papers on progress and achievements. World Health Organization European Office for Europe, Copenhagen, pp. 88–102.

Werna, E., Harpham, T., and Goldstein, G. (1998). *Healthy City Projects in Developing Countries: An international approach to local problems.* Earthscan, London.

Werna, E., Harpham, T., Blue, I., and Goldstein, G. (1999). From healthy city projects to healthy cities. *Envir. Urban.* 11(1):27–39.

Wilkinson, R. (1996). *Unhealthy Societies: The afflictions of inequality.* Routledge, London.

World Bank. (2000). *Entering the 21st century: World Development Report 1999/2000.* Oxford University Press, New York.

World Bank. (2001). *Attacking Poverty: World Development Report 2000/2001.* Oxford University Press, New York.

World Health Organization. (1990). Indoor Environment: Health aspects of air quality, thermal environment, light and noise, Report no. WHO/EHE/RUD/90.2. World Health Organization, Geneva.

World Health Organization. (1992). Our Planet, Our Health: Report of the WHO Commission on Health and Environment. World Health Organization, Geneva.

World Health Organization. (1995). Health in Social Development: WHO Position paper, Report no. WHO/DGH/95.1. World Health Organization, Geneva.

World Health Organization. (1996). The Concept of Health and Environment Geographic Information Systems (HEGIS) for Europe and Requirements for Indicators. Report on a WHO Consultation at Bilthoven, Netherlands, 8-9 November 1994, EUR/HFA target 19. World Health Organization Regional Office for Europe, Copenhagen.

World Health Organization. (1997a). Health and Environment in Sustainable Development: Five years after the Earth Summit, Report no. WHO/EHG/97.8. World Health Organization, Geneva.

World Health Organization. (1997b). *Intersectoral Action for Health: Addressing health and environment concerns in sustainable development.* World Health Organization, Geneva.

World Health Organization. (1997c). City Planning for Health and Sustainable Development, Report no. EUR/ICP/POLC 06 03 05B. World Health Organization Regional office for Europe, Copenhagen.

World Health Organization. (2000a). *The World Health Report 2000: Health Systems: Improving Performance.* World Health Organization, Geneva.

World Health Organization. (2000b). Nutrition for Health and Development, Report no. WHO/NHD/00.6. World Health Organization, Geneva.

World Health Organization. (2000c). Healthy Cities in Action: 5 case-studies from Africa, Asia, Middle East and Latin America, Report no. WHO/SDE/PHE/00.02 World Health Organization, Geneva.

World Health Organization. (2000d). Transport, Environment and Health. World Health Organization European Office WHO Publications, European Series No 89, World Health organization, Europe, Copenhagen.

World Health Organization. (2001). *The World Health Report 2001: Mental Health: New Understanding, New Hope.* World Health Organization, Geneva.

World Health Organization and UNICEF. (2000). Global Water Supply and Sanitation Assessment 2000 Report. World Health Organization and UNICEF, New York.

World Health Organization. (2002). Community Participation in Local Health and Sustainable Development: Approaches and techniques, European Sustainable Development and Health Series no 4. World Health Organization European Office WHO Publications, Copenhagen.

Chapter 25

Building Healthy Cities

Legal Frameworks and Considerations

Wendy C. Perdue

1.0. INTRODUCTION

The physical and social structure of cities is shaped by many factors. These include economic and political conditions, historical and cultural traditions, and weather and topography. However, cities are also importantly shaped by law and government policies and this is true even in cities that seem to be dominated by private property and private enterprises.

Law impacts cities both by what the government regulates and by what it chooses not to regulate. Any decision that a matter should be governed by private choices rather than government regulation is itself a policy choice that can have significant implications on the welfare of residents. For example, the willingness of U.S. courts prior to 1948 to enforce private covenants calling for racial exclusion had important impacts on housing patterns in the U.S. Moreover, many private decisions that seem to be matters solely of private preference may in fact be affected by government intervention. This is particularly true with respect to the built environment. Decisions by private entities about what and where to build are shaped by legal requirements and prohibitions as well as by government created incentives, and the presence or absence of public infrastructure – including roads, transportation networks, parks, and government facilities.

This chapter will explore the range of laws and government policies that have shaped the physical structure of U.S. cities and thereby impacted the health of those cities' residents. This analysis will highlight the many, apparently "private" decisions that have been impacted by government policies. Though some of the laws, policies, prohibitions, and incentives have been formulated explicitly to take into account health considerations, others have unintended effects – both good and bad – on the health of urban populations. Although the chapter focuses on U.S. laws, cities throughout the world are shaped by law and government policy. In some places, it is the absence of regulatory intervention that most dramatically impacts health, as in the case of squalid shanty towns or poorly designed buildings that collapse in the face of earthquakes or high winds. In other places, cities may be the product of very extensive government intervention (Cervero, 1998). Regardless of the intended purpose of laws and policies, any effort to understand or improve the health of urban populations must consider the critical role played by law and government policy.

2.0. THE CONNECTION BETWEEN THE BUILT ENVIRONMENT AND HEALTH

The connection between the built environment and public health became painfully apparent and widely recognized during the industrial revolution of the 19th century. The burgeoning cities were crowded, dirty, unsanitary places. Poor residents lived in tenements with little or no light, ventilation, or sanitation facilities, and frequently located close to noxious industrial uses. Epidemics of infectious disease were all too common. Sanitarians and progressive reformers understood the connection between disease and the physical environment and sought to change that environment (Peterson, 1983; Garb, 2003). Cities were rebuilt with sewers and water systems; tenement housing was improved; parks and recreation spaces were created. All of these physical changes were understood to be important steps in improving public health.

Today, the built environment of our urban centers continues to affect public health, though the primary health concerns have shifted from infectious disease to chronic disease, injuries, and crime. Heart disease, asthma, and diabetes are among the leading causes of death and premature disability in the U.S. (National Center for Health Statistics, 2002). These conditions are affected by a sedentary life style, diet, and poor air quality (National Center for Chronic Disease Prevention, 2003) – all factors that are in turn linked with the built environment. For example, with respect to sedentary life-style, there is a growing body of evidence that links physical activity with the structure of our environment and how easy or hard it is to integrate active living into daily life (Frank, *et al.*, 2003; Frumkin, *et al.*, 2004). Diet is also affected by logistical factors such as a lack of access to stores or farmers markets carrying healthy food options (Morland, *et al.*, 2002) and an ease of access to "fast food" or less healthy food options. Outdoor air quality is linked to roads and transportation systems (Frumkin, *et al.*, 2004); internal air quality is linked with how buildings are built including ventilation and materials used (Samet and Spengler, 2003; National Inst. For Occ. Safety and Health, 1991).

Injuries are also affected by the built environment. Road and sidewalk design affect automobile and pedestrian injuries (Ohland, *et al.*, 2000; Ernst and McCann, 2002). Building design affects injuries from fires and falls (Krieger and Higgins, 2002). Even crime is affected by the built environment. Lighting, visibility, layout, and design can all reduce the incidence of criminal activity and there is a growing interest among architects, planners, and law enforcement in environmental design as a tool in crime prevention (Katyal, 2002; Newman, 1972; Mair and Mair, 2003; Carter, *et al.*, 2003).

As this brief summary highlights, there are important connections between public health and how we build our cities. There are a variety of factors that shape the physical structures of our urban areas including weather, topography and economic conditions. However, a critical influence on the built environment is law and related government policy. The remainder of this chapter focuses on the role that law and government policy plays in shaping our cities.

3.0. THE BASIC LEGAL TOOLS

The laws and policies that determine the physical structure of our cities fall into three basic categories: direct regulation of private parties, economic incentives or subsidies for private parties, and government provisions of facilities or services. These categories are not unique to urban issues, but represent three basic techniques for implementing government policies.

These three different approaches can be illustrated with a simple example. Consider, for example, the public health problem of smoking. One approach is to regulate smoking directly, by prohibiting smoking in particular places and by particular people, i.e., children. A second approach is to provide economic incentives either for individuals to encourage them not to smoke, for example, by raising the price of cigarettes through taxes, or for businesses to encourage them to ban smoking or to offer smoking cessation programs. The third approach is for government itself to provide smoking cessation programs, public information about the harms of smoking, and to ban smoking in government buildings and facilities. These legal techniques vary in their infringement upon individual autonomy and may also vary with respect to cost and effectiveness, but all three are used in connection with urban policy. Each of these approaches is explored below.

The first technique is direct regulation in which government requires or prohibits specific conduct. Direct regulation can be enforced through either criminal or civil sanctions. Direct regulation of private entities is ubiquitous and has a significant role in shaping our urban areas. Zoning and land use regulations prohibit some uses in certain areas. These laws may also require buildings to meet a variety of physical constraints including height, set back and parking requirements. Other types of direct regulations include building code restrictions meant to assure safe buildings, and environmental regulations, which may prohibit the use of certain toxic materials, and require appropriate handling of potential environmental impacts such as storm water run-off.

The second technique – economic incentives and subsidies – is sometimes less obvious but also important in shaping our urban centers. Governments frequently offer tax incentives to encourage investment in housing, or to attract businesses. Such incentives can be an important vehicle for encouraging the private market to build what is needed where it is needed. The tax deduction for home mortgages and tax credits for the construction of low income housing are two examples. In addition, cities may offer a variety of economic incentives in order to attract particular businesses or to encourage redevelopment of particular areas. These incentive programs can also have unintended consequences that can shape urban areas in undesirable ways. For example, the Federal Housing Authority (FHA), which was created in 1934, offered incentives to encourage home construction and renovation, but its rules favored socially homogeneous suburban housing developments and discouraged investment in existing urban neighborhoods, thereby contributing to urban deterioration (Farrell, 2002).

Finally, government is a major direct participant in the building of our urban centers. Most obvious are the roads and transportation networks that provide the skeleton on which our cities grow and are a defining characteristic of each urban area. In addition, other governmental infrastructure such as schools, parks, libraries, and recreation facilities, along with other governmental buildings are important determinants of the character and health of urban areas.

All three of these techniques of government intervention affect the nature and form of our urban areas and reflect fundamental policy choices. These choices may be made taking public health into account, or may be driven primarily by other factors. In an early era, for example, the introduction of public water and sewer systems were major public infrastructure projects undertaken explicitly to improve public health (Peterson, 1983). Parks as well have been understood to have important public health benefits (Peterson, 1983). Today, government intervention through transportation systems or business incentives is intended primarily to promote of economic development. This intervention nonetheless may have important impacts on health. The location and design of roads and transit can affect vehicle miles traveled and the attendant air pollution problems, along with levels of walking and biking, and the numbers of injuries from collisions. Decisions about where businesses and buildings can locate, and what to prohibit or require, encourage or discourage can similarly affect health. Whatever their motivations or articulated goals, government choices about whether and how to intervene in decisions that shape the physical structure of our cities are likely to have important impacts on the health and welfare of the people who inhabit our cities.

4.0. AREAS OF LAW THAT SHAPE OUR CITIES

The forms or techniques of legal intervention described above are not unique to cities or the built environment. However, these techniques are reflected in numerous laws and government policies that affect the built environment and physical shape of our urban centers. The following section explores the specific areas of law that are most significant in shaping our cities. In many of these areas, the relevant laws are promulgated at the state or local level and there are significant variations around the country. Therefore, these areas are described generally by category.

4.1. Zoning and Land Use Laws

In most places, building and development is governed by an array of zoning and land use laws. These laws are generally promulgated locally—at the city or county level—though usually under the authority of state enabling legislation. They are frequently shaped by a process of land use planning intended to lay out an overall plan and vision for the development of the community (Frielich, 1999).

The stated goal of zoning and other land use regulations is to promote "health, safety, morals, or the general welfare of the community" (Standard State Zoning Enabling Act § 1), though some have suggested that many zoning ordinances may have been designed with a priority placed on economic interests than on health (Rodgers, 1998). Traditional zoning ordinances seek to achieve this by dividing the land into different use categories, e.g., residential, commercial, industrial, on the theory that it is better for public health, welfare, and aesthetics to separate these uses. For each category of use, an ordinance usually specifies intensity of use along with other criteria such as minimum lot size, maximum building height and set back requirements. Further development standards may impose additional requirements such as a minimum number of parking spaces; open space, recreation facilities, or public amenity requirements; or requirements to dedicate or build roads or sidewalks (Juergensmeyer and Roberts, 2003). Though most zoning and land use codes are framed in terms of mandates and prohibitions, they may also include incentives as well. For example, codes may allow developers to build more dense projects if the projects include particular desired elements (e.g., affordable housing or a needed grocery store).

Zoning and land use laws impact health in several ways. First, a sedentary lifestyle is one of the most significant controllable risk factors for chronic disease (Frumkin, *et al.*, 2004), and there is a growing body of evidence that levels of physical activity are affected by the design of communities in which people live and work (Ewing, *et al.*, 2003; Frank, *et al.*, 2003; Frumkin, *et al.*, 2004). Neighborhood design characteristics that appear to affect levels of physical activity include how compact development is, whether there is a mix of uses and destinations within an easy walk (King, *et al.*, 2003; Powell, *et al.*, 2003), the pattern of streets, and whether there are sidewalks, bike paths and amenities for walkers and bikers (Frank, *et al.*, 2003; Saelens, *et al.*, 2003).

Unfortunately, the standard approach to zoning is to strictly separate uses, making it less likely that there will be destinations within an easy walk of one's home or business. In addition to separating uses, development standards may require building separations, set backs and parking standards that effectively mandate "strip mall" style developments that are easily accessible to the automobile and quite unconducive to pedestrian activity. Indeed, one study of Illinois municipal zoning codes found that most of those codes impeded rather than facilitated compact, walkable communities (Knapp, *et al.*, 2001). In response to these concerns, some cities have begun revising their zoning codes to encourage mixed-use, compact, and walkable communities (Langdon, 2003a), and the American Planning Association has released a compilation of model provisions for those interested in such revisions (Meck, 2002).

Second, physical layout and design can either facilitate or discourage crime. Careful design can decrease dark and hidden spaces, increase "eyes on the street" (Jacobs, 1961), and affect social norms and a sense of community, all of which can reduce the incidence of at least some crimes. (Katyal, 2002) Zoning law requirements concerning set backs and parking, along with limitations on uses, may make it easier or harder to develop buildings and spaces that discourage crime. Moreover, some zoning or building requirements can discourage redevelopment of older deteriorating neighborhoods and hence contribute to conditions that encourage crime in those neighborhoods (Carter, *et al.*, 2003).

Finally, zoning and land use laws may play a role in diet (Pothukuchi and Kaufman, 2000). In some urban areas, residents have limited access to fruits, vegetables and healthy food alternatives (Sloane, 2004), and this lack of access may correlate with less healthy eating patterns (Morland, *et al.*, 2002; Reidpath, *et al.*, 2002). Zoning or other regulatory obstacles including the requirement to provide vast amounts of parking even in relatively urban settings can make it difficult to develop supermarkets in some areas. More flexible land use rules may also facilitate farmers' markets or community gardens (Schukoske, 1999). On the flip side, zoning and land use laws affect the location and concentration of fast food restaurants (Ashe, *et al.*, 2003).

4.2. Building Codes and Other Regulation of Structures

One of the innovations of the early 20th century progressive movement was the effort to improve safety and sanitation in tenement housing. The landmark 1901 Tenement House Act for the City of New York laid the foundation for subsequent housing and building codes intended to assure that buildings are safe and sanitary.

Further impetus came with the Federal Housing Act of 1954, which required local governments to develop housing and building codes in order to qualify for federal housing and urban renewal programs.

The majority of building codes are adopted as state legislation, though local variations may be permitted, and most are based on model codes developed by private organizations of professionals such as the International Code Council and the National Fire Protection Association. These codes address structural issues along with electrical wiring, plumbing, fire safety, heating, air conditioning and ventilation. Housing codes may specify minimum living area and require that bedrooms have windows or an escape route to the outside. Building codes are nearly always framed as mandates or prohibitions, and, as a result, their effectiveness may depend on the effectiveness of enforcement (Brown, *et al.*, 2001).

These building and housing codes affect public health in several ways. Injuries are the leading cause of death in children ages 1 to 21. Smoke detectors, sprinklers, and safety requirements for electrical and gas systems can reduce fire injuries. Structural requirements can prevent building collapse. Design standards for stairs, railings and window barriers can prevent falls. Adequate ventilation may prevent build up of toxic or combustible compounds. Adequate sanitation may reduce cockroach infestations, a risk factor for asthma (Cummins and Jackson, 2001). On the other hand, codes that are too restrictive can have unintended and undesirable consequences. For example, it can be difficult to retrofit existing buildings to achieve compliance with building codes focused on new construction. This may discourage redevelopment of existing underused buildings which may, in turn, accelerate a decline of older urban neighborhoods and encourage suburban sprawl (McMahon, 2001b). Likewise housing code requirements that go beyond the minimum necessary to assure safety can discourage innovation that could lower housing costs or permit construction of smaller, more affordable units (Kelly, 1996).

4.3. Housing Policy

Adequate housing is one of the most basic human needs and since at least the 1930's, government has been actively involved in encouraging the creation of more housing. The largest government housing programs take the form of economic incentives that encourage housing construction and purchase, but these programs also include direct government provision of housing as well as the use of mandates.

Today, the largest subsidy of housing is through the federal tax system. The total subsidy from deductibility of mortgage interest and real estate taxes, and the exemption from capital gains tax of profits on home sales is estimated to be $100 billion per year (Cunningham, 2003). In addition to these programs that target the broader housing market, the federal government runs other incentive and subsidy programs for low income tenants – both rent subsidies and tax credits to encourage the construction of low-income housing (Cummings and DiPasquale, 1999).

Government involvement in housing is not limited to subsidizing private housing – it also directly provides public housing for citizens in need. In some cities, public housing may represent a significant portion of the housing stock. In Washington, D.C., for example, it is estimated that 5% of the city's population lives in homes owned and operated by the Public Housing Authority – the city's largest single landlord (Cunningham, 2003). Housing policies also take the form of mandates or prohibitions, though some of these may actually discourage rather than encourage certain types of housing. For example, large lot zoning, minimum house size requirements, and the exclusion of multi-family buildings, townhouses or accessory apartments (New Urban News, 2001) or prohibitions on housing built above retail may reduce the availability of lower priced housing (Norquist,1998). On the other hand, some local governments use mandates to increase the supply of affordable housing by requiring that developers of large residential projects set aside a percentage of the units in the project as "moderately priced dwelling units" (Moderately Priced Dwelling Unit Ordinance; Powell, 2003).

Government housing policy affects the health of urban residents in several ways. First, the quality and availability of housing, particularly affordable housing has significant health effects (Krieger and Higgins, 2002). A lack of affordable housing may increase homelessness along with its attendant health problems including higher rates of disease, both chronic (The Urban Institute, 1999) and communicable (Moss, *et al.*, 2000), greater rates of trauma due to victimization and crime (Wenzel, *et al*, 2000), and higher mortality rates than the general population (Barrow, *et al.*, 1999). Likewise, overcrowding has significant health impacts. The greater proximity of people to each other may increase the ease of disease transmission as well as put strains on sanitation and garbage disposal systems. It may also increase psychological stress and the likelihood of violence (Wallace and Wallace, 1998). Moreover, as people are forced to devote more of their income to housing, they are likely to have fewer resources available for other necessities including food and health care (Cummins, 2001).

Second, government policies, including public housing policies, that tend to concentrate poverty in particular neighborhoods, may have adverse health consequences. Studies suggests that even controlling for personal characteristics such as income and education, living in a neighborhood with a high concentration of poverty is associated with a higher incidence of coronary heart disease (Diez Roux, *et al.*, 2001), as well as higher levels of stress and depression (Leventhal and Brooks-Gunn, 2003). In addition, housing projects that are poorly designed and maintained, as many were in the 1950's and 60's (Rybcznski, 1995; Jackson, 1985; Newman, 1972), and lack recreation space, may increase crime in the area and stress for the residents (Quercia and Bates, 2002) as well as decrease the likelihood that residents will walk or that their children will play outdoors.

Finally, policies that encourage large lot, sprawl developments may result in communities that are more likely to be auto dependant rather than pedestrian oriented with the attendant problems of air pollution and sedentary life style (Savitch, 2003). The methodology used for many years by the Federal Housing Authority to appraise homes valued racially segregated, homogenous suburban neighborhoods or new, single-family homes over older, more heterogeneous urban neighborhoods. This both spurred suburbanization and contributed to the deterioration of urban residential neighborhoods (Jackson, 1985). Today, the federal tax treatment of home mortgages and capital gains in residences continues some of this effect because, as economists have argued, these provisions encourage people to purchase larger homes on larger, more suburban lots, and reinforce exclusionary zoning (Voith, 1999; Gyourko and Voith, 1997).

4.4. Transportation

Our transportation infrastructure—roads, transit, sidewalks and bike paths—provides the framework around which our cities are built. Cities allow people to interact physically with many other people and it is our transportation networks that make possible that movement of people to, from, and around the cities. Government is extensively involved in the creation of our transportation systems, primarily by funding and building the systems itself, but also by using economic incentives concerning the use of certain forms of transportation and by imposing mandates on private parties to build transportation components.

One of the most significant government transportation programs was the creation of the interstate highway system. The Federal-Aid Highway Act of 1956 provided for over 40,000 miles of highways, 90% of which were to be funded by the federal government. Although only 15% of the highway miles were to be built in urban areas, the impact of these highways on cities has been dramatic. The highways were designed by road engineers, not urban planners, and were intended to move as many cars as possible as quickly as possible through the city (Altshuler, 1983). As Witold Rybczynski explains: "the highways (usually elevated) wrought physical havoc in the established urban fabric, reducing the older housing stock, creating physical barriers between neighborhoods, and often cutting cities off from their waterfronts. Urban highways also ultimately accelerated central city decline by providing easy access to the suburbs from downtown" (Rybczynski, 1995).

Federal, state and local governments continue to invest heavily in roads. In the year 2000, all levels of government spent a total of $127.5 billion on roads and highways (Federal Highway Admin., 2002). Government also invests in other modes of transportation including public transit, along with pedestrian and bike facilities, but investments in these alternative transportation modes is significantly less than on roads (Surface Transportation Policy Project, 2000).

Cities are affected not only by what is built and where, but also by how transportation projects are built. State and local governments promulgate design standards or "road codes" that specify engineering criteria for roads such as width, curvature, turning radii, tree placements and sidewalks. These codes are generally based on a publication of the American Association of State Highway and Transportation Officials (AASHTO) called A Policy on Geometric Design of Streets and Highways. Although federal law allows AASHTO standards to be applied flexibly, many states and local governments take a more rigid approach. For example, they may require that even residential roads be quite wide, making them harder for pedestrians to cross, (Duany *et al.*, 2000), and may prohibit street trees abutting the roadway thereby making walking less pleasant and possibly less likely.

Transportation demand is affected by a variety of government requirements and incentives. Building and zoning codes can encourage auto-dependant design by requiring extensive amounts of parking. The federal tax code similarly encourages auto use by allowing employers to provide parking benefits of up to $195 tax free, but only $100 in comparable transit benefit. There is no federal tax benefit available to walkers or bikers. On the other hand, disincentives such as higher gas or parking taxes and HOV lanes may discourage driving of single occupancy vehicles.

Our urban transportation networks of roads, sidewalks, bike paths and transit are not built exclusively by government. Private developers may be required to build roads, sidewalks, bus shelters, or bike paths in order to accommodate the increased transportation demands generated by their projects. In the alternative, or where construction of new facilities is not feasible, they may be required to operate "traffic demand management" systems that encourage workers and new residents of their projects to walk, car pool, or take transit so as not to overburden the existing roads.

Transportation systems are linked to health in three critical ways. First, there is the safety of the systems themselves. Roadways, sidewalks and bike paths can be designed and built to reduce the likelihood of injuries. Second, the transportation system can either encourage or discourage active forms of transportation such as walking or biking. Finally, heavy reliance on automobiles has a direct and significant impact on air quality, and air quality is in turn closely linked to a number of health issues including asthma, cancer, respiratory, and cardiovascular diseases (Frumkin *et al.*, 2004).

4.5. Economic Incentives for Redevelopment

Beginning in the 1950s, the federal government began supporting urban "slum clearance" programs, later referred to as "urban renewal." These programs relied on a combination of direct government involvement, incentives, and mandates. Although initially focused on providing better quality housing, the programs were later revised to allow other types of commercial development (Frieden and Sagalyn, 1989). Under these programs, thousands of acres of urban land were cleared and made available for redevelopment, sometimes with the city agreeing to build parking and other infrastructure, along with tax rebates and other incentives. Beginning in the 1970's, there was increasing emphasis on public-private partnerships as vehicles for achieving socially desirable goals. To that end, the federal government made available to local officials several billion dollars as part of the Urban Development Action Grant Program (UDAG) (Frieden and Sagalyn, 1994). The money was used by cities to attract desired developments including downtown retail malls and office developments. Today, state and local governments continue to invest in economic redevelopment projects.

One of the important powers that local governments have in this regard is the power to condemn private land. The condemnation power includes not only taking land necessary for government operations, but also extends to land needed for any "public purpose," including economic development projects (Juergensmeyer and Roberts, 2003). Thus, the U.S. Supreme Court upheld the District of Columbia Redevelopment Act which included the power to condemn "blighted areas" and resell properties to new private owners as part of a redevelopment plan (Berman v. Parker, 1954), although a case curently pending before the Supreme Court could alter the scope of state authority in this area (*Kelo v. City of New London*, 2004).

Not all of the government programs intended to encourage private redevelopment focus on large projects. Many state and local governments have programs that target particular industries or particular locations such as "economic empowerment zones," arts and entertainment districts, or historic areas. Moreover, change is sometimes the result of a series of incentives and regulatory changes. In New York City and elsewhere, for example, the transformation of old industrial space into loft apartments came not as a result of spontaneous demand, but in response to changes in building and zoning codes combined with tax incentives (Frieden and Sagalyn, 1989).

Redevelopment projects have several potential impacts on health. First, health can be affected by whatever the redevelopment project replaces. Projects may be built on and improve sites that are dilapidated, infested with vermin, contaminated with toxic chemicals and may be crime ridden. On the other hand, one of the criticisms of "slum clearance" and urban renewal projects of the 1960's was that they demolished and did not replace large numbers of low income housing units and thereby exacerbated shortages of affordable housing (Frieden and Sagalyn). A second potential health effect stems from what is included in the projects. Redevelopment projects can include elements that themselves contribute to the health of surrounding residents. For example, in areas that are underserved by grocery stores or other sources of nutritious food, governments can require or provide incentives to assure that any redevelopment project in that area includes a grocery store (Burton, 2004; Pennsylvania Dept. of Agriculture, 2004). A final potential health effect of redevelopment projects stems from how the projects are built. Projects can be auto dependant, cut off from the street, and discourage pedestrian activity, or they can include pedestrian amenities and be designed to encourage walking.

4.6. Environmental Protection Laws

The built environment of our urban areas is affected by a number of federal, state and local environmental regulations designed to protect the quality of the air, water, and other environmental conditions. Important federal laws include the Clean Air Act, the Clean Water Act, the Safe Drinking Water Act, the Solid Waste Disposal/Resource Conservation and Recovery Act, the Toxic Substances Control Act, and the Comprehensive Environmental Response, Compensation, and Liability Act of 1980 (CERCLA). State and local laws include regulations concerning storm water management, tree protection requirements, toxic molds, and laws relating to sewer, septic facilities and wells (Nolon, 2002).

Most environmental regulations use mandates and prohibitions to regulate what can be built and where, though some rely on incentives. The Clear Air Act uses a "stick" approach to encourage state and local governments to address air pollution by providing that regions that fail to achieve certain air quality standards may become ineligible for federal highway money. The "Superfund" law (CERCLA), imposes liabilities on site owners of toxic sites in order to fund the clean up of contaminated "brownfields."

The adverse health effects of environmental pollution are well known. Air pollution increases deaths from cardiopulmonary diseases, (Peters and Pope, 2002) and is associated with increases in asthma incidents (Cummins and Jackson, 2001) and infant mortality. (Kaiser, *et al.*, 2004) When traffic was reduced in Atlanta for the 1996 Olympic Games, peak ozone concentrations decreased by 27.9% and the number of asthma medical emergencies fell by 41.6%. (Friedman, *et al.*, 2001) Water can be contaminated with either chemical carcinogens or bacteria (Frumkin, *et al.*, 2004; Savitch, 2000). Indoor toxins such as asbestos, lead from paint, molds, and irritant chemicals can cause cancer, asthma, and learning disabilities or mental impairments (Samet and Spengler, 2003). Finally, toxins from industrial solid waste disposal sites can have significant harmful effects on nearby residents (Lord, 1995).

4.7. Government Facilities

A final set of laws and policies that impact both the physical environments of our urban areas and the health of urban populations are the decisions governments make about what government infrastructure and facilities will be provided and where and how these are built. In addition to roads and transportation systems, discussed above, governments provide parks and recreation facilities, as well as schools, libraries, and numerous government offices. When these facilities are well designed and well placed, they can encourage physical activity through pedestrian access and by creating lively, mixed use communities.

In the late 19th century, planners began to focus on the need for systematic planning concerning parks, civic space and other public facilities. A number of cities responded by creating extensive systems – particularly of parks (Scott, 1969). The most ambitious such plan was Daniel Burnham's 1909 plan for Chicago which called for extensive parks and civic amenities, as well as major improvements to transportation and other commercial facilities (Wrigley, 1983). The city embraced the plan and over the next 20 years invested nearly $300 million in civic improvements. Subsequent residents of Chicago have been the beneficiaries of that foresight and investment.

Today, government entities routinely make choices about what government facilities to build, and where and how to build them. Government decision makers, like their private counterparts, may focus on issues such as keeping down capital and operating expenses, but their decisions in this area do have health implications. First, how buildings are designed may affect levels of physical activity of the users and employees of these facilities. Careful attention to sidewalks, pedestrian amenities, the location of parking (Dallas Morning News, 2003), along with the accessibility and attractiveness of stair ways (Boutelle, *et al.*, 2001), may increase the likelihood that building users will walk. In order to assure attention to pedestrian safety and access, one Maryland community requires that all large government capital projects include a "pedestrian impact statement" (Levine, 2004).

Second, the locations of public facilities can have important implications both on levels of physical activity and on issues such as auto dependency and air pollution. Facilities that are located on large, suburban sites with easy auto access may contribute to sprawl-style development and thereby increase auto use and attendant air pollution problems. In contrast, when facilities are located on more compact sites closer to facilities and destinations, they may contribute to walkable, lively communities (Langdon, 2003b; McMahon, 2001a).

Schools provide a useful illustration of how choices concerning the design and location of government facilities may affect health. Obesity among children is a rising problem (Ogden, *et al.*, 2002). At the same time, the percentage of children who walk to school has declined significantly from about 50% in 1969 to under 10% today (Ernst and McCann, 2003; Savitch, 2003), and mothers of school aged children are spending increasing amounts of time in the car chauffeuring their children (Surface Transportation Policy Project, 2002). While the causes of these changes in behavior are complex, at least one factor may be the size, design, and placement of schools. School acreage requirements have increased over the years, so that today, relying on state and local education department requirements, a high school may require as much as 60 acres. In addition, state funding formulas frequently favor new construction over renovations. The result of these policies is to push schools onto suburban sites that are less accessible by walking or biking (National Trust for Historic Preservation, 2000; McMahon, 2000).

A third implication of decisions concerning government facilities relates to parks and recreation facilities. Proximity to parks and recreation facilities is another factor that correlates with higher levels of physical activity (Huston, *et al.*, 2003). Parks also reduce stress and improve psychological well-being for users (Ho, *et al.*, 2003; Parsons, *et al.*, 1998; Taylor, *et al.*, 1998), as well as contribute to environmental quality. In times of tight budgets, parks and recreation facilities may seem like a luxury, but they can also be understood to be part of our basic health infrastructure.

Fourth, government facilities not only impact the communities in which they are built and the people who use them, their construction presents opportunities for government to lead by example (McMahon, 2001a). Changes and approaches successfully implemented by government can lay the foundation for wider acceptance by the public and by private industry. Finally, the locations of public facilities have important implications not only for health in general, but also for health equity. Public uses that present health hazards such as waste dumps, incinerators or sewage treatment facilities have historically been located in minority neighborhoods (Gelobter, 1994). Conversely, parks and recreation facilities may be disproportionately located in wealthier or non-minority areas (Gelobter, 1994).

5.0. PUBLIC HEATH AND LEGAL CHANGE

The physical form of our cities has been and will continue to be significantly affected by laws and government policies. As Mark Gelfand has written, "federal decisions about interest rates, taxes, military procurement, and scores of other economic matters had a direct and substantial impact upon nearly all facets of urban life" (1975). In addition, state and local decisions about zoning, building codes, street design, transportation systems, parks, and schools, as well as policies concerning economic development all affect not only government contributions to the built environment, but private building and development as well.

In an earlier era, public health practitioners were among the leading voices in discussions about how to shape our cities (Peterson, 1983), but in more modern times these voices have been largely absent (Perdue, *et al.*, 2003). This absence has been significant. As the foregoing section demonstrates, there is a broad array of laws and government policies that affect the built environment in ways that in turn affect health. However, with respect to many of these laws, any health effects were unforeseen or unintended. Even laws intended to improve health and safety sometimes have had other, unanticipated adverse health consequences.

Those interested in building healthier cities may wish to bear in mind the following admonitions:

1. *Be an engaged participant in the full range of policy discussions on matters that affect urban life.* Issues such as health care or smoking policy obviously affect health, but those interested in urban health should look beyond the obvious. As the foregoing analysis highlights, there are important health implications to decisions concerning such diverse matters as transportation and housing policy, zoning laws, and tax incentives.

2. *Bring a broad vision of health impacts.* There are professionals such traffic engineers or fire experts who focus on particular components of health. Though this expertise and focus is very valuable, it sometimes overshadows broader concerns about health and wellbeing. Thus, traffic engineers may design streets with few auto accidents, but which also are so sterile and inhospitable that they have few pedestrians. Public health practitioners and advocates are well situated to focus attention on broader health concerns.

3. *Expand the base of knowledge and bring data to the table.* There is growing recognition of the potential connection between health and the physical and social structure of cities, but further research is needed (Litman, 2003; Dannenberg, *et al.*, 2003; Northridge, *et al.*, 2003). Public health practitioners, with their expertise in

epidemiology and empirical analysis are well situated to provided needed data and analysis.

4. *Think creatively about solutions.* Just as the current structure of cities is the result of a complex array of laws and government policies, changes in the current situation will require a multifaceted response that includes economic incentives and creative government programs. For example, government can sometimes lead by itself becoming a model citizen, e.g., by thoughtful location and design of its own buildings so as to encourage physical activity and a healthy life style by its employees and clients.

5. *Continue to ask: "What will the impact of this policy be on human health?"* Many laws and policies which do not on their face appear to have anything to do with health, may nonetheless have health impacts. However, these impacts may go unnoticed unless those interested in urban health continue to raise the health question.

A greater focus on public health does not guarantee any particular outcome with respect to policy choices. Factors other than health may be given priority. Moreover, sometimes there will be competing health and safety concerns. For example, adding sidewalks and bike paths to encourage physical activity can increase impervious surface and contribute to unhealthy water run-off. Concentrating density may facilitate walking and reduce vehicle miles traveled and overall air pollution levels, but may increase air pollution intensity within certain areas (Frumkin, *et al.*, 2004). Rigorous building codes make buildings safer, but may also discourage reuse of existing dilapidated buildings. In some cases, careful crafting of policy can address the competing claims, as some jurisdictions have done with their road codes (North Carolina Dept. of Transportation, 2000), and building codes (Connolly, 1996). In other cases, the trade-offs will be unavoidable. However, it is only after recognizing the potential health impacts that we can then make the conscious though sometimes difficult choices that good policy decisions require.

6.0. CONCLUSION

This chapter has reviewed the range of laws and government policies that affect the physical form of our cities. These laws and policies include mandates and prohibitions, incentives and subsidies, and direct government involvement, and they touch a broad range of issues including transportation, housing, schools, parks, and economic development. The chapter highlights that the health of urban residents is impacted both directly and indirectly by the built environment in which those residents live and work. As a result, the laws and policies that affect the built environment also affect health.

REFERENCES

Altshuler, A. (1983). The intercity freeway. In: Krueckeberg, D. A. (ed.), *Introduction to Planning History in the United States.* Rutgers University Center for Urban Policy Research, New Jersey, pp. 190-234.

Ashe, M., Jerrigan, D., Kline, R., and Galaz, R. (2003). Land use planning and the control of alcohol, tobacco, firearms, and fast food restaurants. *Am. J. Public Health* 93(9):1404–1408.

Barrow, S. M., Herman, D. B., Cordova, P., and Struening, E. L. (1999). Mortality among homeless shelter residents in New York City. *Am. J. Pubic Health* 89(4):529–534.

Boutelle, K. N., Jeffery, R. W., Murray, D. M., and Schmitz, M. K. H. (2001). Using signs, artwork, and music to promote stair use in a public building. *Am. J. Public Health* 91(12):2004–2006.

Brown, M. J., Gardner, J., Sargent, J. D., Swartz, K., Hu, H., and Timperi, R. (2001). The effectiveness of housing policies in reducing children's lead exposure. *Am. J. Public Health* 91(4):621–624.

Burton, H. (2004). Philadelphia's food trust and supermarket access. *Progressive Planning.* 158:4–6.

Carter, S. P., Carter, S. L., and Dannenberg, A. L. (2003). Zoning out crime and improving community health in Sarasota, Florida: "Crime prevention through environmental design." *Am. J. Public Health* 93(9):1442–1445.

Cervero, R (1998). *The Transit Metropolis: A Global Inquiry.* Island Press, Washington, D.C.

Connolly, W. (1999). Rules that make sense—New Jersey's Rehabilitation Subcode (Online). New Jersey Department of Community Affairs, Trenton (last checked August 8, 2004); http://www.state.nj.us/dca/codes/rehab/pioneerart.shtml.

Cunningham, L. (2003). A structural analysis of housing subsidy delivery systems: Public Housing Authorities' part in solving the housing crisis. *J. Affordable Housing & Community Dev. L.* 13:95–121.

Cummings, J. L., and DiPasquale, D. (1999). The Low-Income Housing Tax Credit: An analysis of the first ten years. *Housing Policy Debate* 10(2):251–307.

Cummins, J. D. (2001). Public interest law: Improving access to justice: Housing matters: Why our communities must have affordable housing. *Wm. Mitchell L. Rev.* 28:197–228.

Cummins, S. K., and Jackson, R. J. (2001). The built environment and children's health. *Pediatr. Clin. of North Am.* 48(5):1241–1252.

Dallas Morning News. (2003). Editorial: The office workout; workforce quietly prodded to healthier lifestyle (October 15, 2003), pp. 20A.

Dannenberg, A.L., Jackson, R.J., Frumkin, H., Schieber, R.A., Pratt, M., Kochitzky, C., and Tilson, H.H. (2003). The impact of community design and land-use choices on public health: a scientific research agenda. *Am. J. Public Health* 93(9):1500–08.

Diez Roux, A. V., Merkin, S. S., Arnett, D., Chambless, L., Massing, M., Nieto, F. J., Sorlie, P., Szklo, M., Tyroler, H. A., and Watson, R. L. (2001). Neighborhood of residence and incidence of coronary heart disease. *N. Engl. J. Med.* 345(2):99–106.

Duany, A., Plater-Zyberk, E., and Speck, J. (2000). *Suburban Nation: The Rise of Sprawl and the Decline of the American Dream.* North Point Press, New York.

Ernst, M., and McCann, B. (2002). Mean Streets 2002 (Online). Surface Transportation Policy Project, Washington, D.C. (August 8, 2004); http://www.transact.org/pdfs/ms2002/meanstreets2002.pdf.

Ewing, R., Schmid, T., Killingsworth, R., Zlot, A., and Raudenbush, S. (2003). Relationship between urban sprawl and physical activity, obesity, and morbidity. *Am. J. Health Promotion* 18(1):47–57.

Farrell, J. L. (2002). The FHA's origins: How its valuation method fostered racial segregation and suburban sprawl. *J. Affordable Housing & Community Dev. L.* 11:374–389.

Federal Highway Admin., U.S. Dept. of Transportation. (2002). Report to Congress: 2002 status of the nation's highways, bridges and transit: conditions and performance, (August 12, 2004); http://www.fhwa.dot.gov/policy/2002cpr

Frank, L. D., Engelke, P. O., and Schmid, T. L. (2003). *Health and Community Design: The Impact of the Built Environment on Physical Activity.* Island Press, Washington, D.C.

Frieden, B. J., and Sagalyn, L. B. (1989). *Downtown, Inc.: How America Rebuilds Cities.* The MIT Press, Massachusetts.

Friedman, M. S., Powell, K. E., Hutwagner, L., Graham, L. M., and Teague, W. G. (2001). Impact of changes in transportation and commuting behaviors during the 1996 Summer Olympic Games in Atlanta on air quality and childhood asthma. *J. Am. Med. Assoc.* 285(7):897–905.

Frielich, R. H. (1999). *From Sprawl to Smart Growth: Successful Legal, Planning, and Environmental Systems.* American Bar Assoc., Chicago.

Frumkin, H., Frank, L., and Jackson, R. (2004). *Urban Sprawl and Public Health: Designing, Planning, and Building for Healthy Communities.* Island Press, Washington, D.C.

Garb, M. (2003). Health, morality and housing: The "tenement problem" in Chicago. *Am. J. Public Health* 93:1420–30.

Gelfand, M. I. (1975). *A Nation of Cities: The Federal Government and Urban America, 1933-1965 (The Urban Life in America Series).* Oxford University Press, Inc., New York.

Gelobter, M. (1994). The meaning of urban environmental justice. *Fordham Urb. L.* J. 21:841–856.

Gyourko, J., and Voith, R. (1997). Does the U.S. tax treatment of housing promote suburbanization and central city decline? Working Paper No. 97-13, Federal Reserve Bank of Philadelphia (September 17, 1997).

Ho, C., Payne, L., Orsega-Smith, E., and Godbey, G. (2003). Parks, recreation and public health. *Parks & Recreation.* April, 2003:18–27.

Huston, S.L., Evenson, K.R., Bors, P.B., and Gizlice, Z. (2003). Neighborhood environment, access to places for activity, and leisure-time physical activity in a diverse North Carolina population. *Am. J. Health Promotion* 18(1):58–69.

Jackson, K. T. (1985). *Crabgrass Frontier: The Suburbanization of the United States.* Oxford University Press, Inc., New York.

Jacobs, J. (1961). *The Death and Life of Great American Cities.* Random House, New York.

Juergensmeyer, J.C., and Roberts, T.E. (2003). *Land Use Planning and Development Regulation Law.* Thompson/West, St. Paul, Minn.

Kaiser, R., Romieu, I., Medina, S., Schwartz, J., Krzyzanowski, M., and Künzli, N. (2004). Air pollution attributable postneonatal infant mortality in U.S. metropolitan areas: A risk assessment study. *Envtl. Health.* 3(1):4.

Katyal, N. (2002). Architecture as crime control. *Yale L. J.* 111:1039–1125.

Kay, J. H. (1997). *Asphalt Nation: How the Automobile Took Over America and How We Can Take It Back.* Crown Publishers, Inc., New York.

Kelly, E. D. (1996). Fair housing, good housing, or expensive housing? Are building codes part of the problem or part of the solution? *John Marshall L. Rev.* 29:349–368.

King, W.C, Brach, J.S., Belle, S., Killingsworth, R. Fenton, M., and Kriska, A.M. (2003). The relationship between convenience of destinations and walking levels in older women. *Am. J. Health Promotion* 18(1):74–82.

Knapp, G., Talen E., Olshanky, R., and Forrest, C. (2001). Zoning, subdivision, and urban development in Illinois (Online). Illinois Dept. of Natural Resources, Springfield (last visited August 8, 2004); http://dnr.state.il.us/orep/NRRC/balancedgrowth/pdfs/zoning.pdf.

Krieger, J., and Higgins, D.L. (2002). Housing and health: Time again for public health action. *Am. J. Public Health* 92(5):758–768.

Langdon, P. (2003a). Zoning reform advances against sprawl and inertia. *New Urban News.* 8(1):1–5.

Langdon, P. (2003b). Public buildings keep town centers alive. *Planning Commissioners J.* 49:10–16.

Leventhal T., and Brooks-Gunn, J. (2003). Moving to opportunity: an experimental study of neighborhood effects on mental health. *Am. J. Public Health* 93(9):1576–82.

Levine, S. (2004). Pedestrian fatalities remain a concern; eight killed in '04 despite safety efforts. *Washington Post.* July 8, 2004 (Montgomery Extra p. 8).

Litman, T. (2003). Integrating public health objectives in transportation decision-making. *Am. J. Health Promotion* 18(1):103–08.

Lord, C. P. (1995). Community initiatives: Environmental justice law and the challenges facing urban communities. *Va. Envtl. L. J.* 14:721–734.

Mair, S., and Mair, M. (2003). Violence prevention and control through environmental modifications. *Annu. Rev. Public Health* 24:209–225.

McMahon, E. T. (2000). School sprawl. *Planning Commissioners J.* 39:16–18.

McMahon, E. T. (2001a). Public buildings should set the standard. *Planning Commissioners J.* 41:3–8.

McMahon, E. T. (2001b). Building codes get smarter. *Planning Commissioners J.* 43:434–435.

Meck, S. (ed.). (2002). Growing smart legislative guidebook: Model statutes for planning and the management of change. American Planning Association.

Morland, K., Wing, S., and Roux, A.D. (2002). The contextual effect of the local food environment on residents' diets: The atherosclerosis risk in communities study. *Am. J. Pub. Health* 92(11):1761–1767.

Moss, A. R. Hahn, J. A., Tulsky, J. P., Daley, C. L., Small, P. M., and Hopewell, P. C. (2000). Tuberculosis in the homeless: A prospective study. *Am. J. Respir. Crit. Care Med.* 162(2 Pt 1):460–464.

National Center for Chronic Disease Prevention and Health Promotion, A Public Health Action Plan to Prevent Heart Disease and Stroke, 2003, Atlanta (August 8, 2004); http://www.cdc.gov/cvh/Action_Plan/.

National Center for Health Statistics, *Health, United States, 2002,* with Chartbook on Trends in the Health of Americans: Tables 32, 70, and 71, 2002, (August 11, 2004); ftp://ftp.cdc.gov/pub/Health_Statistics/NCHS/Publications/Health_US/hus02/.

National Institute for Occupational Safety and Health. (1991). Building air quality: A guide for building owners and facilities managers (Online). National Institute for Occupational Safety and Health Publication No. 91-114, EPA Publication No. 400/1-91/003, Atlanta (August 11, 2004); http://www.cdc.gov/niosh/baqtoc.html.

National Trust for Historic Preservation, Why Johnny can't walk to school, 2000, Washington, D.C. (August 8, 2004); http://www.nationaltrust.org/news/docs/20001116_johnny_cantwalk.html.

New Urban News. (2003). New state rehabilitation codes foster redevelopment of urban centers. *New Urban News* 8(7):13.

New Urban News. (2001). Granny flats add flexibility and affordability. *New Urban News.* 6(8):8–10.

Newman, O. (1972). *Defensible Space: Crime Prevention Through Urban Design.* Macmillan, New York.

Nolon, J. R. (2002). In praise of parochialism: The advent of local environmental law. *Harv. Envtl. L. Rev.* 26:365-416.

Norquist, J. D. (1998). *The Wealth of Cities: Revitalizing the Centers of American Life.* Addison-Wesley, Massachusetts.

North Carolina Dept. of Transportation, Division of Highways. (2000). Traditional Neighborhood Development (TND) guidelines.

Northridge, M., Sclar, E.D., and Biswas, P. (2003). Sorting out the connections between the built environment and health: a conceptual framework for navigating pathways and planning healthy cities. *J. Urban Health* 80(4):556–68.

Ogden, C.L., Flegal, K.M., Carroll, M.D., and Johnson, C.L. (2002). Prevalence and trends in overwieght among US children and adolescents, 1999-2000. *JAMA.* 288(14):1728–32.

Ohland, G., Nguyen, T., and Corless, J. (2000). Dangerous by design: Pedestrian safety in California. Surface Transportation Policy Project.

Parsons, R., Tassinary, L.G., Ulrich, R.S., Hebel, M.R., and Grossman-Alexander, M. (1998). The view from the road: implications for stress recovery and immunization. *J. Envir. Psych.* 18:113–39.

Pennsylvania Dept. of Agriculture, Press release: Pennsylvania officials announce plans to attract supermarkets to underserved areas, 2004, Pennsylvania (August 11, 2004); http://www.agriculture.state.pa.us/agriculture/cwp/view.asp?A=11&Q=131435.

Perdue, W.C., Gostin, L.O., and Stone, L.A. (2003). Public health and the built environment: Historical, empirical, and theoretical foundations for an expanded role. *J. Law Medicine & Ethics* 31:557–66.

Peters, A., and Pope, C.A. III. (2002). Cardiopulmonary mortality and air pollution. *Lancet.* 360(9341):1184–1185.

Peterson, J. (1983). The impact of sanitary reform upon American urban planning, 1840-1890. In: Krueckeberg, D. A. (ed.), *Introduction to Planning History in the United States.* Rutgers University Center for Urban Policy Research, New Jersey, p. 13–39.

Pothukuchi, K., and Kaufman, J. (2000). The food system: A stranger to the planning field. *J. Am. Planning Assoc.* 66(2):113–124.

Powell, J. A. (2003). Opportunity-based housing. *J. Affordable Housing & Community Dev. L.* 12(2): 188-228.

Powell, K.E., Martin, L.M., and Chowdhury, P.P. (2003). Places to walk: convenience and regular physical activity. *Am. J. Public Health* 93(9):1519–21.

Quercia, R. G., and Bates, L. K. (2002). The neglect of America's housing: Consequences and policy responses (Online). Millennial Housing Commission (August 8, 2004); http://www.mhc.gov/papers.html.

Reidpath, D. D., Burns, C., Garrand, J., Mahoney, M., and Townsend, M. (2002). An ecological study of the relationship between social and environmental determinants of obesity. *Health and Place* 8(2):141–145.

Rodgers, D. T. (1998). *Atlantic Crossings: Social Politics in a Progressive Age.* The Belknap Press, Massachusetts.

Rybczynski, W. (1995). *City life: Urban Expectations in a New World.* Scribner, New York.

Saelens, B.E., Sallis, J.F., Black, J.B., and Chen, D. (2003). Neighborhood-based differences in physical activity: an environment scale evaluation. *Am. J. Public Health* 93(9):1552–58.

Samet, J.M. and Spengler, J.D., (2003). Indoor environments and health: moving into the 21st century. *Am. J. Public Health* 93(9):1489–93.

Savitch, H. V. (2003). How suburban sprawl shapes human well-being. *J. Urban Health* 80(4):590–607.

Schukoske, J. E. (1999). Community development through gardening. *N.Y.U. J. Legis. & Pub. Policy* 3:351–392.

Scott, M. G. (1969). *American City Planning Since 1890: A History Commemorating the Fiftieth Anniversary of the American Institute of Planners.* University of California Press, California.

Sloane, D. C. (2004). Bad meat and brown bananas: Building a legacy of health by confronting health disparities around food. *Progressive Planning* 158:1, 7–9.

Standard State Zoning Enabling Act. (1926), reprinted in Rathkopf, A.H. and Rathkopf, D.A. (1975). *The Law of Zoning and Planning.* Vol. 5; app. A. Thompson/West.

Surface Transportation Policy Project. (2000). Changing direction: Federal transportation spending in the 1990's. Washington, D.C., (August 11, 2004); http://www.transact.org/report.asp?id=163

Surface Transportation Policy Project. (2002). High mileage moms—the report. Washington, D.C. http://www.transact.org/report.asp?id=184 (last visited August 11, 2004).

Taylor, A. F., Wiley, A., Kuo, F. E., and Sullivan, W. C. (1998). Growing up in the inner city: Green spaces as places to grow. *Environ. Behav.* 30(1):3–27.

The Urban Institute, Homelessness: Programs and the people they serve, 1999, Washington, D.C., (August 8, 2004); http://www.huduser.org/publications/homeless/homelessness/ch_3.html.

Voith, R. (1999). Does the tax treatment of housing create an incentive for exclusionary zoning and increased decentralization? Working Paper No. 99-22, Federal Reserve Bank of Philadelphia (December 19, 1999).

Wallace, D., and Wallace, R. (1998). Scales of geography, time, and population: The study of violence as a public health problem. *Am. J. Public Health* 88(12):1853–1858.

Wenzel, S. L., Koegel, P., and Gelberg, L. (2000). Antecedents of physical and sexual victimization among homeless women: A comparison to homeless men. *Am. J. Community Psychol.* 28(3):367–390.

Wrigley, R. L., Jr. (1983). The plan of Chicago. In: Krueckeberg, D. A. (ed.), *Introduction to Planning History in the United States.* Rutgers University Center for Urban Policy Research, New Jersey, pp 58–72.

STATUTES AND CASES

Clean Air Act, 42 U.S.C. §7401 et seq.

Clean Water Act, 33 U.S.C. §1251 et seq.

Comprehensive Environmental Response, Compensation, and Liability Act of 1980, 42 U.S.C. §9601 et seq.

Moderately Priced Dwelling Unit Ordinance, Montgomery County Code, Md., Chapter 25A.

Safe Drinking Water Act, 42 U.S.C. §300(f) et seq.

Solid Waste Disposal/Resource Conservation and Recovery Act, 42 U.S.C. §6901 et seq.

Toxic Substances Control Act, 15 U.S.C. §§2661-2671.

Berman v. Parker, 348 U.S. 26 (1954)

Kelo v. City of New London, 125 S.CT.27 (2004) (granting cert.).

Chapter 26

Teaching Urban Health

Nicholas Freudenberg and Susan Klitzman

1.0. INTRODUCTION

Improving the health of urban populations requires a workforce of practitioners, managers, researchers and policy makers with the requisite knowledge and skills. In this chapter, we consider the education of urban health professionals, defined here as practitioners, public health staff, advocates, managers and researchers working to improve the health of urban populations. Our review begins with an examination of the unique characteristics of urban health and its key principles, then, discusses pedagogical approaches to teaching urban health. We propose educational competencies for urban health practitioners and researchers and summarize methods to assess and meet urban health workforce needs. Finally, we examine organizational issues related to educating urban health workers and suggest institutional reforms to improve this education. The chapter is based on our review of the sparse relevant literature, conversations with people teaching urban health, primarily in the U.S. but also in some other countries, and our many years experience teaching urban health at the City University of New York, the largest urban public university in the U.S.

2.0. KEY CONCEPTS IN URBAN HEALTH

Urban health professionals, like other health workers, need education in their own discipline (e.g., medicine, nursing, public health, social work, etc.), in the history, structure and function of the health care delivery and public health systems, and in the broader social and natural sciences. It is worth noting that urban health professionals include both entry-level practitioners who happen to be practicing in cities (but have no special training for this setting) and those with advanced training in urban health. Both groups require preparation for their work in urban areas and it is this unique need that is the focus of this chapter.

What's different about the demands of the urban setting? Several features of the urban environment distinguish it in character or degree from other settings. These differences constitute the foundation for a consideration of those elements of teaching about urban health that are distinct from teaching about health in general.

First, urban settings are complex. Political, social, and economic factors operate at the individual, family, community, municipal, regional, national and global levels to influence health. Multiple systems including health care, education, criminal justice, environmental protection, housing and employment interact to shape the urban living conditions that determine health. Population density amplifies the effect of any single influence (e.g. an outbreak of infectious disease) and population heterogeneity demands that any response to health problems must be tailored to the diverse populations that comprise modern cities. Urban health professionals must have the conceptual capacity to appreciate and analyze this complexity, distinguish primary from secondary factors, and use these insights to implement appropriate interventions.

Many researchers have suggested that ecological models may be useful tools for understanding complexity (Lawrence, 1999; Diez-Roux, 2000; Krieger, 2000). These models organize variables of interest into appropriate levels of biological (e.g., cell, organism and population) and social (e.g. individual, community, and municipality) organization and may provide a useful intellectual foundation for the study of urban health (Lawrence, 2002; Galea, *et al.*, 2005; Duhl and Hancock, 1988).

Second, urban populations are diverse. Compared to non-urban areas, cities have higher proportions of immigrants than other areas, more ethnic and lifestyle variability, and greater disparities in socioeconomic status. Urban health professionals need the cultural and communications skills, the anthropological knowledge, and the epidemiological evidence to work effectively with the many constituencies that comprise urban communities.

Third, cities have unique assets and problems. For example, cities use energy more efficiently, tolerate better differences in values and behavior, and have a richer array of health, social service and community-based organizations than rural or suburban communities. For some health conditions and in some places, urban residents are healthier than their non-urban counter-parts. But cities also have higher rates of many illnesses, more access to health-damaging resources (e.g., drugs and guns), and higher levels of the income disparities associated with poor health. To be effective, urban health professionals need the tools to identify these unique strengths and weaknesses and the skills to use the assets to address the problems.

Fourth, urban context matters. Every health problem is embedded in a broader biological, social and political context. Urban health professionals must be able to analyze how human biology, time (a historical perspective), space (a geographical perspective), and culture (an anthropological perspective), among other factors, influence the patterns of health and disease at the individual and populations levels. Developing this capacity to consider simultaneously both foreground (the health outcome of interest) and background (the environment in which disease unfolds) is a critical challenge for the education of urban health professionals.

Finally, solving the health problems that face cities requires scientific, technical, organizational and political skills. Scientific knowledge offers frameworks for understanding how variables at different levels combine within cities to influence health and disease. Technical knowledge includes the ability to measure, assess and intervene effectively within the urban environment. Organizational knowledge yields the ability to make institutional decisions that change practices and policies, and build coalitions for urban health. Political knowledge produces the capacity to mobilize resources to achieve health objectives. By achieving competencies in each of these dimensions of knowledge, urban health professionals can develop the skills they need to improve the health of city dwellers.

What are the educational implications of these unique characteristics of urban settings? We suggest that professional preparation programs for urban health professionals should be interdisciplinary, educate students to observe, analyze and intervene at several levels of social organization, equip them to understand and communicate with people from different cultures, prepare them to advocate policies and programs that protect health and ensure that graduates have scientific, technical, organizational and political competencies.

In the literature, the terms multidisciplinary, interdisciplinary and transdisciplinary are sometimes used interchangeably. Stokols *et al.*, (2003) propose that unidisciplinary research relies solely on the methods, concepts and theories of a single discipline; multidisciplinary research combines methods, concepts and theories from several disciplines; and transdisciplinary research integrates methods, concepts and theories from two or more disciplines. The Institute of Medicine Report *The Future of the Public's Health* (Committee on Assuring the Health of the Public, 2003) distinguishes between multidisciplinary and interdisciplinary research, using the latter to describe research or education that integrates subject matters across disciplines. In this chapter, we use the term interdisciplinary in this sense.

3.0. PEDAGOGICAL APPROACHES TO TEACHING URBAN HEALTH

To prepare health professionals with the specific competencies needed to work effectively in cities requires the development of pedagogical methods suited to these aims. Pedagogy includes learners, students, academic settings, and the methods and content of teaching. We review here methods to recruit students and faculty particularly suited for this work, approaches to interdisciplinary teaching, experiential and service learning, and various formats for organizing urban health education. The urban health workforce includes diverse layers of job categories – from outreach workers to administrators to specialized nurses and physicians; each must master specific competencies. Some of the pedagogical approaches described here are relevant to many job categories; others may apply to only a few.

3.1. The Students

The opening question for any educational program is, "Who is in the classroom?". No field of study exists in a vacuum and *who* gets trained in urban health influences practice and research as much as the *content* of the training. In the U.S. and most other nations, socioeconomic class, ethnicity and income (Educational Testing Service, 2004) limit access to higher and professional education. Acknowledging this reality, some health professional training programs have made special efforts to recruit students who better represent excluded populations, including low-income urban residents. As we shall see, the rationale for these efforts is that compared to outsiders, students from under-served urban communities are more likely to return there for practice, to understand better the life circumstances of their clients, and to communicate effectively with patients and communities. Recruitment methods include targeted outreach to under-represented populations, affirmative action and other admissions policies, scholarships and loan forgiveness programs, scheduling to meet the needs of working people with families, remedial and basic education programs, and partnerships with secondary schools or community college in targeted communities (Tekian, 2000; Thurmond and Kirch, 1998; Pathman, *et al.*, 2000; Burns, 2002). For example, the Urban Health Program at the University of Illinois at Urbana and Champaign was created in the 1970s to assist in lessening health disparities in communities of color by increasing the pool of students of color matriculating and graduating from medical schools (UIC Urban Health Program, 2004). As well as targeted recruitment, the program offered summer enrichment courses for incoming students designed to allow them to overcome previous disparities in educational opportunities.

Another approach has been to prepare urban community residents to serve as community health or outreach workers, lay health advisers or peer educators (Eng and Young, 1992; Zuvekas, 1999; La Pierre, *et al.*, 1995). By recruiting and training people who themselves live in low income urban neighborhoods and are connected to local social networks, it is believed that health care programs can better reach and engage these populations.

Several rationales are proposed for these varying efforts to change who is educated. First, evidence suggests that at least for physicians, those recruited from low-income disadvantaged neighborhoods are more likely to return to those areas for professional practice and may be perceived by their patients to be more caring and understanding (Komaromy, *et al.*, 1996). Thus, these programs may help to reduce disparities in health care. Second, some advance moral reasons for special recruitment. Limiting access to higher education based on class, race, or ethnicity is wrong and educators have an obligation to reduce such discrimination. Third, some educators argue that students from more privileged backgrounds benefit from diversity and learn important lessons from their peers (Bowen and Bok, 2000). This argument may be especially relevant for health professionals, where students with more privileged or homogeneous experiences may learn from their peers how to communicate with people from different class or cultural backgrounds, identify resources within urban communities, and appreciate the impact of urban living conditions on health.

3.2. The Teachers

Deciding who sits in front of the class is also important. Hiring faculty who reflect the diversity of their students and the populations students are expected to serve after they graduate may increase the likelihood that students will develop the cultural and communications skills they need (Wright and Carresse, 2003). Faculty from disadvantaged backgrounds can serve as role models and mentors for students with similar characteristics and may help all students to understand better the impact of poverty, discrimination and disadvantage on health. In the U.S., evidence suggests that many health professional training programs, including those in medicine, public health and dentistry, do not yet have a faculty diversity that represents the broader population (Palepu, *et al.*, 1998, Healton, 1999; Logan, 1997).

Disciplinary faculty diversity is also important. For students to appreciate the value of other disciplines to the study of urban health, they should be taught by faculty from these disciplines. Ideally, some classes should be taught by faculty members from two or more disciplines, with the integration of theories, concepts and methods from the two an explicit topic of discussion. In practice, organizational and professional imperatives often thwart this objective. Few institutions have well-established procedures for team teaching and many disciplines often insist that all faculty have doctorates in that profession, limiting students' exposures to other perspectives. At a minimum, students preparing for urban health professional careers should receive instruction from faculty in the natural, social, and health sciences, and have at least a few opportunities to analyze urban health problems from several disciplinary perspectives.

3.3. Experiential Learning

Educational research suggests that having the opportunity to practice skills and apply concepts to real world settings increase the likelihood that learning can be generalized to practice. To achieve this, many urban health training programs have designed experiential learning including service learning, internships, fieldwork and practicums. These experiences allow students to appreciate the complexity of urban communities, to interact with community residents and other professionals, to apply skills and concepts learned in the classroom and to identify gaps in their education. A few examples illustrate the range of approaches. At the Johns Hopkins University, for example, the School of Nursing established an undergraduate track in urban community health nursing specifically designed for returning Peace Corps volunteers (Shiber, 1999). The program acknowledged students' prior experiences, placed students in a service setting while they were enrolled in school where they are assisted to integrate their Peace Corps experience into nursing practice, and added non-hospital clinical rotations to placement opportunities. Students were also given the opportunity to earn a stipend by serving as community outreach workers in the faculty community practice.

In New York City, several medical schools, community health centers, and neighborhood organizations collaborated in the 1980s to create clinical preceptorships in community settings, to offer community projects for medical students and to design a special course on community-oriented primary care and community health diagnosis (Boufford and Shonubi, 1986). Some of these efforts continue two decades later. Other medical schools have also offered clinical practicums designed to prepare students for urban practice (Yu and Towns, 1997; Gemson, *et al.*, 1995).

At three Urban Research Centers funded by the US Centers for Disease Control and Prevention, medical, public health, nursing and social work students joined participatory research teams in Seattle, Detroit and New York City. The teams included neighborhood residents, community leaders, service providers, and researchers, who used community-based participatory research methods to study such issues as social stress and family health, asthma, substance abuse, and immigrant health (Metzler, *et al.*, 2003). These experiences provided students an opportunity to collect data on urban community health problems, learn from community residents, plan interventions, and interact with researchers from several disciplines.

3.4. Special Programs in Urban Health

Another approach to studying urban health has been to offer special courses, degrees, and programs on urban health topics. South Bank University in

London, for example, offers a PhD program in Urban Health. Faculty members include geographers, public health researchers, architects, planners, and social scientists and students have advisers from at least two disciplines (Harpham, 2004). Each student develops a tailored program to correspond to their interests.

Hunter College in the City University of New York combined three previously separate programs in community health education, environmental and occupational health and nutrition into a single Masters in Urban Public Health Program. Its mission is to educate public health professionals who can promote health and prevent disease among diverse urban populations. Students continue to take courses in one of the three specialization areas as well as the core public health courses and they are also required to take two courses in urban health and concepts and principles of urban health are integrated into many other courses.

At the City University of New York, we have also developed special undergraduate, Masters and doctoral level courses in urban health. In the late 1990s, an undergraduate course *Multidisciplinary Perspectives on the South Bronx* focused on a single low-income neighborhood, located within the then poorest Congressional district in the U.S. The course reviewed the health and social problems in the South Bronx, invited community leaders, activists, and service providers to lecture on community resources and needs, and required students to investigate a problem of their choice. About a quarter of the students lived or worked in the South Bronx, offering other students the opportunity to learn about community conditions and history. A more recent course on *Health, Wealth and Social Justice in New York City* reviewed data on health disparities in New York City and asked students to investigate a specific health problem in one community, and then compare their findings to another community's experience with that condition. Both these undergraduate courses also served to introduce basic concepts of urban health and to recruit students into graduate health professional programs.

City University of New York also established a pathway between its MPH programs, including the Hunter program in urban health, and its social science PhD programs. Sociology, anthropology or psychology doctoral students with interests in urban health work towards an MPH degree while pursuing their doctoral studies. This program prepares students to work in two or more disciplines and to gain experience in the classroom and in field placements interacting with public health professionals engaged in addressing urban health problems.

3.5. Continuing Education

The discussion so far has focused on preservice education. In recent years, however, health workforce development specialists have also emphasized the importance of continuing education, offered to health staff already employed (Committee on Assuring Health, 2003; Lichtveld, *et al.*, 2001; Kennedy and Moore, 2001). Continuing education enables employers to develop their staff's skills, fill in gaps in their prior education, meet emerging needs, or use resources more effectively. From a pedagogical perspective, continuing education often borrows principles and approaches from adult education, where the focus is on practical skills, short-term courses, and methods that engage learners with multiple competing demands. In urban health, continuing education is a valuable tool for strengthening the capacity of an entire agency, meeting an emerging health need such as HIV infection or diabetes, or teaching new technologies, e.g., a new MIS system or rapid HIV testing.

In Allegheny County (Pittsburgh), Pennsylvania, for example, the county health department worked with the University of Pittsburgh School of Public Health to offer its employees the opportunity to participate in a 10 session course called "Practical Professional Skills: Cross-Cutting Competencies for the 21st Century Public Health Workforce." (Potter, *et al.*, 2003; Pennsylvania and Ohio Public Health Training Center, 2003). Seventy-seven staff attended the course designed to improve planning skills, develop cultural competencies, and teach research and evaluation methods. The goal was to develop a cadre of leaders throughout the organization who could help the health department better meet the health needs of this urban county.

In New York City, the growing prevalence of a more aggressive form of diabetes led the city health department and public hospital system to team up to offer a continuing education initiative. It was designed both to provide clinicians with the latest information on medical management of Type II diabetes but also to engage learners in developing practical diabetes protocols for their institution. In this case, the continuing education served as a vehicle for bringing people together for institutional change.

4.0. COMPETENCIES FOR URBAN HEALTH PROFESSIONALS

Defining an intellectual framework for urban health and developing appropriate pedagogical methods for teaching this framework set the stage for identifying specific competencies for urban health professionals. Some competencies are required for all categories of workers; others are appropriate for particular groups such as clinicians, public health personnel, managers and researchers. Once again, the discussion here focuses on the competencies needed to address the urban context; they supplement the additional professional competencies that each discipline requires.

4.1. Generic Urban Health Competencies

All urban health professionals should be able to explain the various theories and evidence on how city living affects health, describe multiple levels of influence on health behavior and health status, identify the contributions of various disciplines and professions to urban health research and intervention, explain the influence of class, ethnicity, culture and gender, among others, on health, and communicate effectively with people of different backgrounds. In addition, since the content of health sciences is constantly changing, students need to learn how to find information using available technologies.

4.2. Competencies for Urban Clinicians

Physicians, nurses, dentists, psychologists, and other urban clinicians should be able to describe how different types and levels of exposure to urban living conditions affect well-being. Depending on their discipline and specialty area, they should also be able to explain how urban living influences the clinical course and management of common illnesses (e.g., asthma, depression, hypertension, diabetes, influenza), characterize significant disparities in health within urban populations, and explain the roles of health providers in reducing such disparities, identify sources of formal and informal social support for health promotion and disease management for their patients and their families, find community resources to assist their patients to improve their health, connect their clinical practice to other levels of intervention that improve community health (e.g., support community campaigns to increase access to healthy food and safe places to exercise), and advocate for health and other policies that will improve the health of their patients.

4.3. Competencies for Urban Public Health Professionals

Public health professionals working in cities should be able to identify the social determinants of the health and health behavior of residents and develop multilevel interventions to mitigate or reverse health-damaging urban conditions or behaviors (Geronimus, 2000). They should be also be able to conduct comprehensive assessments of the health of urban communities, describe the interactions between the urban physical and social environments, and explain the roles and responsibilities of various municipal sectors (e.g., education, welfare, criminal justice, sanitation, environmental protection) in health and their relationship to the public health system. Finally, they should be able to mobilize diverse urban constituencies to promote health and prevent disease at the community, municipal and regional levels.

4.4. Competencies for Urban Health Managers and Administrators

Managers of urban health agencies should be able to identify and apply for support from the funding streams that support health care and public health, plan, implement and evaluate urban health programs, interact effectively with different municipal sectors and systems, understand how urban politics affects operation of health and public health systems, and work in coalitions and networks to achieve their institutional objectives.

4.5. Competencies for Urban Health Researchers

Urban health researchers should be able to frame meaningful questions on how city living affects health and how to intervene to improve the well-being of urban populations. They should also be able to design and implement studies to answer these questions and to evaluate the impact of interventions. Researchers should be able to use multiple quantitative and qualitative methods and to work effectively on multidisciplinary research teams) to study the health of urban populations; they should be capable of integrating and synthesizing findings from different types of research. They should be able to describe the history of urban health research and main findings from previous studies of the differences between urban and rural health, among different cities and types of cities, and among different populations or neighborhoods within cities. They should know how to keep abreast of current research developments and controversies in public health. Urban health researchers should be able to use participatory and community-based research methods. Finally, researchers should be able to find financial support for their studies.

4.6. Evaluation of Urban Health Competencies

Evaluation of educational programs enables faculty, administrators, student and employers to determine whether the identified competencies have been achieved. While traditional evaluation methods of testing and writing papers are often used, other approaches deserve consideration. Some academic programs have introduced "capstone projects" that require students to synthesize knowledge and competencies and to demonstrate mastery of critical skills. Others have employed a portfolio approach, in which students assemble different types of evidence including clinical or community reports, academic papers, journals and program plans (Gordon, 2003; Scholes, *et al.*, 2004). While capstone projects and portfolios require more time and faculty resources to evaluate, they may be more suitable to the assessment of the ecological, interdisciplinary, and cross-cultural competencies urban health professionals are expected to develop.

In summary, urban health professionals need the competencies to use multilevel and multidisciplinary methods, to communicate across boundaries and systems, and to operate effectively in scientific, organizational and political arenas. They also need to know how and where to find the financial, human and scientific resources needed to address recurring and emerging urban public health issues. The competencies proposed here derive from our reading of the literature and our own experience. As such, they constitute a work in progress, the opening of a dialogue, rather than a prescriptive mandate. Their ultimate value lies in their contribution to the development of curricula and programs that can educate competent urban health professionals.

5.0. INSTITUTIONAL CHANGE

To produce the health professionals needed to create healthier cities will require institutional as well as pedagogical and intellectual transformations. Among the institutions that will need to change are universities, professional accreditation bodies, and health departments. A brief review of the structures and processes now used to address the education of urban health professionals within these institutions helps to identify possible targets for reform.

5.1. Universities and Professional Training Programs

Currently, universities use various organizational forms to focus institutional resources on urban health. These include traditional academic departments, special interdisciplinary programs, research/service centers, and more informal collaboratives and networks. Each form has unique advantages and disadvantages. In this section, we describe each of these forms briefly, provide two examples and highlight some of the strengths and weaknesses.

Academic departments in urban health prepare health professionals to work in urban settings. Two previously mentioned examples are the PhD program in urban health at South Bank University in London and the Masters of Public Health in Urban Health at Hunter College, City University of New York. The South Bank degree attracts students from both developed and developing nations and takes about three years to complete. Its faculty are based in several disciplines and students are expected to involve faculty from different disciplines in their dissertation research (Harpham, personal communication, 2004). The Hunter program prepares Masters level public health professionals for urban practice, with a focus on meeting the needs of the New York metropolitan region. Affiliations with more than one hundred agencies, including local and state health departments, offices of local elected officials, other municipal agencies, hospitals, health centers, voluntary and advocacy health associations, for-profit consulting groups, and community-based organizations provide students with opportunities for field work, internships and independent study in diverse urban settings. Most courses require some field assignments, e.g., students in the required public health policy course interview an urban elected officials or public health advocates; those in the community organization for health course volunteer with a community-based or health advocacy group for some organizational tasks in exchange for access to the group for a required semester paper. The MPH program has close ties with the local municipal health department – more than a fifth of its recent graduates are employed there and several faculty members sit on health department advisory boards or expert panels, faculty conduct research and intervention studies in partnership with or funded by the health department, and several senior managers are graduates of the Hunter academic program. No Hunter student graduates without multiple encounters with the health department: using its data and technical reports for class assignments, interviewing health department staff, completing field placements at its facilities, or working in a group on a class project with other students employed by the health department.

To achieve the interdisciplinary perspectives needed for urban health practice, the Hunter program uses several methods to expose its students to various disciplines and professions. A third of the courses include students from the three specialization tracks, community health education, nutrition and environmental and occupational health sciences, requiring students to work together and learn from each other. Many courses also include students from nursing, urban planning and social science doctoral programs. MPH students also have the opportunity to take elective courses in these and other departments within the larger City University. Finally, the 16 full-time faculty have graduate degrees in several disciplines, including public health, epidemiology, nutrition, food sciences, physics, biochemistry, environmental sciences, health education, social psychology, anthropology, and human ecology.

What are the advantages of a department or program in urban health? Perhaps most importantly, this structure provides an academic home for the field, allowing the unit to hire, promote, and tenure faculty based on criteria that can take into account the special needs of urban health such as disciplinary diversity and applied research (Harpham, 2004; Vlahov and Galea, 2003). Urban health researchers in more traditional departments sometimes report that their chairs complain of "disciplinary drift" or research interests that are "too broad". In addition, focused urban health departments can recruit the type of students they want, plan and implement their own curricula, and attain the status of a university department or program, often the prerequisite for resources and prestige in academic settings.

Within schools or programs in public health, medicine, or other disciplines, an "urban health" unit may also help to break down the barriers among the various specialization areas. In many schools of public health, for example, students and faculty from epidemiology, environmental health, and health education rarely study or teach together, making it more difficult for students to integrate these approaches in professional practice. An urban health unit can help to model such integration.

The disadvantages of this structure are that creation of a department or program often requires significant time and effort and may encounter opposition from other disciplines that fear encroachment on their turf (Guyer and Gibbons, 2004). Moreover, few institutions have the range of expertise to offer separate degrees in urban health. Finally, some health researchers and social scientists question whether "urban health" is a sufficiently robust or developed concept to warrant its own department (Guyer and Gibbons, 2004). Choosing this path in the face of such opposition may diminish the likelihood of success.

An alternative approach to the creation of a separate department or program is to create a dual degree program or a sub-program within an existing department. Several U.S. universities offer dual degrees in urban planning and public health, in effect creating urban health specialists. At the University of North Carolina in Chapel Hill, for example, students can pursue a dual degree in city and regional planning and public health. In this program, planning students learn about "the public health impacts of planning and how public health professionals can be allies in achieving shared goals" while public health students learn "how to shape the physical and social urban community in health-enhancing ways. This combination of skills will help forge broader and more powerful alliances that promote public health, safety and livability in American communities." (Program in City and Regional Planning at University of North Carolina – Chapel Hill, 2003).

Still another option is to combine related academic programs into a single unit that enables interdisciplinary collaboration. At Portland State University, for example, the schools of government, urban studies and planning, and community health joined to form the College of Urban and Public Affairs. The College works closely with local and state government and encourages collaborative research on the issues facing the Portland metropolitan region (College of Urban and Public Affairs, 2003).

5.2. Centers or Institutes on Urban Health

Other universities have chosen to create institutes or centers on urban health. These organizations usually include researchers and sometimes practitioners from several disciplines, conduct research and service projects within urban settings, and often offer continuing education, academic courses, and fieldwork opportunities. Unlike academic departments, they usually do not offer degrees or academic tenure to their faculty. Often, they rely heavily on grants and contracts for financial support, making them vulnerable to the vagaries of funding fashions. The focus of the discussion here is on the role of urban health centers in the education of urban health personnel.

For example, The Johns Hopkins University's Urban Health Institute (UHI), was created in 2000 with support from virtually all the schools that constitute the university, based in part on the advice of the Urban Health Council, an advisory group representing community, university and local government constituencies. The UHI's mission is "to marshal the resources of the Johns Hopkins Institutions as well as other external resources to improve the health and well-being of the residents of East Baltimore and Baltimore City and to promote evidence-based interventions to solve urban health problems nationwide." (Urban Health Initiative, 2002). The Institute serves as a focal point for the establishment of participatory research studies that bring together university faculty and staff with community organizations to define and carry out studies to improve community health. It organizes community-based service learning opportunities for Hopkins students in various disciplines and it offer courses on urban health for students at different levels in several disciplines.

A second example is the World Health Organization's Collaborating Centre for Urban Health, a partnership that includes the School of Public Health at the University of Witwatersrand, the Health and Development Research Group at the Medical Research Council of South Africa, and the Greater Johannesburg Metropolitan Council. The Centre participates in international Healthy Cities projects, sponsors research projects on urban health and offers special courses on urban health. For example, in partnership with the University of the Western Cape, the Centre offered a 2-week course on urbanization and health, designed for public health workers from around Africa (Centre for Urban Health, 2000).

The Center for Urban Epidemiological Studies (CUES) at the New York Academy of Medicine illustrates yet another approach. Although CUES is primarily a research rather than a teaching institution, it offers placements to students from various disciplines at many levels of education. By providing students with the opportunity to participate in multidisciplinary, multilevel research and intervention studies, it exposes them to the practice of urban health and supplements the gaps in education at a variety of universities (CUES, 2004).

Centers offer several organizational advantages for addressing urban health. Their express purpose is to meet needs and seize opportunities not addressed by traditional academic departments. They are thus more flexible and often more open to interdisciplinary approaches and Center activities are also less likely to elicit hostile reactions from turf-defending departments. For educators, centers also provide opportunities to offer courses that transcend traditional boundaries. Urban health centers have offered continuing education courses for practicing professionals, certificates for community health workers, special programs for high school students, and seminars for researchers and doctoral students. This ability to operate at several educational levels in a variety of settings simultaneously – a capacity most academic departments lack – provides centers the ability to address urban health problems, e.g., expanding HIV testing and counseling or improving asthma or diabetes self-management capacity, rapidly and comprehensively.

Centers may also be a useful vehicle for faculty development in urban health. The Institute for Urban Health Research at Northeastern University in Boston, for example, provides research support to faculty from throughout the university who want to begin research in urban health. The Center provides release time from teaching, consultation with faculty in other disciplines, access to research staff, and availability of mentoring with senior faculty (Amaro, personal communication; Institute on Urban Health Research, 2003).

The disadvantages of centers are the mirror image of their strengths. Their reliance on soft money, their location on the periphery of academia, and their focus on the application of research to emerging issues often make it difficult for centers to sustain their efforts or to become institutionalized within the fabric of higher education. Centers have a shorter average life span than academic departments and may not be able to make long term commitments to preparing the urban health professionals needed in coming decades.

5.3. Collaboratives and Networks

Less formal than departments or centers are urban health collaboratives or networks. These groupings bring together researchers, teachers, staff and students with interest in urban health from different disciplines to exchange information, develop common research or intervention projects, or plan courses. The City University of New York Urban Health Collaborative (UHC), for example, brings together faculty, staff and students from more than a dozen departments at CUNY's 16 campuses. For the last three years, the UHC sponsored a faculty development seminar that brought together 50-75 faculty five or six times a year to explore topics of common interest such as developing multidisciplinary research methods in urban health or exploring the links between urban health and social justice. These sessions enabled faculty, who rarely had the opportunity for intellectual discussions, with faculty from such diverse disciplines to exchange ideas, learns new approaches, and, on several occasions, to meet colleagues who then became research partners. The Collaborative created a list serve that eventually included more than 200 individuals within CUNY and distributed each semester a schedule and description of CUNY courses related to urban health at the different campuses. The UHC Steering Committee also planned the previously described MPH-PhD pathway program and successfully convinced the University administration to approve a "cluster hire" of several new tenure track faculty with interests in environmental and urban health.

This approach has the advantage of requiring only modest resources and having an open structure that allows a wide range of participants to select varying levels of involvement. Its informal structure allows human resources to be dedicated to intellectual rather than administrative pursuits and it does not necessarily require approval from university or departmental administrators. The limitations of this approach are that it lacks the resources, institutional commitment, or prestige needed to make long-term changes in curricula, degrees, or faculty hiring and tenure practices. Its reliance on mostly volunteer participation limits its ability to provide high level coordination to the disparate activities related to urban health that occur within many universities.

In summary, universities have a variety of organizational structures through which to plan and carry out education for urban health. Each has distinct benefits and constraints and some institutions may use more than one approach. The collaborative model, for example, could serve as a starting point for planning a center or a new academic program in urban health. Faculty interested in developing education in urban health at their institution need to identify unmet urban health workforce needs in their region (see the next section), inventory the intellectual and financial resources that are available, assess the available level of administrative and external support for various options, then set realistic goals for the institutional change that will best support their objectives.

5.4. Accrediting Bodies

Most health professional educational programs are accredited by one or more accrediting organizations. These bodies set standards for curriculum, faculty credentials, student admissions procedures, and other educational and administrative tasks. Most identify specific educational competencies that students in a particular degree program are expected to achieve. In recent decades, these accrediting organizations have played a growing role in shaping health professional education.

They influence the education of urban health professionals in several ways. On the positive side, accreditation helps to set standards and ensure the quality of educational programs. It provides both graduates and their employers with some assurances that students have learned what professional leaders have determined to be the important concepts and skills.

On the other hand, existing accreditation guidelines can cause problems for urban health education. Many accrediting agencies mandate a significant portion of the curriculum, leaving students limited options for pursuing an interest such as urban health or taking several courses in a second discipline. Some accreditors require all or most courses to be taught by faculty with a doctorate in the discipline (e.g. nursing, law, or social work), reducing a department's ability to hire the interdisciplinary faculty suited to urban health. Accrediting agencies may also set admissions requirements, limiting entry to the field to students from disadvantaged backgrounds or making it more difficult to recruit the diversity needed for an adequate urban health workforce. While accreditation guidelines may state the value of diverse students, their procedures usually focus on non-discriminatory admissions procedures, a far narrower conception of the issue.

Finally, in recent years, some health accrediting bodies have raised the requirements for entry into the professions from a Bachelors degree to a Masters or even a clinical doctorate (e.g., physical therapy, audiology, and pharmacology). While the expressed intention of these increasing requirements is to improve quality of care, some observers fear that this inflation of credentials may limit access to care, especially for low income urban populations, increase the costs of care and exclude from professional training programs those most likely to practice in underserved urban areas.

To ensure that requirements for accreditation help to improve the quality of services without serving as an obstacle to meeting the workforce needs of urban areas, urban health professionals, faculty, researchers and policy makers should raise this issue for discussion within their accrediting and professional organizations. Recent reports by the Institute of Medicine identifying the need for new competencies for 21st century health professionals provide a positive model for revisiting credentialing standards. Topics the IOM suggested for additional emphasis in public health professional education included the importance of ecological, multilevel models, community-based participatory research, opportunities for supervised fieldwork and cultural competence, all key areas within urban health (Committee on Educating Public Health Professionals for the 21st Century, 2003). By joining or testifying before national, state, and local bodies reviewing health professional education, urban health professionals can help to make accreditation standards a positive force for change.

5.5. Departments of Health

Urban departments of health are a primary consumer of the products of health educational programs, i.e., health professionals, and they are also the bodies accountable for the health of urban populations. Thus, they are key stakeholders in the development of the urban health workforce. To date, however, municipal health departments have not had a defined role or a strong voice in professional education. More often, their role has been limited to providing internships, sponsoring continuing education for their employees (Potter, *et al.*, 2003), or helping to coordinate the educational responses to emerging needs, e.g., the HIV epidemic or bioterrorism.

In our view, health departments could play a more central role in the education of urban health professionals, both by contributing more to preservice education, as recommended in the IOM report on the Future of Public Health (Committee on Assuring the Health of the Public, 2003), and by playing a lead role in conducting comprehensive assessments of urban health workforce needs. While local health departments cannot and should not take on this task single handedly, they are the sole agency with accountability for population health and with the mandate and capacity to collect the data needed to identify current and emerging needs. Other stakeholders that need to be involved in such assessments are educational institutions including high schools, community and four-year colleges, research universities and the various health professional training programs, local health care providers, community representatives, and elected officials. The London Health Policy and Research Resources (Health Workforce Policy and Research Resource for London, 2003), described below, provides one example of a collaborative approach to assessing urban health workforce needs.

6.0. ASSESSING URBAN HEALTH WORKFORCE AND EDUCATIONAL NEEDS

The education of urban health professionals is shaped by the existing intellectual and conceptual frameworks for urban health, by the pedagogical approaches that educators employ and by the requirements of accrediting bodies and the structure of schools and programs of various disciplines. Another critical influence comes from assessments of workforce needs. In any given time and place, the content and structure of urban health workforce education results from the interactions of these influences.

In the last several years, health planners have developed new methods for assessing the workforce needs of a region (Kennedy and Moore, 2001; Chauvin, *et al.*, 2001). Some of these assessments take place at the national level (Gebbie, 1999) but those that look specifically at urban health usually focus on smaller regions or municipalities. In general, the approach is to inventory existing health personnel, and using empirical or theoretical standards, identify either types of personnel or geographic areas that are experiencing shortages, and then recommend changes in educational programs to meet these needs (Gebbie, 1999; Fraser, 2003). Ironically, despite the concentration of the U.S. population and ill health in metropolitan regions and especially central cities, health workforce issues in rural areas have attracted more attention in the literature than have urban workforce needs (Rosenblatt, *et al.*, 2002).

An example from London, England, shows one approach to workforce needs assessment. Ongoing problems with recruitment and retention of health professionals led to the creation of the Health Workforce Policy and Research Resource for London (2003). Its goals are to analyze the unique dynamics of the city health labor force and to make specific recommendations for meeting unmet and emerging needs. Participants in the process include five local London Workforce Development Confederations, a network of London human resource managers, the Health and Social Care Directorate, and the King's Fund, a philanthropic organization. Among the recommendations are the establishment of "skills escalator" training programs in which health staff can add skills throughout their career and move into new positions as they acquire the necessary competencies (Factsheet on Work Force Development, 2003)

Another type of assessment looks at the unique needs of a specific community or population. In low-income urban areas such assessments often find shortages of specific types of personnel such as primary care practitioners. In the U.S. such a finding can lead to the designation of a medically underserved area, making institutions eligible for certain types of federal support and graduates who choose to work in these areas able to apply for cancellation of loans for medical education. At a higher policy level, these findings can lead educational institutions to establish special programs to meet these needs. At City University of New York, for example, the Sophie Davis Biomedical Center was created to increase the supply of physicians willing to work in under-served urban communities (Geiger, 1980)

An ongoing challenge is to identify who has responsibility for undertaking this task; failure to identify a lead agency may lead to many uncoordinated assessment projects where institutional imperatives rather than regional needs drive decisions about education and workforce policy.

7.0. CONCLUSION

This review has suggested priorities for the education of urban health professionals. First, researchers, practitioners and policy makers need to define the scope of the field of urban health and encourage the development of theories, models and concepts that bring together the diverse disciplines working to improve the health of urban populations. Second, universities and other training programs should broaden the diversity of the students they educate to be urban health professionals and the faculty who teach them. Third, teachers should continue to develop pedagogical strategies uniquely suited to developing the competencies that urban health professionals will need to master. Fourth, universities need to consider various organizational frameworks for teaching urban health and select the options that best match their resources and mission and meet the personnel needs of the region they serve. Finally, universities, health departments and accrediting agencies need to identify new opportunities for collaboration to create the health workforce needed to improve the health of urban populations in the 21st century.

REFERENCES

American College of Physicians. (1997). Inner-city health care. *Ann. Intern. Med.* 127:485–490.

Boufford, J.I., and Shonubi, P.A. (1986). Community-Oriented Primary Care Training for Urban Practice. Praeger, New York, NY.

Bowen, W.G., and Bok, D. (2000). *The Shape of the River.* Princeton University Press, Princeton, NJ.

Burns, E.R. (2002). Anatomy of a successful K-12 educational outreach program in the health sciences: eleven years experience at one medical sciences campus. *Anat. Rec.* 269(4):181–93.

Center for Urban Epidemiological Studies (CUES), 2003, New York, (August 24, 2004); http://www.nyam.org/initiatives/cues-training.shtml

Centre for Urban Health, Medical Research Council, 2000, South Africa, (June 21, 2004); http://www.mrc.ac.za/urbanbulletin/december2000/course.htm.

Chauvin, S.W., Anderson, A.C., and Bowdish, B.E. (2001). Assessing the professional development needs of public health professionals. *Journal of Public Health Management and Practice.* 7(4):23–37.

College of Urban and Public Affairs, Portland State University, (2003). Oregon, (July 6, 2004); http://www.upa.pdx.edu/schools.htm.

Committee on Assuring the Health of the Public in the 21st Century (2003) *Future of the Public's Health in the 21st Century.* National Academy Press, Washington D.C.

Committee on Educating Public Health Professionals for the 21st Century. (2003) *Who will keep the public healthy? Educating public health professionals for the 21st Century.* National Academy Press, Washington D.C.

Corburn, J. (2004) Confronting the challenges in reconnecting urban planning and public health *Am. J. Public Health* 94:541–6.

Diez-Roux, A. V. (2000). Multilevel analysis in public health research. *Annu. Rev. Public Health 21:*171-192.

Duhl, L., and Hancock T. (1988). *Health in an Urban Setting*. WHO Europe, Copenhagen, Denmark

Educational Testing Service. (2004).Toward Inequality: Disturbing Trends in Higher Education, (July 5, 2004); http://www.ets.org/research/pic/twsec4.html

Eisinger, A.A., Viruell-Fuentes, E.A., Gheisar, B., Palermo, A.G., and Softley, D. (2003). Addressing urban health in Detroit, New York City, and Seattle through community-based participatory research partnerships. *Am. J. Public Health* 93(5):803–11.

Eng, E., and Young, R. (1992). Lay health advisers as community change agents. *J. Family and Comm. Health* 15:24–40.

Factsheet on Workforce Development (2003). United Kingdom. (June 24, 2004) http:// www.kingsfund.org. uk/pdf/workforce_factsheet.pdf

Fraser, M.R. (2003). The local public health agency workforce: research needs and practice realities. *J. Public Health Manag. Pract.* 9(6): 496–9.

Frumkin, H. (2002). Urban sprawl and public health. *Public Health Rep.* 117:201–217.

Galea, S., Freudenberg, N., and Vlahov, D. (2005). Cities and population health *Soc. Sci. Med.* 60(5):1017–1033.

Gebbie, K.M. (1999). The public health workforce: key to public health infrastructure. *Am. J. Public Health* 89:660– 661.

Geiger, H.J. (1980) Sophie Davis School of Biomedical Education at City College of New York prepares primary care physicians for practice in underserved inner-city areas. *Public Health Rep.* 95(1):32–7.

Gemson, D.H., Ashford, A.R., Dickey, L.L., Raymore, S.H., Roberts, J.W., Ehrlich, M.H., Foster, B.G., Ganz, M.L., Moon-Howard, J., and Field, L.S. (1995). Putting prevention into practice. Impact of a multifaceted physician education program on preventive services in the inner city. *Arch. Intern. Med.* 155(20):2210–6.

Geronimus, A.T. (2000). To mitigate, resist, or undo: addressing structural influences on the health of urban populations. *Am. J. Public Health* 90(6):867–72.

Gordon, J. (2003). Assessing students' personal and professional development using portfolios and interviews. *Med. Educ.* 37(4):335–40.

Guyer, B., and Gibbons, M.C. (2004). Urban health—discipline or field – does it matter? *J. Urban Health* 81:165–167.

Harpham, T. (2004). Urban health: a future focus for career development *J. Urban Health* 81:168.

Health Workforce Policy and Research Resource for London. (2003). United Kindom, (June 24, 2004); http://www.kingsfund.org.uk/HealthCarePolicy/health_workforce.html.

Healton, C.G. (1999). The shape of our river. *Am. J. Prev Med.* 116(3 Suppl):1–4.

Institute on Urban Health Research.(2003). Northeastern University. (September 17,2004) http://www.iuhr.neu.edu/

Kennedy, V.C., and Moore, F.I. (2001). A systems approach to public health workforce development. *J. Public Health Mana. Prac.* 7(4): 7–22.

Krieger, N. (2000). Epidemiology and social sciences: towards a critical re-engagement in the 21st century. *Epidemiol Rev.* 11:155–163.

Komaromy, M., Grumbach, K., Drake, M., Vranizan, K., Lurie, N., Keane, D., and Bindman, A.B. (1996). The role of black and Hispanic physicians in providing health care for underserved populations. *N. Engl J. Med.* 334(20):1305–10.

Lapierre, J., Perreault, M., and Goulet, C.(1995). Prenatal peer counseling: an answer to the persistent difficulties with prenatal care for low-income women. *Public Health Nurs.* 12(1):53–60.

Lawrence, R.J. (2002). Inequalities in urban areas: innovative approaches to complex issues. *Scan. J. Public Health* 30:34–40

Lawrence, R.J. (1999). Urban health: an ecological perspective. *Rev. Environ. Health 14*(1):1–10.

Lichtveld, M.Y., Cioffi, J.P., Baker, E.L. Jr., Bailey, S.B., Gebbie, K., Henderson, J.V., Jones,D.L., Kurz, R.S., Margolis, S., Miner, K., Thielen, L., and Tilson, H.(2001). Partnership for front-line success: a call for a national action agenda on workforce development. *J. Public Health Manag. Pract.*7(4):1–7.

Logan, N.S. (1997). Promoting the recruitment and retention of minority faculty. *J. Dent. Educ.* 61(3):273–6.

Metzler, M.M., Higgins, D.L., Beeker, C.G., Freudenberg, N., Lantz, P.M., Senturia, K.D., Northridge, M., Sclar, E., and Biswas, P.(2003). Sorting out the connections between the built environment and health: a conceptual framework for navigating pathways and planning healthy cities. *J. Urban Health* 80(4):556–68

Palepu, A., Carr, P.L., Friedman, R.H., Amos, H., Ash, A.S., and Moskowitz, M.A. (1998). Minority faculty and academic rank in medicine. *JAMA.* 280(9):767–71.

Pathman, D.E., Taylor, D.H. Jr., Konrad, T.R., King, T.S., Harris, T., Henderson, T.M., Bernstein, J.D., Tucker, T., Crook, K.D., Spaulding, C., and Koch, G.G. (2000). State scholarship, loan forgiveness, and related programs: the unheralded safety net. *JAMA.* 284(16):2084–92.

Pennsylvania and Ohio Public Health Training Center. (2003). Training Curriculum. (June 22, 2004); http://www.pophtc.pitt.edu.

Potter, M.A., Ley, C.E., Fertman, C.I., Eggleston, M.M., and Duman, S. (2003). Evaluating workforce development: Perspectives, processes and lessons learned. *J. Public Health Manag. Pract.* 9:489–495.

Program in Public Health and Planning, University of North Carolina (2003), Chapel Hill, (July 6, 2004); http://www.planning.unc. edu/program/jointHealth.htm.

Rosenblatt, R.A., Casey, S., and Richardon, M. (2002). Rural-urban differences in the public health workforce: Local health departments in 3 rural Western states *Am. J. Public Health* 92:1102–5.

Scholes, J., Webb, C., Gray, M., Endacott, R., Miller, C., Jasper, M., and McMullan, M. Making portfolios work in practice. *J. Adv. Nurs.* 46(6):595–603.

Shiber, S. (1999). Expanding urban learning experiences for non-traditional students. *Public Health Nurs.* 16:228–232.

Stokols, D., Fuqua, J., Gress, J., Harvey, R., Phillips, K., Baezconde-Garbanati, L., Unger, J., Palmer, P., Clark, M.A., Colby, S.M., Morgan, G., and Trochim, W. (2003). Evaluating transdisciplinary science. *Nicotine Tob. Res.* 5(Suppl 1):S21–S39.

Tekian, A. (2000). Minority students, affirmative action, and the admission process: a literature review, 1987-1998. *Teach. Learn. Med.* 12(1):33–42.

Thurmond, V.B., and Kirch, D.G. (1998). Impact of minority physicians on health care. *South Med J.* 91(11):1009– 13.

UIC Urban Health Program, 2004, New York, (September 17, 2004) http://www.med.uiuc.edu/sa/uhp/).

University of Illinois-Urbana Champaign, 2004, Illinois, (June 24, 2004); http://www.med.uiuc.edu/sa/uhp/The%20Urban%20Health%20Program%20at%20UIUC.htm.

University of Western Cape. (2000). Republic of South Africa, (June 24, 2004); http://www.mrc.ac.za/urbanbulletin/december2000/course.htm

Urban Health Institute, Johns Hopkins University, 2002, Baltimore, MD, (June 21, 2004); http://www.hopkinsmedicine.org/community/urbanhealth.html.

Vlahov, D., and Galea, S. (2002). Urbanization, urbanicity, and health. *J. Urban Health* (79 Suppl 1):S1–S12.

Vlahov, D., and Galea, S. (2003). Urban health: a new discipline. *Lancet.* 362(9390):1091-2.

Wright, S.M., Carrese, J.A. (2003). Serving as a physician role model for a diverse population of medical learners. *Acad Med.* 78(6):623–8.

Yu, M., Hawley, C., and Towns, A.B. (1997). A year-long longitudinal third-year clerkship in an inner-city health center designed to maximize continuity. *Acad Med.* 72(5):439–40

Zuvekas, A., Nolan, L., Tumaylle, C., and Griffin, L. (1999). Impact of community health workers on access, use of services, and patient knowledge and behavior. *J. Ambul. Care Manage.* 22:33–44.

Chapter 27

Strategies that Promote Health in Cities

A Local Health Department's Perspective

Mary T. Bassett, Thomas R. Frieden, Deborah R. Deitcher, and Thomas D. Matte

1.0. INTRODUCTION

The health of those living and working in a city is influenced by many factors: the physical, social, and economic environment; access to quality medical care; availability of lucid, understandable health information; presence of programs that promote health; and adoption, by individuals, of healthy behaviors. While these factors deserve consideration in any locale, urban or otherwise, they present considerable challenges for the urban public health practitioner. Deteriorating housing stock in older, urban neighborhoods – with its concomitant peeling paint and pest infestations – has implications for lead poisoning control and asthma management (Leighton, *et al.*, 2003; Rosenstreich, *et al.*, 1997). The relative dearth of outdoor recreation areas and the perception that urban parks are unsafe discourage physical activity (Estabrooks, *et al.*, 2003; Parks, *et al.*, 2003), and thus may be associated with greater risk of disease. The clustering of new immigrant populations in urban areas presents language and cultural challenges that affect health care delivery and health education efforts (Kandula, *et al.*, 2004). And poverty itself – a defining characteristic of vulnerable urban populations (Geronimus, 2000) – is strongly associated with decreased life expectancy (Lin, *et al.*, 2003; Wong, *et al.*, 2002). Strategies that promote health in cities must consider these and other variables to succeed.

This chapter's focus is the role of a municipal health department in setting and implementing an urban health agenda, specifically drawing on the experiences and approach of the New York City Department of Health and Mental Hygiene (DOHMH). Several relevant DOHMH health promotion efforts are also described.

2.0. SETTING THE AGENDA: THE ROLE OF THE MUNICIPAL HEALTH DEPARTMENT.

While acute, communicable diseases once accounted for most illness and death in the U.S., today's leading public health concerns are largely chronic and noncommunicable. As a result, the roles of health departments nationwide are shifting – albeit slowly. While still responsible for such traditional public health functions as investigating outbreaks, disease surveillance, diagnosing and treating tuberculosis and sexually transmitted diseases, and enforcing laws and regulations that protect health and ensure safety, health agencies are now confronted with the need to develop and implement an agenda responsive to the current burden of disease. Reasons for the slow embrace of a chronic disease action plan are many: (1) chronic diseases do not present as crises, and given their long latency periods, it is difficult to generate enthusiasm for interventions with few short-term impacts; (2) the public is more concerned about involuntary (e.g., living next to a hazardous waste site) than what are perceived as voluntary (e.g., smoking) risks; (3) many local health agencies do not have chronic disease and risk factor surveillance systems necessary for identifying priorities and evaluating interventions; and (4) insufficient resources have been made available for chronic disease prevention efforts (Brownson, *et al.*, 2004).

In recent years, the DOHMH has intensified its efforts to create and set into motion an urban health agenda responsive to the needs and concerns of the city's residents – a large component of which is devoted to chronic disease prevention and control activities. Below we discuss the steps taken and factors considered in developing and implementing this agenda.

2.1. Identify Public Health Needs and Affected Populations

New York City's health agenda is a response to the burden of disease of its populace. Priority setting is data driven, informed by morbidity, mortality and risk factor data – and complemented by community perceptions about health and causes of disease. In New York City, a unique data source is the Community Health Survey, a neighborhood-level adaptation and enhancement of the Behavioral Risk Factor Surveillance System (BRFSS), which has been conducted annually since 2002. The distribution of disease and risk factors for disease also shapes the agenda, with resources directed at communities and population groups disproportionately affected. In developing an action plan, emphasis has been placed on high-burden conditions that are amenable to prevention efforts, i.e., those health problems for which evidence-based interventions exist.

As an example of how data can inform the establishment of public health priorities, consider New York City mortality data. Cardiovascular disease, followed by cancer, are the city's leading killers, accounting for, respectively, 41.1% and 23.0% of all deaths in 2002. Many of these deaths can be directly attributed to cigarette smoking, which kills approximately 10,000 New Yorkers per year, making it the leading preventable cause of death. A further examination of these mortality data reveals, for example, that for both heart disease and colon cancer, black New Yorkers die at younger ages than white New Yorkers (Figure 1, Figure 2), which may indicate missed opportunities for prevention, early detection and treatment among blacks. Similar patterns can be detected when examining another leading cause of death among New Yorkers – HIV/AIDS. While mortality rates have been declining over time, differences among racial/ethnic and income groups exist

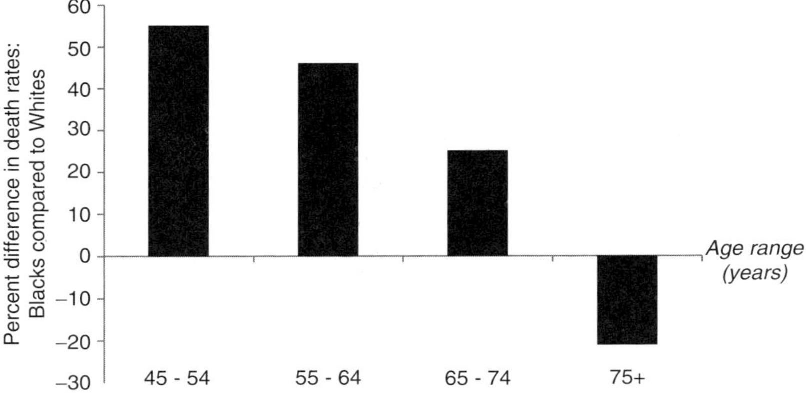

Sources: Bureau of Vital Statistics, NYC DOHMH, 1999-2001; U.S. Census 2000/NYC Department of City Planning.

Figure 1. Racial Disparities in Cardiovascular Disease Mortality, New York City.

(Figure 3), with blacks and those living in very low-income neighborhoods most likely to die from AIDS – perhaps reflecting differential access to life-prolonging medical treatment (Karpati, *et al.*, 2004). Data such as these help establish priorities, determine intervention strategies and identify populations and neighborhoods to be targeted.

2.2. Promote Evidence-Based Interventions

Tackling priority health concerns requires an appreciation of the conditions that underlie them. For example, an examination of "actual" causes of death, i.e., external, modifiable factors that contribute to death, reveals that, in 2000, approximately half of all deaths in the U.S. could be attributed to largely preventable behaviors and exposures; heading the list were tobacco and poor diet/physical inactivity, accounting for 18.1% and 16.6% of all deaths nationwide, respectively (Mokdad, *et al.*, 2004). Thus, if the public health community hopes to have an impact on preventable deaths, effective interventions to address tobacco use, physical inactivity and poor diet are needed.

The Task Force on Community Preventive Services—a non-federal, independent panel of experts convened by the Centers for Disease Control and Prevention—is systematically reviewing the scientific literature to identify community interventions that are effective in promoting health and preventing disease (Truman, *et al.*, 2000). The product of this undertaking, *The Community Guide to Preventive Services,* found at www.thecommunityguide.org is a valuable resource to local health agencies engaged in developing health agendas and corresponding action plans. The DOHMH often consults the *Community Guide,* and its recommendations have been incorporated into community program planning efforts – resulting, for example, in enhanced physical activity programs in New York City schools and parks in at-risk communities and increased school-based dental sealant activities.

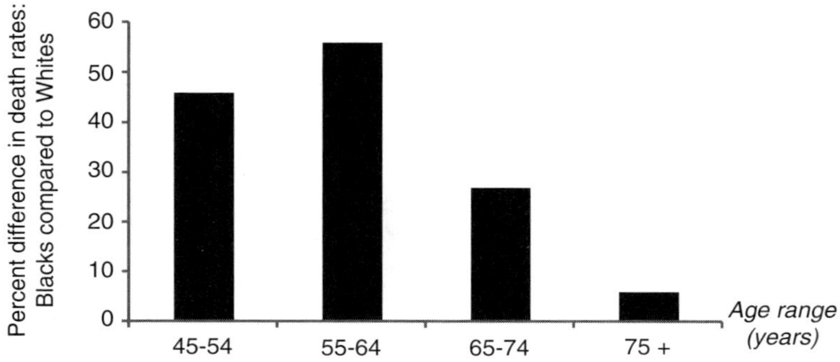

Sources: Bureau of Vital Statistics, NYC DOHMH, 1999-2001; U.S. Census 2000/NYC Department of City Planning

Figure 2. Racial Disparities in Colon Cancer Mortality, New York City.

2.3. Promote Coordination of Services

For an intervention to be successful, a coordinated effort is often required. In large urban areas where coordination can be complex, health departments can play an important convening role. Additionally, local health agencies need to look within and identify internal obstacles to providing a coordinated effort. Development and maintenance of an organizational culture that encourages cooperation and collaboration across programs is key (Brownson, *et al.*, 2004).

2.4. Foster Diverse Partnerships

Closely linked with coordinating services is the need to engage a diverse array of organizations – including community-based and nonprofit organizations, health care providers, faith-based organizations, businesses, unions, media, and local and state government – in the development and launch of often large, multi-faceted interventions. Involvement of many sectors of the community is believed to increase the likelihood of success for collaborative efforts (Israel, *et al.*, 2001). Also critical to the success of a partnership and the project it spearheads are a clearly articulated mission, strong leadership, a well-conceived action plan, and good communication (Kegler, *et al.*, 1998). Again, health departments – which often are experienced in coalition building and in working with communities to address health concerns – can assume a central role in fostering such partnerships and providing leadership; such a role is recommended by the National Public Health Performance Standards Program, a collaborative, CDC-initiated effort that has created performance standards for local public health systems found at www.phppo.cdc.gov/nphpsp.

2.5. Advocate for Broader Social and Economic Change

In the pursuit of population-wide health, there are many social and economic forces to be addressed, many of which are not within the exclusive purview of the local health department. Still, health departments can be important advocates for change. By arming communities with health data and facilitating community dialogue, local health systems can influence policy development, enabling informed

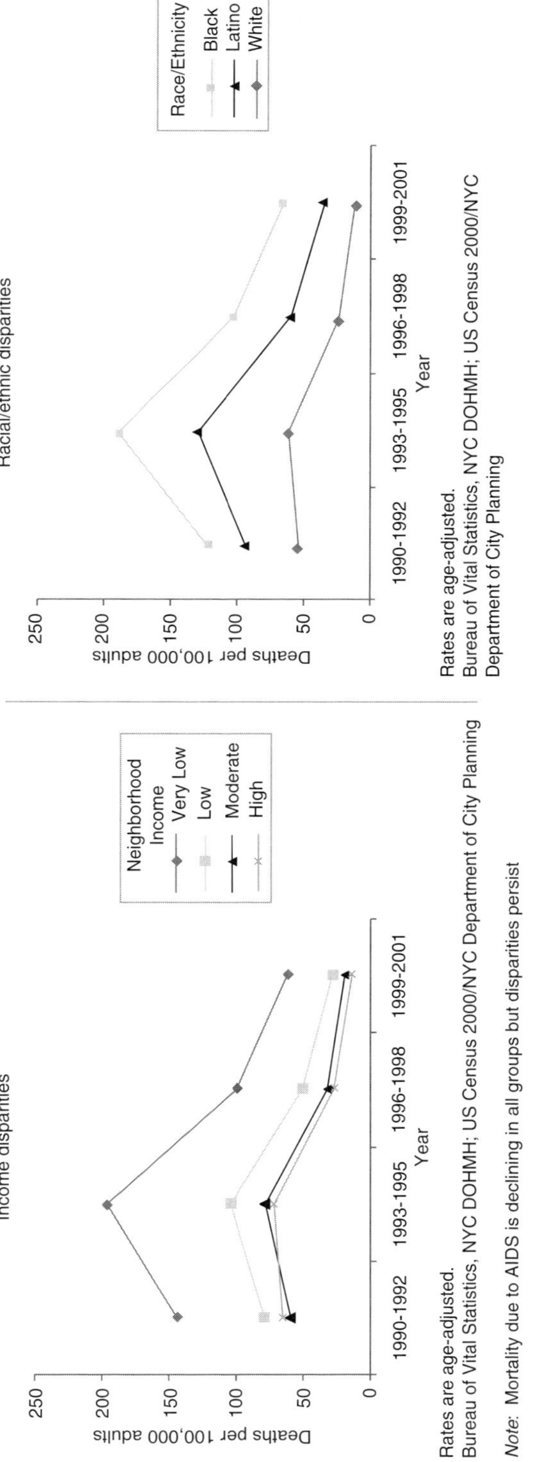

Figure 3. Income and Racial/Ethnic Disparities in AIDS Mortality, New York City.

decisions to be made concerning issues related to the public's health. Leading by example is another important role to be assumed by health departments. Through identifying and modeling best practices, health departments can shift attention (and ultimately, public investments) from acute medical care to broader measures aimed at protecting health and preventing disease – particularly targeting those populations that bear a disproportionate burden of morbidity and mortality. (Baxter, 1998)

3.0. NEW YORK CITY'S EXPERIENCE

Serving the most populous city in the U.S., the DOHMH's public health agenda is vast and varied. What follows are some examples of programs and initiatives that reflect the agency's commitment to evidence-based health promotion strategies that target a variety of sectors, including the health care setting, physical environment, schools, high-risk communities and the policy environment.

3.1. Strategies Directed at the Health Care Setting

In 2004, the DOHMH introduced Take Care New York (TCNY), an initiative that aims to prioritize areas of intervention for the agency – with an emphasis on prevention (www.nyc.gov/healh/tcny). While the scope of TCNY extends beyond the health care setting, encompassing businesses and community and non-profit organizations, one priority area is the clinical encounter as an opportunity for prevention. TCNY focuses on disseminating information on best practices to clinicians, equipping the public with the knowledge needed to better negotiate the clinical visit, and advocating for policies that are supportive of health.

An underlying assumption of TCNY is that more can be done in the clinical setting to promote health. Nearly 15% of the U.S. gross domestic product is spent on health care (Levit, *et al.*, 2004). And yet, many do not receive optimal care, with a recent study revealing that those residing in the U.S. receive only about half of recommended medical care (McGlynn, *et al.*, 2003). TCNY aims to improve the clinical encounter through a variety of interventions, providing clinicians with better access to up-to-date treatment guidelines and facilitating communication between providers and patients.

Ten priority action areas – with accompanying messages for providers, consumers, policymakers, and others – have been identified, based on the burden of disease and the amenability to intervention (New York City Department of Health Mental Hygiene, 2004a). These key messages are: (1) have a regular doctor or other health care provider; (2) be tobacco-free; (3) keep your heart healthy; (4) know your HIV status; (5) get help for depression; (6) live free of dependence on alcohol and drugs; (7) get checked for cancer; (8) get the immunizations you need; (9) make your home safe and healthy; and (10) have a healthy baby. Below we provide details about several of these action areas.

3.1.1. Have a Regular Doctor or Other Health Care Provider

Having a regular doctor decreases the overall cost of medical care, reduces disease burden and prolongs life (Franks, *et al.*, 1998). However, 1.5 million adult New Yorkers (about 1 in 4) do not have a regular doctor. More than a quarter of those without health coverage said they were unable to obtain needed medical care at least once in the past year.

Among New Yorkers ages 18 to 64 who do not have a regular doctor, almost 70% have health insurance. Many people may be unaware that they have health coverage through an employer group insurance plan, while others may not know how to utilize these benefits. For those who are uninsured or underinsured, New York City offers several Medicaid public health insurance plans, and the City's public hospital facilities and community health clinics have additional capacity to provide medical care.

Among the activities in which the DOHMH and its partners are engaged are: (1) providing information on accessing health services to those with insurance; (2) assisting New Yorkers who are uninsured but qualify for public health insurance programs to enroll and stay enrolled; (3) assisting uninsured New Yorkers who do not qualify for public insurance to obtain a doctor at a public hospital or community health clinic; (4) assisting private insurance carriers with efforts to encourage covered individuals to utilize preventive care appropriately; (5) advocating for simpler Medicaid managed care enrollment and recertification processes; (6) identifying barriers to obtaining regular medical care among insured and uninsured populations and proposing solutions; and (7) advocating for health insurance coverage of routine preventive care at no charge to patients, as well as investigating the possibility of requiring companies that contract with New York City to provide employees with at least basic health coverage.

3.1.2. Keep Your Heart Healthy

Cardiovascular disease (CVD) is the leading cause of death among New Yorkers, with 27,000 CVD-related deaths reported each year (New York City Department of Health and Mental Hygiene, 2004b). One quarter of New York City adults have been diagnosed with high blood pressure, and a similar number have been diagnosed with high cholesterol, with many more remaining undiagnosed. One-sixth of New York City adults are obese, and three-fourths of New Yorkers do not get at least 30 minutes of physical activity four or more days per week. More than 500,000 adult New Yorkers (9%) have been diagnosed with diabetes, a 2½-fold increase in the past decade. Another 250,000 New Yorkers may have diabetes and not know it, and close to a million more with pre-diabetes are likely to eventually develop diabetes.

Blood pressure and cholesterol can be controlled with diet, exercise and medications. Control of blood pressure with medications significantly reduces the incidence of stroke, heart attack and heart failure (Neal, *et al.*, 2000). Treatment of high cholesterol reduces deaths by 25% (LaRosa, *et al.*, 1999). Most overweight people are capable of achieving a healthier weight, and increased physical activity lowers mortality even in the absence of weight loss. Even modest weight loss (5-10%) and increased physical activity reduces the risk of developing diabetes by 60% in people at high risk (Knowler, *et al.*, 2002).

Among the activities in which the DOHMH and its partners are engaged are: (1) disseminating print and online materials, including a "Passport to Your Health," to assist New Yorkers in tracking their vital signs (blood pressure, cholesterol, weight) and taking actions supportive of good health; (2) offering screenings at municipal hospitals and through partner organizations, and providing appropriate counseling or treatment as indicated; (3) promoting better screening of people who are overweight for pre-diabetes, pre-hypertension and other early indicators of developing CVD; (4) promoting better diabetes management through partnering with health care providers and disseminating treatment information through public health detailing efforts; (5) partnering with large employers in initiating worksite wellness programs and advocating for policies that provide incentives to employers who subsidize employee health club memberships; (6) advocating for reduced prescription drug costs, particularly blood pressure- and cholesterol-lowering medications; (7) advocating for mandatory performance standards for managed care and Medicaid providers; (8) advocating for the development of a comprehensive network of bicycle lanes and walking paths; and (9) exploring the feasibility of developing nutritional labeling guidelines for restaurants and other establishments providing prepared foods.

3.1.3. Know Your HIV Status

New York City has the highest AIDS case rate of any city in the U.S. (Centers for Disease Control and Prevention, 2001); AIDS is the seventh leading cause of death among all New Yorkers and the leading cause of death for New Yorkers aged 25–44 (New York City Department of Health and Mental Hygiene, 2004b). More than 100,000 New Yorkers are living with HIV/AIDS; as many as 25,000 are HIV-positive but do not know their status. More than 5,000 New Yorkers are newly diagnosed with HIV infection each year, with one in four first learning they are HIV positive at the time they are diagnosed with AIDS (New York City Department of Health and Mental Hygiene, 2003).

HIV is preventable through reduction in risky behaviors, use of latex or polyurethane condoms, and not sharing needles for injection drug use (Centers for Disease Control and Prevention, 1992; 2001; 2004). Increased awareness of HIV status and improved risk reduction initiatives can substantially reduce risky behaviors, HIV transmission, HIV-related illness, and AIDS deaths. Syringe exchange programs reduce HIV transmission among intravenous drug users, with no increase in crime or drug use (Gibson, *et al.*, 2001). Effective medical treatment of people with HIV infection, coupled with appropriate housing and social support, can suppress viral load, prevent hospitalizations, prevent drug resistance, prolong life, improve quality of life, and reduce the risk of HIV transmission (Centers for Disease Control and Prevention, 1992; 2001; 2004).

Among the activities in which the DOHMH and its partners are engaged are: (1) providing free, confidential HIV testing (including expanded use of HIV rapid testing) and counseling at public health clinics and public hospitals, with expanded outreach to pregnant women to prevent HIV transmission to their babies; (2) strengthening partner notification programs; (3) providing free condoms to community-based and non-profit organizations for distribution, as well as to businesses with high numbers of customers with HIV risk factors (e.g., gay bars, sex venues); (4) working to increase availability of syringe exchange and other harm reduction programs to injection drug users; (5) providing and/or ensuring access to high-quality treatment and case management services to people living with HIV/AIDS, including improved quality and efficiency of housing and other social services; (6) advocating for increased Ryan White funding for care services and expanded housing support; (7) requiring Medicaid managed care plans to provide free and expanded HIV testing; (8) advocating for full coverage of HIV/AIDS treatment by all public and private health insurance plans; and (9) advocating for local community boards to support the creation of syringe exchange programs in underserved neighborhoods (local community board support is a pre-requisite for establishment of syringe exchange programs in New York State).

3.1.4. Get Checked for Cancer

Each year more than 1,500 New Yorkers die of colon cancer, more than 1,200 New York City women die of breast cancer and more than 150 die of cervical cancer (New York City Department of Health and Mental Hygiene, 2004b). Only half of New Yorkers age 50 and older report ever having undergone colon cancer screening via sigmoidoscopy or colonoscopy. One in four women aged 40 and older has not had a mammogram in the past two years, and one in seven women report never having had a Pap smear.

Colon cancer is among the most preventable cancers. Colonoscopy not only prevents colon cancer, but also completely removes pre-cancerous adenomatous polyps and the majority of early-stage cancers before they can spread (Walsh, *et al.*, 2003). Almost all cervical cancer deaths can be prevented through screening and early detection, and breast cancer survival improves with early detection (Centers for Disease Control and Prevention, 1992). Risk for many types of cancer (including colorectal, cervical and breast) is greatly reduced by not smoking, maintaining a healthy diet, and engaging in regular physical activity (Jemal, *et al.*, 2004).

Among the activities in which the DOHMH and its partners are engaged are: (1) expanding colon cancer screening efforts in high-prevalence neighborhoods through partnerships with public hospitals and the American Cancer Society, including community outreach, professional education and public health detailing activities; (2) coordinating citywide resources to expand colon cancer screening capacity, educating the public and health care providers on appropriate colon cancer screening guidelines, and monitoring use of colonoscopy procedures to document the increase in utilization; (3) promoting free or low-cost colon, breast and cervical cancer screenings; (4) implementing media campaigns to increase public awareness of the value of cancer screening; (5) promoting reimbursement policies to increase numbers of colonoscopies performed; (6) examining the feasibility of making outpatient colonoscopy a reportable procedure in order to better monitor citywide performance and capacity; and (7) advocating for full coverage of cancer screenings (i.e., colonoscopies, Pap smears and mammograms) by public and private health insurers.

3.1.5. Future Directions

The intent of TCNY was to identify a limited number of key areas for which interventions were clear and achievable. The focus is on "winnable battles" – the biggest population health problems for which feasible, evidence-based interventions exist. As a result, there are many important conditions not targeted by TCNY, such as obesity and musculoskeletal disorders. In choosing just ten action areas, the DOHMH sought to assure focus and promote action. To succeed, the DOHMH has begun the task of building partnerships with the city's health care providers, as the agency's own role in providing health care services, particularly primary health care, has diminished over time (Duffy, 1968). How should a health department engage clinicians in the management of chronic disease? In the control of communicable disease, health departments took on both a service and a regulatory role (Rosner, 1995). They served as a provider of last resort, a distributor of free vaccines, and a source of technical advice, while at the same time mandating reporting. To be effective, health departments face the challenge of identifying analogous incentives and monitoring strategies in the control of non-communicable disease. Tracking chronic disease management and assessing the impact on a population of patients will require electronic medical records and/or disease registries (Bodenheimer, *et al.*, 2002). How health departments can support and accelerate adoption of these tools is an important future challenge.

3.2. Strategies Directed at the Physical Environment

The urban physical environment affects a wide range of health domains. These impacts can be direct, such as lead poisoning from deteriorated paint in housing, or more complex, such as ready access to parks and recreation facilities promoting physical activity. The DOHMH has a history of significant success in prevention programs focused on the physical environment. The largest long-standing program, as at many urban health departments, is childhood lead poisoning prevention and, as elsewhere, New York City's program has focused on correcting hazards in homes of lead-poisoned children. In addition, DOHMH has worked in partnership with New York City's Department of Housing Preservation and Development to improve compliance with housing codes requiring the elimination of lead paint hazards. From 1995 to 2002, the number of New York City children newly identified with elevated blood lead levels declined by 77%, but the 4,876 children identified in 2002 indicates that lead poisoning remains a significant problem in the city. Another historical success is DOHMH's role in education and enforcement to reduce window fall fatalities from 217 in 1973, when a law requiring window guards was enacted, to 6 in 2003.

Past successes, while notable, have touched on only some of the health problems related to New York City's physical environment. In expanding the scope and effectiveness of its efforts in this domain, the DOHMH has been confronted with certain challenges faced by most urban health departments. First, local departments typically have authority and capacity to effectively regulate only a limited number of the environmental conditions that can impact on health. Second, resource constraints may limit a health department's ability to enforce regulations in all places where violations may occur. Third, disparities in physical conditions are typical; low-income neighborhoods most often have more adverse conditions, such as deteriorated housing, and fewer health-promoting physical assets, such as safe and attractive parks. Fourth, the economic conditions in poor communities limit the extent to which private, voluntary action to improve physical conditions can occur. For example, resources and incentives to invest voluntarily in improvements – such as safe housing renovation that can reduce lead paint hazards or construction of playgrounds to encourage physical activity – are scarce.

To address these challenges, the DOHMH has begun to develop programs to intervene on health-related physical environment factors in a way that complements the more reactive, enforcement-based programs and to focus resources where they will have the most benefit. Key strategies employed by these programs, as illustrated below, include: partnerships with other city agencies; incorporation of physical environment activities into other existing programs; employing staff in new roles suited to their skills and experience; and using data to define target populations and focus resources.

3.2.1. Shape Up New York

Others have noted how urban "sprawl" can increase dependence on automobiles for transportation and decrease physical activity in the form of walking and biking (Ewing, *et al.*, 2003). But older and more traditional high-density urban neighborhoods can vary in their accessibility to parks, recreation facilities and other places to exercise. Increasing neighborhood access to physical activity opportunities has been shown to increase physical activity (Task Force on Community Preventive Services, 2002).

New York City's Department of Parks and Recreation operates more than 1,700 parks, playgrounds and recreation facilities across the city's five boroughs. These facilities represent an underutilized resource for promoting physical activity, especially in low-income neighborhoods where use of private gyms and health clubs is not an option. The DOHMH developed *Shape Up New York*, a year-round, free family fitness program, in partnership with the NYC Department of Parks and Recreation, which runs the program. The program is designed to provide participants of varying fitness levels with an opportunity to exercise in a supportive social environment. In the summer of 2004, the program was offered at nine sites in low-income communities and included cycling, walking, and stretching classes, as well as education on how to incorporate exercise into a daily routine. A pilot program, on which the *Shape Up* program is based, successfully reached overweight or obese people (77% of adult participants), and 87% of *Shape Up* participants reported an increase in physical activity compared to the previous summer (NYCDOHMH, unpublished data).

3.2.2. The Newborn Home Visit Program

The connections between housing quality and health are important and complex (Matte and Jacobs, 2000). For many housing-related health concerns, very young children are at increased risk because their size and behavior causes more exposure, their metabolism causes greater uptake of toxicants, and their developing bodies mean greater vulnerability to certain effects. To direct more home environmental intervention resources at this vulnerable population, the DOHMH has incorporated a home environment assessment protocol into its *Welcome Newborn* program. In this program, public health advisors conduct home visits to first-time mothers in New York City neighborhoods with high rates of poverty and health problems such as infant mortality. *Welcome Newborn* staff provides health education and referrals on a wide range of issues, including safe sleep position, infant nutrition, immunization, lead hazards and other home environment issues.

The home assessment protocol includes observation for immediately hazardous conditions, such as lack of heat, hot water, electricity and dangerous structural defects. Staff advises and assists mothers in contacting the landlord and/or New York City's Housing Emergency Repair Program, as appropriate. For other conditions, such as peeling paint, the absence of window guards, absent or nonfunctioning smoke detectors and rodent and/or roach infestation, staff advises mothers of relevant regulations and assists them in advising the landlords of their legal responsibilities.

3.2.3. Future Directions

While past and more recent DOHMH programs illustrate the potential for urban departments of health to contribute to a healthier physical environment, many aspects of the physical environment remain to be addressed. Among the initiatives being considered by DOHMH are building on a successful pilot program to expand the use of integrated pest management for roach and rodent control in public and private housing, expanding availability of healthy food choices, encouraging the use of stairwells instead of elevators to promote increased physical activity, and enhancing enforcement of no-idling regulations for school buses and other diesel-powered vehicles.

3.3. Strategies Directed at the School Setting

The school setting offers the only ready opportunity for sustained direct contact with young people in large numbers. In 2002, projected enrollment in U.S. elementary and secondary schools stood at over 53 million in more than 120,000 schools. For 13 years, between the ages of 5 and 17, students spend six hours per day, five days per week in school for some 40 weeks each year, providing a setting for ongoing, incremental intervention. Although young people are generally healthy, these are years when many key health-related habits of adult life are established (Grunbaum, *et al.*, 2004). By modifying the pattern of risk factors that underlie chronic disease (mainly tobacco use, physical inactivity and nutritional habits) and other causes of premature mortality (risky sexual behavior, violence), subsequent injury and ill health can be averted (Kolbe, 2004).

The New York City public education system is the largest in the nation, with 1.2 million students who attend some 1,300 schools. The Office of School Health has focused efforts on monitoring health risks, strengthening health services, and promoting physical education and health education. A restructuring of school oversight in 2001 offered an opportunity to address the organizational structure of the school health program. For the first time, school health activities of the DOHMH and the Department of Education were placed under a single management structure, encompassing health services and curriculum-based activities (health and physical education).

3.3.1. Risk Factor Surveillance and Medical Room Utilization

The CDC Youth Risk Behavioral Surveillance System (YRBSS), established in 1990 and conducted biannually, measures the high school (grades 9–12) prevalence of risk behavior in six key areas: intentional and unintentional injury, tobacco use, alcohol and other drug use, sexual activity, diet and physical activity. Surveys typically permit citywide estimates and analysis by gender and race/ethnicity, but sample sizes are too small to examine by geographic area within cities, which may be important for local planning. A modest increase in financial support to increase the sample size permitted calculation of New York City borough-specific estimates (Fornek, *et al.*, 2004). The DOHMH also conducted a special survey of heights and weights among elementary students that highlighted the extent and magnitude of obesity and overweight (Thorpe, *et al.*, 2004).

In contrast to well-established surveillance of behavioral risks, the monitoring of the approximately one million annual visits to the elementary school medical room was limited to simple manual tallies. Because these encounters were documented on a paper record, there was no ready way to generate reports by type of complaint or diagnosis, view other data about students during a consultation (such as attendance, vision screening, immunization records), or track students over time, especially if the student moved within the school system, a relatively common occurrence. To address this, an ambitious effort was undertaken to automate the school health record. The Automated School Health Record (ASHR) also produces reports, so that the nurse can generate, for example, a list of all children who failed the vision exam, or have asthma or diabetes.

3.3.2. Health Services

To expand beyond the "first aid" function that a walk-in service offers, the program targets two important conditions that can be effectively addressed in schools: asthma and impaired vision. To better manage asthma, nurses are being trained to assess asthma severity and appropriateness of medication, so that when appropriate, they can advocate for regimen review to both the parent and the child's physician. To better identify those with impaired vision and especially those at risk for amblyopia, vision screening teams now focus on younger children. Although large numbers of children are tested, documented follow-up has been patchy. The principal, classroom teacher and parent liaison staff have all been rallied to inform parents that untreated amblyopia will lead to blindness and to help the Department monitor for adequate follow-up. A public education campaign in schools will support vision screening.

3.3.3. Curriculum-Based Programs

The pressure to devote school time to examinable academic subjects has led to the marginalization of non-examinable activities. Although New York State education laws contain explicit guidelines on classroom time for health education – including sex education, information about HIV/AIDS and physical education – there is concern that these goals are not being met (Stringer, 2003). Nationally, too, the amount of school time devoted to physical education is minimal and has declined substantially in the past ten years (Gerberding, *et al.*, 2004). In New York City, efforts are underway to invigorate school-based physical activity and health education programming, with the selection of a single curriculum for each and identification of regional physical education coordinators. The physical activity curriculum includes a fitness report to parents that will allow students and parents to track progress. In aggregate, these data (which include BMI measurements) will allow tracking of program impact.

3.3.4. Future Directions

Key issues for a school health program include coordinating diverse partners within the schools and across agencies, optimizing the impact of a health service geared toward screening and diagnosis, and building support for health-related activities in schools that are struggling to meet educational goals. Urban areas offer special challenges because schools are large, students are poor, and many face a wide range of social disadvantages.

While New York City has made considerable progress in a variety of areas (Waller and Goldman, 1993; De Simone Eichel, 2001), some very important issues have yet to be effectively addressed. The YRBSS data suggest that many students are troubled and unhappy, but there is, at present, no clear strategy to improve behavioral health. Dental health remains a central health concern in poor communities; while a DOHMH dental sealant program targets vulnerable children, budget constraints have limited its reach. A recent revamping of New York City's school meals program has led to improved, nutrition-conscious offerings, but implementation and oversight citywide continue to present challenges.

3.4. Strategies Directed at Communities with Greatest Need

Urban communities are typically diverse, characterized by neighborhoods that share social, ethnic and economic characteristics. In the U.S., non-whites are disproportionately low-income and the residential patterns are segregated, resulting in a concentration of the black and latino poor in geographically demarcated communities. The U.S. Census calculates a "dissimilarity index" (DI) to measure racial dispersion (Iceland, *et al.*, 2002). By this index, of 312 metropolitan areas, New York City ranks among the most segregated in the nation. Indeed, nearly 85% of New York City whites would have to move in order to achieve an even black-white distribution. Nearly all U.S. metropolitan areas would be considered at least moderately segregated.

These residential patterns result in the geographic clustering of vulnerable populations. Health disparities, which occur strikingly by race-ethnic group and income level, also occur among neighborhoods (Karpati, *et al.*, 2004). In 2003, in an effort to reduce excess morbidity and mortality in neighborhoods where poor health outcomes aggregate, the DOHMH established three District Public Health Offices (DPHOs) in Harlem, the South Bronx and North-Central Brooklyn. If mortality rates in these targeted areas were the same as in New York's wealthiest neighborhoods, more that 4,000 deaths would be averted each year. Disparities in mortality are complemented by marked differences in individual risk factors reported by residents. New York City is able to document such variation at the neighborhood level with data available from the Community Health Survey. High rates of smoking, HIV infection, sexually transmitted disease, obesity and physical inactivity also cluster in these three communities. This targeting is not perfect. There are geographic communities elsewhere in New York with poor health outcomes. Staten Island, with a population concentration of white, blue-collar workers, has the highest smoking rates. Parts of Jamaica, Queens are poor and have poor health outcomes. Acquisition of HIV infection remains higher in the Manhattan neighborhood of Chelsea than in other New York neighborhoods, reflecting the presence of large numbers of men who have sex with men. The selection of just three communities out of the scores of New York City neighborhoods reflects the DOHMH effort to target the neediest communities as its main approach to eliminating health disparities.

The three DPHOs provide community infrastructure for DOHMH activities. In establishing these offices, the DOHMH, for the first time in many years, deployed senior staff (Assistant Commissioners or higher) to communities of need, rather than to lower Manhattan, the seat of city government. This redeployment occurs in the context of a long DOHMH history of district health work. Always conceived as a way to bring services closer to those most in need, earlier efforts were based on the notion of decentralization and direct service provision (Widdemer, 1932). Decades of struggle between the vertically-organized, centrally-managed bureaus and the

District Health Centers ended with the dismantling of district services and the eventual elimination of most clinical services delivered by the DOHMH (Duffy, 1968). The DPHO effort is more limited in scope. Not all communities are in need of a DOHMH presence. Some of New York's wealthiest neighborhoods had, in 2000, already achieved many of the goals laid out in Healthy People 2010, the federal health target-setting document (U.S. Department of Health and Human Services, 2000). High-cost public health interventions, many of which require one-on-one contact with individuals, should be limited to communities that need them most.

DPHO activities fall under three general headings: (1) implementation of health promotion activities, both those launched by DPHO staff and those developed by other agency bureaus but housed in the DPHO; (2) local coordination of agency-wide activities, as well as those of other governmental agencies and community-based organizations; and (3) provision of health information and technical assistance to local community groups.

The DPHO also provides a strategic framework for the entire agency that promotes the targeting of scarce programming resources to communities most in need. Some activities are envisioned as based only in the DPHO. Other activities eventually suitable for citywide implementation can first be piloted in the DPHO. Each DPHO is autonomous and, while all three DPHOs have a similar operational structure, budget and staffing plan, each has a unique public health agenda that reflects specific community needs. The full-time DPHO staff number between 15 and 20. In addition to the District Public Health Officer, there is a program director, epidemiologist and administrator. Other staff are tasked to specific sectors, such as schools, community-based organizations or health services, or smaller geographic areas within the target area.

The catchment area for each DPHO ranges between 225,000 and 500,000. East and Central Harlem comprises about 225,000 residents. Most residents are black (56%) or latino (35%) and poor, with 37% living in poverty (as compared to the citywide average of about 20%) (Karpati, *et al.*, 2003). Its health profile reveals a high rate of obesity, diabetes and childhood asthma. Initial activities identified by the DPHO staff include better management of childhood asthma and the promotion of physical activity. Staff have partnered with the New York City Department of Parks and Recreation to offer *Shape Up New York*, a free family exercise program. Asthma activities have focused on the development of an asthma registry in schools.

The North-Central Brooklyn DPHO covers a geographic area with a population of about 250,000. With a mostly 19th and early 20th Century housing stock (in contrast to East and Central Harlem, where 25% of the population live in post-World War II government apartment buildings), disproportionate numbers of lead-poisoned children reside here. Thus, the DPHO has focused on housing and health; a home visiting program has been launched to identify peeling paint and pest infestations and make appropriate referrals for remediation. The Brooklyn office, like the Harlem DPHO, has also worked closely with the Parks Department to support the *Shape Up New York* program.

The Bronx DPHO covers the largest area and population, about 500,000 people. A predominantly latino (62%) and black (33%) community, it is also younger than the Harlem or Brooklyn DPHO areas. Forty percent (40%) of the population is under the age of 20, compared to 28% citywide. Because teen pregnancy rates are 50% higher in this community than in the rest of New York City, the Bronx DPHO has focused on promotion of contraceptive access for teenagers. Much of this work has been done in collaboration with the 11 public high schools located within the target area, which enroll over 10,000 teens. Although contraceptives are not dispensed or prescribed in schools, condoms are available in health resource rooms. The program has aimed to assure that all students know about these resource rooms, and all rooms are stocked with condoms. In addition, the DPHO is working to ensure that community providers are "teen friendly" and community pharmacies stock drugs for emergency contraception. In addition, the Bronx DPHO has promoted physical activity through both *Shape Up New York* in neighborhood parks and a program to train day care providers to lead physical activity sessions for young children.

In their role as coordinator of public health activities within the community, the DPHOs have housed and provided support to the agency's public health detailing program, a door-to-door direct marketing program for prevention targeting health care settings. In the last year, this effort has promoted flu shots, colon cancer screening and tobacco cessation, providing doctors with brief messages and tools that facilitate best practices for prevention. For a DOHMH rodent control initiative, DPHO staff coordinated the distribution of garbage cans. A billboard public education campaign to promote awareness of emergency contraception and other forms of contraception targeted DPHO neighborhoods, with staff providing assistance in identifying suitable advertisement placement locations. In its role as convener, the Harlem DPHO, for example, brought together organizations involved in improving asthma management in the schools; an activity plan was developed and roles for all involved organizations were delineated, ensuring that efforts were complementary rather than duplicative.

A subcommittee of the DOHMH health advisory council, comprised of many of the Department's key community partners, advises the department on the DPHOs, reviewing plans and providing advice. DPHO efforts to build community relationships have included participating in such events as community health fairs and local planning board meetings and providing testimony at public hearings convened by local political leaders. The DOHMH has a rich repository of city health information, and the DPHOs have tapped into this resource to help build health awareness and provide communities with information that supports advocacy for services.

3.4.1. Future Directions

At a time of budget cutbacks, the DPHOs offer a framework for targeting scarce DOHMH community outreach resources to New York's most vulnerable communities. The DPHOs, though, are not wholly responsible for these highest-risk populations; they are rightly the responsibility of every program in the DOHMH, with the DPHOs assuming a coordinating role. Also, policy and regulatory efforts, which can be enormously effective in improving the health of large numbers of people, necessarily occur at a higher level – well beyond the boundaries of the DPHO communities. For example, although Central Harlem has high smoking rates, the policy interventions to reduce smoking occur primarily at the citywide level. Harlem-based efforts might focus on tobacco sales to minors by local retail outlets (Gemson, *et al.*, 1998), but addressing smoking in the workplace requires a broader strategy. A - challenge, then, is simultaneously working on policy approaches that redress disparities while focusing community-based efforts on New York City's disadvantaged populations.

3.5. Strategies Directed at the Policy Environment

The DOHMH approach to tobacco control demonstrates the key role that policy interventions can play in health promotion (Orleans and Cummings, 1999). In 2002, the DOHMH estimated that tobacco accounted for 10,000 deaths per year in New York City, of which about 1,000 were due to secondhand smoke exposure. Citywide, about one in five adults reported that they smoked (22%), although in some communities this rose to one in three adults. To address this leading preventable cause of death, the DOHMH implemented a five-point strategy: (1) taxation; (2) legislation; (3) cessation; (4) public education; and (5) evaluation. These strategies reflected the national and international experience in tobacco control, where policy interventions, including taxation and legislation, became crucial complements to public education and cessation efforts.

Increasing the unit price of cigarettes both reduces smoking initiation and increases cessation (Task Force on Community Preventive Services, 2001). The DOHMH had long advocated for excise tax increases, and in 2002, the tobacco excise tax in New York City rose twice. First, New York State raised its excise tax from \$1.11 to \$1.50 per pack, followed by an increase in New York City's excise tax from \$0.08 to \$1.50 – resulting in a combined tax of \$3.00 and a pack price ranging from \$7.00 to \$7.50 – at the time, the highest price in the nation.

Smoke-free air or clean indoor air legislation has been shown effective in reducing exposure to secondhand smoke and encouraging smokers to quit (Task Force on Community Preventive Services, 2001). In 1995, New York City enacted clean air legislation that prohibited smoking in many workplaces and public areas, including larger restaurants. However, this bill exempted bars and small restaurants, and allowed designated smoking areas in many non-residential settings. In March 2003, with the DOHMH's active support, the New York City Smoke Free Air Act (SFAA) took effect, providing further protection to employees by eliminating smoking in virtually all establishments with employees, including all retail businesses, bars, restaurants and office buildings (Chang, *et al.*, 2004). Compared to the year prior to its implementation, 110,000 fewer New Yorkers reported secondhand smoke exposure at work, and a statewide study of nonsmoking bar and restaurant employees, conducted just prior to and post-implementation of the New York State Clean Indoor Air Act in July 2003, showed an 85% reduction in cotinine blood serum levels (New York City Department of Finance, *et al.*, 2004). The effective implementation and enforcement of the law was facilitated by the DOHMH's ability to rapidly train its large and experienced workforce in SFAA enforcement and, thereby, inspect more than 22,000 establishments as part of routine inspections after the law took effect. Legal requirements to post no-smoking signs prominently and to remove ashtrays have greatly facilitated implementation of the law.

The legislative approach has also been effective in reducing tobacco sales to minors. Such sales were widespread in New York City, especially in poor communities (Gemson, *et al.*, 1998). The Tobacco Product Regulation Act (New York City Administrative Code §§17-616–626) originally became effective in April 1993 and was last amended effective August 2000. Provisions of this law forbid the sale of tobacco products to minors. It also forbids sales of unpackaged, single cigarettes ("loosies") and the sale of tobacco products by anyone under the age of 18, unless that person is under the direct supervision of another employee who is of age and on the premises. The retailer must post specifically worded signs indicating that sales to minors are prohibited and must also request to see a photo ID from the prospective buyer, unless the purchaser reasonably appears to be at least 25 years of age. Also forbidden is the use of any tobacco product on school premises. The DOHMH, in collaboration with the New York City Department of Consumer Affairs, conducts routine "sting" operations, in which underage youth attempt to purchase tobacco products at retail outlets.

Strategies that combine education with efforts to affect the scope of health-related choices always encounter political opposition. This has been true of the DOHMH tobacco control strategy, which engaged the agency in a concerted effort to explain and promote the change in taxation and legislation. This strategy, while making it easier for New Yorkers not to smoke, has its opponents. Despite data to the contrary (New York City Department of Finance, *et al.*, 2004), some restaurant and bar owners have continued to argue that their businesses have suffered because of the smoking ban. A health department's pursuit of policy change is seldom without controversy, particularly if such change in policy is accompanied by enforcement, through legislation or taxation.

4.0. CONCLUSION

Urban health departments share the challenges of modern public health generally: a disease burden dominated by chronic disease, much of it noncommunicable. The underlying causes of this pattern are embedded in the way we live. Tobacco use, physical inactivity and poor diet – rather than a single causative agent – are largely responsible for morbidity and mortality trends. Important communicable diseases, notably HIV-related illness, have also acquired a chronic character, to be managed rather than cured. To this, the urban setting brings its particular social and physical environment, characterized by dense population settlements, substantial poverty and a highly built environment with deteriorating housing stocks. To succeed, the public health enterprise requires not only government, but a range of partners (Institute of Medicine, 2003). Among the roles of the local urban health department are to serve as community convener, spearhead the development of a focused strategy directed at current disease burden, harness the potential of secondary prevention, ensure that resources are directed to the most vulnerable, and advocate for policy changes supportive of healthy choices.

REFERENCES

Baxter, R.J. (1998). The roles and responsibilities of local public health systems in urban health. *J. Urban Health* 75(2):322–329.

Bodenheimer, T., Wagner, E.H., and Grumbach, K. (2002). Improving primary care for patients with chronic illness: the chronic care model, part 2. *JAMA.* 288(15):1909–14.

Brownson, R.C., and Bright, F.S. (2004). Chronic disease control in public health practice: looking back and moving forward. *Public Health Rep.* 119:230–238.

Centers for Disease Control and Prevention. (2001). HIV/AIDS surveillance report, 2001; 13(2). CDC, Atlanta, GA.

Centers for Disease Control and Prevention. (2004). Division of HIV/AIDS Prevention, 2004, Atlanta, GA, (May 2004); http://www.cdc.gov/hiv/pubs.htm.

Centers for Disease Control and Prevention (1992). Update: National Breast and Cervical Cancer Early Detection Program, July 1991-July 1992. *MMWR.* 41(40):739–743.

Chang, C., Leighton, J., Mostashari, F., McCord, C., and Frieden, T.R. (2004). The New York The New York City Smoke-Free Air Act: second-hand smoke as a worker health and safety issue. *Am. J. Ind. Med.* 46(2):188–95.

Centers for Disease Control and Prevention, 2004, National Public Health Performatnce Standards Program, Atlanta GA, (October 1, 2004); www.phppo.cdc.gov/nphpsp.

Community Guide to Preventive Services, Atlanta, GA, (October 1, 2004); www.thecommunityguide.org

Department of Health and Mental Hygiene, Take Care New York, New York, NY, (October 1, 2004); www.takecarenewyork.org. or nyc.gov/health/tcny

De Simone Eichel, J., and Goldman, L. (2001). Safety makes sense: a program to prevent unintentional injuries in New York City public schools. *J. Sch. Health* 71(5):180–183.

Duffy, J. (1968). *A History of Public Health in New York City.* New York: Russell Sage Foundation.

Estabrooks, P.A., Lee, R.E., and Gyurcsik, N.C. (2003). Resources for physical activity participation: does availability and accessibility differ by neighborhood socioeconomic status. *Ann. Behav. Med.* 25(2): 100–104.

Ewing, R., Schmid, T., Killingsworth, R., Zlot, A., and Raudenbush, S. (2003). Relationship between urban sprawl and physical activity, obesity, and morbidity. *Am. J. Health Promot.* 18: 47-57.

Fornek, M.L., Thorpe, L.E., Platt, R., Mostashari, F., and Henning, K. (2004). Risky business? Health behaviors of New York City high school students. *NYC Vital Signs.* 3(2):1–4.

Franks, P., and Fiscella, K. (1998). Primary care physicians and specialists as personal physicians. Health care expenditures and mortality experience. *J. Fam. Pract.* 47(2):105-9.

Gemson D.H., Moats H.L., Watkins B.X., Ganz M.L., Robinson S., and Healton E. (1998). Laying down the law: reducing illegal tobacco sales to minors in central Harlem. *Am. J. Public Health* 88(6):936–9.

Gerberding, J.L., and Marks, J.S. (2004). Making America fit and trim – steps big and small. *Am. J. Public Health* 94:1478–1479.

Geronimus, A.T. (2000). To mitigate, resist, or undo: addressing structural influences on the health of urban populations. *Am. J. Public Health* 90(6):867–872.

Gibson, D.R., Flynn, N.M., and Perales, D. (2001). Effectiveness of syringe exchange programs in reducing HIV risk behavior and HIV seroconversion among injecting drug users. *AIDS* 15(11):1329–1341.

Grunbaum, J., Kann, L., and Kinchen, S.A. (2004). Youth Risk Behavioral Surveillance – United States 2003. *MMWR.* 53(2):1–96.

Iceland, J., Weinberg D.H., and Steinmetz, E. (2002). Racial and Ethnic Segregation in the United States: 1980-2000. U.S. Census Series CENSR-3. U.S. Government Printing Office, Washington, D.C.

Institute of Medicine (2003). *The future of the public's health in the 21st century.* Washington DC: The National Academies Press.

Israel, B.A., Schulz, A.J., Parker, E.A., and Becker, A.B. (2001). Community-based participatory research: policy recommendations for promoting a partnership approach in health research. *Educ. Health* 14(2):182–197.

Jemal, A., Tiwari, R.C., Murray T., Ghafoor, A., Samuels, A., Ward, E., Feuer, E.J., and Thun, M.J. (2004). Cancer statistics, 2004. *C.A. Cancer J. Clin.* 54(1):8–29.

Kandula, N.R., Kersey, M., and Lurie, N. (2004). Assuring the health of immigrants: what the leading health indicators tell us. *Annu. Rev. Public Health* 25: 357–376.

Karpati, A., Kerker, B., Mostashari, F., Singh, T., Hajat, A., Thorpe, L., Bassett, M., Henning, K., and Frieden, T. (2004). Health disparities in New York City. New York: New York City Department of Health and Mental Hygiene.

Karpati, A., Lu, X., Mostashari, F., Thorpe, L., and Frieden, T.R. (2003). The health of Central Harlem. *NYC Comm. Health Profiles* 1(5,17)1–12.

Kegler, M.C., Steckler, A., McLeroy, K., and Malek, S.H. (1998). Factors that contribute to effective community health promotion coalitions: a study of 10 Project ASSIST coalitions in North Carolina. *Health Educ. Behav.* 25(3):338–353.

Kolbe, L., Kann, L., Patterson, B., Wechsler, H., Osorio, J., and Collins, J. (2004). Enabling the nation's schools to help prevent heart disease, stroke, cancer, COPD, diabetes and other serious health problems. *Public Health Rep.* 119(3):286–302.

Knowler, W.C., Barrett-Connor E., Fowler, S.E., Hamman, R.F., Lachin, J.M., Walker, E.A., and Nathan, D.M. (2002). Reduction in the incidence of type 2 diabetes with lifestyle intervention or metformin. *N. Engl. J. Med.* 346(6):393–403.

LaRosa, J.C., He, J., and Vupputuri, S. (1999). Effects of statins on risk of coronary disease: a meta-analysis of randomized clinical controlled trials. *JAMA.* 282(24):2340– 2346.

Leighton, J., Klitzman, S., Sedlar, S., Matte, T., and Cohen, N.L. (2003). The effect of lead-based paint hazard remediation on blood lead levels of lead poisoned children in New York City. *Environ. Res.* 92(3):182–190.

Levit, K., Smith, C., Cowan, C., Sensenig, and Catlin, A. (2004). Health spending rebound continues in 2002. *Health Aff.* 23(1):147–159.

Lin, C.C., Rogot, E., Johnson, N.J., Sorlie, P.D., and Arias, E. (2003). A further study of life expectancy by socioeconomic factors in the National Longitudinal Mortality Study. *Ethn. Dis.* 13(2):240–247.

Matte, T.D., and Jacobs, D.E. (2000). Housing and health – current issues and implications for research and programs. *J. Urban Health* 77(1):7–25.

Marx, M.A., Crape, B., Brookmeyer, R.S., Junge, B., Latkin, C., Vlahov, D., and Strathdee, S.A. (2000). Trends in crime and the introduction of a needle exchange program. *Am. J. Public Health* 90(12):1933–1936.

McGlynn, E.A., Asch, S.M., Adams, J., Keesey, J., Hicks, J., DeCristofaro, A., and Kerr, E.A. (2003). The quality of health care delivered to adults in the United States. *N. Engl. J. Med.* 348:2635–2645.

Mokdad, A.H., Marks, J.S., Stroup, D.F., and Gerberding, J.L. (2004). Actual causes of death in the United States, 2000. *JAMA.* 291(10):1238–1245.

Neal, B., MacMahon, S., and Chapman, N. (2000). Effects of ACE inhibitors, calcium antagonists, and other blood-pressure lowering drugs: results of prospectively designed overviews of randomized trials. *Lancet* 356(9246):1955–1964.

New York City Department of Finance, New York City Department of Health and Mental Hygiene, New York City Department of Small Business Services, and New York City Economic Development Corporation, 2004, The state of smoke-free New York City: a one-year review, New York, NY (October 1, 2004); http://archive.naccho.org/documents/Smoke-Free-Law.pdf

New York City Department of Health and Mental Hygiene, 2003, HIV/AIDS Surveillance and Epidemiology Program fourth quarter report, New York, NY, (May 2003); http://www.nyc.gov/html/doh/pdf/dires/qtr4-2003.pdf.

New York City Department of Health and Mental Hygiene, 2004a, Take Care New York: A Policy for a Healthier New York City. New York, NY (October 1, 2004); http://www.nyc.gov/html/doh/pdf/tcny/tcny-policy.pdf.

New York City Department of Health and Mental Hygiene, 2004b, Summary of Vital Statistics 2003, the City of New York, New York, NY, (December 2004); http://www.nyc.gov/html/doh/pdf/vs/2003sum.pdf.

New York City Department of Health and Mental Hygiene, Take Care New York, New York, NY, (October 1, 2004); www..nyc.gov/health/tcny

Orleans, C.T., and Cummings, K.M. (1999). Population-based tobacco control: progress and prospects. *Am. J. Health Promot.* 14:83–91.

Parks, S.E., Housemann, R.A., and Brownson, R.C. (2003). Differential correlates of physical activity in urban and rural adults of various socioeconomic backgrounds in the United States. *J. Epidemiol. Comm. Health* 57:29–35.

Rosen, G. (1998). *A History of Public Health.* Baltimore: The Johns Hopkins University Press.

Rosenstreich, D.L., Eggleston, P., Kattan, M., Baker, D., Slavin, R.G., Gergen, P., Mitchell, H., McNiff-Mortimer, K., Lynn, H., Ownby, D., and Malveaux, F. (1997). The role of cockroach allergy and exposure to cockroach allergen in causing morbidity among inner-city children with asthma. *N. Engl. J. Med.* 336(19):1356–1363.

Rosner, D. (ed.). (1995). *Hives of Sickness: Public Health and Epidemics in New York City.* New Brunswick: Rutgers University Press.

Stringer, S. (2003). *Failing grade: health education in NYC schools. An analysis of K-8 health education in New York City's public school system.* New York, Report no. June 2003, 67th AD.

Task Force on Community Preventive Services.(2002). Recommendations to increase physical activity in communities. *Am. J. Prev. Med.* 22(4S): 67–72.

Task Force on Community Preventive Services. (2001). Reviews of evidence regarding interventions to reduce tobacco use and exposure to environmental tobacco smoke. *Am. J. Prev. Med.* 20(2S):16–66.

Thorpe, L.E., List, D.G., Marx, T., May, L., Helgerson, S.D., and Frieden, T.R. (2004). Childhood obesity in New York City elementary school students. *Am. J. Public Health* 94: 1496–1500.

Truman, B.I., Smith-Akin, C.K., Hinman, A.R., Gebbie, K.M., Brownson, R., Novick, L.F., Lawrence, R.S., Pappaioanou, M., Fielding, J., Evans, C.A., Guerra, F.A., Vogel-Taylor, M., Mahan, C.S., and Fullilove, M. (2000). Developing the Guide to Community Preventive Services – overview and rationale. *Am. J. Prev. Med.* 18(1S):18-26.

US Department of Health and Human Services. (2000). *Healthy People 2010: understanding and improving health, Second edition.* Government Printing Office, Washington D.C.

Waller, J.V., and Goldman, L. (1993). Bringing comprehensive health education to the New York City Public Schools: a private-public success story. *Bull. N. Y. Acad. Med.* 70(3):171-187.

Walsh, J.M., and Terdiman, J.P. (2003). Colorectal cancer screening: scientific review. *JAMA* 289(10):1288–1296.

Widdemer, K.D. (1932). *A decade of district health center pioneering: ten year report of the East Harlem Health Center. A demonstration in coordinated health and welfare work in a defined city area undertake by the Department of Health, City of New York and twenty-one cooperating voluntary agencies.* New York City: East Harlem Center, Inc. and the New York Center of the American Red Cross, New York, NY.

Wong, M.D., Shapiro, M.F., Boscardin, W.J., and Ettner, S.L. (2002). Contribution of major diseases to disparities in mortality. *N. Engl. J. Med.* 347(20):1585–1592.

Chapter 28

Providing Health Services to Marginalized Urban Populations

Anita Palepu and Mark W. Tyndall

1.0. INTRODUCTION

Part I of this book highlighted the diversity of urban populations. We learned that the residents of an urban core often differ widely in terms of income, age, education, chronic health conditions, physical ability and mental capacity. They can range from homeless people to ethnic minorities to the upper classes and the elderly, and each subgroup has its own set of unique health challenges. To add further complexity to this, the methods of delivery of health services in urban centers vary with respect to their funding structures; publicly funded services are often rationed by wait-lists, whereas private services are rationed by the user's ability to pay (Alter, *et al.*, 1999; Detsky and Naylor, 2003; Iglehart, 2000). General principles of delivering quality health care (Chassin and Galvin, 1998) suggest that the provision of services must be tailored to address the predominant health concerns and social environment of the target subpopulation being served (Vlahov and Galea, 2002). Good examples of this are the numerous interventions that address child health issues in urban settings, such as immunizations, nutrition and asthma (Lara, *et al.*, 1999; McCormick, *et al.*, 1997; Tallon and Sandman, 1998; D. Wood, *et al.*, 1994). These approaches consider the complex life situations that many urban children and families face. Another group who are challenging to provide comprehensive health services to in the urban setting are persons who are homeless and persons with severe and persistent mental illness. They face barriers to accessing conventional health care and adhering to treatment plans thus requiring a modified delivery approach (Barkin, *et al.*, 2003; Hwang and Bugeja, 2000; Hwang, *et al.*, 2001; Kushel, *et al.*, 2001; Prevention of Homelessness, 1998).

The tailoring of health services in an urban context is often related to the social and physical environment in which people live. (Vlahov and Galea, 2002). Even within an urban center, the social and physical environments can be varied and often reflect the income and education of the persons residing in these neighborhoods. One important aspect of urban health includes the health issues faced by persons of lower socioeconomic status and visible minority groups, particularly in the U.S. where they are over-represented and experience numerous barriers to quality health care (Vlahov and Galea, 2002). We recognize that there are many advantaged urban populations who have access to some of the best health care services in the world, however, we will describe a model of health services delivery to disadvantaged urban populations.

In this chapter, we focus on one of the marginalized urban sub-populations, namely drug users, since many of the challenges faced by this group are issues that are relevant to other disadvantaged populations in urban areas. Drug users face particular complexities that can provide a helpful model in considering the issues of health service provision to other marginalized urban populations. This will be highlighted by the challenges of providing comprehensive health services to these persons who have numerous medical and mental health complications of their drug use. We recognize the funding of health care in other settings differ from the universal, publicly funded health care in Canada, however, we offer a description of providing a spectrum of health services to marginalized persons including illicit drug users drawing from the setting and services in Vancouver, British Columbia as a practical example of service delivery to this population. By studying these challenges and methods employed to meet their needs, we hope to provide a useful model that can be applied to other marginalized populations in our cities.

2.0. HEALTH NEEDS OF DRUG USERS

The health status of drug users is typically poor, as described in more detail in an earlier chapter. As a direct consequence of their drug use, individuals may suffer from symptoms of withdrawal, intoxication and overdose. The most worrying consequence, however, is that drug users are at great risk of contracting HIV and Hepatitis C. In 1997, the incidence of HIV infection among injection drug users reached 18%, which was the highest rate in the Western world (Strathdee, *et al.*, 1997). The prevalence of HIV and Hepatitis C among injection drug users is 30% and 90%, respectively (Tyndall, *et al.*, 2001).

In addition to these serious viral infections and their associated complications, injection drug users are susceptible to a range of bacterial infections due to unhygienic injection practices and the lack of clean water (Kerr and Palepu, 2001). These include soft-tissue infections (cellulitis and abscess) bacterial pneumonia, endocarditis, septic arthritis and osteomyelitis (Ebright and Pieper, 2002; Kak and Chandrasekar, 2002; O'Connor, *et al.*, 1994; Palepu, *et al.*, 2001). Adding further complexity to the medical needs of drug users is the high prevalence of concurrent psychiatric diagnoses, such as mood disorders, personality disorders, post-traumatic stress disorders and psychosis (O'Connor, *et al.*, 1994; Palepu, *et al.*, 2001; Stein, 1999).

The myriad and severity of physical and mental health issues faced by injection drug users highlights the complexity of health care they require. It is important to note that there is a substantial overlap between the health needs of drug users and the issues facing homeless people and those living with severe and persistent mental illness. Clearly, these groups share a common need for innovative approaches to health services delivery.

3.0. DETERMINING THE OBSTACLES TO HEALTH CARE ACCESS

The list of obstacles to health care access for disadvantaged urban groups is long (Freudenberg, 2000). Perhaps the most significant barrier in most countries is the lack of health care insurance for marginalized populations (Newacheck, *et al.*, 1998). Without the ability to pay for the services they simply go without. But even in Canada, a society where universal health care is a fundamental tenet, drug users and homeless persons still face a variety of additional barriers when it comes to accessing these services (Cheung and Hwang, 2004).

Again, it is important to note that many of the obstacles described in the following sections also apply to other disadvantaged urban subpopulations, such as homeless people and those with severe and persistent mental illness. In addition, minority groups are often over-represented in urban centers and require special consideration. Aboriginal people in some Canadian cities and black people in cities throughout the U.S. are consistently found to have substantially worse health outcomes when compared to white residents (Craib, *et al.*, 2003). Ethno-cultural practices and beliefs must be taken into consideration when developing programs for these groups (Benoit, *et al.*, 2003).

3.1. Social Obstacles

Perhaps the most troubling obstacle for drug users seeking treatment is that, historically, the response to drug addiction in North America has been one of *law enforcement*. Addiction is seen as a criminal issue rather than a health issue. Accordingly, drug users may be reluctant to seek medical services because they fear criminal repercussions to their actions and there is evidence that police presence may reduce the willingness of drug users to access available health services (Wood, *et al.*, 2003). Viewing the issue of addiction through the lens of health rather than enforcement permits a broader approach to providing health services to this vulnerable population.

Along with fears of criminal prosecution, drug users also face the *social stigma* that accompanies addiction. They may feel discriminated against for their habits and lifestyle and therefore not seek the help they need. In some cases, the potential for discrimination is enough to keep individuals away from public health support, but in others cases the social isolation resulting from addiction is a very real and psychologically debilitating obstacle.

Individuals in this marginalized population often suffer from extremely *low self-esteem*. They are commonly embarrassed by their health issues and their poverty and do not seek help for fear of further injuring their self-worth. In addition, health care workers who are under-trained and lack addiction experience can sometimes act antagonistically towards drug users, which contribute further to their low self-esteem. By judging them instead of welcoming them, inexperienced health care providers can increase the chance that an addicted individual will avoid public services in the future.

Another significant reason for health care avoidance is the *low level of awareness* within the drug-using community about the medical issues associated with injection drug-use (Metzger and Navaline, 2003). Without access to education programs, individuals may not recognize the severity of their situations until they have reached a crisis-point. Awareness of the importance of detecting the early warning signs of various complications may increase their willingness to seek health care when these symptoms arise.

Finally, the *transience* of many marginalized groups limits their ability to access proper medical care and follow-up. Without proper housing opportunities, they are unable to settle in one place, adding a further handicap to their uptake of health care services (Lewis, *et al.*, 2003).

3.2. Institutional Obstacles

Many health care services for drug users are *"high-threshold" services* (Appel, *et al.*, 2004). This means they are programs that are based on abstinence and require individuals to stop using the drugs they are addicted to. These programs are problematic, however, and they symbolize a common misconception about drug addiction therapy. Many abstinence programs do not recognize the long-term, comprehensive process by which an injection drug user successfully gains control over their addiction. A large part of a successful treatment plan involves "preparing" the individual to quit (i.e., through education, motivation, raising self-esteem, etc.) and may be conducted while the individual is still using drugs. Unfortunately, the majority of drug users who enter abstinence programs do not have this background. They are not properly prepared to quit, and so they often drop out.

3.3. Continuity-of-Care

Continuity-of-care is also a challenging problem (Chan, *et al.*, 2002). For many, the hospital emergency room is their first and only point of contact with the medical system. It is also clear that many of the people who frequent emergency rooms also make frequent visits to primary care (Byrne, *et al.*, 2003). The transition between acute hospital care and community follow-up is sub-optimal because primary care clinics are not readily accessible, and those that do exist are unable to provide the requisite level of diagnostic testing and treatment. This is not sufficient for chronic illnesses such as drug addiction and HIV infection, both of which require long-term, consistent care. The result is a pattern of "crisis-based" medical interventions without a focus on early-detection, prevention or follow-up.

The traditional model for medical service requires patients to make *appointments* and arrive on time. However, for many active drug users, the chaotic nature of their lifestyle makes it difficult for them to adhere to specific meeting times. Therefore, the inflexibility of scheduled appointments limits the level of uptake of health services by these individuals. In addition, drug addicted people are unlikely to persevere through the typically *long wait times* in emergency rooms. They often leave the hospital without being seen because they do not want to wait, which results in frustration for both the addicted individuals and the health care providers.

4.0. MODELS OF HEALTH SERVICE DELIVERY

Now that we have determined the obstacles that drug users and other marginalized groups face with respect to health care access, we can discuss some of the ways in which those obstacles can be overcome. The most important point to recognize is that traditional methods to medical service are probably not going to be effective with these groups. We need flexible, innovative programs if we want to reach these people. The facilities used to administer health care must be flexible and welcoming to those who are being served. In the case of people using illicit drugs and other marginalized groups, this may be very different than traditional models of care. The location of the office, expected waiting times, hours of operation, and the ancillary services offered are critical considerations in this setting. In addition, many people on society's margins do not actively pursue health care when faced with the immediate concerns of obtaining illicit drugs, and securing housing, food and money.

Given that addiction is the underlying health problem in these cases, health services must always consider the addiction when addressing the attendant medical conditions. As we stated earlier, medical programs for drug-dependent people can be categorized as high-, medium- or low-threshold. "Threshold" refers to the eligibility criteria for participation (i.e., the ability of individuals to meet program demands) and the amount of organizational structure involved. The higher the threshold, the more demands and long-term expectations are placed on the participant. As threshold decreases, the treatment environment becomes less rigid and the focus shifts to short-term goals and contracts.

Low threshold programs can be a major point of contact for drug dependent individuals. Accordingly, a significant percentage of the medical community's efforts in Vancouver are directed towards these innovative initiatives. In recognition of the complex life situations of many drug users, the programs are multidisciplinary in their approach. They combine the expertise of people from a variety of fields such as education, psychology and social work within the context of medical service in order to help participants overcome the long list of obstacles they face.

The key to these programs is well-trained, highly skilled staff. They must be able to de-escalate tense situations, set realistic expectations and boundaries and show empathy and respect towards the participants. These skill sets are critical given the nature of addiction as a chronic relapsing illness and are necessary attributes for low-threshold health services to succeed.

We advocate multi-disciplinary public health and clinical programs that help people manage social issues as well as health concerns (Galea and Vlahov, 2002). There are alternate models of care that can successfully engage marginalized individuals in a process that will see substantial improvements in their social and health situation. Below, we provide examples of health care delivery models that can attract, sustain, and benefit urban populations who are not engaged in care.

4.1. Community Drop-In Centers

Community drop in centers offer a range of social services in addition to health care. The scope of the services varies, but access to experienced social and health professionals in a casual setting is a prerequisite. These facilities are often managed by community members and encourage the participation of peer workers and volunteers. They often have extended hours of operation to accommodate those who have difficulty attending during regular daytime appointments and services are provided on a drop-in basis. Contact and trust is developed over time and health interventions are introduced slowly. Community-based facilities such as these can be the only viable entry point for many individuals. These initiatives are based on a long-term vision for their community that involves a commitment to low-threshold programs, and it is vital that they resist becoming institutionalized.

4.2. Food Programs

Food programs offer an excellent point of contact and can attract people who may not otherwise attend health clinics. Along with a nutritional meal, participants have the opportunity to connect with health care professionals in a casual setting. Many meal programs have participants who attend on a regular basis. This provides an opportunity to develop trusting relationships between participants and health workers. For the regular attendees there is an opportunity to dispense medications. In Vancouver, a successful food program exists that provides antiretroviral therapies on a daily basis for those who are not able to take their medications on a consistent basis.

4.3. Needle Exchange Programs (NEPs)

NEPs are very effective as points of contact for marginalized individuals who are using injection drugs. Although most NEPs are designed to be hassle-free and provide a quick exchange, they can also serve to direct participants to health care professionals. Some NEPs are affiliated with health care facilities that can provide rapid access to care if the staff are able to identify clients in need of attention as well as offer important interventions (Stein, *et al.*, 2002; Stein, *et al.*, 2002a; Strathdee, *et al.*, 1999). The NEPs are also an important venue to distribute educational materials and promote vaccines and other health interventions. They provide a way to rapidly disseminate information about changes in drug purity, drug contamination and other suspicious observations regarding street drugs.

4.4. Opiate Replacement Therapy

Opiate replacement therapy with methadone and buprenorphine has been shown to reduce the adverse health impacts associated with opiate addiction and to improve health outcomes (Barnett, *et al.*, 2001; Zaric, Barnett, and Brandeau, 2000). The daily dispensing of methadone provides an opportunity for ongoing contact and relationship building and can be linked to ongoing medical care and monitoring. The dispensing of antiretroviral medications along with daily methadone is convenient and acceptable to many HIV seropositive individuals (Conway, *et al.*, 2004).

4.5. Outreach Nursing

Outreach nursing has become an important health delivery model in many urban settings. Community-based nurses are able to provide critical health interventions to highly marginalized groups in locations far from traditional clinics. Visits to apartments, hotels, shelters, recovery houses and street-based contacts require a flexible team of nursing professionals equipped with a range of skills and equipment. Educational messages, vaccination programs, STD screening and medication delivery are examples of initiatives that can be conducted through outreach nursing. Some of these services can be delivered out of *mobile health vans* that can be used as small clinics where minor procedures can be performed, such as dressing changes for abscesses and foot care.

4.6. Peer Involvement

Peer involvement is an important and under-explored concept in health service delivery to marginalized populations. Many hard-to-reach individuals may only respond to peer contacts who have an intimate understanding of the obstacles to accessing health care. Successful collaboration with outreach teams has been developed in Vancouver, with a street-nurse program that includes past and present drug users. Similar outreach teams have also been used to attract and support a wide range of other marginalized urban subpopulations (Broadhead, *et al.*, 2002).

North America's first *Supervised Injection Site* (SIS) was opened in Vancouver in September 2003 (Wood, *et al.*, 2004). Although the primary impetus to open the facility was the issue of drug-dependent people injecting in public spaces, there is an excellent opportunity to link the SIS with health and counseling services. There are already nurses on the premises to deal with injection-related complications as well as a counselor to provide on-site addiction counseling. Links to public health interventions and detoxification programs are also in place.

5.0. STAFF SAFETY AND SECURITY

In order to connect with marginalized people and have the opportunity to improve health in urban environments, an emphasis has been placed on accessibility to health care programs and acceptance by the health care team. A major barrier to working in this environment is personal safety concerns on the part of the staff. This must be addressed in all low-threshold programs. The establishment of clear rules of conduct for the clients, including appropriate sanctions on those who are not willing to comply with these expectations, not only improve the working environment for the staff but are supported by the vast majority of clients, who also value a respectful and safe environment.

6.0. INTEGRATION OF CLINICAL SERVICES

There is no substitute for establishing relationships between health care providers and their clients. Multi-disciplinary models offer the best chance for success as they can provide a range of services and can include members who are not commonly involved with health care delivery. Traditional physician-based models of care are less successful as they are often clinic based and do not provide the services that are required.

Screening, diagnostic testing, and medical treatment is at the core of health care provision, and well-equipped facilities must be available within the communities. People are unlikely to travel long distances to receive care, and transportation is an obstacle faced by many. The provision of comprehensive primary care can prevent some of the more catastrophic illness that requires hospital care and preempt "crisis-based" care.

Substance misuse contributes to poor health in many ways and is the major determinant of low uptake of health services. Therefore, addiction counseling and treatment programs must be readily available and of high quality. Addiction counselors have an important role to play in attracting people to medical care and in encouraging their persistence. The integration of substance abuse treatment, detoxification and harm reduction services with primary care can improve access to primary medical care and adherence to recommended interventions (Broadhead, *et al.*, 2002; Heller, *et al.*,2004; Samet *et al.*, 2003; Sweeney, *et al.*, 2004).

A pharmacy is another important component to health care delivery. A health facility with a pharmacy on-site is ideal as the medicine can be provided directly to the patient. In addition, pharmacists can explain the expected effects of the medications and answer any questions the individual might have. In some cases, medications can be dispensed from the pharmacy on a daily basis in order to enhance adherence and identify adverse events.

A one-stop approach to receiving medical assistance is optimal but not always possible. The size of the facility and the resources that are available will ultimately determine what each site can offer. If resources permit, financial services can also be an important addition to any health-related facility since finances are often a major concern for many marginalized people. The amount of social assistance available is related to health status, and if an individual is unable to fill out the appropriate forms they may not receive the level of help they need. Housing assistance is also a valuable service and can be an important determinant of health. Unstable housing situations can make it difficult to attend follow-up appointments, take regular medications, and eat properly (Hwang, 2001; Hwang and Bugeja, 2000; Hwang, *et al.*, 2003).

7.0. GOALS AND MEASURABLE OUTCOMES

Program evaluation is a critical component of any health intervention. Many innovative and successful programs aimed at marginalized populations have gone unnoticed and un-replicated because they have not been adequately evaluated. Likewise, resources continue to be invested in programs that are not effective because they have not been critically assessed.

Due to the "hidden" nature of the urban, drug-dependent population, a major obstacle to evaluating the impact of an intervention is determining the number of people who are in need of medical services. In this case there is a tendency for a relatively small proportion of the population to be responsible for a large percentage of the health service uptake, while the majority of individuals do not participate. These kinds of artifacts in the data must be kept in mind when dealing with specific subpopulations.

There are several methods of data collection that allow us to evaluate the current situation as well as the success of specific programs over time.

7.1. Databases at Health Care Facilities

Databases at health care facilities provide a crude measure of health care uptake and are probably the best resources available. Databases have been used to assess STD prevalence, HIV prevalence and infective endocarditis. However, simply counting the number of individuals who present with a particular illness tends to underestimate the true scope of the problem. Of course, these types of observations are needed in order to launch more rigorous investigations. As existing electronic databases are improved and new ones are implemented, these records become more useful in determining individual and community health service uptake. For example, the province of British Columbia established a centralized database that records all antiretroviral prescriptions. These data have proved invaluable in determining who is accessing therapy for HIV as well as response to treatment (Hogg, *et al.*, 2001).

7.2. Sentinel Disease Surveillance

Sentinel disease surveillance gives an indication of the burden of disease within the population. Examples of this include standardized surveillance programs for STDs,

HIV, tuberculosis and overdose deaths. This type of analysis can show trends of disease burden over time. Therefore, correlations can be made between these trends and specific health care interventions to determine their impact. This type of data collection can be limited by a failure to access some of the higher risk groups.

7.3. Rapid Assessment Surveys

Rapid Assessment Surveys target specific health outcomes and can be implemented to determine the needs within a community (Fitch, *et al.*, 2004). These surveys are best conducted by persons who are familiar with the community and can gain access to hard-to-reach places and people. For example, housing surveys can be performed within specific neighborhoods and health outcomes that are associated with homelessness can be determined (Hwang, *et al.*, 2003).

7.4. Prospective Cohort Studies

Prospective studies in which a representative sample of people are monitored to track health concerns and diagnostic testing, is also a good way to measure outcomes. These cohort studies are expensive to initiate and sustain but they can contribute important information over time. In Vancouver, the Vancouver Injection Drug Users Study (VIDUS) was instrumental in identifying a major outbreak of HIV and continues to influence policy by providing important information on the course of the HIV epidemic (Strathdee, *et al.*, 1997).

There are also a number of measurable health outcomes that can be monitored to assess needs, evaluate progress and determine the impact of health interventions in urban settings. In the case of illicit drug users, we can examine *HIV testing statistics* to determine the proportion of individuals that have been tested in the past six months. For those who test HIV positive, the CD4 and viral load measures can also be monitored every three months. We can also look at the uptake of *antiretroviral therapy* among injection drug users as another good measure of health care coverage (in many urban centers the uptake is sub-optimal due to inadequate services and support). We can analyze the number of *annual Pap smears* to determine the level of screening in women, and we can examine the number of influenza and pneumococcal *vaccinations* within specific groups to provide additional measures of primary care uptake.

Finally, we can also look at adverse outcome statistics (i.e., *emergency room visits, drug overdoses, injection-related infections*, etc.) to determine the health of the community. One important adverse outcome that is sometimes overlooked is the level of *public disorder* within the community. Public order and safety are intimately linked to individual health and well-being. Communities that are able to improve the health status of their residents invariably see improvements in order and safety.

8.0. CONCLUSION

In this chapter, we have provided an overview of providing health services to a marginalized group who live in an urban setting. It is clear that the context that the target population is living in must be considered in designing and implementing health care services. Understanding the health needs and barriers to care are crucial in planning and implementing health services to various urban populations.

In many North American cities the approach to health care among marginalized groups in urban centers has been paradoxical. While there is intense public and political scrutiny of poverty and poor health outcomes in inner cities, there is also a severe lack of resources to improve services and reach those in need. Although each community requires unique approaches to confront the challenges of poor health outcomes, inadequate housing, entrenched poverty and substance misuse are consistent features of inner city environments.

There are a number of general lessons that can be learned from the observations and research to date. First, there are no "quick-fixes" for many of the people who are out of care and living in urban centers. Realistic goals must be set and each situation requires an innovative approach to improve health. Second, the generational cycle of poverty and poor health needs to be broken. A renewed focus on youth, young mothers and minority groups should be promoted in any program. Third, multidisciplinary teams are required to address the needs of the community. Success will come when these teams begin to operate outside of the traditional models of health care delivery. Fourth, the community itself must be involved in programming to ensure that the interventions are needed and appropriate and to promote buy-in from those that are expected to benefit from the program. Finally, a system of evaluation is required so that the outcomes can be measured and successful interventions can be expanded and replicated.

Designing health services for marginalized urban subpopulations requires ingenuity, persistence and compassion. It is a holistic approach – one that considers the specific health concerns and barriers facing individuals within these groups – that is most likely to yield a positive, practical and sustainable health service environment in our cities.

REFERENCES

Alter, D. A., Naylor, C. D., Austin, P., and Tu, J. V. (1999). Effects of socioeconomic status on access to invasive cardiac procedures and on mortality after acute myocardial infarction. *N. Engl. J. Med.* 341:1359–1367.

Appel P.W., Ellison A.A., Jansky H.K., and Oldak R. (2004). Barriers to enrollment in drug abuse treatment and suggestions for reducing them: opinions of drug injecting street otureach clients and other system stakeholders. *Am. J. Drug Alcohol Abuse* 30: 129–153.

Barkin, S. L., Balkrishnan, R., Manuel, J., Andersen, R. M., and Gelberg, L. (2003). Health care utilization among homeless adolescents and young adults. *J. Adolesc Health 32*: 253–256.

Barnett, P. G., Zaric, G. S., and Brandeau, M. L. (2001). The cost-effectiveness of buprenorphine maintenance therapy for opiate addiction in the United States. *Addiction* 96: 1267–1278.

Benoit, C., Carroll, D., and Chaudhry, M. (2003). In search of a healing place: Aboriginal women in Vancouver's Downtown Eastside. *Soc. Sci. Med.* 56:821–833.

Broadhead, R. S., Heckathorn, D. D., Altice, F. L., van Hulst, Y., Carbone, M., Friedland, G. H., Connor, P.G., and Selwyn, P.A. (2002). Increasing drug users' adherence to HIV treatment: results of a peer-driven intervention feasibility study. *Soc. Sci. Med., 55*(2):235–246.

Byrne, M., Murphy, A.W., Plunkett, P.K., McGee, H.M., Murray, A., and Bury, G. (2003) Frequent attenders to an emergency department: a study of primary health care use, medical profile and psychosocial characteristics. *Ann. Emerg. Med.* 41:309-318.

Chan, B.T., and Ovens, H.J. (2002). Frequent users of emergency departments. Do they also use family physicians' services? *Can. Fam. Physician* 48:1654–1660.

Chassin, M. R., and Galvin, R. W. (1998). The urgent need to improve health care quality. Institute of Medicine National Roundtable on Health Care Quality. *JAMA. 280*:1000–1005.

Cheung, A.M., and Hwang, S.W. (2004). Risk of death among homeless women: a cohort study and review of the literature. *CMAJ.* 170:1243–1247.

Conway, B., Prasad, J., Reynolds, R., Farley, J., Jones, M., Jutha, S., Smith, N., Mead, A., and DeVlaming, S. (2004). Directly observed therapy for the management of HIV-infected patients in a methadone program. *Clin. Infect. Dis. 38*: S402-408.

Craib, K. J. P., Spittal, P. M., Wood, E., Laliberte, N., Hogg, R.S., Li, K., Heath, K., Tyndall, M.W., O'Shaughnessy, M.V., and Schechter, M.T. (2003). Risk factors for elevated HIV incidence among Aboriginal injection drug users in Vancouver. *CMAJ.* 168:19–24.

Detsky, A. S., and Naylor, C. D. (2003). Canada's health care system–reform delayed. *N. Engl J. Med.* 349: 804–810.

Ebright, J. R., and Pieper, B. (2002). Skin and soft tissue infections in injection drug users. *Infect. Dis. Clinic. North Am.* 16:697–712.

Fitch, C., Stimson, G.V., Rhodes, T., and Poznyak, V. (2004). Rapid assessment: an international review of diffusion, practice and outcomes in the substance use field. *Soc. Sci. Med.* 59(9):1819-1830.

Freudenberg, N. (2000). Health promotion in the city: a review of current practice and future prospects in the United States. *Annu. Rev. Public Health* 21:473–503.

Galea, S., and Vlahov, D. (2002). Social determinants and the health of drug users: Socioeconomic status, homelessness, and incarceration. *Public Health Rep.* 117: S135–S145.

Heller, D., McCoy, K., and Cunningham, C. (2004). An invisible barrier to integrating HIV primary care with harm reduction services: philosophical clashes between the harm reduction and medical models. *Public Health Rep.* 119: 32–39.

Hogg, R.S., Yip, B., Chan K.J., Wood, E., Craid, K.J., O'Shaughnessy M.V., and Montaner, J.S. (2001). Rates of disease progression by baseline CD4 cell count and viral load after initiating triple-drug therapy. *JAMA.* 286(20):2568-77.

Hwang, S. W. (2001). Homelessness and health. *CMAJ.* 164: 229–233.

Hwang, S. W., and Bugeja, A. L. (2000b). Barriers to appropriate diabetes management among homeless people in Toronto, *CMAJ.* 163:161–165.

Hwang, S. W., Martin, R. E., Tolomiczenko, G. S., and Hulchanski, J. D. (2003). The relationship between housing conditions and health status of rooming house residents in Toronto. *Can. J. Public Health* 94:436–440.

Hwang, S. W., O'Connell, J. J., Lebow, J. M., Bierer, M. F., Orav, E. J., and Brennan, T. A. (2001). Health care utilization among homeless adults prior to death. *J. Health Care Poor Underserved* 12:50–58.

Iglehart, J. K. (2000). Revisiting the Canadian health care system. *N. Engl. J. Med.* 342:2007-2012.

Kak, V., and Chandrasekar, P. H. (2002). Bone and joint infections in injection drug users. *Infect Dis. Clin. North Am.* 16:681–695.

Kerr, T., and Palepu, A. (2001). Safe injection facilities in Canada: is it time? *CMAJ.* 165: 436-437.

Kushel, M. B., Vittinghoff, E., and Haas, J. S. (2001). Factors associated with the health care utilization of homeless persons. *JAMA.* 285: 200–206.

Lara, M., Allen, F., and Lange, L. (1999). Physician perceptions of barriers to care for inner-city Latino children with asthma. *J. Health Care Poor Underserved* 10:27–44.

Lewis, J.H., Andersen, R.M., and Gelberg, L. (2003). Health care for homeless women. *J. Gen. Intern. Med.* 18:921–928.

McCormick, L. K., Bartholomew, L. K., Lewis, M. J., Brown, M. W., and Hanson, I. C. (1997). Parental perceptions of barriers to childhood immunization: results of focus groups conducted in an urban population. *Health Educ. Res.* 12:355–362.

Metzger, D.S., and Navaline, H. (2003). HIV Prevention among injection drug users: the need for integrated models. *J. Urban Health.* 80(Suppl 3):iii59–66.

Newacheck, P.W., Stoddard, J.J., Hughes, D.C., and Pearl, M. (1998). Health insurance and access to primary care for children. *N. Engl. J. Med.* 338:513–519.

O'Connor, P. G., Selwyn, P. A., and Schottenfeld, R.S. (1994). Medical care for injection-drug users with human immunodeficiency virus infection. *N. Engl. J. Med.* 331:450–459.

Palepu, A., Tyndall, M. W., Leon, H., Muller, J., O'Shaughnessy, M. V., Schechter, M. T., and Anis, A.H. (2001). Hospital utilization and costs in a cohort of injection drug users. *CMAJ. 165*: 415–420.

Prevention of Homelessness. (1998); http://www/cotu/vamcpiver/bc/ca/commsvcs/housing/sochous/1council/1998/98-12-17.htm

Samet, J. H., Larson, M. J., Horton, N. J., Doyle, K., Winter, M., and Saitz, R. (2003). Linking alcohol- and drug-dependent adults to primary medical care: a randomized controlled trial of a multi-disciplinary health intervention in a detoxification unit. *Addiction* 98: 509–516.

Stein, M. D. (1999). Medical consequences of substance abuse. *Psychiatr. Clin. North Am.* 22: 351–370.

Stein, M. D., Anderson, B., Charuvastra, A., Maksad, J., and Friedmann, P. D. (2002). A brief intervention for hazardous drinkers in a needle exchange program. *J. Subst. Abuse Treat.* 22: 23–31.

Stein, M. D., Charuvastra, A., Maksad, J., and Anderson, B. J. (2002a). A randomized trial of a brief alcohol intervention for needle exchangers (BRAINE). *Addiction* 97:691–700.

Strathdee, S. A., Celentano, D. D., Shah, N., Lyles, C., Stambolis, V. A., Macalino, G., Nelson, K., and Vlahov, D. (1999). Needle-exchange attendance and health care utilization promote entry into detoxification. *J. Urban Health 76*: 448-460.

Strathdee, S. A., Patrick, D. M., Currie, S. L., Cornelisse, P. G., Rekart, M. L., Montaner, J. S., Schechter, M.T., and O'Shaughnessy, M.V. (1997). Needle exchange is not enough: lessons from the Vancouver injecting drug use study. *AIDS.* 11:F59–65.

Sweeney, L. P., Samet, J. H., Larson, M. J., and Saitz, R. (2004). Establishment of a multidisciplinary Health Evaluation and Linkage to Primary care (HELP) clinic in a detoxification unit. *J. Addict. Dis.* 23:33–45.

Tallon, J. R., Jr., and Sandman, D. (1998). Health care coverage and access for children in an urban state: the New York perspective. *J. Urban Health* 75: 693–701.

Tyndall, M. W., Craib, K. J., Currie, S., Li, K., O'Shaughnessy, M. V., and Schechter, M. T. (2001). Impact of HIV infection on mortality in a cohort of injection drug users. *J. Acquir. Immune Defic. Syndr.* 28: 351–357.

Vlahov, D., and Galea, S. (2002). Urbanization, urbanicity, and health. *J. Urban Health. 79*(Suppl 1):S1–S12.

Wood, D., Halfon, N., Sherbourne, C., and Grabowsky, M. (1994). Access to infant immunizations for poor, inner-city families: what is the impact of managed care? *J. Health Care Poor Underserved* 5:112-123.

Wood, E., Kerr, T., Montaner, J. S., Strathdee, S. A., Wodak, A., Hankins, C. A., Schechter, M.T., and Tyndall, M.W. (2004). Rationale for evaluating North America's first medically supervised safer-injecting facility. *The Lancet Infectious Diseases* 4:301–306.

Wood, E., Kerr, T., Small, W., Jones, J., Schechter, M. T., and Tyndall, M. W. (2003). The impact of a police presence on access to needle exchange programs. *J. Acquir. Immune Defic. Syndr.* 34:116–118.

Zaric, G. S., Barnett, P. G., and Brandeau, M. L. (2000). HIV transmission and the cost-effectiveness of methadone maintenance. *Am. J. Public Health* 90:1100–1111.

Chapter 29

Integrative Chapter

Training and Practice for Promoting Health in Cities

The Editors

The preceding six chapters in many ways are the most optimistic chapters of this book. These chapters offer practical examples of interventions that have been implemented in cities that have the potential to improve population health (ranging from city-wide efforts to local, small-scale interventions). They also present focused theoretic frameworks that can help guide our thinking about how we can conceive of, and implement interventions to improve urban health. These chapters then offer suggestions for how urban environments and the health of urban populations can be improved in spite of the complexity of the task at hand.

However, implicit in the chapters in this last section is a recognition, in line with the discussions in Sections I and II, that the urban environment is a complicated determinant of health and that the factors that shape the urban environment are themselves complex. For example, while one chapter presents a discussion of a specific local health department intervention, it still recognizes how this intervention is part of a much larger whole that is the fundamental target of health department activities. This is perhaps most easily illustrated in the chapter that considers the legal and regulatory frameworks that underpin many of the determinants of health in cities. The author makes it amply clear that the success of interventions that target more proximal determinants of health (e.g., local street quality) depends as much on the intervention itself as it does on the more upstream laws and regulations that may enable, facilitate, or obviate an intervention. Therefore, interventions in the urban context need to consider factors at multiple levels that may, as discussed in the previous two sections, affect the health of urban populations.

Promoting health in cities requires an appreciation of the multiple levels of determinants that shape population health and also practitioners with the skills to develop and implement programs that take these multiple levels of determinants into account. As such, teaching students urban health is the essential first step in any effort that aims to improve urban health in the long-term. The chapter on teaching urban health offers clear suggestions about how this may be, and is being achieved, in some settings. However, as we also discussed in chapters 12 and 22, one of the primary insights that we have drawn from the chapters in this book is that there is much to be learned and that it is unlikely that any single discipline, as currently constituted, can train professionals who have the breadth and depth necessary to embrace the full range of theoretic, empiric, and practical skills needed to improve health in cities.

What this last section and indeed the entire book projects however, is that urban health practice is not waiting for advanced theory or methods development; practitioners have to move forward to address current and projected problems. An assumption in this book is that urban health practice can, and should, be empirically based. In essence, the science needs to catch up to practice if we are truly to have empiric based urban health practice. As our knowledge of health and disease outcomes grows, the task of those interested in the health of urban populations is to catalogue the array of exposures involving physical and social influences at the micro-, meso-, and macro-levels that independently and jointly affect different populations and manifest as health, well-being, and disease. We have shown here some appreciation of the complexity that this task involves. Understanding and improving urban health will require expertise that crosses disciplines and the flexibility to adapt this mastery to develop interventions that target multiple levels of influence in rapidly changing urban contexts. Conceptual frameworks to guide our construction are being refined. Multi-level analytic tools to more carefully disentangle a multitude of factors are evolving. More nuanced thinking to consider transition from etiologic analyses to intervention strategies is starting. Building a cadre of scholars and practitioners to move forward this agenda is happening. The intent of this book has been to bring together a range of scholars and practitioners in one volume that together can stimulate the important next steps that can help public health practitioners address the unrelenting global demographic shift toward city living. With half of the world's population becoming urban as this book is published, and more rapid growth of cities projected, we have an important opportunity not simply to react to immediate crises, but to aggressively think, learn, plan, and act to improve the health of urban residents. The urgency of rising to this challenge and embracing this opportunity provides a vision of the city that can be a healthier place to live.

Index

H

I

J

K

L

M

O

P

Q

R

S

T

U

V

W

Y

Z